Assad Movahed, Gopinath Gnanasegaran, John R. Buscombe, Margaret Hall

Integrating Cardiology for Nuclear Medicine Physicians

Assad Movahed, Gopinath Gnanasegaran,
John R. Buscombe, Margaret Hall

Integrating Cardiology for Nuclear Medicine Physicians

A Guide to Nuclear Medicine Physicians

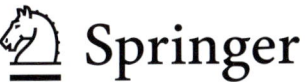

Assad Movahed MD, FACP, FACC
Section of Cardiology
Department of Medicine
The Brody School of Medicine
East Carolina University
600 Moye Blvd.
Greenville, NC 27858-4354
USA

Gopinath Gnanasegaran, MBBS, MSc, MD
Department of Nuclear Medicine
Guy's & St Thomas' Hospital NHS Foundation Trust
St. Thomas Street
London, SE1 9RT
UK

John R. Buscombe, MBBS, MSc, MD, FRCP, FRCPEd, FEBNM
Department of Nuclear Medicine
Royal Free Hospital
Pond Street
London, NW3 2QG
UK

Margaret Hall, MB ChB, MSc, FRCP
Department of Nuclear Medicine
Royal Free Hospital
Pond Street
London, NW3 2QG
UK

ISBN 978-3-540-78673-3   e-ISBN 978-3-540-78674-0

DOI 10.1007/978-3-540-78674-0

Library of Congress Control Number: 2008940028

© 2009 Springer-Verlag Berlin Heidelberg

This work is subject to copyright. All rights are reserved, wether the whole or part of the material is concerned, specifically the rights of translation, reprinting, reuse of illustrations, recitation, broad-casting, reproduction on microfilm or any other way, and storage in data banks. Duplication of this publication or parts thereof is permitted only under the provisions of the German Copyright Law of September 9, 1965, in it current version, and permission for use must always be obtained from Springer. Violations are liable to prosecution under the German Copyright Law.

The use of general descriptive names, registed names, trademarks etc. in this publication does not imply, even in the absence of a specific statement, that such names are exempt from the relevant protective laws and regulations and therefore free for general use.

Product liability: the publishers cannot guarantee the accuracy of any information about dosage and application contained in this book. In every individual case the user must check such information by consulting the relevant literature.

Cover design: Frido Steinen-Broo, eStudio Calamar, Spain
Reproduction, typesetting and production: le-tex publishing services oHG, Leipzig, Germany

Printed on acid-free paper

9 8 7 6 5 4 3 2 1

springer.com

Preface

Nuclear cardiology has become the mainstay of many departments of nuclear medicine, driving what was once an academic and sometimes eccentric specialty into what is today the centre of many patients' lives. As nuclear cardiology has matured our concerns have shifted from how can we do this to how can we do this better. Many of the most recent publications in nuclear cardiology have focused upon how imaging and reporting quality can be improved, i.e. how to be more consistent in what we do and how to be more reliable with regard to our diagnoses.

Coronary artery disease and Ischaemic heart disease affects people from all countries and all social strata. The idea that it is a disease only of the affluent West has been shown to be untrue and as a consequence, nuclear cardiology has become a truly global specialty. This is reflected in the fact that the number of practitioners in nuclear cardiology is increasing and despite the arrival of cardiac CT and cardiac MRI, demand continues to grow. In response to the importance of the subject we have brought together experts not only from Europe and North America but also from the emerging centres of excellence in Asia to produce a book with a truly global perspective on the role of nuclear cardiology in patients with heart disease.

The editors have worked closely with cardiovascular physicians around the globe to produce a book that will be essential reading for those practising nuclear cardiology, as it provides information on basic anatomy and physiology, on the technical aspects of the methodology and how the results can affect clinical management. All this they could not do themselves. The editors therefore wish to thank the authors for their contributions, the team at Springer for bringing the disparate manuscripts into a single text and those who read the manuscripts for providing us with insightful comments, which enabled us to improve the text. The editors also wish to thank those AVA/medical illustration units worldwide producing high quality illustrations including the AVA unit at the Royal Free Hospital for their skills in graphics.

The editors hope that you enjoy the efforts of all these professionals and hope that you will read this text, learn from it and apply something new and beneficial for the care of your patients.

Assad Movahed
Gopinath Gnanasegaran
John Buscombe
Margaret Hall

Contents

Part I Basic Sciences

1. The Heart: Anatomy, Physiology and Exercise Physiology 3
   Syed Shah, Gopinath Gnanasegaran, Jeanette Sundberg-Cohon, and John R Buscombe

2. Pathophysiology of Coronary Artery Disease ... 23
   Shahid Mahmood

3. Pathology of Coronary Artery Disease and Ischemic Heart Disease 31
   Usha Kini and Shalini Mullick

4. Pathophysiology of Diabetic Vascular Complications 45
   Francis Estrada and John R. Buscombe

Part II Conventional Investigation of Coronary Artery Disease and Ischaemic Heart Disease

5. Clinical Assessment and Evaluation of the Cardiovascular System 53
   Jeanette Sundberg-Cohon, Nivedita Gauthaman, Gopinath Gnanasegaran and Margaret Hall

6. The Plain Chest Radiograph in the Assessment of Cardiac Disease 65
   Nicola Mulholland

7. Ischaemic and Inflammatory Biomarkers in Cardiovascular Disease 77
   Gopinath Gnanasegaran, Gregory Shabo and John R. Buscombe

8. Electrocardiography and Exercise Stress Test ... 87
   Humayun Bashir, Gopinath Gnanasegaran and John R. Buscombe

9. Ambulatory Electrocardiography, Transient Event Monitors, and Continuous Loop Recorders 113
   R. Wayne Kreeger, John Brooks and Assad Movahed

10. Echocardiography and Contrast Echocardiography 117
    Firas A Ghanem, Jaffar Ali Raza, Ishtiaque H. Mohiuddin and Assad Movahed

11. Dobutamine Stress Echocardiography 127
    Satish C. Govind and S. S. Ramesh

12. Transesophageal echocardiography 137
    Satish C. Govind and S. S. Ramesh

13. Clinical Cardiac Electrophysiology – An Overview 145
    Senthil Thenappan, Jaffar Ali Raza, R. Wayne Kreeger and Assad Movahed

14. Cardiac Catheterization and Selective Coronary Angiography: Current Status and Limitations 155
    Matt Cummings, Aravinda Nanjundappa and Assad Movahed

15. Emerging Role of Multi-detector CT Imaging ... 163
    Shahid Mahmood and John Hoe

16. Current Status of Cardiovascular MR Imaging 177
    Shahid Mahmood and Robert Kwok

Part III Nuclear Cardiology

17. Principles of Myocardial SPECT Imaging ... 191
    Kathryn Adamson

18	Radionuclides in Nuclear Cardiology: Current Status and Limitations .... 213 *Richard Fernandez*		30	First Pass Studies – Current Status and Limitations .... 355 *Radhakrishnan Jayan and Linda Smith*	
19	Planar and SPECT Radiopharmaceuticals in Nuclear Cardiology: Current Status and Limitations .... 221 *Gopinath Gnanasegaran, Akhtar Ahmed, Jilly Croasdale and John R. Buscombe*		31	Cardiac PET: Physics and Methodology ..... 363 *Lefteris Livieratos*	
			32	PET Radiopharmaceuticals in Nuclear Cardiology: Current Status and Limitations .... 379 *James R. Ballinger*	
20	Myocardial Perfusion Imaging for Risk Stratification in Suspected or Known Coronary Artery Disease: Current Status and Limitations .... 231 *Firas A. Ghanem and Assad Movahed*		33	Cardiac PET Imaging: Current Status and Limitations .... 387 *Ishtiaque H Mohiuddin and Assad Movahed*	
21	Imaging Protocols in Myocardial Perfusion Scintigraphy .... 237 *Shobhan Vinjamuri*		34	Paediatric Nuclear Cardiology .... 401 *Pietro Zucchetta*	
22	Pharmacological Stress Myocardial Perfusion Imaging: Current Status and Limitations .... 245 *Gopinath Gnanasegaran, Francis Sundram, Margaret Hall and John R Buscombe*		35	Cardiac Adrenergic Imaging .... 409 *Shinichiro Fujimoto, Shohei Yamashina and Junichi Yamazaki*	

Part IV Management of Coronary Artery Disease and Ischaemic Heart Disease

23	Gated Single Photon Emission Computed Tomography (SPECT) Imaging: Current Status and Limitations .... 261 *Sagir Ahmed and Assad Movahed*	
36	Prevention of Coronary Heart Disease ...... 419 *Firas A Ghanem and Assad Movahed*	
24	Myocardial Perfusion Scintigraphy in the Assessment of Post-Revascularization – Current Status and Limitations .... 275 *Jaffar Ali Raza and Assad Movahed*	
37	Cardiovascular Medications: Pharmacokinetics and Pharmacodynamics .. 425 *Jaffar Ali Raza, Wayne Kreeger and Assad Movahed*	
25	Nuclear Cardiology in Women .... 287 *A. Muhammad Umar Khan and John R. Buscombe*	
38	Anti-Arrhythmic Drugs: Pharmacokinetics and Pharmacodynamics .... 453 *R. Wayne Kreeger, Jaffar Ali Raza and Assad Movahed*	
26	Myocardial Perfusion Scintigraphy in Acute Chest Pain: Current Status and Limitations .. 299 *Priya Velappan and Assad Movahed*	
39	Coronary Angioplasty and Newer Interventional Strategies .... 463 *Aravinda Nanjundappa, Pabitra Saha and Assad Movahed*	
27	Myocardial Perfusion Scintigraphy in Diabetes: Current Status and Limitations 305 *John O. Prior*	
28	Artefacts and Pitfalls in Myocardial Perfusion Imaging .... 325 *Iulia Heinle and Qaisar H. Siraj*	
40	Coronary Artery Bypass Surgery: Science and Practice .... 471 *Michael W. A. Chu, W. Randolph Chitwood Jr and T. Bruce Ferguson*	
29	Multiple Gated Equilibrium Blood Pool Imaging (MUGA) .... 343 *Rakesh Kumar*	
41	Minimally Invasive Cardiac Surgery .... 487 *L. Wiley Nifong and W. Randolph Chitwood Jr*	

42 **Transmyocardial Revascularization** 497
*Jay Jayakumar, Wai Weng Woon
and Peter L. C. Smith*

43 **Prevention of Re-Stenosis
of Coronary Arteries by Radionuclides** 511
John R. Buscombe

44 **Cardiac Transplantation:
Current Status and Limitations** 517
Sheetal Kaul and Assad Movahed

Subject Index 525

List of Contributors

Kathryn Adamson
Department of Nuclear Medicine
Guy's & St. Thomas' Hospital NHS Foundation Trust
St. Thomas Street
London, SE1 9RT
UK

Akhtar Ahmed
Nuclear Institute of Medical Radiotherapy (NIMRA)
Liaquat University of Medical & Health Sciences
Jamshoro
Pakistan

Sagir Ahmed
Section of Cardiology
East Carolina University
Brody School of Medicine
Greenville, NC 28858-4354
USA

James R. Ballinger
Nuclear Medicine Department
Guy's & St. Thomas' Hospitals
St. Thomas Street
London, SE1 9RT
UK

Humayun Bashir
Department of Nuclear Medicine
Guy's & St. Thomas' Hospital NHS Foundation Trust
St. Thomas Street
London, SE1 9RT
UK

John Brooks
Section of Cardiology
Department of Medicine
The Brody School of Medicine
East Carolina University
Greenville, NC 28858-4354
USA

John R. Buscombe
Department of Nuclear Medicine
Royal Free Hospital
Pond Street
London, NW3 2QG
UK

W. Randolph Chitwood
Division of Cardiovascular and Thoracic Surgery
Department of Surgery
Brody School of Medicine
East Carolina University
Greenville, NC 28858-4354
USA

Michael W. A. Chu
Division of Cardiac Surgery
University of Western Ontario
B6–106 University Hospital
339 Windermere Road
London Health Sciences Centre
London, Ontario, N6A 5AS
Canada

Jilly Croasdale
Department of Nuclear Medicine
City Hospital
Birmingham
UK

Matt Cummings
Section of Cardiology
Department of Medicine
The Brody School of Medicine
East Carolina University
Greenville, NC 28858-4354
USA

Francis Estrada
Department of Nuclear Medicine
Royal Free Hospital
Pond Street
London, NW3 2QG
UK

T. Bruce Ferguson
Division of Cardiovascular and Thoracic Surgery
Department of Surgery
Brody School of Medicine
East Carolina University
Greenville, NC 28858-4354
USA

Richard Fernandez
Department of Nuclear Medicine
Guy's & St. Thomas' Hospital NHS Foundation Trust
St. Thomas Street
London, SE1 9RT
UK

Shinichiro Fujimoto
Division of Cardiovascular Medicine
Department of Internal Medicine
Ohmori Hospital, Toho University School of Medicine
Tokyo, 143-8541
Japan

Nivedita Gauthaman
Royal Free Hospital
Pond Street
London, NW3 2QG
UK

Firas A. Ghanem
Section of Cardiology
Department of Medicine
The Brody School of Medicine
East Carolina University
Greenville, NC 28858-4354
USA

Gopinath Gnanasegaran
Department of Nuclear Medicine
Guy's & St. Thomas' Hospital NHS Foundation Trust
St. Thomas Street
London, SE1 9RT
UK

Satish C. Govind
Heart Centre Vivus
Bhagwan Mahaveer Jain Hospital
Millers Road
Bangalore 560052
India

Margaret Hall
Department of Nuclear Medicine
Royal Free Hospital
Pond Street
London, NW3 2QG
UK

Iulia Heinle
Nuclear Medicine Department
Royal Hospital Haslar, Gosport and St Mary's Hospital
Portsmouth
UK

John Hoe
Department of Diagnostic Radiology
Mount Elizabeth Hospital
3-Mt Elizabeth
Singapore

Jay Jayakumar
Guy's & St. Thomas' Hospital NHS Foundation Trust
St. Thomas Street
London, SE1 9RT
UK

Radhakrishnan Jayan
Department of Nuclear Medicine
Royal Liverpool University Hospital
Liverpool L7 8XP
UK

Sheetal Kaul
Division of Cardiology
Department of Internal Medicine
Brody School of Medicine at East Carolina University
2100 Stantonsburg Road
Greenville NC 27834
USA

A. Muhammad Umar Khan
Shankat Khanum Memorial Cancer Hospital &
Research Centre
Lahore
Pakistan

Usha Kini
Department of Pathology
St John's Medical College and Hospital
Bangalore 560034
India

R. Wayne Kreeger
Section of Cardiology
Department of Medicine
The Brody School of Medicine
East Carolina University
Greenville, NC 28858-4354
USA

Rakesh Kumar
All India Institute of Medical Sciences
E-81, Ansari Nagar (EAST)
New Delhi, 110029
India

Robert Kwok
Department of Diagnostic Radiology
Mount Elizabeth Hospital
3-Mt Elizabeth
Singapore

Lefteris Livieratos
Nuclear Medicine Department
Guy's & St. Thomas' Hospitals
St. Thomas Street
London, SE1 9RT
UK

Shahid Mahmood
Singapore PET and Cardiac Imaging Centre
Singapore, 238859

Ishtiaque H. Mohiuddin
Section of Cardiology
Department of Medicine
The Brody School of Medicine
East Carolina University
Greenville, NC 28858-4354
USA

Assad Movahed
Section of Cardiology
Department of Medicine
The Brody School of Medicine
East Carolina University
Greenville, NC 28858-4354
USA

Nicola Mulholland
Department of Nuclear Medicine
King's College Hospital
Pond Street
London, NW3 2QG
UK

Shalini Mullick
Department of Pathology
St John's Medical College and Hospital
Bangalore
India

Aravinda Nanjundappa
Section of Cardiology
Department of Medicine
The Brody School of Medicine
East Carolina University
Greenville, NC 28858-4354
USA

L. Wiley Nifong
Department of Cardiovascular Sciences
East Carolina Heart Institute
Brody School of Medicine
East Carolina University
Greenville, NC 28858-4354
USA

John O. Prior
Nuclear Medicine Department
Centre Hospitalier Universitaire Vaudois
(CHUV University Hospital)
Rue du Bugnon 46
Lausanne, CH-1011
Switzerland

S. S. Ramesh
Heart Centre Vivus
Bhagwan Mahaveer Jain Hospital
Millers Road
Bangalore 560052
India

Jaffar Ali Raza
Department of Interventional Cardiology
Lenox Hill Heart and Vascular Institute
130 East 77th Street, 9th Floor
New York, NY 10021
USA

Pabitra Saha
Section of Cardiology
Department of Medicine
The Brody School of Medicine
East Carolina University
Greenville, NC 28858-4354
USA

Gregory Shabo
Department of Nuclear Medicine
Guy's & St. Thomas' Hospital NHS Foundation Trust
St. Thomas Street
London, SE1 9RT
UK

Syed Shah
Department of Nuclear Medicine
Guy's & St. Thomas' Hospital NHS Foundation Trust
St. Thomas Street
London, SE1 9RT
UK

Qaisar H. Siraj
Nuclear Medicine Department
Royal Hospital Haslar, Gosport and St Mary's Hospital
Portsmouth
UK

Linda Smith
Department of Nuclear Medicine
Royal Liverpool University Hospital
Prescot Street
Liverpool L7 8XP
UK

Peter L. C. Smith
Hammersmith Hospital
London
UK

Jeanette Sundberg-Cohon
Guy's, Kings and St. Thomas School of Medicine
St. Thomas Street
London, SE1 9RT
UK

Francis Sundram
Department of Nuclear Medicine
City Hospital
Birmingham
UK

Senthil Thenappan
Section of Cardiology
Department of Medicine
The Brody School of Medicine
East Carolina University
Greenville, NC 28858-4354
USA

Priya Velappan
Section of Cardiology
Department of Medicine
The Brody School of Medicine
East Carolina University
Greenville, NC 28858-4354
USA

Sobhan Vinjamuri
Department of Nuclear Medicine
Royal Liverpool NHS Foundation Trust
Prescot Street
Liverpool, L7 8XP
UK

Wai Weng Woon
Royal London Hospitals
London
UK

Shohei Yamashina
Division of Cardiovascular Medicine
Department of Internal Medicine
Ohmori Hospital, Toho University School of Medicine
Tokyo, 143-8541
Japan

Junichi Yamazaki
Division of Cardiovascular Medicine,
Department of Internal Medicine,
Ohmori Hospital, Toho University School of Medicine
Tokyo, 143-8541
Japan

Pietro Zucchetta
Medicina Nucleare
Universita di Padova
Padiglione Giustinianeo
Via Giustiniani 2
35128 Padova
Italy

Part I Basic Sciences

The Heart: Anatomy, Physiology and Exercise Physiology

Syed Shah, Gopinath Gnanasegaran, Jeanette Sundberg-Cohon, and John R Buscombe

Contents

1.1	Introduction	3
1.2	Anatomy of the Heart	3
1.2.1	Chamber and Valves	4
1.2.2	Cardiac Cell and Cardiac Muscle	4
1.2.3	Coronary Arteries and Cardiac Veins	6
1.2.4	Venous Circulation	6
1.2.5	Nerve Supply of the Heart	9
1.2.6	Conduction System of the Heart	10
1.3	Physiology of the Heart	11
1.3.1	Circulatory System: Systemic and Pulmonary Circulation	11
1.3.2	Conduction System of the Heart (Excitation Sequence)	11
1.3.3	Action Potential (AP)	11
1.3.4	Mechanism of Excitation and Contraction Coupling of Cardiac Myocytes	13
1.3.5	Autonomic Nervous System and Heart	16
1.3.6	Cardiac Cycle	16
1.3.7	Physiology of Coronary Circulation	17
1.3.8	Coronary Collaterals	17
1.4	Exercise Physiology	18
1.4.1	Gender and Exercise Performance	19
1.4.2	Age and Exercise Performance	19
1.5	Conclusion	20
	References	20

1.1 Introduction

The impact of anatomy on medicine was first recognised by Andreas Vesalius during the 16th century [1] and from birth to death, the heart is the most talked about organ of the human body. It is the centre of attraction for people from many lifestyles, such as philosophers, artists, poets and physicians/surgeons. The heart is one of the most efficient organs in the human body and heart disease is one of the commonest causes of morbidity and mortality in both developing and developed countries. Understanding the anatomy and pathophysiology is very important and challenging. With innovative changes in the imaging world, the perception of these has changed radically and applied anatomy and physiology plays an important role in understanding structure and function.

1.2 Anatomy of the Heart

The heart is located in the chest, directly above the diaphragm in the region of the thorax called mediastinum, specifically the middle mediastinum. The normal human heart varies with height and weight (Table 1.1). The tip (apex) of the heart is pointed forward, downward, and toward the left. The (inferior) diaphragmatic surface lies directly on the diaphragm. The heart lies in a double walled fibroserous sac called the pericardial sac, which is divided into (a) fibrous pericardium, and (b) serous pericardium. The fibrous pericardium envelops the heart and attaches onto the great vessels [2]. The serous pericardium is a closed sac consisting of two layers – a visceral layer or epicardium forming the outer lining of the great vessels and the heart, and a parietal layer forming an inner lining of the fibrous pericardium [2–4]. The two layers of the serous pericardium contain the pericardial fluid, which prevents friction between the heart and the pericardium [2–4].

Table 1.1 Anatomical facts about the human heart

Normal human heart varies with height and weight
Weighs approximately 300–350 grams in males
Weighs approximately 250–300 grams in females
Right ventricle thickness is 0.3–0.5 cm
Left ventricle thickness is 1.3–1.5 cm
Divided into four distinct chambers
Composed of three layers (epicardium, myocardium and endocardium)
Contains two atria (left and right)
Contains two ventricles (left and right)
Contains four valves (aortic, mitral, tricuspid, pulmonary)

The wall of the heart is composed of three layers: (a) epicardium; (b) myocardium; and (c) endocardium (Fig. 1.1) [5, 6]. The epicardium is the outer lining of the cardiac chambers and is formed by the visceral layer of the serous pericardium. The myocardium is the intermediate layer of the heart and is composed of three discernable layers of muscle [5, 6] that are seen predominantly in the left ventricle and inter-ventricular septum alone and includes a subepicardial layer, a middle concentric layer and a subendocardial layer. The rest of the heart is composed mainly of the subepicardial and subendocardial layers [7, 8]. The myocardium also contains important structures such as excitable nodal tissue and the conducting system. The endocardium the innermost layer of the heart is formed of the endothelium and subendothelial connective tissue [5, 6].

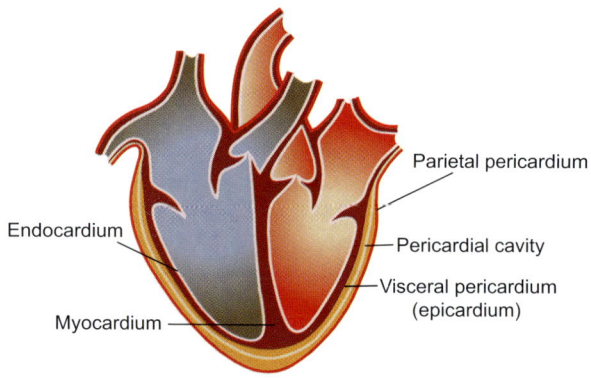

Fig 1.1 Layers of the heart

1.2.1
Chamber and Valves

The heart is divided into four distinct chambers with muscular walls of different thickness [2, 4, 9]. The left atrium (LA) and right atrium (RA) are small, thin-walled chambers located just above the left ventricle (LV) and right ventricle (RV), respectively. The ventricles are larger thick-walled chambers that perform most of the work [2, 4, 9] (Table 1.2). The atria receive blood from the venous system and lungs and then contract and eject the blood into the ventricles. The ventricles then pump the blood throughout the body or into the lungs. The heart contains four valves and the fibrous skeleton of the heart contains the annuli of the four valves, membranous septum, aortic intervalvular, right, and left fibrous trigones [3, 4, 6, 10, 11] (Fig. 1.2, Table 1.3). The right trigone and the membranous septum together form the central fibrous body, which is penetrated by the bundle of His [3, 4, 6, 10, 11]. The fibrous skeleton functions not only to provide an electrophysiological dissociation of atria and the ventricles but also provides structural support to the heart [8, 12, 13]. Each of the four valves has a distinctive role in maintaining physiological stability [3].

1.2.2
Cardiac Cell and Cardiac Muscle

The cardiac cell contains bundles of protein strands called myofibrils. These myofibrils are surrounded by sarcoplasmic reticulum, which contains cysternae (dilated terminals) [6, 10, 11, 14–16]. The sarcomeres are the contractile unit of myofibrils and the T tubules are continuations of the cell membrane located near the Z-lines, which conduct the action potential (AP) to the interior of the cell [6, 14]. The T tubules connect the sarcolemma to the sarcoplasmic reticulum in the skeletal muscle and the cardiac muscle [14, 15].

Cardiac muscle is an involuntary striated muscle, which is mononucleated and has cross-striations formed by alternate segments of thick and thin protein filaments, which are anchored by segments called Z-lines. Cardiac muscle is relatively shorter than skeletal muscle [6, 10, 11, 14–16] and actin and myosin are the primary structural proteins. When the cardiac muscle is observed by a light microscope, the thinner actin filaments appear as lighter bands, while thicker myosin filaments appear as darker bands [8, 12, 13, 15]. The dark bands are actually the region of overlap between the actin and myosin filaments and the light bands are the region of actin filaments [8, 12, 13, 15]. The thinner actin flaments contain two others proteins called troponin and tropomyosin, which play an important role in contraction [6, 14, 15]. Cardiac muscle also contains dense bands (specialised

Table 1.2 Cardiac atrial and ventricular chambers [2, 4–6, 9]

Left ventricle (LV)

1. Made of an inlet portion comprised of mitral valve apparatus, subaortic outflow portion and a trabeculated apical zone
2. Three times thicker than the RV and most muscular
3. Thickest towards the base and thinnest towards the apex
4. LV free wall and septal thickness is three times the thickness of the RV free wall
5. Mitral and aortic valves share fibrous continuity
6. LV apex is relatively less trabeculated than the RV apex

Right ventricle (RV)

1. Comprised of inlet and outflow segments
2. Inlet extends from tricuspid annulus to the insertions of the papillary muscles
3. Apical trabecular zone extends inferiorly beyond the papillary muscle attachment toward the ventricular apex and halfway along the anterior wall.
4. Outflow portion (conus) is a muscular subpulmonary channel
5. Arch shaped muscular ridge separates the tricuspid and pulmonary valves

Right atrium (RA)

1. Thinnest walls of the four chambers
2. Forms the right border of the heart
3. Gives off the right auricular appendage
4. Receives the superior vena cava, inferior vena cava and coronary sinus
5. Discharges into right ventricle through the tricuspid valve

Left atrium (LA)

1. Forms base of the heart (posterior surface)
2. Gives off the left auricular appendage.
3. Receives two right pulmonary veins (sometimes three) and two left pulmonary veins (sometimes one)
4. Discharges into the left ventricle through the mitral valve

Ventricular septum

1. Intracardiac partition having four parts (inlet, membranous, trabecular and infundibular)
2. Divided into muscular and membranous septum
3. Membranous septum lies beneath the right and posterior aortic cusps and contact mitral and tricuspid annuli

Atrial septum

1. Composed of interatrial and atrioventricular regions when viewed from right
2. Composed of entirely interatrial regions when viewed from the left
3. Interatrial region is characterised by fossa ovalis
4. Atrioventricular portion separates the right atrium from the left ventricle

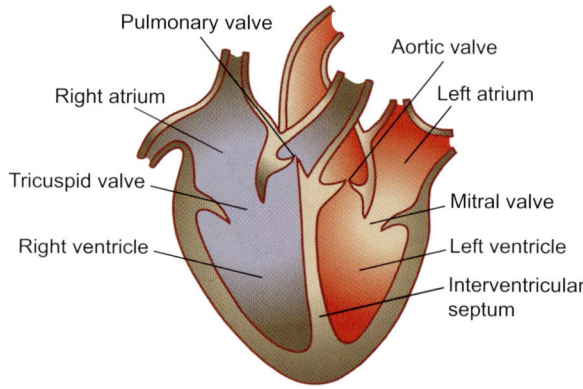

Fig 1.2 Cardiac chambers and valves

cell junctions) called intercalated discs that separate individual cells from one another at their ends [6, 14, 15] and these discs consist of a transverse and a lateral portion. The transverse portion of the disc acts as a zone of firm adhesion and a route of transmission of contractile force and the lateral portion of the disc acts as a gap junction across which propagation of electrical impulses between the adjacent cardiac cells occurs [6, 14, 15]. This in effect allows the individual cells of the heart to act as a syncytium [8, 12–15].

1.2.3
Coronary Arteries and Cardiac Veins

The heart receives blood from left coronary arteries (LCA) and right coronary arteries (RCA) [17] (Fig. 1.3, Table 1.4). The left coronary artery arises from the left aortic sinus (at an acute angle from the aorta) [2, 3, 6, 8] as a single short main artery (left mainstem). The LCA bifurcates to form the left anterior descending artery (LAD) and left circumflex (LCx) [2, 3, 6]. The LAD anastomoses with the posterior descending artery (PDA) a branch of the right coronary artery (RCA) [2, 3, 6]. The LAD supplies the interventricular septum (anterior two-thirds), the apex, and the anterior aspects of the right and left ventricle. The LCx has a major branch, the left marginal artery, and in around 10–15% of the population, the LCx anastomoses with the RCA to give rise to the PDA [2, 3, 6–8]. In general, the LCx supplies the posterior aspect of the left atrium and superior portion of the left ventricle [2, 3, 6–8].

The RCA arises from the right aortic sinus and has major branches such as the PDA (supplying the posterior third of the interventricular septum and AV node [6, 7], the nodal artery (supplying the right atrium and the SA node), and the right marginal artery (supplying a portion of the right ventricle, the inferior left ventricular wall, and the PDA). In the majority (80–90%) of cases, the RCA supplies the atrioventricular node (AV node). Finally, the coronary arteries branch into small arteries and arterioles. These vessels terminate in end arteries that supply the myocardial tissue with blood [2, 3, 6–8].

In general, the RCA is dominant in 60–65% of cases because it gives off a PDA branch (balanced coronary circulation) [2, 3, 6–8]. In about 10–15% of cases, the LCx gives rise to the PDA (left predominant circulation). In 20–25% of cases, the RCA, in addition to supplying the PDA, crosses the posterior interventricular septum to reach as far as the left marginal artery and thereby supply the diaphragmatic surface of the left ventricle (right predominance) [2, 3, 8]. However, this term does not distinguish this condition from balanced coronary circulation (Table 1.5) [7].

1.2.4
Venous Circulation

The venous circulation of the heart is from the coronary sinus, anterior cardiac veins and the lesser cardiac (thebesian) veins [6]. The coronary sinus receives most of the venous return from the epicardium and myocardium [6] and it opens into the right atrium between the opening of the inferior vena cava and the right AV valve [2, 3, 5, 6]. The coronary sinus gives rise to tributaries such as the great cardiac vein, middle cardiac vein, smaller cardiac vein and oblique vein. The great cardiac vein drains the anterior portion of the interventricular septum and anterior aspects of both ventricles [2–6].

The middle cardiac vein drains the posterior portion of the interventricular septum and posterior aspect of

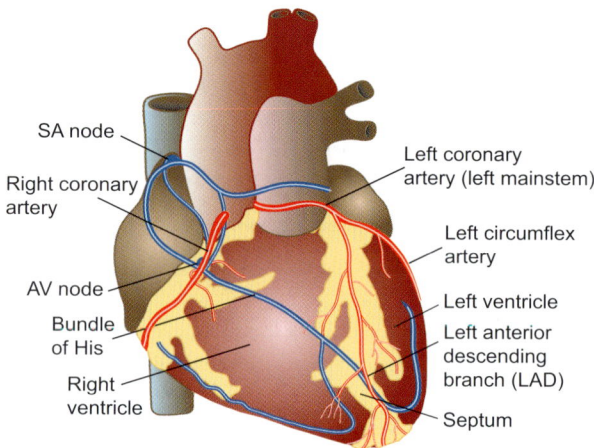

Fig 1.3 Coronary arteries

Table 1.3 Cardiac valves and cardiac skeleton [2, 4–6, 8, 9]

Tricuspid valve

1. Tricuspid valve (right atrioventricular valve) connects the right atrium and the right ventricle
2. Composed of five components (annulus, leaflets, commissures, chordae tendineae, papillary muscles)
3. Anterior tricuspid leaflet is the largest (most mobile) and the posterior leaflet is the smallest
4. Tricuspid valve has a triangular orifice

Mitral valve

1. Mitral valve (left atrioventricular valve) connects the left atrium to the left ventricle
2. Composed of five components (annulus, leaflets, commissures, chordae tendineae, papillary muscles)
3. Composed of two leaflets only
4. Anterior tricuspid leaflet is large, semicircular and twice the height of posterior leaflet
5. Posterior leaflet is rectangular and is divided into three scallops
6. Mitral valve has an elliptical orifice

Aortic valve

1. Aortic valve (semilunar valve) opens between the left ventricle and the aorta
2. Composed of three components (annulus, cusps, commissures)
3. Composed of three semilunar cusps

Pulmonary valves

1. Pulmonary valve (semilunar valve) regulates flow between the right ventricle and the pulmonary artery
2. Composed of three components (annulus, cusps, commissures)

Cardiac grooves

1. Atrioventricular (AV) groove separates the atria from the ventricle
2. Anterior and posterior interventricular (IV) grooves separate the ventricles
3. Right coronary arteries (RCA) travel in the right atrioventricular groove
4. Circumflex artery (Cx) travels in the left atrioventricular groove
5. The left anterior descending artery (LAD) travels along the anterior interventricular groove
6. Posterior descending artery (PDA) travels along posterior interventricular groove

Cardiac crux (external and internal)

1. External cardiac crux is the intersection between the AV, posterior IV and interatrial (IA) grooves
2. Internal cardiac crux is the posterior intersection between the mitral and tricuspid annuli and the atrial and ventricular septa

Cardiac margins

1. Acute margin – junction between anterior and inferior wall of the right ventricle
2. Obtuse margin – rounded lateral wall of left ventricle

Table 1.4 Coronary blood supply [2, 3, 6, 8]

Coronary arterial circulation

A. Left coronary artery (LCA)

1. Ostium of the left coronary artery originates from the left aortic sinus.

2. LCA arises at an acute angle from the aorta.

3. LCA courses to the left and anteriorly (Left anterior descending artery – LAD) and after variable length gives rise to left circumflex artery (LCx).

4. Diagonal artery may arise between LAD and LCx or from the LAD.

5. LAD continues towards the septum and gives rise to septal perforator branches.

B. Right coronary artery

1. Arises from the right aortic sinus.

2. Major branches are nodal, right marginal, PDA.

3. Supplies the RA, SA node, part of RV, posterior third of the interventricular septum, AV node and right branch of the AV bundle (of His).

C. Left circumflex artery (LCx)

1. Originates from the LAD and course is variable.

2. May terminate into one or more large obtuse marginal branches.

3. May continue as a large artery and give rise to posterior descending artery (PDA).

4. When the left circumflex artery supplies the major PDA, it is referred to as a dominant artery.

Coronary venous circulation

1. Composed of the coronary sinus, cardiac veins, and thebesian venous system.

2. Great cardiac vein and other cardiac veins (left posterior and middle) drain into the coronary sinus and finally empties into the right atrium.

3. Rarely, the coronary sinus drains directly into the left atrium.

Coronary collaterals

1. Provide communication between major coronary arteries and branches.

2. May dilate and provide blood supply beyond the obstructed/stenosed epicardial vessel.

3. May develop between the terminal extension of two arteries, between side branches of two arteries, between branches of same artery or within the same branch.

4. Most common in the ventricular septum, ventricular apex, anterior right ventricular free wall, anterolateral left ventricle free wall, cardiac crux and atrial surfaces.

Cardiac lymphatics

1. Lymphatics drain towards the epicardial surface and they merge to form the right and left channels.

2. Left and right channels travel in a retrograde fashion with their respective coronary arteries.

3. The left and right channels travel along the ascending aorta and merge before draining into the pretracheal lymph node.

4. The merged single lymphatic chain travels through a cardiac lymph node and finally empties into the right lymphatic duct.

Table 1.4 *(continued)* Coronary blood supply [2, 3, 6, 8]

Great vessels
1. Subclavian and internal jugular veins join together bilaterally to form right and left innominate (brachiocephalic) veins.
2. Right and left (longer) innominate veins join together to form superior vena cava (SVC).
3. SVC receives azygous vein before draining into the right atrium.
4. Thoracic aorta arises at the level of aortic valve and is made up of the ascending aorta (sinus and tubular portions), aortic arch and descending aorta.
5. Aortic arch gives rise to the innominate, left common carotid and subclavian arteries.
6. Descending aorta lies adjacent to the left atrium, oesophagus and vertebral column.

Table 1.5 Regions supplied by coronary arteries [7]

Right coronary artery	Left coronary artery (Left anterior descending)	Left coronary artery (Left circumflex artery)
Right ventricle	Anterior and lateral wall of LV	SA node (40–45%)
Right atrium	Most of the left ventricle	Left atrium
Diaphragmatic surface/inferior wall of left ventricle (LV)	Interventricular septum (anterior 2/3rd)	AV node and bundle of His (10%)
	Right and left bundle branches	Lateral wall of LV
Posterior wall of left ventricle (90%)		Posterior wall of left ventricle (10%)
Posterior third of interventricular septum (90%)		Posterior third of interventricular septum (10%)
SA node (55–60%)		
AV node and bundle of His (80–90%)		

both ventricles [4, 6] and the smaller cardiac vein drains the marginal aspect of the right ventricle [11]. The thebesian veins drain the endocardium and the innermost layers of the myocardium directly into the underlying chamber [11].

1.2.5
Nerve Supply of the Heart

The sympathetic and parasympathetic autonomic nervous supplies to the heart form the cardiac plexus, which is located close to the arch of the aorta. The fibres from the cardiac plexus accompany the coronary arteries and reach the heart, with most of them terminating at the SA node, AV node and a much less dense supply to the atrial and ventricular myocardium [11]. In general, the parasympathetic vagal fibres are inhibitory and reduce the heart rate and stroke volume. The sympathetic nerves act as accelatory nerves increasing both the heart rate and stroke volume [11]. The afferent nerves run along sympathetic pathways via both cardiac accelerator nerves and thoracic splanchnic nerves to reach the intermediolateral horn of T1–T4 of the spinal cord [11]. The noradrenergic or the sympathetic nervous system is mainly involved with increasing the heart rate (chronotropy), contractility (ionotropy) and the speed of conduction (dromotropy) in the cardiac muscle fibres and the conduction tissue; and the transmitter involved is mainly nor-epinephrine [6]. The SA node receives most of it nerve fibres from the right-sided thoracic sympathetic ganglia and the right vagus [8]. The AV nodes and ventricles receive their nerve supply form the left-sided thoracic sympathetic ganglia and the left vagus, which is mainly because SA node develops from the structures on the right side of the embryo and the AV node develops from the structures on the left side of the embryo [8].

The sympathetic effects are mediated mainly by the adrenergic receptors, which includes β-1 and β-2 adrenergic receptors [2, 11]. β-1 receptors are found mainly in the SA node and AV node, and the ventricular myocardium acts via activation of adenylate cyclase and an increase in cAMP (cyclic adenosine monophosphate) concentration in the cell to mediate the above mentioned sympathetic effects [2, 11]. β-2 receptors are mainly found in the vascular smooth muscles in addition to the bronchial smooth muscle and wall of the GI tract and the bladder. The mechanism of action is same as that of β-1 receptors, i.e., increase in cAMP levels but they cause relaxation of the vascular smooth muscle and are involved in regulation of blood flow and systemic blood pressure [2, 11].

The cholinergic or the parasympathetic nervous system effects in the heart are opposite to the ones mentioned above and the transmitter involved is mainly acetylcholine [8, 12, 13]. The vagi supply the parasympathetic fibres to the heart via the cardiac plexuses. The parasympathetic effects are mediated via the muscaranic receptors, which act by inhibition of adenylate cyclase and hence decrease the intracellular cAMP levels and result in a decrease in heart rate, contraction and conduction velocity [8, 12, 13].

The autonomic centres in the CNS, mainly the vasomotor centre of medulla and the hypothalamus regulate the balance between the level of sympathetic and the parasympathetic output to the cardiovascular system, depending on the afferent inputs from the periphery and the CNS [7, 8, 12, 13]. There is normally a tonic vagal discharge in humans, which overrides the moderate tonic discharge in the cardiac sympathetic nerves [7, 8, 12, 13]. Both the sympathetic and the parasympathetic fibres in the splanchnic thoracic nerves and the vagi carry afferent input mediated via baroreceptors and chemoreceptors to the autonomic centres in the CNS, in addition to the efferent output from the CNS. These afferents and efferents are involved in mediation of cardiovascular reflexes as baroreceptor and chemoreceptor reflexes [7, 8, 12, 13].

The receptors of the autonomic nervous system to the heart are the target of numerous drugs used in the treatment of various cardiovascular disorders in both acute and chronic settings [8, 12, 13].

1.2.6 Conduction System of the Heart

The cardiac conduction system consists of highly specialised cells, which are mainly involved in the conduction of impulses to the different regions of the myocardium [19, 20]. It has been seen to be composed of three types of morphologically and functionally distinct cells, which include P-cells (Pale/Pacemaker-cells), transitional cells and Purkinje cells [19, 20]. These are important in maintaining the heart's electrical activity in an orderly fashion. The conduction system consists of sinus node, internodal tracts, AV node, AV (His) bundle,

Table 1.6 Conduction system of the heart [2, 6, 9]

Sinoatrial (SA)/sinus node
1. Heart's normal pacemaker automatically initiates impulses/contraction cycle at a rate of approximately 72 depolarisations per minute
2. Located by the right atrium (cista terminalis) near the superior vena cava
3. Supplied by the nodal branch of RCA
4. Innervation is principally by the parasympathetic nervous system (slows the autorhythmicity)
5. Blood supply arises from RCA in 55–60% of people (close contact with right atrial appendage and SVC)
6. Blood supply arises from left circumflex in 40–45% of people (lies close to left atrial appendage)

Atrioventricular (AV) node/node of Tawara
1. Located in the right atrium along the lower part of the inter-atrial septum
2. Autorythmic with approximately 40 depolarisations per minute
3. In majority, supplied by RCA
4. It gives rise to the AV bundle

AV Bundle of His
1. Band of nerve fibres that originates from AV node and cross the A-V ring
2. AV bundle is closely related to the annuli of aortic, mitral and tricuspid valves
3. AV bundle receives dual blood supply (AV nodal artery and first septal perforator of LAD)
4. Divides into right and left bundle branches that are continuations of the bundle of His
5. These right and left bundles extend along the right and left sides of the inter-ventricular septum to the tips of the two ventricles

Purkinje fibres
1. Terminal branching of the right and left bundle (thousands of fibrils extending between myocardial fibres).

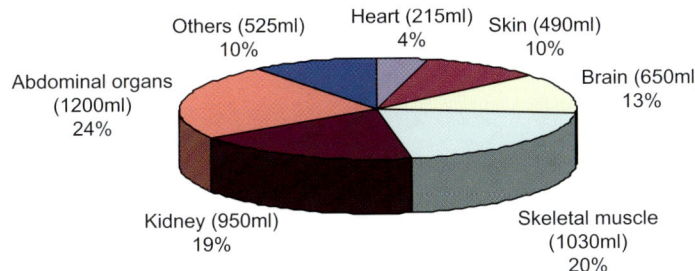

Fig 1.4 Distribution of systemic blood flow to various organs of the body during rest (adapted from Widmaier et al. [14])

right and left bundle branches and Purkinje fibres [4, 18] (Table 1.6).

1.3 Physiology of the Heart

1.3.1 Circulatory System: Systemic and Pulmonary Circulation

The cardiovascular system delivers oxygen and nutrients to the tissues and carries away waste materials to be eliminated by organs such as lungs, liver and kidneys [1, 4] (Fig. 1.4). This system is required to function under various normalised and diseased conditions. The pulmonary and systemic circulations together help in fulfilling this role. Pulmonary circulation is a low resistance, high capacitance bed, and systemic circulation, in comparison, is a relatively high resistance vascular bed [4, 11, 14, 21] (Fig. 1.5).

The deoxygenated blood from the superior vena cava (from upper extremities, head, and chest wall), inferior vena cava (trunk, abdominal organs and lower extremities) and the coronary sinuses (from myocardium) reaches the RA [1, 4, 6, 11]. The RA is filled with deoxygenated blood, increasing pressure in the atrial chamber. When the atrial pressure exceeds the pressure in the RV, the tricuspid valve opens allowing this blood to enter the RV [1, 4, 6, 11]. As a result of this filling, and as the RV starts to contract the pressure in the RV builds up forcing the tricuspid valve to close and the pulmonic valve to open, thereby ejecting the blood into the pulmonary arteries and lungs [1, 4, 6, 11].

The oxygenated blood from the lungs reaches the LA via the pulmonary veins and as a result, pressure in LA builds up and when it exceeds that of the LV, the mitral valve opens, allowing the blood to enter the LV [1, 4, 6, 11]. When the blood fills the LV, and as the LV starts to contract, the LV chamber pressure increase forces the mitral valve to close and aortic valve to open, thus ejecting blood into the aorta, to be distributed throughout the body [1, 4, 6, 11].

1.3.2 Conduction System of the Heart (Excitation Sequence)

The cardiac myocytes have a unique ability of automatic impulse generation, which results in automatic rhythmicity. Normally the electrical impulse begins in the SA node, as it has the fastest impulse generation ability and hence drives the heart. The impulse then spreads to the rest of the right atrial walls directly, to the left atrium by the interatrial conducting fibres and then to the AV node (AV junctional tissue) [6] (Fig. 1.6). The AV node conducts the impulse with a delay and propagates through the ventricular myocardium via the AV bundle of His and Purkinje fibres [1, 3, 6, 8–13, 18]. From the Purkinje fibres, the excitation impulse then continues through myocardial cells outside the specialised conduction pathway to reach the subendocardial surface. This rapid, simultaneous and coordinated spread of excitation through the ventricles produces a coordinated contraction of both ventricles, thus ensuring efficient pumping of blood to the pulmonary and systemic circulations [1, 3, 6, 8–13, 18].

1.3.3 Action Potential (AP)

Ventricles, atria and the Purkinje system have a stable resting membrane potential of about −90 mV, determined mainly by K^+ conductance [12, 13]. The action potential is of long duration about 300 ms, which is prolonged in comparison with the action potential of the rest of the cells in the body. The action potential of the myocardial cells excluding the nodal tissue is initiated by a sudden transient inward increase in the membrane conductance of the Na^+ ion, referred to as the upstroke of the action potential or phase 0 (Figs. 1.7 and 1.8) [12, 13]. This is followed by a brief transient outward increase in K^+ ion membrane conductance resulting in a brief period of initial repolarisation. The decreasing Na^+ ion conductance also plays a part in this initial repolarisation phase and is referred to as phase 1 of action po-

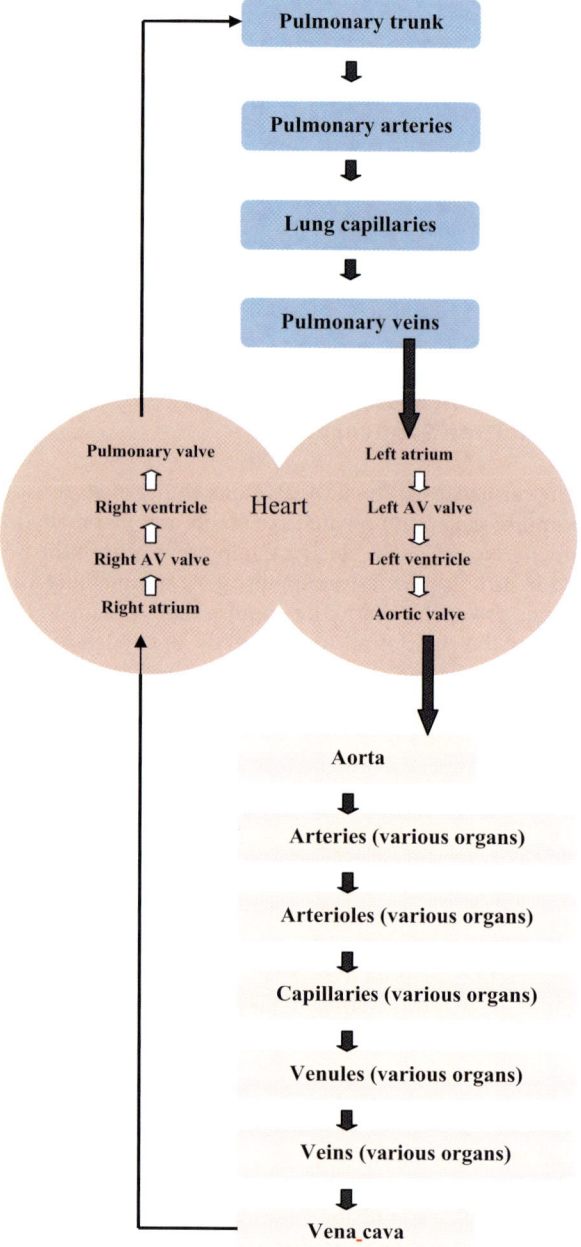

Fig 1.5 Circulatory pathway of the cardiovascular system [8]

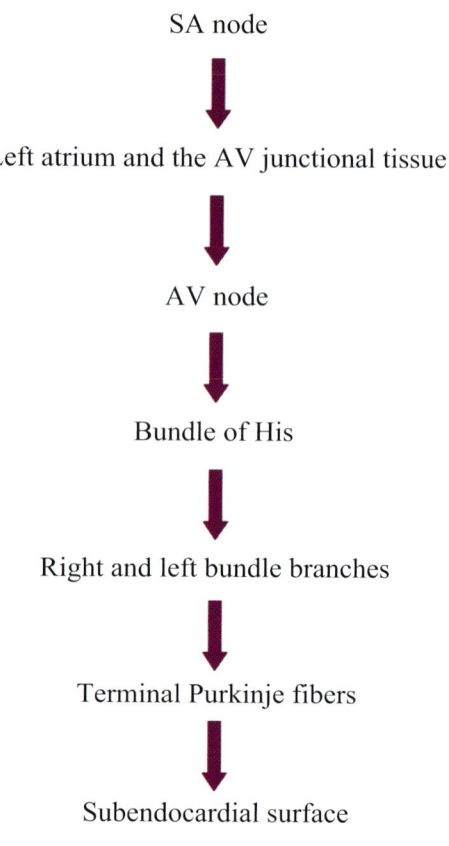

Fig 1.6 Conducting system of the heart

tential [12, 13]. After this phase comes the plateau phase or phase 2 of action potential, which is characterised by the transient increase in inward Ca^{++} ion conductance, accompanied by an increase in outward K^+ ion conductance [12, 13]. These outward and inward currents are such that they maintain the membrane potential in the plateau phase. The plateau phase is followed by the repolarisation phase of the action potential or phase 3, which results from the declining inward Ca^{++} ion conductance and an increase in the outward K^+ ion conductance [12, 13]. This outward K^+ ion conductance hyperpolarises the membrane towards K^+ ion equilibrium and brings about the repolarisation or phase 4 [12, 13].

The SA node action potential is different from the rest of the conducting system and the myocardium. It is characterised by an unstable resting membrane potential or phase 4. This results from an increased Na^+ ion conductance resulting in inward Na^+ current [12, 13]. The inward Na^+ current is triggered by the repolarisation of the preceding action potential. In addition, the phase 0 of the action potential in the SA node is the result of inward Ca^{++} ion conductance in contrast to Na^+ ion, as in the rest of the myocardium [12, 13]. In addition, the SA node action potential lacks the plateau or phase 2 of the myocardial cell action potential [12, 13]. The upstroke of the action potential in the AV node is also due to the Ca^{++} ion conductance as in the SA node. The conduction velocity is fastest in the Purkinje system and slowest in the AV node [12, 13].

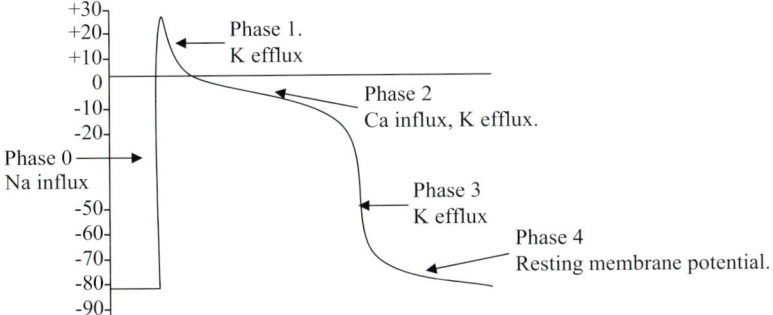

Fig 1.7 Cardiac action potential

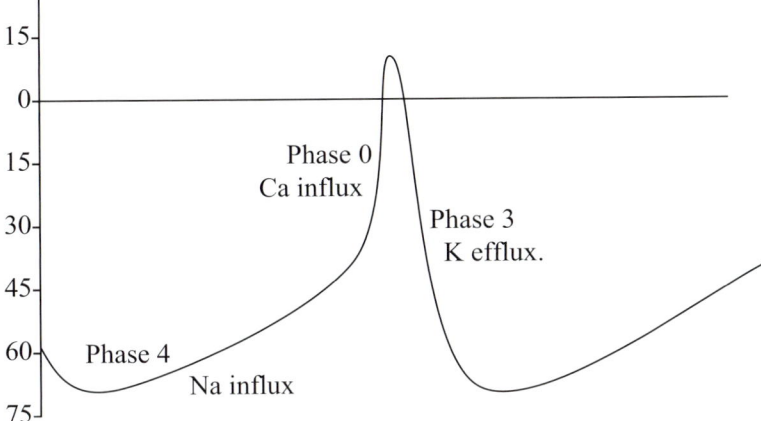

Fig 1.8 SA nodal action potential

1.3.4
Mechanism of Excitation and Contraction Coupling of Cardiac Myocytes

The regulation of cardiac muscle contraction has neural, hormonal and intrinsic components. The heart is composed of cylindrical cardiac cells and stimulation of one cardiac cell initiates stimulation of adjacent cells [7, 22]. In general, the cardiac cells are of two types (a) electrical cells and (b) myocardial cells [7]. The electrical cells are specialised myocardial cells that have essentially lost the ability to contract but have become specialised in the conduction of cardiac impulses.

The myocardial cells have two specific properties: contractility (ability of the cells to shorten and return to their original length) and extensibility (cell filaments' ability to stretch) [22]. The contraction mechanism contains numerous steps and "excitation–contraction coupling" is the term used to define the events that translate the depolarisation of the cardiac cell membrane to the contraction of the muscle fibres [5, 6, 11] (Fig. 1.9). The contractile filaments actin and myosin in the myocardium are responsible for the contraction. In the cardiac cell, the sarcoplasmic reticulum and the cisternae contains high concentrations of ionised Ca^{++} and depolarisation of the T tubules, which is an extension of the cell membrane, causes the release of Ca^{++} from these structures [5, 6, 11]. In general, an action potential precedes each contraction, and between contractions the Ca^{++} within the cell is very low. The cardiac action potential is unique in that it has a plateau phase, which is maintained by the inward Ca^{++} influx (current) [5, 6, 11]. It is this inward Ca^{++} current that triggers release of further Ca^{++} from the sarcoplasmic reticulum. The amount of Ca^{++} released depends on the strength of the inward Ca^{++} current. Compared with the resting or basal conditions, the concentration of Ca^{++} is ten times higher during an AP [5]. When the concentration of the Ca^{++} is high, the troponin-C is bound by four Ca^{++} ions per molecule and this changes the shape of troponin [6, 7, 11]. This change in shape allows the tropomyosin to uncover the cross-bridge sites, which allows the formation of cross bridges between actin and myosin filaments [6, 7, 11]. In the resting state, the troponin molecules shield the cross-bridges.

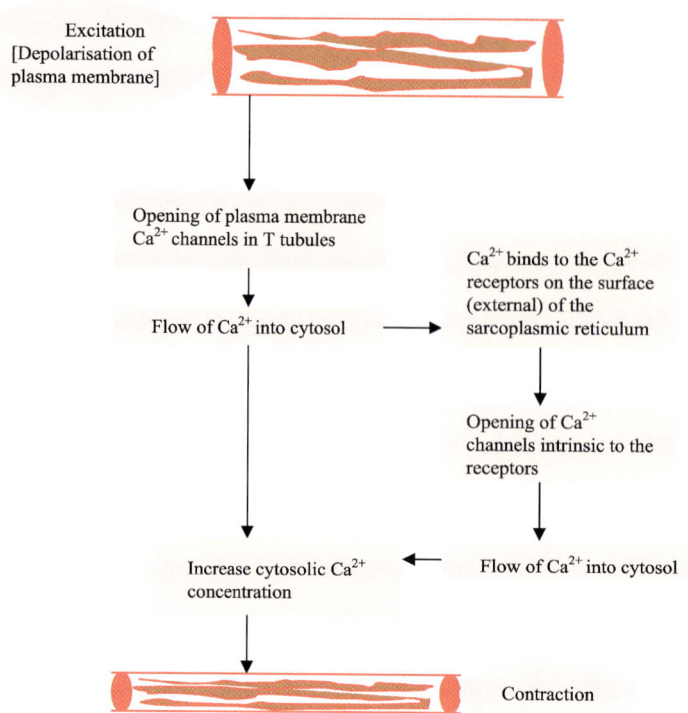

Fig 1.9 Excitation contraction coupling

The presence of adenosine triphosphate (ATP) is important in the contractile process. The actin–myosin cross-bridges are formed in the presence of ATP, which later hydrolyses. The energy derived from ATP hydrolysis leads to changes in the myosin head configuration so that actin can be detached from myosin (10 nm/cycle). Finally, ATP is required for relaxation of the muscle by dissociating the cross-bridges [6]. In general, an increase in the number of bridges causes an increase in the force of contraction, which is proportional to the intracellular Ca^{++} concentration [6]. Relaxation occurs when the intracellular Ca^{++} is re-sequestered back into the sarcoplasmic reticulum by the Ca^{++}-ATPase pump. Administration of drugs like epinephrine, norepinephrine, and digitalis and sympathetic nerve stimulation increases the intracellular Ca^{++} levels, which results in forceful contraction [6]. Norepinephrine not only causes forceful contraction but also shortens the AP and contraction by causing more rapid uptake of Ca^{++} by the sarcoplasmic reticulum [6]. The contractility can be quantified by calculating the ejection fraction (EF), which is defined as the ratio of stroke volume (SV) to end-diastolic volume (EDV) ($EF = SV/EDV$) [11, 23, 24].

The electrical cells are special cardiac cells of the conducting system [22]. These cells are primarily responsible for the formation and conduction of the impulses. They have some specific properties such as (a) conductivity (ability to transmit electrical impulse from one cell to another), (b) excitability (ability of the cell to respond to electrical impulses) and (c) automaticity (ability of the cell to spontaneously generate and discharge an electrical impulse) [7, 22]. The depolarisation (electrical activation), contraction and repolarisation (Fig. 1.10) of cardiac cells is due to the ability of the electrical cells to generate and conduct electrical impulses. The flow of positively charged ions across the cardiac cell membranes results in the formation of these electrical impulses [7, 22]. The extracellular fluid surrounding the cardiac cells contains positively and negatively charged ions. However, the composition of these ions in the extra- and intracellular spaces is different [7]. The intracellular space contains positively charged potassium ions in high concentration and positively charged sodium in lower concentration. The extracellular space contains the positively charged sodium and negatively charged chloride in high concentration and a lower concentration of potassium [7]. The movement of the primary intracellular ion (potassium) and primary extracellular ion (sodium) mediates the regulation of electrical charges. The cyclical shift of ions changes the electrical field inside the cell leading to depolarisation and repolarisation [7, 22]. In part, the ionic shift is dependent on the pores or channels present on the cell membrane, and partly on the opening and closing of channels which is

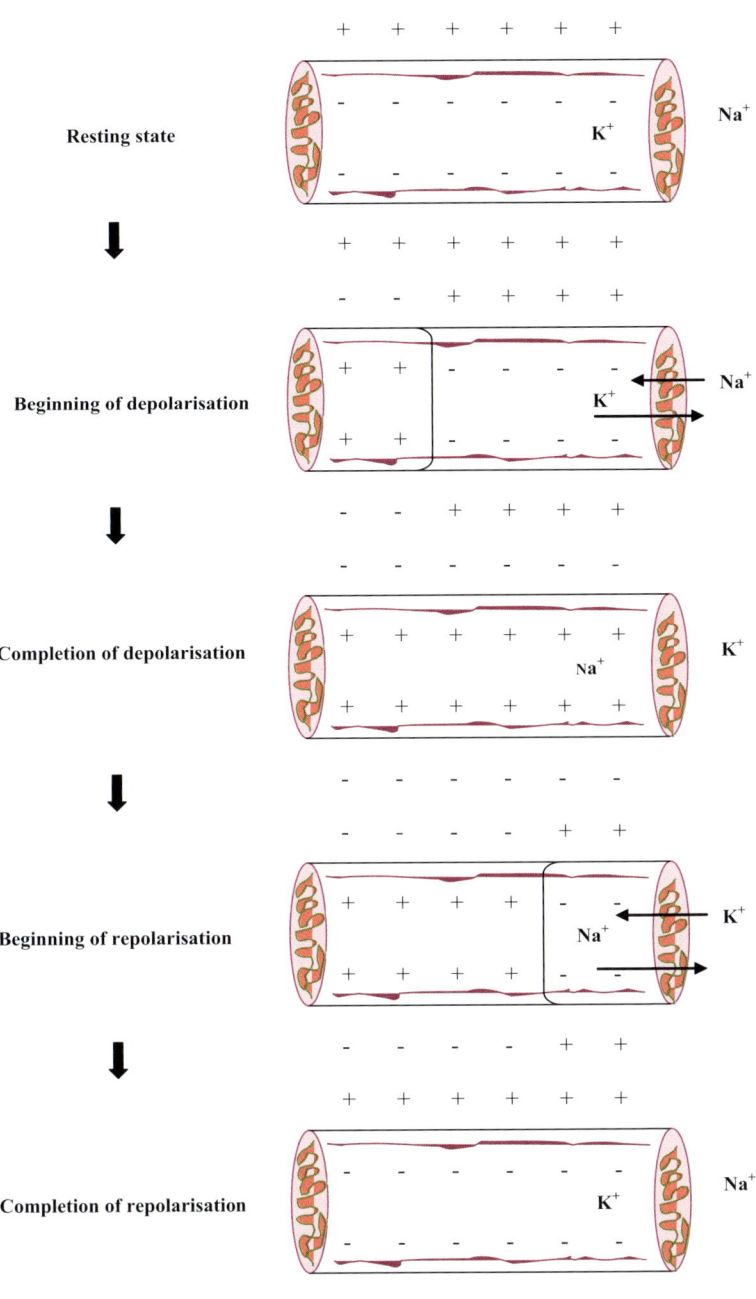

Fig 1.10 Cardiac cell depolarisation and repolarisation [7]

regulated by electrical, mechanical or chemical stimuli [7]. Furthermore, the concentration gradient affects the ion distribution across the cell membrane [7].

In the resting state of the cell, the electrical activity is more positive outside the cell and more negative inside the cell and no electrical activity occurs [7, 22]. When the cell is stimulated, the permeability of the membrane changes allowing sodium to enter the cell [7]. This results in the inside of the cell becoming more positive than the outside, resulting in a depolarised state [7]. Once depolarisation is complete, the membrane allows sodium to exit, once again making the cell more negative inside. This end result is called repolarisation (cell recovery) [7].

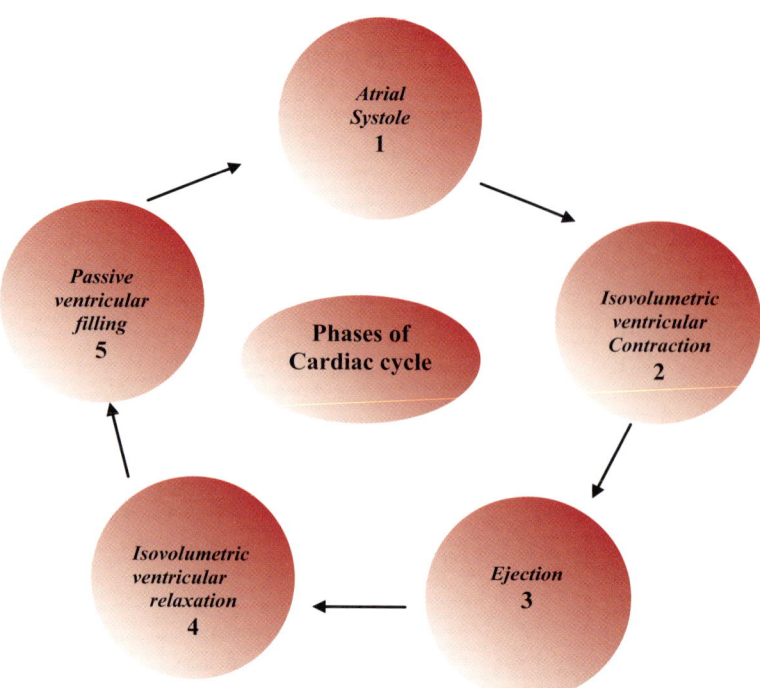

Fig 1.11 Phases of cardiac cycle

1.3.5
Autonomic Nervous System and Heart

The autonomic nervous system has both cardioacceleratory and cardioinhibitory effects on the heart, which are manifest both in the resting state and in times of stress [4–6, 8, 11–14]. The noradrenergic or the sympathetic nervous system is mainly involved with increasing the heart rate (chronotropy), contractility (ionotropy) and the speed of conduction (dromotropy) in the cardiac muscle fibres and the conduction tissue; and the transmitter involved is mainly nor-epinephrine [4–6, 8, 11–14]. The sympathetic effects are mediated mainly by the adrenergic receptors, which includes β-1 and β-2 adrenergic receptors. β-1 receptors are found mainly in the SA node, AV node and ventricular myocardium, and operate via activation of adenylate cyclase and increase in cAMP (cyclic adenosine monophosphate) concentration in the cell to mediate the above mentioned sympathetic effects [4–6, 8, 11–14]. β-2 receptors are mainly found in the vascular smooth muscles in addition to the bronchial smooth muscle and wall of the GI tract and the bladder [4–6, 8, 11–14]. The mechanism of action is same as that of β-1 receptors i.e, increase in cAMP levels but they cause relaxation of the vascular smooth muscle and are involved in regulation of blood flow and systemic blood pressure [4–6, 8, 11–14].

The cholinergic or the parasympathetic nervous system effects in the heart are opposite to the ones mentioned above and the transmitter involved is mainly acetylcholine [4–6, 8, 11–14]. The vagi supply the parasympathetic fibres to the heart via the cardiac plexuses. The parasympathetic effects are mediated via the muscaranic receptors, which act by inhibition of adenylate cyclase and hence decrease the intracellular cAMP levels and result in a decrease in heart rate, contraction and conduction velocity [4–6, 8, 11–14].

The autonomic centres in the CNS, mainly the vasomotor centre of medulla and the hypothalamus regulate the balance between the level of sympathetic and the parasympathetic output to the cardiovascular system depending on the afferent inputs from the periphery and the CNS [4–6, 8, 11–14]. There is normally a tonic vagal discharge in humans which overrides the moderate tonic discharge in the cardiac sympathetic nerves [12,13]. Both the sympathetic and the parasympathetic fibres in the splanchnic thoracic nerves and the vagi carry afferent input mediated via baroreceptors and chemoreceptors to the autonomic centres in the CNS, in addition to the efferent output from the CNS [12, 13]. These afferents and efferents are involved in mediation of cardiovascular reflexes such as baroreceptor and the chemoreceptor reflexes [4–6, 8, 11–14].

1.3.6
Cardiac Cycle

The cardiac cycle consists of contraction and relaxation of both atria and ventricles (Fig. 1.11). The heart does not contract or relax as a single unit [11]. The cardiac cycle consists of cyclic structural and functional changes which the heart under goes every 0.8 s on average to maintain the blood flow through the body. The cycle starts with an atrial systole, which is preceded by an impulse generated in the SA node and is spread across the atria corresponding to a P-wave on the electrocardiogram [11]. The atrial systole contributes to, but is not essential for, ventricular filling, but it does become an important factor in a diseased heart [11, 14]. Filling of the ventricles by atrial contraction causes the fourth heart sound, this is not normally audible in adults. During this phase, the AV valves are open and the ventricles are relaxing. The semilunar valves (SL) are closed, which prevents re-entry of blood from the pulmonary artery or the aorta. The isovolumetric ventricular contraction (start of ventricular systole while the SL valves are closed) follows the atrial systole, during which the ventricular volume remains constant [6, 11, 14]. The isovolumetric ventricular contraction is preceded by the spread of the electric impulse from the AV node to the rest of the ventricular myocardium, and this is seen as the QRS complex on an electrocardiogram [6, 11, 14]. When the ventricular pressure becomes greater than the atrial pressure, the AV valves close, corresponding to the first heart sound, with the mitral valve closing fractionally before the tricuspid valve. The semilunar (SL) valves open as the pressure in the ventricles exceeds that of the pressure in the aorta and the pulmonary artery, resulting in rapid ventricular ejection. This results in a dramatic reduction in the ventricular volume as most of the ventricular blood (stroke volume) is ejected during this phase. The atria also begin to fill during this phase. The end of ventricular contraction corresponds to the onset of the T-wave on the electrocardiogram [6, 11, 14]. Towards the end of the ventricular contraction the ejection of blood from the ventricles is slower as the ventricular pressure starts to drop. This is followed by isovolumetric ventricular relaxation marked by closure of the aortic and pulmonic valves. The closure of the semilunar valves corresponds to the second heart sound. The AV valves are closed and the ventricular volume remains constant. The pressure in the ventricles is reduced rapidly [6, 11, 14]. When the ventricular pressure becomes less than the atrial pressure, the AV valves open marking the end of the isovolumetric phase of ventricular relaxation and the onset of rapid ventricular filling. During the beginning of this phase of ventricular relaxation, there is passive filling of the ventricles with the blood from the atria, which is rapid [6, 11, 14]. The rapid flow of blood from the atria into ventricles causes the third heart sound, which is normal in children but in adults is associated with disease. Reduced ventricular filling sometimes referred to as diastasis, which is the longest period of the cardiac cycle, follows the rapid filling. Most of the myocardium receives its blood supply during this phase of the cardiac cycle [6, 11, 14].

1.3.7
Physiology of Coronary Circulation

The primary function of the coronary circulation is to meet the metabolic demand of the heart. Coronary blood flow increases from the baseline or resting level to the maximum depending on myocardial oxygen requirements [25–27]. An adequate increase of coronary blood flow is required to meet myocardial oxygen consumption. During strenuous exercise or metabolic demand, the coronary blood flow increases up to 4–6 times [25–27]. In conditions such as left ventricular hypertrophy (LVH), myocardial ischaemia, and diabetes mellitus (DM) the normal increase in coronary flow can be blunted. The epicardial conduit resistance is produced by atherosclerotic stenosis and the distal vascular bed maintains satisfactory blood flow by dilating. The maximal increase in coronary flow above resting levels is defined as coronary flow reserve (CRF) [27,28]. The major determinants of myocardial oxygen consumption are heart rate (HR), myocardial wall tension/stress (after-load) and inotropic state (contractility) of the myocardium [27, 29]. Vascular resistance also plays an important role in coronary circulation and is mainly determined by myocardial oxygen consumption, and modulated mainly by local metabolic factors (vasoactive autacoids) with some contribution from neural stimuli, and circulating vasoactive substances [27].

1.3.8
Coronary Collaterals

The initial documentation of coronary collaterals in humans was not made until 1964, although their presence was considered as far back as the 16th century [21, 30]. There are few and small collateral vessels and they may develop into a major vascular network in patients with obstructive coronary artery disease [21]. It is generally believed that the collateral vessels, or network, develop only when the occlusive disease or stenosis is severe enough to produce a substantial transstenotic pressure drop [21]. When collaterals are present in patients with severe or significant occlusive CAD, the part of the myocardium supplied by the stenotic vessel seems to have better contractile function than in patients without collaterals [31]. Further, it is hypothesised that pre-existing collaterals may also play an important role by decreasing the extent and degree of myocardial damage at the time or during an acute coronary episode [21]. In general, the

Table 1.7 Physiological changes and cardiovascular response to moderate exercise [33, 35–38]

Physiological response and cardiovascular changes during moderate exercise	Contributing factors to fatigue during prolonged exercise	Contributing factors to muscle fatigue during exercise
Heart rate increases	Fatigue	Muscle fatigue
Increased sympathetic stimulation	Reduction in muscle glycogen	Acidosis
Decreased parasympathetic stimulation	Hyperthermia	Central nervous system (CNS) factors
CO increases	Dehydration	Increased NH_3
SV increases	Hypoglycaemia	Electrochemical changes
EDV increases	Muscle damage	Cell phosphorylation potential
Pulse pressure increases	Electrolyte imbalance	ATP Reduction
MAP (mean arterial pressure) increases	CNS/neuromuscular junction and muscle electrochemical abnormalities	Increased ADP
TPR decreases		Increased free inorganic phosphate
Oxygen extraction increases		
Blood flow to heart, muscle and skin increases		
Blood flow to brain increases (slightly)		
Blood flow to other viscera decreases		

coronary collaterals are capable of preserving the function and structure in a resting myocardium, however, the coronary flow per gram in a collateral-dependent myocardium is reduced when compared with the normally perfused myocardium. One reason for this could be the change in pressure gradient across the collateral vessels (arterial pressure is lower than aortic pressure in the collateralised segment) [21, 32].

1.4
Exercise Physiology

Exercise physiology is a branch of physiology, which studies how exercise alters the structure and function of the body. Exercise is now used as a therapy during rehabilitation from various injuries or illness and it is used as a preventive strategy to delay the onset and progression of atherosclerotic cardiovascular disease [33–35]. Exercise testing using a treadmill or bicycle ergometer is commonly used in the cardiology department to assess the exercise tolerance and diagnosis of ischaemic heart disease. However, exercise tolerance and capacity depends on multiple factors such as age, sex, physical/mental conditioning, medications, disease status, etc. [33–35].

During exercise, multiple physiological changes are encountered (Table 1.7). In general, cardiac output (CO) increase is due to a larger increase in heart rate (HR) and a smaller increase in stroke volume (SV). During exercise, the CO may increase to a maximum value of 35 L/min (baseline 5 L/min) [14]. Most of the increased cardiac output goes to the exercising muscle and part of it goes to the skin (to dissipate heat) and heart [14]. The increase in flow to these organs is due to vasodilatation and the flow to the gastrointestinal organs and kidneys decreases (secondary to increased sympathetic activity) [36–39].

The total peripheral resistance to blood flow is reduced due to the arteriolar vasodilatation in the skeletal muscle, skin, and cardiac muscle. The net result is a decrease in total peripheral resistance (TPR) [14]. In addition, there is increased venous return because of increased muscular activity, which in turn further increases the cardiac output. The cardiovascular and muscular changes in blood flow with exercise is also controlled by various factors including but not limited to (a) exercise centres in the brain, (b) local chemical changes in the muscle, (c) mechanoreceptors and chemoreceptors in muscle, and (d) arterial baroreceptors [14] (Fig. 1.12).

1.4.1
Gender and Exercise Performance

Gender differences relating to the cardiovascular system in terms of body composition, metabolism, muscle morphology and endocrine responses are well reported and documented in the medical literature [40]. Women have smaller lung volume and pulmonary capillary volume than men, resulting in lower maximum pulmonary ventilation [40]. Women also have a smaller heart, with a lower filling volume, lower maximum stroke volume and lower cardiac output [40]. Women are reported to have a lower haemoglobin concentration, haematocrit and total blood volume; therefore, they are at a relative disadvantage for transport of oxygen to skeletal muscle during exercise. However, gender differences become less notable when cardiovascular parameters are expressed relative to body surface area and mass [40] (Table 1.8).

Research on men and women runners indicates that women tend to have smaller amounts of slow twitch fibres type in the gastrocnemius muscle. The greater lean body mass in men is a major determinant of greater muscle strength [40]. Maximum oxygen consumption is different for men and women and men seem to have higher maximal oxygen consumption [40]. However, when these are expressed in relation to lean body mass, there appears to be little significant difference between the sexes [40]. Finally, there are considerable endocrine or hormonal differences between men and women. In women who train very aggressively or too hard, the luteal phase of the menstrual cycle is shortened and eventually the cycle is lost (athletic amenorrhoea) [33, 40].

1.4.2
Age and Exercise Performance

Aging is a normal biological process, which is inevitable. Aging has been defined as a progressive loss of physiological capacities that culminates in death [40–42].

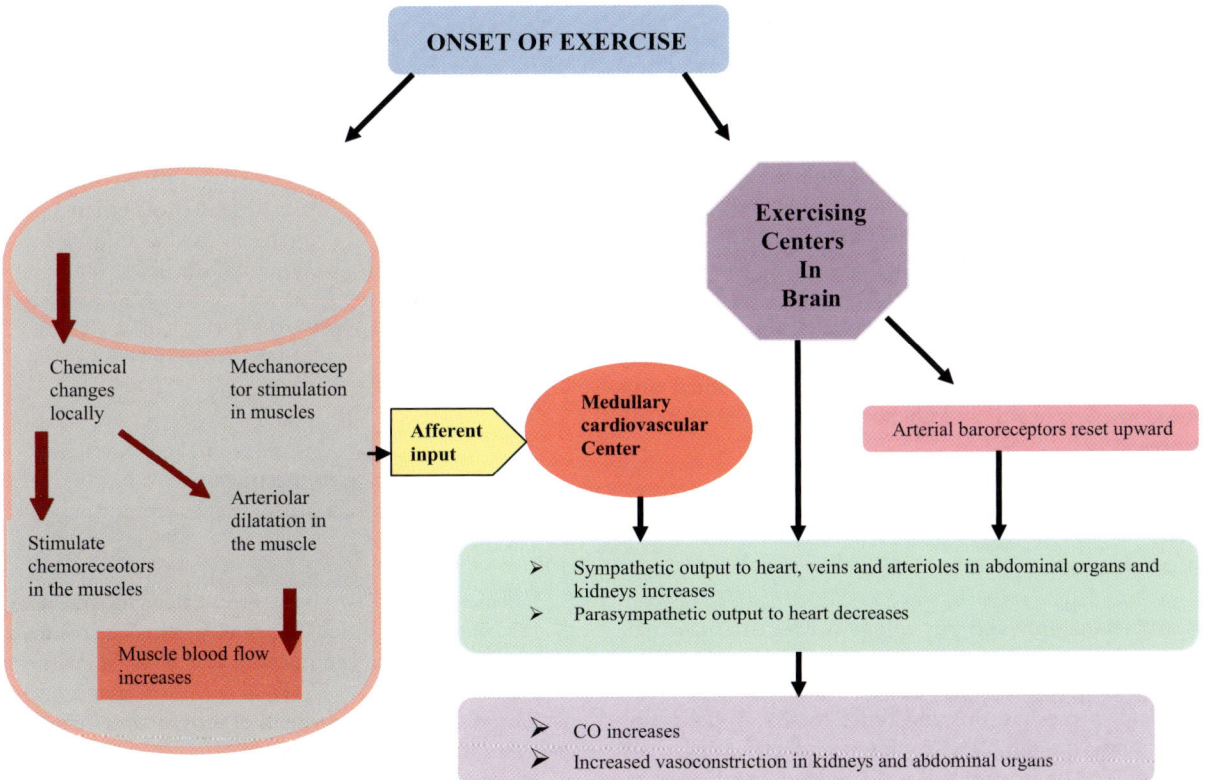

Fig 1.12 Changes in cardiovascular system during exercise [14]

Table 1.8 Gender, cardiovascular system and exercise physiology [40]

Females have higher percentage of body fat and is more often distributed around hips and thighs, as compared to males' body fat which tends to be distributed at the waist and stomach
Males have larger lean body mass and are generally taller than the average female
Males have a narrower pelvic region than females
Females have fewer sweat glands than males
Females have smaller hearts than males
Females have smaller lung volume and pulmonary capillary volume than males
Females have lower percentage of slow twitch motor unit than males
Females have a smaller blood volume than males
Females have lower haemoglobin concentration than males
Females have a lower haematocrit than males
Females have ovaries and they produce estrogen and progesterone
Men have testes and they produce testosterone

Table 1.9 Effect of aging on the cardiovascular system [40–42]

Maximum oxygen consumption	Reduced
Maximum heart rate	Reduced
Cardiac output	Reduced
Blood pressure	Increased
Vascular resistance	Increased
Total cholesterol	Increased
Triglycerides	Increased
LDL	Increased
HDL	Reduced
Maximum ventilation	Reduced
Respiratory muscle strength	Reduced
Vital capacity	Reduced
Expiratory flow rate	Reduced
Muscle strength, endurance, flexibility	Reduced
Pulmonary diffusion	Reduced
Alveolar surface area	Reduced
Chest wall structures	Altered
Alveolar elastic recoil	Altered
Pulmonary blood volume	Reduced
Lean body mass	Reduced
Adipose tissue	Increased
Basal metabolic rate	Reduced
Sleep	Reduced
Cognitive function	Reduced

Various natural and pathophysiological changes occur during the course of life [41, 42] (Table 1.9). The commonest of these are loss of height, greying hair, changes in vision, reduction in lean body mass, wrinkling of skin, etc. [41, 42]. Many interesting theories have been implicated to explain the process of aging. However, how long an individual lives depends on multiple factors including heredity, environment, individual attitude towards health and life and finally access to health services [41, 42].

1.5 Conclusion

Cardiac anatomy and physiology is extensive, fascinating and exciting. However, exploiting their role in clinical practice requires a thorough understanding of basic principles, mechanisms and functionality. Appreciating and understanding the anatomy and physiology and recognising their changes will help not only in anticipation of disease but also in appreciating the signs and symptoms produced by them.

References

1. Callahan JA, Kay JD (1991) Foundations of cardiology. In Giuliani ER et al. (eds), Cardiology Fundamentals and Practice, Vol. 1, 2nd edn. Mosby-Year Book, St Louis, pp. 3–25.
2. Edwards WD (1984) Anatomy of the Cardiovascular System; Clinical Medicine, Vol. 6. Harper & Row, Philadelphia, pp. 1–24.
3. Malouf JF, Edwards WD, Tajil AJ, Seward JB (2001) Functional anatomy of the heart. In Fuster F, Alexander RW,

O'Rourke RA (eds), Hurst's: The Heart, 10th edn. McGraw-Hill Inc., pp. 19–62.
4. Boulpaep EL (2005) Organisation of Cardiovascular System. Boron WF, Boulpaep EL, updated version. Elsevier Saunders, pp. 423–507.
5. Tortora GJ, Grabowski SR (1996) Principles of Anatomy and Physiology, 8th edn. HarperCollins College Publishers, New York, pp. 598–600.
6. Bullock J, Boyle J III, Wang MB (1991) Physiology, The National Medical Series for Independent Study, 2nd edn. Williams and Wilkins, pp. 93–148.
7. Huff J (2002) ECG Workout Exercise in Arrhythmia Interpretation, 4th edn. Lippincott.
8. Gray's PG (1995) In Gray's Anatomy, 38th edn. Churchill Livingston, New York, p.1498.
9. Edwards WD (1995) Cardiac anatomy and examination of cardiac specimens. In Emmanouilides G et al. (eds). Moss & Adams Heart Diseae in Infants, Children and Adolescents, 5th edn. Williams & Wilkins, Baltimore, pp. 70–105.
10. Edwards WD (1991) Applied anatomy of the heart. In Guiliani ER et al. Cardiology Fundamentals and Practice, Vol. 1, 2nd edn. Mosby-Year Book, St Louis, pp. 47–112.
11. Thibodeau GA, Patton KT (1996) Anatomy of the cardiovascular system. In Anthony's Textbook of Anatomy and Physiology, 15th edn, pp. 614–657.
12. Ganong WF (2003) Lange Review of Medical Physiology, 21st edn. McGraw-Hill.
13. Ganong WF (2005) Lange Review of Medical Physiology, 22nd edn. McGraw-Hill.
14. Widmaier EP, Raff H, Strang KT (2006) Cardiovascular physiology. In Vanders Human Physiology – The Mechanism of Body Function, 10th edn. McGraw-Hill, pp. 387–476.
15. Apkon M (2005) Cellular physiology of skeletal, cardiac and smooth muscle. In Boron WF, Boulpaep EL (eds), Medical Physiology. Elsevier Saunders, pp. 230–254.
16. Edwards WD (1984) Anatomic basis for tomographic analysis of the heart at autopsy. Cardiol Clin 2:485–506.
17. Katz AM (2006) Physiology of the Heart, 4th edn. Lippincott Williams & Wilkins, Philadelphia..
18. Lederer WJ (2005) Cardiac electrophysiology and electrocardiogram. In Boron WF, Boulpaep EL (eds), Medical Physiology. Elsevier Saunders, updated version, pp. 483–507.
19. Opic LH (2004) The Heart: Physiology, from Cell to Circulation, 4th edn. Lippincott Williams & Wilkins, Baltimore, MD.
20. Kurachi Y, Terzic A, Cohen M, Sperelakis N (2001) Heart Physiology and Pathophysiology, 4th edn. Academiv Press.
21. Klocke FJ, Ellis AK (1990) Physiology of the coronary circulation. In Parmley WW, Chatterjee K (eds), Cardiology. Philadelphia:, JB Lippincott Co., pp.1–16.
22. Seward W (1994) Transoesophageal echocardiograhic anatomy. In Feeman W, Seward J et al. (eds), Transeosophageal Echocardiography. Little, Boaston, pp. 55–101.
23. Boulpaep EL (2005) Heart as a pump. In Boron WF, Boulpaep EL (eds), Medical Physiology. Elsevier Saunders, updated version, pp. 509–533.
24. Boulpaep EL (2005) Regulation of arterial pressure and cardiac output. In Boron WF, Boulpaep EL (eds), Medical Physiology. Elsevier Saunders, updated version, pp. 534–557.
25. Porenta G, Cherry S, Czernin J, Brunken R, Kuhle W, Hashimoto T, Schelbert HR. (1999) Noninvasive determination of myocardial blood flow, oxygen consumption and efficiency in normal humans by carbon-11 acetate positron emission tomography imaging. Eur J Nucl Med 26:1465–74.
26. Pitkanen OP, Nuutila P, Raitakari OT et al. (1999) Coronary flow reserve in young men with familial combined hyperlipidemia. Circulation 99:1678–84.
27. Maseri A et al. (2001) Coronary blood flow and myocardial ischaemia. In Fuster F, Alexander RW, O'Rourke RA (eds), Hurst's: The Heart, 10th edn. McGraw-Hill, pp.1109–1131.
28. Vassalli G, Hess OM (1998) Measurement of coronary flow reserve and its role in patient care. Basic Res Cardiol 93:339–53.
29. Braunwald E. (1999) 50th anniversary historical article. Myocardial oxygen consumption: the quest for its determinants and some clinical fallout. J Am Coll Cardiol 34:1365–8.
30. Fulton WFW (1965) The Coronary Arteries. Charles C. Thomson, Springfield IL.
31. Schwarz F, Flameng W, Ensslen R et al. (1978) Effects of collaterals. Am Heart J 95:570.
32. Arani DT, Greene DG, Bunnell IL et al. (1984) Reductions in coronary flow under resting conditions in collateral-dependant myocardium of patients with complete occlusion left anterior descending coronary artery. J Am Coll Cardiol 3:668–2005.
33. McArdle WD, Katch FI, Katch V (2006) The cardiovascular system. In Exercise Physiology – Energy, Nutrition, Human Preference, 6th edn. Lippincott, William and Wilkins, pp. 313–332.
34. McArdle WD, Katch FI, Katch VL (2006) Physical activity health and aging. In Exercise Physiology – Energy, Nutrition, Human Preference, 6th edn. Lippincott, William and Wilkins, pp. 883–924.
35. Wilmore JH, Costill DL (2004) Cardiovascular control during exercise. In Physiology of Sport and Exercise, 3rd edn. Human Kinetics, pp. 206–241.
36. Roberts RA, Roberts SO (1997) Factors contributing to fatigue during exercise. In Exercise Physiology (Exercise, Performance & Clinical Application), Mosby, pp. 546–563.

37. Roberts RA, Roberts SO (1997) Cardiovascular function and adaptation to exercise. In Exercise Physiology (Exercise, Performance & Clinical Application), Mosby, 268–293.
38. Wilmore JH, Costill DL (2004) Cardiovascular and respiratory adaptations to training. In Physiology of Sport and Exercise, 3rd edn, Human Kinetics, pp. 270–305.
39. McArdle WD, Katch FI, Katch VL (2006) Cardiology regulation integration. In Exercise Physiology – Energy, Nutrition, Human Preference, 6th edn. Lippincott, William and Wilkins.
40. Roberts RA, Roberts SO (1997) Gender and exercise performance. In Exercise Physiology (Exercise, Performance & Clinical Application), Mosby, pp. 564-577.
41. Roberts RA, Roberts SO (1997) Exercise and aging. In Exercise Physiology (Exercise, Performance & Clinical Application). Mosby, pp. 578–599.
42. Wilmore JH, Costill DL (2004), Aging in sports and exercise. In Physiology of Sport and Exercise, 3rd edn, pp. 538–565.

Further Reading

1. Boron WF, Boulpaep E (2005) In Medical Physiology: a Cellular and Molecular Approach. Elsevier/Saunders, updated version, pp. 423–507.
2. Thibodeau GA, Patton KT (1996) Anthony's Textbook of Anatomy and Physiology, 15th edn. Mosby, pp. 614–657.
3. Ganong WF (2003) Lange Review of Medical Physiology, 21st edn. McGraw-Hill.
4. Gray's Anatomy 38th edn (1995) Churchill Livingston, New York.
5. Bullock J, Boyle J III, Wang MB (1991) Physiology, The National Medical Series for Independent Study, 2nd edn. Williams and Wilkins, pp. 93–148.

Pathophysiology of Coronary Artery Disease

Shahid Mahmood

Contents

2.1	Incidence	23
2.2	Introduction	24
2.3	Pathophysiology	24
2.3.1	Endothelial Dysfunction and Atherosclerosis	25
2.3.2	Inflammation and Atherosclerosis	27
2.3.3	Race and Genetics	27
2.3.4	Collateral Circulation and Angiogenesis	27
2.3.5	Apoptosis	28
	References	28

2.1 Incidence

Coronary artery disease (CAD), also called coronary heart disease (CHD) is the most common form of heart disease and is a serious health problem worldwide, leading to cardiovascular disability and death. It is the leading cause of mortality in the UK [1, 2] (Table 2.1). One recent estimate is that approximately 2.65 million people in the UK are suffering from CAD, and of these 1.2 million have had a myocardial infarction. There were an estimated 275,000 heart attacks in the UK in 2001, and 335,000 new cases of angina are diagnosed each year [2]. According to data from the Centre for Disease Control and Prevention (CDC) in the USA, 761,085 Americans died due to heart diseases in 1981 and 700,142 in 2001 (Table 2.2). The slight decline in mortality is most likely related to improved therapeutic options and better preventive strategies. Approximately, two million Europeans die from coronary artery disease each year.

Table 2.1 Comparison of number of deaths due to heart diseases in 1998

Total deaths	555,000
Circulatory diseases	226,700
Malignancies	138,300

(Source: London Deaths: 1998. Office of National Statistics (1999), Mortality Statistics by Cause in 1998, HMSO)

Table 2.2 Comparison of number of deaths due to heart diseases in 1980 and 2001 using CDC data based on death certificates

	1980	2001
Total deaths	1,989,841	2,416,425
Diseases of the heart	761,085	700,142
Malignancies	416,509	553,768

According to the World Health Organization, in 1996, 29.0% of worldwide deaths were due to cardiovascular diseases [3]. Mortality rate has already doubled due to coronary artery disease in an upcoming economy like China, more marked in the younger age group [4]. Over the last 40 years; the incidence has increased six-fold in the Indian urban population [5]. It has been predicted that by 2020 there will be an overall 9.1% reduction of mortality due to all diseases combined. However, the cardiovascular disease mortality rate will increase by 16.2% (predominantly coronary artery disease) particularly in developing countries [6]. While most people are scared of HIV, the incidence and mortality of coronary artery disease are higher.

2.2
Introduction

Clinical CAD is due to atherosclerosis, in which arteries become narrow and hardened due to gradual cholesterol plaque build-up [7]. In Greek, Athere (gruel) means "focal accumulation of" and Sclerosis (hardening) means "thickening of intima". The disease develops silently and progresses over decades and remains unnoticed until it produces symptoms (Fig. 2.1). The blood components aggregation on the surface of these plaques results in thrombi formation [8–11].

Extensive research has been carried out to understand the pathophysiology and complications of coronary artery disease. A landmark historical study was initiated in Framingham (Massachusetts, USA), known as the "Framingham Study", in 1948. The study lasted thirty years and involved 5127 asymptomatic people, providing in-depth information about different aspects of coronary heart disease [12, 13]. Today, the causes of heart disease are well known. Further investigations have been carried out to understand both the modifiable (high blood cholesterol, hypertension, smoking, diabetes, obesity, sedentary life style, and stress) and unmodifiable risk factors (gender, family history, race, and genetics [14–20]).

2.3
Pathophysiology

It is important to understand pathophysiology, in order to envisage the current and future scope of radioisotope imaging in coronary artery disease. It is conceived that radioisotope imaging will be able to demonstrate different aspects of pathophysiology, biology and on-going humeral changes, in order to prevent and monitor progression of the disease.

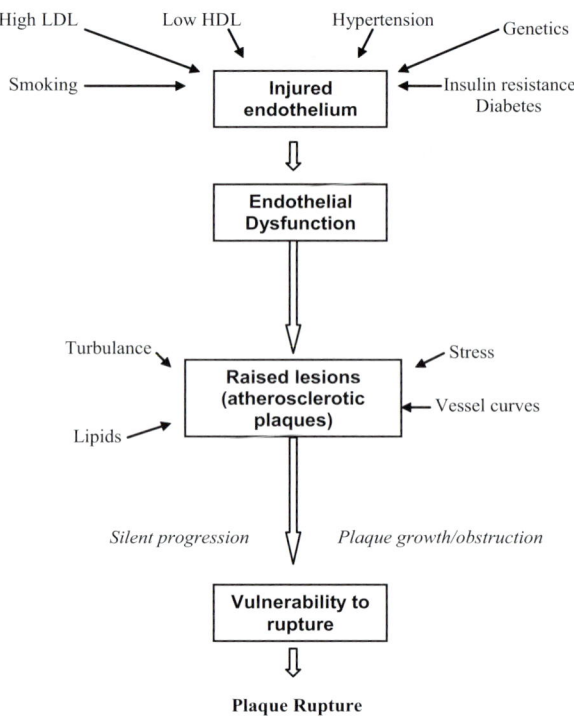

Fig. 2.1. Sequence of events in coronary artery disease (HDL = high-density lipoprotein, LDL = low-density lipoprotein, MI = myocardial infarction)

Coronary artery disease ultimately leads to myocardial ischaemia, myocardial infarction or heart failure and at times to sudden death [7] (Fig. 2.2). An imbalance between oxygen demand and supply causes myocardial ischaemia [21–24]. Increased demand may occur simply by increased heart rate or other physiological phenomena, such as left ventricular contraction, systolic wall tension, catecholamines and myocardial metabolism [22–25]. The reduced supply occurs mostly due to coronary spasm or obstruction and in coronary artery disease, myocardial ischaemia mostly occurs as a result of both. Clinically, it is manifested as angina pectoris, with or without ST-segment changes on the ECG.

The pathophysiology of atherosclerosis encompasses a complex interaction between endothelial cells, smooth muscle cells, platelets, and leucocytes [7, 9]. The vascular inflammation, lipid buildup, calcium and cellular debris within the intimal walls lead to plaque formation. This contributes to vascular remodeling, luminal obstruction, abnormalities in blood flow, and reduced oxygen supply to the myocardium.

The earliest pathologic lesions of atherosclerosis are "fatty streaks" in the intimal layer of the vessel wall,

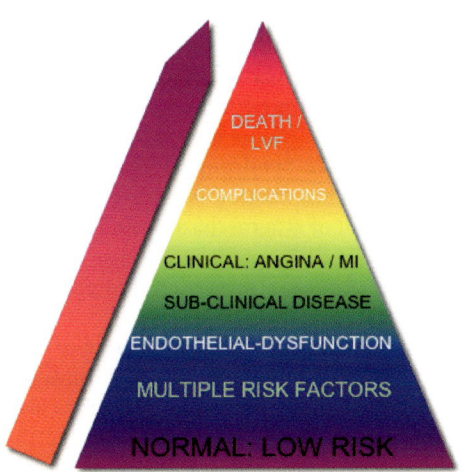

Fig. 2.2 Coronary artery disease cascade

feron), and nitric oxide play an important role in proliferation and migration of smooth muscle cells.

This early stage of atherogenesis is progressed further, with associated endothelial dysfunction. The fibrous plaque leads to vascular remodeling, progressive narrowing and abnormal flow (Fig. 2.3). The rupture of the protective fibrous cap due to weakness or denudation of the overlying endothelium results in exposure of the thrombogenic material from the plaque to the circulating blood. This exposure forms an advanced or complicated lesion. Inflammatory cells localize to the shoulder region of the vulnerable plaque. A plaque rupture may result in thrombus formation, partial or complete occlusion of the vessel, or organization of the thrombus within the plaque leading to further progression of the atherosclerotic lesion.

2.3.1 Endothelial Dysfunction and Atherosclerosis

and predominantly contain lipid-laden macrophages, T lymphocytes, and smooth muscle cells. These streaks are found both in the aorta and coronary arteries at a much younger age. In one study of 2876 autopsies of accident victims between the age of 15 and 34 years, fatty streaks were seen in 99.93% and there was some evidence of the presence of atherosclerosis in 50% of teens between 15 and 19 years of age [11]. The fatty streak may progress to form a fibrous plaque, due to progressive lipid accumulation and proliferation of smooth muscle cells. The smooth muscle cells proliferation within the intima makes up the substantial bulk of the atherosclerotic lesion, rising several millimeters above the surrounding level. A number of molecular factors, such as growth factors (e.g., platelet-derived growth factor, or PDGF), eicosanoids (hydrolyzing cholesteryl esters), cytokines (e.g., tumor necrosis factor, interleukin-1 and inter-

Marcello Malpighi (1628–1694), an Italian physician described the presence of an inner vascular lining known as "vascular endothelium". In a person with a body weight of 70 kg, the endothelium covers approximately an area of 700 m^2 and weighs approximately 1 to 1.5 kg [26]. This internal lining of the endothelial cells is a vasoactive organ [27, 28], regulating vascular tone through production of a variety of factors. It secretes potent vasodilators and vasoconstrictors [28–34] (Table 2.3). In the normal healthy vascular bed, the vasodilatation predominates over vasoconstriction. However, alterations in myocardial oxygen balance lead to sudden changes in the coronary vascular resistance [25–27, 31].

Nitric oxide, prostaglandins, carbon dioxide, Adenosine and the presence of hydrogen ions are some of the important mediators responsible for maintaining vascular tone [31–36]. The most important endothelium

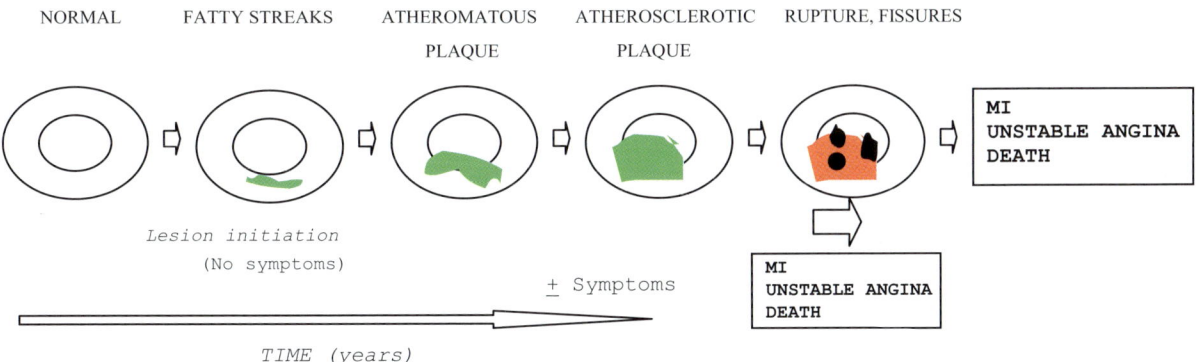

Fig. 2.3 Pathophysiology of coronary artery disease

Table 2.3 Important chemicals released by the endothelium. Endothelial cells release both vasodilators and vasoconstrictors to maintain tone. Acetylcholine produces vasodilatation only in the presence of endothelium. In the absence of endothelium, acetylcholine causes vasoconstriction.

a. Vasodilators

- Endothelium-derived relaxing factor (EDRF)
- Nitric Oxide (NO)
- Prostacyclin
- Bradykinin
- Substance P
- Serotonin, Histamine

b. Vasoconstrictors:

- Endothelin-1 (ET-1)
- Endothelium 1,2 and 3
- Angiotensin II
- Thromboxane A2
- Prostaglandin (PGH2)

relaxing factor (EDRF) is nitric oxide [37–39]. Under normal conditions, nitric oxide is continuously released, helping to maintain a vasodilator status, thereby inhibiting platelet aggregation and adhesion as well as inhibition of proliferation and migration of vascular smooth muscle cells. In endothelial dysfunction, there is loss of nitric oxide bioavailability, due to both reduced synthesis as well as accelerated breakdown of nitric oxide. Most of the risk factors such as cigarette smoking, diabetes mellitus, dyslipidaemias, hypertension, old age, menopause and hyperhomocystinemia, lead to impairment of the endothelium-dependent vasodilatation, mutations in the enzyme nitric oxide synthetase messenger RNA (mRNA) and post-transcriptional destabilization of mRNA. The reduction in the levels of nitric oxide leads to increased platelet adhesion and tissue factor and decreased plasminogen activator and thrombomodulin, leading to enhanced platelet thrombus formation.

Adenosine is another molecule of interest [32, 33] for its potent capability as a pharmacological stress agent in myocardial perfusion imaging. Elevated interstitial concentration of adenosine increases the coronary blood flow.

The earliest changes that precede the formation of lesions of atherosclerosis also take place in the endothelium [40]. In the initial stages, there is increased endothelial permeability to lipoproteins and other plasma constituents. The impairment of endothelial function with the presence of risk factors not only plays an important role in subsequent development of acute coronary syndromes (Fig. 2.4), but also in microvascular ischaemic syndromes (like "syndrome X") [41, 42]. Loss of endothelium-dependent dilation is probably the first step in the development of atherosclerosis. Radioisotope imaging with SPECT or PET holds the promise of demonstrating perfusion abnormalities, related to endothelial dysfunction [43].

The Acute Coronary Syndromes (unstable angina, myocardial infarction) have fissured or ruptured plaques, with platelet aggregation and thrombus formation. Rupture of the fibrous cap or ulceration of the plaque can rapidly lead to thrombosis. and it usually occurs at sites of thinning of the cap covering advanced lesions. Patients with complex plaques have elevated circulatory serotonin, being released by the aggregated platelets. Any reduction in the level of nitric oxide will lead to further increased vasoconstriction, with increased chances of destabilization. It appears that nitric oxide (NO) is probably the most important molecule, and helps to regulate a broad range of physiological processes like vasodilatation, inflammation and immune function. Nitric oxide has also been demonstrated to be involved in the regulation of apoptosis [38, 39].

It is now well recognized that insulin resistance and its cluster of associated abnormalities are also responsible for endothelial dysfunction and are important risk factors, due to their effects in more than one way. Modification of the risk factors improves both endothelial function and coronary artery disease outcomes [40, 41, 44].

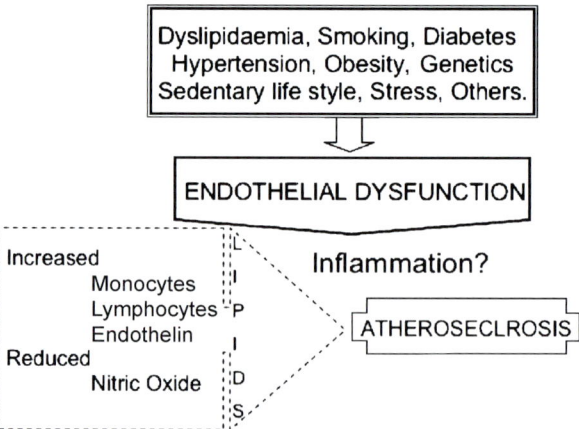

Fig. 2.4 Mechanism of atherosclerosis

Abnormalities associated with insulin resistance/hyperinsulinaemia are as below:
a. **Endothelial dysfunction**
   Increased mononuclear cellular adhesion
   Decreased endothelial-dependent vasodilatation
b. **Glucose intolerance**
   Impaired fasting glucose and glucose tolerance
c. **Abnormal uric acid metabolism**
   Increased Plasma uric acid concentration with decreased clearance
d. **Dyslipidaemia**
   Elevated triglycerides
   Lower HDL
e. **Haemodynamic**
   Increased sympathetic activity
   Hypertension
f. **Haemostatic**
   Elevated plasminogen activator inhibitor 1 and fibrinogen levels

2.3.2
Inflammation and Atherosclerosis

Inflammation has been implicated in the pathogenesis of coronary artery disease [45–47]. Inflammation is the common response of endothelial cells to different factors that attack arterial intima. Elevated levels of inflammation markers, particularly C-reactive protein (CRP) support this concept indirectly [45–47]. CRP has been shown to predict the risk of first myocardial infarction, ischaemic stroke and peripheral vascular disease [48]. CRP level also appears to be a strong predictor of short-term mortality and future cardiac events in cases of unstable angina.

The protective effects of aspirin and lipid lowering drugs have also been related to the markers of inflammation. The protective effect of aspirin is more pronounced in patients with higher levels of CRP, probably due to its anti-platelet and anti-inflammatory effects. Moreover, combined assessment of CRP and lipid parameters appears to have a prognostic advantage over the lipid status alone, including total cholesterol to HDL ratio [49].

Chronic infections particularly with Chlamydia pneumoniae and cytomegalovirus (CMV) have also been related with atherosclerosis [50, 51]. The pathologic tissue specimens in various studies have demonstrated the presence of viral antigen, however, no exact relation has been established yet. Many serologic studies have also demonstrated the presence of Chlamydia organisms in atherosclerotic material [52]. The level of anti-chlamydial antibodies has also been shown to be related to the risk of future coronary events.

In middle-aged British men with coronary artery disease, and baseline levels of plasma C reactive protein, serum amyloid A protein, and leucocyte counts, no association has been found with Helicobacter pylori seropositivity, Chlamydia pneumoniae titers, or plasma homocysteine levels [53]. This again suggests that inflammatory processes of unknown etiology could also be associated with subsequent coronary heart disease.

2.3.3
Race and Genetics

It is well known that people with a family history of CAD, are more prone to develop coronary artery disease. Similarly, racial differences also occur. Indians in the UK appear to have a three times higher risk of CAD.

One gene has been discovered in a few people living in Iceland, related to the inflammation of the artery walls known as the FLAP gene [54]. Similarly, patients with Tangier disease, living in Tangier Island, have almost no HDL, and are at increased risk of future cardiac events. The culprit gene in this case is ABC1, also known as ABCA1.

Due to the multi-factorial and complex nature of atherosclerosis, it is apparent that there may be many genes responsible for triggering atherosclerosis, yet to be discovered.

2.3.4
Collateral Circulation and Angiogenesis

The formation of new coronary vessels (collateral circulation) has been known since 1956 [55, 56]. In patients with coronary artery disease, obstruction leads to a drop in distal pressure and opening up of pre-existing non-functional epicardial vessels, which enlarge and form new vessels and collaterals. However, several factors and mechanisms, such as diabetes, severity of occlusion, stress, inflammation and vascular endothelial growth factors (VEGF) contribute to the development of a collateral mesh [57–60].

Collateral circulation potentially offers an important alternative source of blood supply when the original vessel is haemodynamically critically obstructed. The incidence of infarction in patients with well-developed collaterals is relatively lower than in those without good collaterals. Good collaterals can also mitigate the severity of coronary artery disease by improving flow, thereby reducing infarct size, and improving survival rate in myocardial infarction [61–63].

The collaterals formation includes three major steps of vasculogenesis, angiogenesis and arteriogenesis. The initial event of migration, localization and differentiation of the endothelial cell precursors (angioblasts) is called vasculogenesis. The subsequent growth, and remodeling into a mature vascular network is called angiogenesis [57, 58, 64]. The term arteriogenesis is limited to the transformation of preexisting (collateral) arterioles into functional (muscular) collateral arteries, with vasoelastic and vasomotor properties. Angiogenesis may also result in formation of subendocardial collaterals, besides epicardial vessels. Therapeutic angiogenesis has attracted great interest during the last decade [65, 66]. In therapeutic angiogenesis, genes encoded with growth factors are administered to stimulate neovascularization in severely ischaemic myocardium [67, 68]; different delivery systems have been attempted [69, 70]. Therapeutic angiogenesis is a promising treatment for patients with coronary artery disease, unlikely to benefit from standard revascularization procedures. The effectiveness of therapeutic angiogenesis can be assessed with myocardial perfusion imaging [71].

While reporting a myocardial perfusion scan, it is important to consider the contribution of collateral circulation. In cases of total occlusion with an area of prior infarct, depicting reversible ischaemia may represent collateral insufficiency under stress, rather than ischaemia related to the main coronary artery itself, as that is completely obstructed.

2.3.5
Apoptosis

Apoptosis (or programmed cell death) is a physiological phenomenon of cell replacement in certain adult tissues (e.g., the thymus). In contrast to necrosis, apoptosis occurs in isolated cells, without inflammation [72, 73].

It is now widely accepted that apoptosis does occur in the heart [73–75]. Heart failure has been characterized morphologically by a 232-fold increase in myocyte apoptosis and biochemically by DNA laddering (an indicator of apoptosis) [76, 77].

Elevated sphingolipids (from spinx in Greek: part woman and part lion) is an important pathway contributing to apoptosis [78]. In an acute coronary event, there are excessively higher amounts of sphingolipids present which are cardiotoxic, contributing to myocyte dysfunction and death. Therefore an inhibitor that stops the production or action of these sphingolipids, as an adjunct to current therapies, could prevent or reduce heart damage related to ischaemic events.

The molecular biology of myocyte apoptosis will permit inhibition or prevention of apoptosis (anti-apoptotic) as one potentially new and attractive future therapeutic option for treating cardiac disease [79]. Imaging with new radiopharmaceuticals would be of great help in monitoring such therapies. The current therapies, such as beta-blockers and ACE inhibitors, have demonstrated some anti-apoptic properties. However, the degree of apoptosis contributing to the initiation and progression of cardiac disease is yet to be determined. The amount of myocardium that can be salvaged and impact on cardiac function and prognosis, using an anti-apoptotic approach has also to be evaluated. It is possible that prevention of myocyte apoptosis might not necessarily mean full functional recovery.

References

1. Office of National Statistics (1999) London Deaths: 1998. Mortality Statistics by Cause in 1998. HMSO.
2. National Institute for Clinical Excellence (2003) Final Appraisal Determination. Myocardial perfusion scintigraphy for the diagnosis and management of angina and myocardial infarction. October.
3. WHO (1997) The World Health Report 1997. Conquering, suffering, enriching humanity. Geneva, World Health Organization.
4. WHO (2002) The World Health Report 2002. Reducing risks, promoting healthy life. Geneva, World Health Organization.
5. Reddy KS (2004) Cardiovascular disease in the non-western countries. NEJM 350(24):2438–2440.
6. Murray CJL, Lopez AD (1996) The global burden of disease: a comprehensive assessment of mortality and disability from diseases, injuries and risk factors in 1990 and projected to 2020. Harvard School of Public Health on behalf of WHO and the World Bank, USA.
7. Tokin A (ed.) (2003) Atherosclerosis and Heart Disease. Martin Dunitz, New York
8. Libby P (1995) Molecular bases of the acute coronary syndromes. Circulation 91:2844–2850.
9. Libby P (1996) Atheroma: more than mush. Lancet 348:S4–S7.
10. Kolodgie FD, Gold HK, Allen P. Burke AP et al. (2003) Intraplaque hemorrhage and progression of coronary atheroma. NEJM 349:2316–2325.
11. Strong JP et al. (1999) JAMA 281:725–735.
12. Myers RH, Kiely DK, Cupples LA, Kannel WB (1990) Parental history is an independent risk factor for coronary artery disease: the Framingham Study. Am Heart J 120(4):963–969.
13. Feng DaLi, Lindpaintner K, Larson GM et al. (2001) Platelet glycoprotein iiia pla polymorphism, fibrinogen, and platelet aggregability: the Framingham Heart Study. Circulation 104:140–144.

14. Kannel WB, McGee DL (1979) Diabetes and cardiovascular risk factors: the Framingham study. Circulation 59:8–13.
15. Levine GN, Keaney JF, Vita JA (1995) Cholesterol reduction in cardiovascular disease – clinical benefits and possible mechanisms. N Engl J Med 332:512–521.
16. Manolio T (2003) Novel risk markers and clinical practice. N Engl J Med 349:1587–1589.
17. Galobardes B, Costanza MC, Bernstein MS et al. (2003) Trends in risk factors for lifestyle-related diseases by socioeconomic position in Geneva, Switzerland, 1993-2000: health inequalities persist. Am J Public Health 93:1302–1309.
18. Lee J, Heng D, Chia, KS et al. (2001) Risk factors and incident coronary heart disease in Chinese, Malay and Asian Indian males: the Singapore Cardiovascular Cohort Study. Int J Epidemiol 30:983–988.
19. Raitakari OT, Adams MR, Celermajer DS (1999) Effect of Lp(a) on the early functional and structural changes of atherosclerosis. Arterioscler Thromb Vasc Biol 19(4):990–995.
20. Ridker PM, Buring JE, Shih J et al. (1998) Prospective study of C-reactive protein and the risk of future cardiovascular events among apparently healthy women. Circulation 98(8):731–733.
21. Selwyn AP, Kinlay S, Libby P, Ganz P (1997) Atherogenic lipids, vascular dysfunction, and clinical signs of ischemic heart disease. Circulation 95(1):5–7.
22. Braunwald E (1971) Control of myocardial oxygen consumption: physiologic and clinical considerations. Am J Cardiol 27(4):416–432.
23. Braunwald E (2000) Myocardial oxygen consumption: the quest for its determinants and some clinical fallout. J Am Coll Cardiol 35(Suppl B):45B–48B.
24. Takaoka H, Takeuchi M, Odake M et al. (1993) Comparison of hemodynamic determinants for myocardial oxygen consumption under different contractile states in human ventricle. Circulation 87(1):59–69.
25. Austin RE Jr, Smedira NG, Squiers TM, Hoffman JI (1994) Influence of cardiac contraction and coronary vasomotor tone on regional myocardial blood flow. Am J Physiol 266(6 Pt 2):H2542–H2553.
26. Cryer A (1983) Scale and diversity of interaction at the vascular endothelium. In Biochemical Interactions of the Endothelium. Elsevier, Amsterdam, pp. 1–3.
27. Chilian WM (1997) Coronary microcirculation in health and disease. Circulation 95(2):522–528.
28. Embrey RP, Brooks LA, Dellsperger KC (1997) Mechanism of coronary microvascular responses to metabolic stimulation. Cardiovasc Res 35(1):148–157.
29. Furchgott RF, Zawadzky JV (1980) The obligatory role of endothelial cells in the relaxation of arterial smooth muscle by acetylcholine. Nature 288:373–376.
30. Simionescu M, Simionescu N (1986) Functions of the endothelial cell surface. Annu Rev Physiol 48:279–304.
31. Furchgott RF (1996) The discovery of endothelium-derived relaxing factor and its importance in the identification of nitric oxide. JAMA 276(14):1186–1188.
32. Yada T, Richmond KN, Van Bibber R et al. (1999) Role of adenosine in local metabolic coronary vasodilation. Am J Physiol 276(5 Pt 2):H1425–H1433.
33. Belardinelli L, Linden J, Berne RM (1989) The cardiac effects of adenosine. Prog Cardiovasc Dis 32(1):73–97.
34. Palmer RMJ, Ferrige AG, Moncada S (1987) Nitric oxide release accounts for the biological activity of endothelium-derived relaxing factor. Nature 327:524.
35. Seo B, Oemar BS, Siebermann R, von Segesser L, Luscher TF (1994) Both ETA and ETB receptors mediate contraction to endothelin-I in human blood vessels. Circulation 89:1203–1208.
36. Panza JA, Casino PR, Kilcoyne CM, Quyyumi AA (1993) Role of endothelium-derived nitric oxide in the abnormal endothelium-dependent vascular relaxation of patients with essential hypertension. Circulation 87:1468–1474.
37. Smits P, Williams SB, Lipson DE et al. (1995) Endothelial release of nitric oxide contributes to the vasodilator effect of adenosine in humans. Circulation 92(8):2135–2141.
38. Maxwell AJ, Cooke JP (1999) The role of nitric oxide in atherosclerosis. Coronary Artery Dis 1999:277–286.
39. Quyyumi AA, Dakak N, Mulcahy D et al (1997) Nitric oxide activity in the atherosclerotic human coronary circulation. J Am Coll Cardiol 29(2):308–317.
40. Mombouli JV, Vanhoutte PM (1999) Endothelial dysfunction: from physiology to therapy. J Mol Cell Cardiol 31(1):61–74.
41. Kinlay S, Ganz P (1997) Role of endothelial dysfunction in coronary artery disease and implications for therapy. Am J Cardiol 80(9A):11I–16I.
42. Maseri A, Crea F, Kaski JC, Crake T (1991) Mechanisms of angina pectoris in syndrome X. J Am Coll Cardiol 17(2):499–506.
43. Hasdai D, Gibbons RJ, Holmes DR Jr et al. (1997) Coronary endothelial dysfunction in humans is associated with myocardial perfusion defects. Circulation 96(10):3390–3395.
44. Anderson TJ, Meredith IT, Yeung AC et al. (1995) The effect of cholesterol-lowering and antioxidant therapy on endothelium-dependent coronary vasomotion. N Engl J Med 332(8): 488–493.
45. Ross R (1999) Atherosclerosis – an inflammatory disease. N Engl J Med 340(2):115–126.
46. Vorchheimer DA, Fuster V (2001) Inflammatory markers in coronary artery disease. Let prevention douse the flames. JAMA 286:2154–2156.
47. Blake GJ, Ridker PM (2001) Novel clinical markers of vascular wall inflammation. Circulation Res 89:763–771.

48. Lagrand WK, Visser CA et al. (1999) C-reactive protein as a cardiovascular risk factor: more than an epiphenomenon? Circulation 100:96–102.
49. Ridker P, Glynn R, Hennekens C (1998) C-reactive protein adds to the predictive value of total and HDL cholesterol in determining risk of first myocardial infarction. Circulation 97:2007–2011.
50. Epstein SE, Zhou YF et al. (1999) Infection and atherosclerosis: emerging mechanistic paradigms. Circulation 100:e20–e28.
51. Kuvin JT, Kimmelstiel CD (1999) Infectious causes of atherosclerosis. Am Heart J 137:216–226.
52. Gupta S, Leatham EW et al. (1997) Elevated Chlamydia pneumoniae antibodies, cardiovascular events, and azithromycin in male survivors of myocardial infarction. Circulation 96:404–407.
53. Danesh J, Whincup P, Walker M et al. (2000) Low grade inflammation and coronary heart disease: prospective study and updated meta-analyses. BMJ 321:199–204.
54. Helgadottir A, Manolescu A, Thorleifsson G et al. (2004) The gene encoding 5-lipoxygenase activating protein confers risk of myocardial infarction and stroke. Nature Genetics 36:233–239.
55. Baroldi G, Mantero O, Scomazzoni G (1956) The collaterals of the coronary arteries in normal and pathologic hearts. Circulation Res. 4:223–229.
56. Koerselman J, Graaf YVD, Jaegere P et al. (2003) Coronary collaterals: an important and underexposed aspect of coronary artery disease. Circulation 107:2507.
57. Carmeliet P (2000) Mechanisms of angiogenesis and arteriogenesis. Nat Med 6:389–395.
58. Conway EM, Collen D, Carmeliet P (2001) Molecular mechanisms of blood vessel growth. Cardiovasc Res 49:507–521.
59. Buschmann I, Schaper W (2000) The pathophysiology of the collateral circulation (arteriogenesis). J Pathol 190:338–342.
60. Shweiki D, Itin A, Soffer D, Keshet E (1992) Vascular endothelial growth factor induced by hypoxia may mediate hypoxia-initiated angiogenesis. Nature 29:843–845.
61. Charney R, Cohen M (1993) The role of the coronary collateral circulation in limiting myocardial ischemia and infarct size. Am Heart J 126(4):937–945.
62. Sabia PJ, Powers ER, Ragosta M et al. (1992) An association between collateral blood flow and myocardial viability in patients with recent myocardial infarction. N Engl J Med 327:1825–1831.
63. Fukai M, Ii M, Nakakoji T et al. (2000) Angiographically demonstrated coronary collaterals predict residual viable myocardium in patients with chronic myocardial infarction: a regional metabolic study. J Cardiol 35:103–111.
64. Lee SH, Wolf PL, Escudero R et al. (2000) Early expression of angiogenesis factors in acute myocardial ischemia and infarction. N Engl J Med 342(9):626–633.
65. Henry TD (1999) Therapeutic angiogenesis. BMJ 318:1536–1539.
66. Rosengart TK (2003) Commentary: Gene therapy: true promise fulfilled. Nature 10.
67. Rosengart TK, Patel SR, Crystal RG (1999) Therapeutic angiogenesis: protein and gene therapy delivery strategies. J Cardiovasc Risk 6:29–40.
68. Syed JS, Sanborn TA, Rosengart TK (2004) Therapeutic angiogenesis: a biologic bypass. Cardiology 101:131–143.
69. Schlach P, Rahman GF, Patejunas G et al. (2004) Adenoviral-mediated transfer of vascualr endothelial growth factor 121 cDNA enhances myocardial perfusion and exercise performance in the nonischemic state J Thorac Cardiovasc Surg 127:535–540.
70. Lopez JJ, Laham RJ, Stamler A et al. (1998) Therapeutic angiogenesis in chronic myocardial ischemia: intracoronary vs. extracoronary delivery strategies. Cardiovasc Res 40:272–281.
71. Udelson JE, Dilsizian V, Roger J et al. (2000) Therapeutic angiogenesis with recombinant fibroblast growth factor-2 improves stress and rest myocardial perfusion abnormalities in patients with severe symptomatic chronic coronary artery disease. Circulation 102:1605–1610.
72. Majno G, Joris I (1995) Apoptosis, oncosis, and necrosis. An overview of cell death. Am J Pathol 146(1): 3-15.
73. Colucci WS (1996) Apoptosis in heart. N Engl J Med 335:1224–1226.
74. Kang PM, Izu S (2000) Apoptosis and heart failure: a critical review of the literature. Circulation Res 86:1107–1111.
75. Yaoita H, Ogawa K, Maehara K et al. (2000) Apoptosis in relevant clinical situations: contribution of apoptosis in myocardial infarction. Cardiovasc Res 45:630–641.
76. Gill C, Mestril R, Samali A (2002) Losing heart: the role of apoptosis in heart disease – a novel therapeutic target? FASEB J. 16:135-146.
77. Olivetti G, Abbi R, Quaini F (1997) Apoptosis in the failing human heart. New Engl J Med 336:1131–1141.
78. O'Brien NW, Gellings N et al. (2003) Factor associated with sphingomyelinase activation and its role in cardiac cell death. Circulation Res 92:589–591.
79. Haunstetter A, Izumo S (2000) Toward antiapoptosis as a new treatment modality. Circulation Res 86:371–376.

Pathology of Coronary Artery Disease and Ischemic Heart Disease

Usha Kini and Shalini Mullick

Contents

3.1	Introduction	31
3.2	Pathology of Coronary Artery Disease	31
3.2.1	Atherosclerosis	31
3.2.2	Localization of Plaques	32
3.2.3	Morphological Evaluation of Atherothrombotic Lesions	32
3.2.4	Phases of Atherothrombosis	33
3.2.5	Lesions with Thrombi	37
3.3	Pathology of Coronary Interventions	38
3.3.1	Angioplasty	38
3.3.2	Intracoronary Stents	38
3.4	Pathology of Coronary Artery Bypass Grafts	38
3.4.1	Saphenous Venous Bypass Grafts (SVBG)	38
3.4.2	Internal Mammary Artery Grafts	39
3.5	Non-Atheromatous Coronary Artery Disease	39
3.5.1	Congenital Anomalies of Coronary Arteries	39
3.5.2	Spontaneous Dissection of Coronary Arteries	39
3.5.3	Aneurysms of the Coronary Arteries	39
3.6	Pathology of Ischemic Heart Disease	39
3.6.1	Mechanisms of Myocardial Ischemic Injury	39
3.6.2	Pathology of Myocardial Ischemia	40
3.6.3	Patterns of Myocardial Infarction	40
3.6.4	Location of Infarcts	40
3.6.5	Macroscopic Characteristics of Myocardial Infarcts	40
3.6.6	Evolution of Microscopic Characteristics of Myocardial Infarcts	41
3.6.7	Infarct Expansion and Infarct Extension	41
3.7	Pathological Complications of Myocardial Infarction	42
3.8	Chronic Ischemic Heart Disease	42
3.9	Pathology of Reperfusion	43
	References	43

3.1 Introduction

Atherosclerotic coronary artery disease and acute coronary syndromes are a leading cause of mortality and morbidity all over the world. As a result of intensive investigation over decades, a detailed understanding of the pathophysiology of these conditions has resulted in advances in their therapeutics as well as prevention.

3.2 Pathology of Coronary Artery Disease

3.2.1 Atherosclerosis

Atherosclerotic coronary artery disease is well known to be a leading cause of mortality in the western world and is now being recognized as a major health problem in the rest of the world as well. While acute coronary syndromes lead to different clinical conditions, therapies and prognosis, they share a similar pathophysiology characterized largely by atherothrombotic coronary artery occlusion due to plaque rupture and superimposed thrombosis.

While the lesions of atherosclerosis were identified by anatomical pathologists as early as 1829, when Jean Lebstein first used the term [1], in the past 20 years, much new knowledge regarding its pathogenesis, pathophysiology and clinical correlates has been discovered, leading to the transformation of cardiovascular pathology into a dynamic and rapidly evolving branch of surgical pathology.

The incrustation hypothesis and the lipid hypothesis in the late 19th century focused on fibrin deposition, extracellular matrix formation and lipid accumulation in the pathogenesis of atherosclerosis. Virchow later linked inflammation to the disease and it is now well known that chronic inflammation is intimately linked to the early phases of the disease and also to plaque rupture and thrombosis. Aschoff identified two distinct components, lipid and fibrous, and distinguished between atherosis in infants and adolescents and atherosclerosis in adults. He was also among the initial investigators to recognize a sequential development of these lesions.

The role of thrombosis, lipid metabolism and inflammation has been investigated at the cellular and molecular level resulting in important new diagnostic and therapeutic strategies. Detailed morphological and clinicopathological studies in the last two decades by anatomic pathologists provided very important new insights leading to the use of the term *atherothrombosis*, which unifies and integrates these concepts [2]. The characterization of the role of blood flow induced shear stress and the recognition of the endothelium as a crucial integrator of normal and abnormal vascular biology have provided further insights. Finally, the role of adult stem cells, or bone marrow derived endothelial precursor cells in the maintenance and regeneration of the endothelium has opened up a new area of vascular research which has an important impact on the diagnosis, treatment and prevention of acute coronary syndromes [3].

Atherothrombosis is defined as a systemic disease of large and medium sized arteries (external diameter >2 mm) and is characterized by the formation of individual lesions called plaques. The main components of atherothrombotic plaques are extracellular matrix, including collagen and proteoglycans; cholesterol, cholesteryl esters, and phospholipids; cells such as monocyte-derived macrophages, T-lymphocytes, and smooth-muscle cells; and thrombotic material with platelets and fibrin deposition. Varying proportions of these components are found in different plaques, thus giving rise to a spectrum of lesions.

These components chiefly affect the intima, but secondary changes also occur in the media and adventitia. Atherosclerosis progresses through lipid core expansion and macrophage accumulation at the edges of the plaque, potentially leading to fibrous cap rupture.

3.2.2 Localization of Plaques

Characterized by a focal distribution, plaques are more commonly seen just proximal to branching points of vessels, which are areas of low shear rates. Shear rates refer to velocity gradients between the layers of fluid in close proximity to the endothelial surface. Low shear rate areas have prolonged contact between platelets and endothelial surfaces, thereby increasing the tendency for receptor mediated adhesion.

3.2.3 Morphological Evaluation of Atherothrombotic Lesions

In 1995, the Committee on Vascular Lesions of the Council on Arteriosclerosis formed by the American Heart Association (AHA) histologically classified human atherosclerotic lesions and designated them by Ro-

Table 3.1 Current AHA classification of atherosclerotic lesions [4]

Type of lesion	Terminology in histological classification	Other terms often used	
Early lesions			
I	Initial lesion	Fatty dot/Streak	
II a	Progression-prone Type II lesion	Fatty dot/Streak	Early Lesion
II b	Progression-resistant Type II lesion	Fatty dot/Streak	
III	Intermediate lesion (preatheroma)		
Advanced lesions			
IV	Atheroma	Atheromatous plaque, fibrolipid plaque, fibrous plaque	
V a	Fibroatheroma (Type V) lesion		
Complicated lesions			
V b	Calcific lesion (Type VII) lesion	Calcified plaque	Advanced Lesions, Raised Lesions
V c	Fibrotic lesion (Type VIII) lesion	Fibrous plaque	
VI	Lesion with surface defect and/or hematoma/hemorrhage and/or thrombotic deposit.	Complicated lesion/ Complicated plaque	

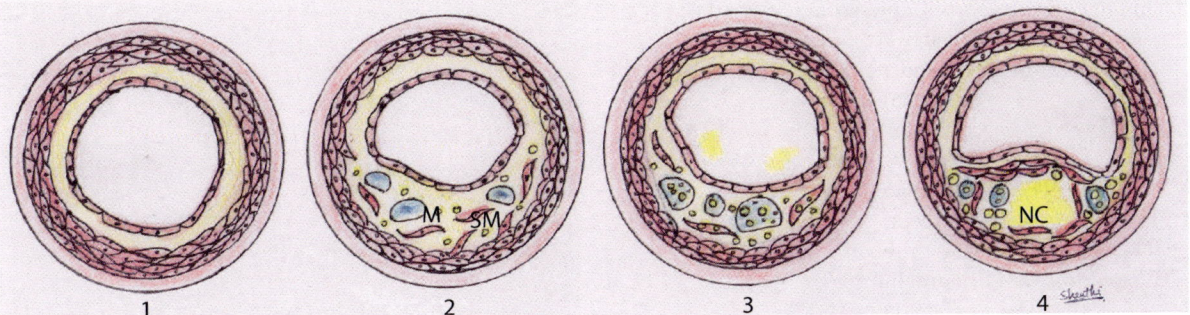

Fig. 3.1 Diagrammatic representation to describe the sequence of events in the pathogenesis of an atheromatous plaque: 1. normal coronary artery; 2. macrophages (M) and smooth muscle cells (SM) in the intima; 3. smooth muscle cell proliferation into the intima; 4. A well developed plaque with a central necrotic core (NC)

man numerals, which indicated the usual sequence of lesion progression (Table 3.1) [4]. This classification also attempted to correlate the appearance of lesions noted in clinical imaging studies with histological lesion types and corresponding clinical syndromes.

3.2.4 Phases of Atherothrombosis

3.2.4.1 Early Lesions (Phase 1)

Lesions are small, and are not associated with any symptoms. They are categorized into three types, as follows (Fig. 3.1):

- **Type I lesions** consist of macrophage-derived foam cells that contain lipid droplets. This lesion contains enough atherogenic lipoprotein to elicit an increase in macrophages and formation of scattered macrophage foam cells (Fig. 3.2).
- **Type II lesions** consist of both macrophages and smooth-muscle cells and mild extracellular lipid deposits and include lesions grossly designated as *fatty streaks* (Figs. 3.3 and 3.4).
- **Type III lesions** are the intermediate stage between Type II and Type IV (*atheroma*, a lesion that is potentially symptom-producing). In addition to the lipid-laden cells of Type II, Type III lesions contain scattered collections of extracellular lipid droplets and particles that disrupt the coherence of some intimal smooth muscle cells. This extracellular lipid is the immediate precursor of the larger, confluent, and more disruptive core of extracellular lipid that characterizes Type IV lesions.

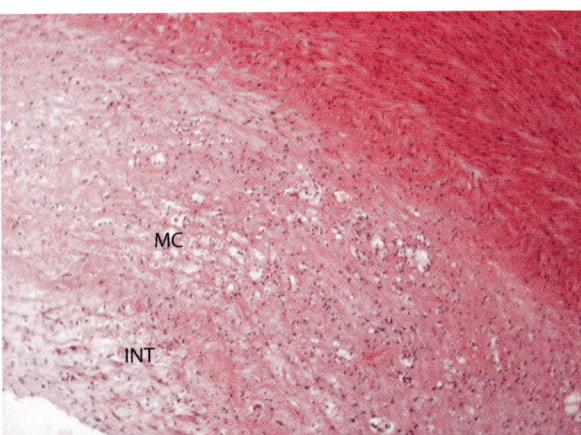

Fig. 3.2 Type I lesion of atherosclerosis showing numerous macrophages (M) in the thickened intima (INT) of the coronary artery (×400)

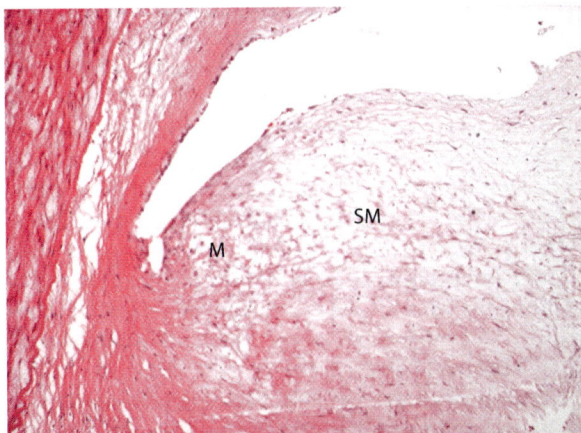

Fig. 3.3 Type II lesion of atherosclerosis (fatty streak) consisting of both macrophages (M) and smooth muscle cells (SM) along with extracellular lipid (×40)

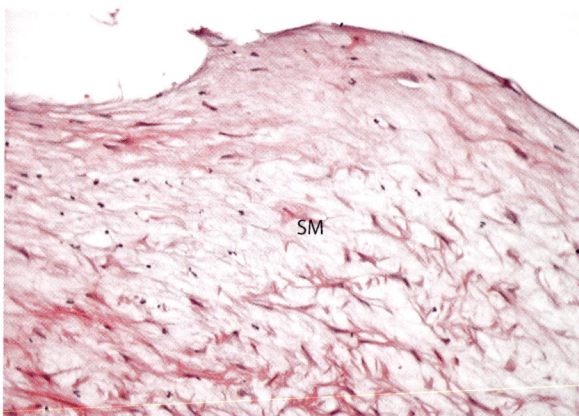

Fig. 3.4 Higher magnification of Type II lesion highlighting the smooth muscle cells (SM) (×400)

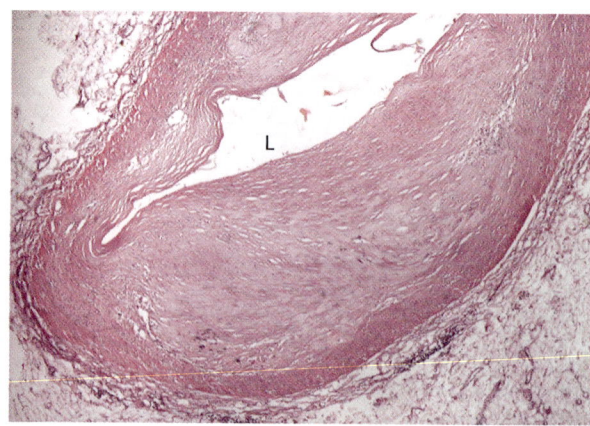

Fig. 3.5 Type III lesion of atherosclerosis showing an eccentric lumen (L) with a spectrum of atherosclerotic lesions (×20)

3.2.4.2 Advanced Lesions (Phase 2)

These lesions, although not necessarily stenotic, can evolve to acute Phases 3 and 4 and may be prone to rupture (Figs. 3.5, 3.6 and 3.7). These plaques are categorized morphologically as one of two variants:

- Type IV lesions consist of confluent cellular lesions with a dense accumulation of extracellular lipid known as the lipid core. There is usually no increase in fibrous tissue and defects of the surface or thrombosis are not present. The type IV lesion is also known as atheroma. Type IV is the first lesion considered advanced in the histological classification because of the severe intimal disorganization caused by the lipid core. The potential clinical significance of Type IV lesions can be great, even though this advanced lesion may not cause much narrowing of the lumen. Because, the region between the lipid core and the lesion surface contains proteoglycans and macrophage foam cells, isolated smooth muscle cells and minimal collagen, it may be susceptible to formation of fissures (Type VI lesion). The periphery of advanced lesions, particularly Type IV, may be vulnerable to rupture because macrophages are generally abundant in this location.
- Type V lesions are lesions with abundant new fibrous tissue formation. Type Va lesions possess an extracellular lipid core covered by a fibrous cap and are called fibroatheromas. A type V lesion in which the lipid core and other parts of the lesion are calcified may be referred to as Type Vb. A type V lesion in which a lipid core is absent and lipid content is minimal may be referred to as Type Vc. In these lesions, the normal intima is replaced and thickened by fibrous connective tissue, while lipid is minimal or even absent. Type Vb and Vc lesions have also been called Type VII and Type VIII lesions, respectively.

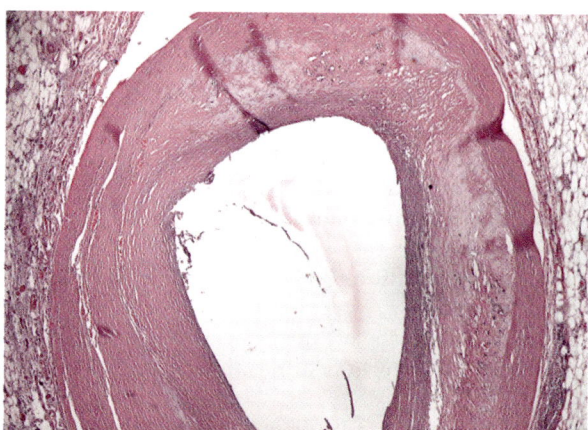

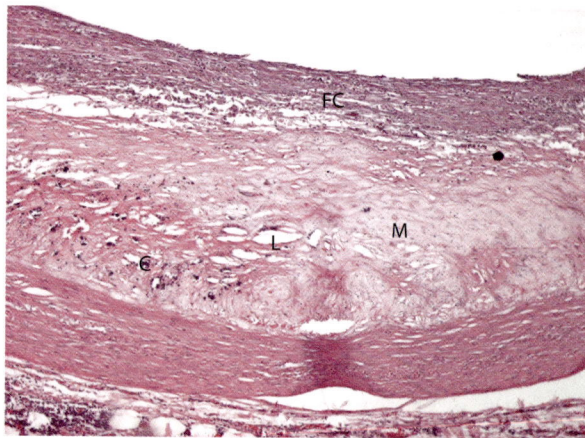

Figs. 3.6 and 3.7 Low (×40) and high (×200) magnification views of advanced (Type V) lesions of atherosclerosis with luminal narrowing, characterized by a core of extracellular lipid (L), foci of calcification (C), macrophages (M) and a fibrous cap (FC)

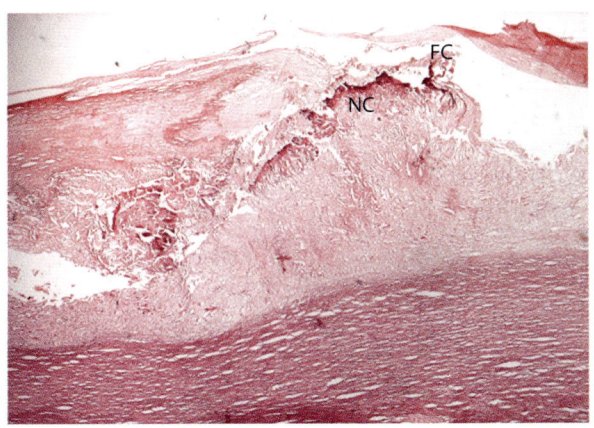 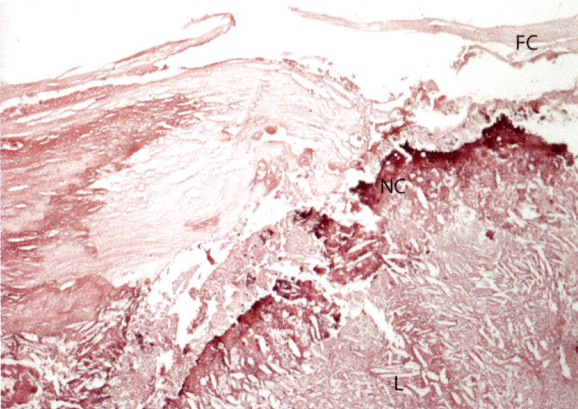

Figs. 3.8 and 3.9 Low (×40) and high (×200) magnification views of a Type VI lesion of atherosclerosis (complicated lesion) showing rupture of the fibrous cap (FC), with the underlying necrotic core (NC) and extensive exracellular lipid (L) seen as needle like crystals

3.2.4.3 Phase 3 Lesions

Comprises of Type VI lesions or complicated lesions that are characterized by disruptions of the lesion surface (plaque rupture) (Figs. 3.8 and 3.9), hematoma or hemorrhage, and thrombotic deposits in Type IV and Type V lesions and are a significant cause of morbidity and mortality from atherosclerosis.

3.2.4.4 Phase 4 Lesions

These lesions are characterized by acute complicated Type VI lesions, with fixed or repetitive occlusive thrombosis. This process becomes apparent in the form of an acute coronary syndrome but it may also be clinically silent.

3.2.4.5 Phase 5 Lesions

These lesions are characterized by Type Vb (calcific) or Type Vc (fibrotic) lesions (Fig. 3.10) that may cause angina; however, if the myocardium happens to be protected by collateral circulation, such lesions may then be silent.

As mentioned earlier, the AHA classification of atherosclerosis is based on an orderly linear progression of these lesions. However, the limitation of most of current clinical imaging methods with respect to anatomic pathology is that they visualize the vessel lumen as opposed to the vessel wall. Thus, the analysis of human arteries from a histological point of view is highly dependent on autopsy studies. Over the last decade or so, autopsies conducted largely on patients who died of sudden cardiac death have brought up new concepts that are not entirely consistent with the belief that the rupture of a Type IV lesion is the single histological determinant of sudden occlusion and atherosclerotic death [5]. It has been established that the presence of a plaque rupture does not always imply a causal association with the thrombus that occluded the lumen and that non-fatal lesions can also contain areas of rupture. Moreover, the documentation of non-ruptured but fatal lesions suggests that coronary thrombi can arise without rupture. Based on these observations, Lafont et al. have proposed to extend the concept of the vulnerable plaque [6], which earlier referred to a plaque prone to rupture (Muller et al.) [7] to a "plaque prone to thrombose". Also, some new histological clinically significant entities have been described like those of plaque erosion or the Thin Cap Fibroatheroma (TCFA).

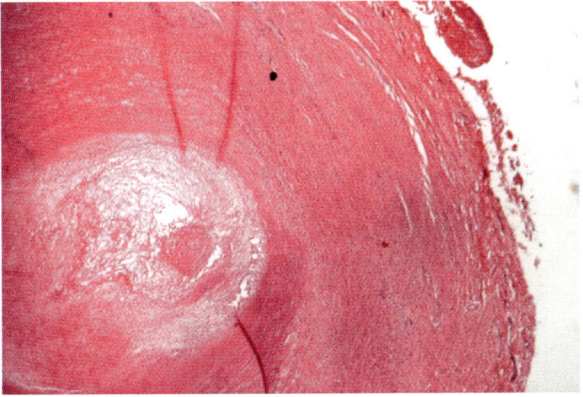

Fig. 3.10 Coronary artery showing near total luminal occlusion due to a Type Vc fibrotic lesion (×40)

Table 3.2 Modified AHA classification [5]

Lesion	Morphological description	Thrombosis
Non-atherosclerotic intimal lesions		
Intimal thickening	The normal accumulation of smooth muscle cells in intima without lipid or macrophage foam cells.	Absent
Intimal xanthoma/Fatty streak	Luminal accumulation of foam cells without a necrotic core or a fibrous cap.	Absent
Progressive atherosclerotic lesions		
Pathological Intimal Thickening	Smooth muscle cells in a proteoglycan rich matrix with areas of extracellular lipid accumulation without necrosis.	Absent
Erosion	Luminal thrombosis, Plaque same as above.	Thrombus mostly mural, infrequently occlusive
Fibrous cap atheroma	Well formed necrotic core with an overlying fibrous cap.	Absent
Erosion	Luminal thrombosis, plaque same as above; no communication of thrombus with necrotic core.	Thrombus mostly mural, infrequently occlusive
Thin fibrous cap atheroma	A thin fibrous cap infiltrated by macrophages and lymphocytes with rare smooth muscle cells and underlying necrotic core.	Absent, may contain intraplaque hemorrhage and fibrin
Plaque rupture	Fibroatheroma with cap disruption, luminal thrombus communicates with necrotic core.	Thrombus usually occlusive
Calcified nodule	Eruptive nodular calcification with underlying fibrocalcific plaque.	Thrombus, usually non-occlusive
Fibrocalcific plaque	Collagen-rich plaque with significant stenosis and large areas of calcification and few inflammatory cells.	Absent

Taking into account these new concepts, a different classification including these two categories has been proposed by Virmani et al. (Table 3.2) [5]. This modification discusses mainly the AHA Type IV, V and VI lesions and includes seven morphological types of lesions, focusing on the status of the fibrous cap. These categories include intimal xanthoma, intimal thickening, pathological intimal thickening, fibrous cap atheroma, thin fibrous cap atheroma, calcified nodule, and the fibrocalcific plaque.

- **Intimal thickening**: The normal accumulation of smooth muscle cells (SMCs) in the intima in the absence of lipid or macrophage foam cells.
- **Intimal xanthomata (fatty streak)**: Focal accumulation of lipid-laden macrophages. There is no fibrous cap or necrotic core. Most of these lesions regress spontaneously.
- **Fibrous cap atheromata**: These lesions have a "fibrous cap" defined as a distinct layer of connective tissue completely covering the lipid core. The fibrous cap may be a thick or thin one overlying a lipid-rich core.
- **Thin cap fibrous atheroma**: Based on morphometric studies, a "thin" fibrous cap is defined as one which is less than 65 mm thick [8]. The thin, fibrous cap is characterized by the loss of smooth muscle cells, extracellular matrix, and inflammatory infiltrate (Fig. 3.11). The necrotic core underlying the thin fibrous cap is usually large; hemorrhage and/or calcification is often present and intraplaque vasa vasorum are abundant.
- **Fibrocalcific plaque**: This is a collagen-rich plaque with significant stenosis; usually contains large areas of calcification with few inflammatory cells. A necrotic core may be present (Fig. 3.12).

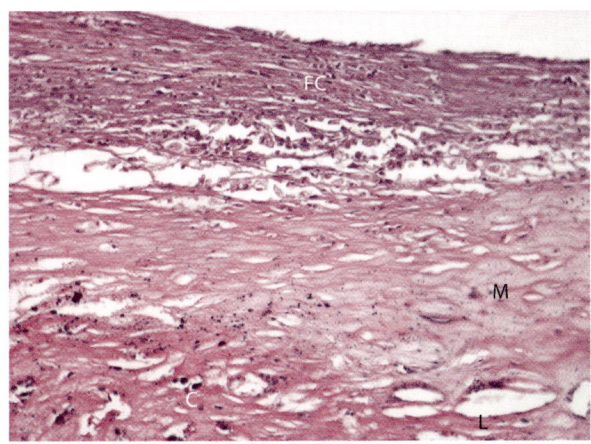

Fig. 3.11 The thin cap fibrous atheroma showing a well defined fibrous cap (FC), inflammatory infiltrate, macrophages (M), extracellular lipid (L) and calcification (C). (×400)

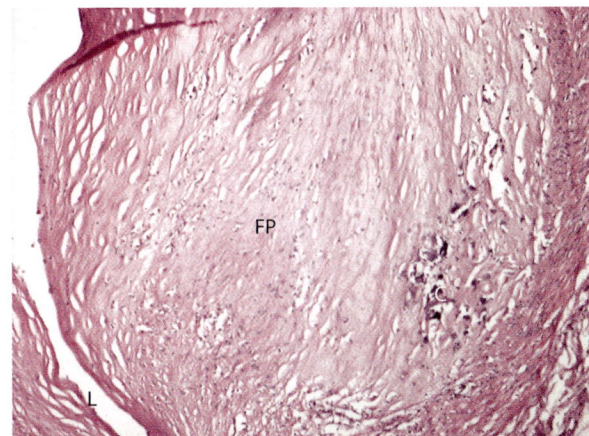

Fig. 3.12 Coronary artery showing marked luminal (L) narrowing, due a fibrotic plaque (FP) with calcification (C) (×400)

3.2.5
Lesions with Thrombi

The modified classification considers lesions with thrombi as being affected principally by three distinct processes: rupture, erosion, and, less frequently, the calcified nodule. These processes can occur in the setting of a fibrous cap atheroma or, in the case of erosion, pathological intimal thickening. A single lesion may contain morphological evidence of both rupture and erosion (Fig. 3.13).

3.2.5.1 Plaque Rupture

Plaque rupture is seen in about 60% of sudden cardiac death. More common in young males and postmenopausal females, it is clinically associated with hypercholesterolemia and low HDL levels. The concept of plaque rupture is based on the disruption of the cap of the fibroatheromatous lesion exposing the circulating blood to the potentially thrombogenic underlying large necrotic lipid core. The disrupted fibrous cap is infiltrated by macrophages and lymphocytes and smooth muscle is typically sparse. The most extensive hypothesis to explain rupture is that proposed by Libby et al. [9]. This hypothesis proposes that inflammation-derived cytones stimulate the expression of proteases and obstruct the actions of proteolytic inhibitors. It is also suggested that specific antigens elicit a T-cell response and that disease progression may be stimulated by autoimmune responses to oxidized lipoproteins.

3.2.5.2 Plaque Erosion

This is identified when serial sectioning of a thrombosed arterial segment fails to reveal fibrous cap rupture. The endothelium is absent at the erosion and the eroded plaque is rich in smooth muscle cells and proteoglycans [10]. Inflammation is minimal. Plaque erosions are more common in young women and men, and are associated with smoking, especially in premenopausal women. The mechanisms underlying erosion are yet to be fully elucidated but apoptosis is believed to be a major contributor.

3.2.5.3 Plaque Calcification (Calcified Nodules)

This term refers to a lesion with fibrous cap disruption and thrombi associated with eruptive, dense, calcific nodules. Calcified nodules are plaques with luminal thrombi showing calcific nodules protruding into the lumen through a disrupted thin fibrous cap. There is absence of an endothelium at the site of the thrombus, and inflammatory cells (macrophages, T lymphocytes) are absent. The origin of this lesion is not precisely known, but it appears to be associated with healed plaques and is a relatively less common cause of thrombotic occlusion.

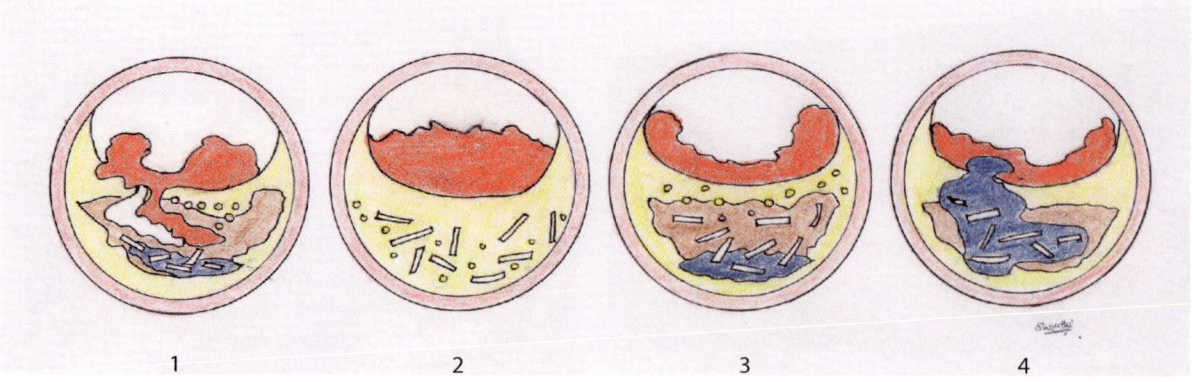

Fig. 3.13 Diagrammatic representation of complicated plaques with thrombi (red) showing 1. rupture; 2. erosion; 3. erosion with a focus on calcification (blue); 4. calcific nodule

3.3
Pathology of Coronary Interventions

Percutaneous coronary interventions (PCI) are an important group of non-surgical procedures used to treat blocked coronary arteries. While, initially, these were largely limited to percutaneous transluminal coronary angioplasty (PTCA), PCI now includes other new techniques capable of relieving coronary narrowing such as rotational atherectomy, directional atherectomy, extraction atherectomy, laser angioplasty, implantation of intracoronary stents and other catheter devices. Most commonly performed among these are the use of intracoronary stents and PTCA.

3.3.1
Angioplasty

The use of a balloon to increase the luminal area of a stenosed vessel by inflating it has been done for almost 25 years now, but the mechanisms underlying this increase in luminal diameter are becoming clearer only now. Even less study has focused on the histopathological changes in vessels which have been subjected to angioplasty, even though histomorphometric studies indicate that remodeling of the vessel wall, and not only neointimal formation, determine the long-term outcome of PTCA [11]. The morphological changes include rupture of the plaque, or extending beyond it, dissections (fissures), intra-plaque hemorrhage, plaque emboli and thrombosis. While fibro-intimal proliferation is a characteristic finding in these vessels, the histopathological appearance of older and more recent fibrous lesions is different. Older lesions contain more collagen and elastin fibres, whereas recent ones are more cellular with loosely arranged connective tissue.

3.3.2
Intracoronary Stents

Intravascular stents are intraluminal metallic prostheses which, when expanded, provide a scaffolding for the diseased vessel to maintain long-term patency. Many of these are coated with polymers and drugs to allow slow drug release over extended periods of time.

As these stents are very pliable, ideally examination of these specimens should be carried out in a well equipped reference laboratory. 2–3 mm cross-sections of the stents can be obtained using specialized scissors, for examination under a dissecting microscope. The wires can then be removed for routine paraffin embedding. Alternatively, the whole stented segment of the artery can be embedded in methylmethacrylate and cut into proximal, middle and distal parts and examined histologically for the presence of any thrombi over the stent wires, fibrointimal proliferation and destruction of the media. Any other injury to the media such as inflammation, especially with a dominance of eosinophils, foreign body giant cell reaction and presence of granulomas, are documented. These have been seen to be more common with the drug-eluting stents and may be seen in all the vessel wall layers [12].

3.4
Pathology of Coronary Artery Bypass Grafts

3.4.1
Saphenous Venous Bypass Grafts (SVBG)

The use of Saphenous veins as aorto-coronary bypass conduits have revolutionized interventional cardiology. However, they have a high failure rate mostly due to re-occlusion by the atherosclerotic process. Clinically, both graft-dependent factors (age and location of graft) and graft-independent factors (left ventricular dysfunction, patient age, etc.) determine the progression and prognosis of SVBG failure. However the pathophysiology is characterized by the three time-dependent, but to some extent overlapping processes of thrombosis, fibrointimal hyperplasia and, finally vein graft atherosclerosis. The morphology of vein graft atherosclerosis is distinct from that of native coronary atherosclerosis in that it involves the graft in a diffuse and concentric fashion. Also, atheromatous plaques in saphenous venous grafts are characterized by a weak or absent fibrous coat and a rich inflammatory cell infiltrate, inclusive of lipid-laden giant cells [13]. This exposure of lipid debris and foam cells to circulating blood creates a fragile and friable lesion at risk of embolism of atherosclerotic debris, especially during re-operation or angioplasty.

3.4.2
Internal Mammary Artery Grafts

Grafts from the left internal mammary artery (LIMA) have been shown to have a significantly higher patency rate and are now the preferred grafts for revascularization especially in left ventricular ischemia. The sternum, usually supplied by this artery can withstand a significant decrease in blood flow making this artery one of the few which can be removed. Also it has been shown to have a better endothelial cell function than saphenous vein, making it less prone to atherosclerosis. Furthermore, its own nourishment is independent of its vasa vasorum due to a thin media. Other structural characteristics which have made it popular are a luminal diameter corresponding to that of the coronary arteries and the absence of valves and varicosities.

3.5
Non-Atheromatous Coronary Artery Disease

While coronary atherosclerosis is the major significant determinant of myocardial ischemia, the coronary arteries can show evidence of other congenital and acquired pathologies.

3.5.1
Congenital Anomalies of Coronary Arteries

The term coronary artery anomaly refers to a wide range of congenital abnormalities involving the origin, course, and structure of epicardial coronary arteries. By definition, these abnormalities occur in less than 1% of the general population. In adults, the clinical interest in coronary anomalies relates to their occasional association with sudden death, myocardial ischemia, congestive heart failure, or endocarditis.

3.5.2
Spontaneous Dissection of Coronary Arteries

Dissecting aneurysms of the ascending aorta may extend into the coronary arteries, more commonly the right coronary artery. Dissection may also occur as a complication of procedures like endarterectomy and angioplasty or be entirely spontaneous. Coronary artery dissections are characterized by a subadventitial hematoma and dissection usually occurs in the plane between the media and the adventitia, compared with aortic aneurysms, which have a plane of separation within the media.

3.5.3
Aneurysms of the Coronary Arteries

Coronary artery aneurysms are a relatively infrequent abnormality. The diagnosis of coronary artery aneurysm became more frequent after the advent of coronary angiography. Atherosclerotic lesions account for the majority of cases of coronary artery aneurysms. Other etiologies include congenital, dissection, infection, vasculitis, post-coronary intervention, and other inflammatory lesions. The etiology may vary according to the geographic location (e.g., Kawasaki disease in Japan or atherosclerosis in North America).

3.6
Pathology of Ischemic Heart Disease

Ischemic heart disease is a group of closely related syndromes resulting from myocardial ischemia, usually a consequence of atherosclerotic coronary artery occlusion. Clinically, these may be expressed as any one of the following clinical syndromes

- Acute myocardial infarction
- Angina pectoris
- Chronic ischemic heart disease
- Sudden cardiac death

3.6.1
Mechanisms of Myocardial Ischemic Injury

Impairment in coronary perfusion, relative to the myocardial demand leads to functional and biochemical changes in the myocardium, which progress from reversible to irreversible and are reflected in the morphological evolution of the infarction. Oxygen deficiency results in cessation of mitochondrial oxidative phosphorylation, and thus, of ATP production. This altered metabolic milieu of reduced ATP and pH and lactate accumulation in ischemic myocytes leads to impaired membrane transport and increased intracellular calcium, eventually resulting in cytoskeletal damage. Both apoptosis (characterized by cell injury and shrinkage) and oncosis (cell injury with swelling) are implicated in cardiomyocyte ischemic injury [14]. Apoptosis is an energy-dependent process and thus, the rate and magnitude of ATP depletion determines which of the two is chiefly responsible for the progression of cell injury.

3.6.2
Pathology of Myocardial Ischemia

Myocardial infarction is characterized by necrosis of myocytes due to ischemia. Myocardial infarction begins in the subendocardium as blood flow in the myocardium occurs inwards from the epicardium to the endocardium. It then progresses as a wavefront of necrosis from the subendocardium to the subepicardium over a time, depending on the duration of occlusion and the availability of pharmacological or mechanical thrombolytic therapy.

3.6.3
Patterns of Myocardial Infarction

Infarcts may involve predominantly the *subendocardial* portion of the myocardium (Fig. 3.14) or they may be *transmural*. Also, the ischemic changes may be *regional* (localized to the area of perfusion of a major coronary artery) or *diffuse*. Subendocardial infarcts affect the inner third or half of the left ventricular wall. As they are usually a result of generalized myocardial hypoperfusion, they are diffuse or multifocal and patchy in distribution. They may, however, also be regional. Transmural infarcts, commonly the result of occlusion of a major coronary artery, are usually regional and involve the entire thickness of the left ventricular wall.

3.6.4
Location of Infarcts

The location of ischemic manifestations resulting from the occlusion of any one of the three major epicardial coronary arteries can be predicted by the areas of supply of these blood vessels (Table 3.3). Infarcts involve the left ventricle much more commonly and extensively than the right ventricle. This is partly due to the greater thickness of the left ventricular wall and the greater workload on the left ventricle. Infarction of the posterior right ventricle occurs in a percentage of right coronary artery occlusions but isolated right ventricular infarcts are rare.

3.6.5
Macroscopic Characteristics of Myocardial Infarcts

Experimental animal studies have demonstrated that functional changes can be detected as early as 10 seconds after the ligation of a coronary artery. The myocardium stops contracting and becomes cyanotic and bulges outwards. Contractions usually resume if the obstruction is rapidly relieved. However, sometimes contractility may be depressed in post-ischemic tissue even for many hours after the obstruction. This phenomenon is called a *stunned myocardium*.

Grossly, an infarct is not identifiable within the first 12–18 hours. However, histochemical demonstration by the dye triphenytetrazolium chloride (TTC) can be done to highlight the area of necrosis as early as 2–3 hours after the infarct. This dye stains non-infarcted myocardium because the dehydrogenases are preserved. The infarcted area, characterized by cell membrane injury with the leakage of enzymes, remains unstained. The cut surface of the infarct shows pallor in about 24 hours and the infarct gradually acquires a mottled appearance. The outline of the infarct becomes sharply defined with a hyperemic border of highly vascularized granulation tissue by 3–7 days, and by 2–3 weeks, the infarcted region becomes depressed and soft. Over the next few weeks, a fibrous scar develops.

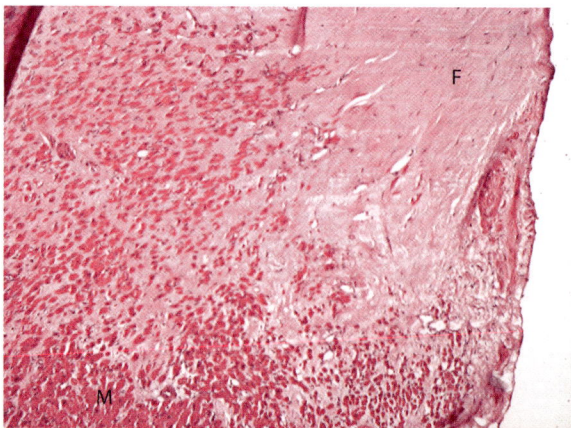

Fig. 3.14 Healed subendocardial infarct showing fibrosis (F) replacing the myocardium (M) beneath (×200)

Table 3.3 Sites of myocardial infarction based on vessel

Infarct	Occluded vessel	Site
Posterolateral infarct	Left circumflex artery	Posterolateral wall of left ventricle
Anterior infarct	Left anterior descending branch of left coronary artery	Anterior wall of left ventricle and adjacent two-third of interventricular septum
Posterior or diaphragmatic infarct	Right coronary artery	Posterior wall of left ventricle including posterior one-third of septum and papillary muscle

3.6.6 Evolution of Microscopic Characteristics of Myocardial Infarcts

3.6.6.1 Electron Microscopy

The earliest morphological changes in myocardial infarction can be detected at the ultra structural level, as early as a few minutes to one hour after onset of ischemia in the form of relaxation of the myofibrils, glycogen depletion and mitochondrial swelling.

3.6.6.2 Light Microscopy

The changes that can be seen using light microscopy become detectable in about 4–12 hours, in the form of coagulation necrosis. The coagulation necrosis continues over the next 12–24 hours. The periphery of the infarct is characterized by the presence of *wavy fibres* and *myocytolysis* (vacuolar degeneration). The necrotic muscle initiates an acute inflammatory response and an interstitial neutrophilic infiltrate can be seen in the infarct after 12–24 hours but is most marked at 2–3 days (Fig. 3.15). After this the acute inflammation is replaced by a chronic infiltrate characterized by macrophages, which phagocytose necrotic myocytes This response is maximal at about 5–10 days, and is followed by progressive establishment of granulation tissue (maximally developed at 10–14 days). Over the next 2–8 weeks this granulation tissue becomes gradually replaced by collagen and becomes more fibrous, and a dense collagenous scar develops (Figs. 3.16 and 3.17).

3.6.7 Infarct Expansion and Infarct Extension

Two common but distinct processes often observed after infarction are extension and expansion of the infarct.

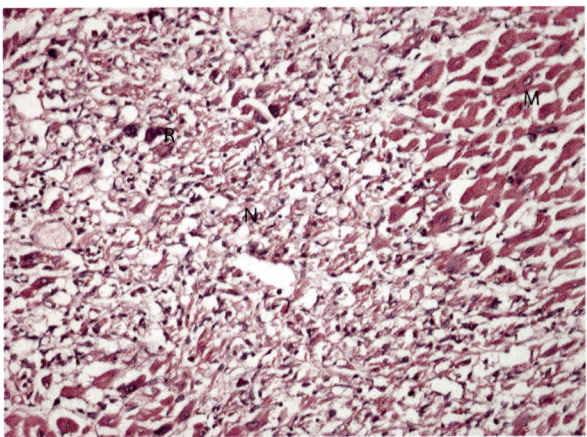

Fig. 3.15 Recent myocardial infarction of about 2–3 days duration showing necrosed myocardium (N) in contrast to viable myocardium (M). Note the associated inflammation with regenerating myocytes (R) (×400)

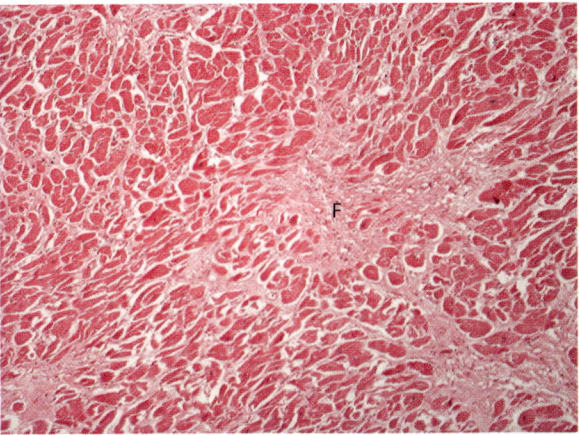

Fig. 3.16 Healed myocardial infarct showing fibrotic bands (F) between viable cardiac muscle fibres (×200)

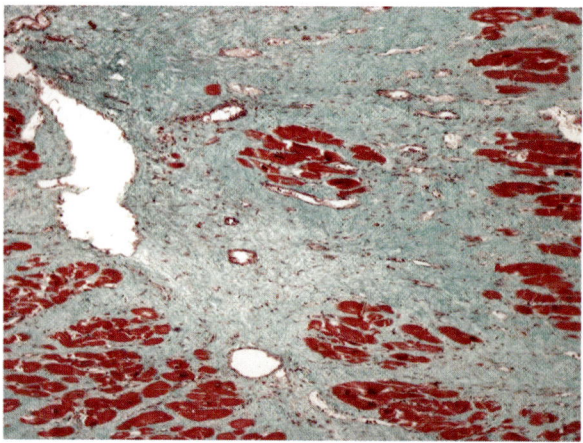

Fig. 3.17 Masson Trichrome stain of the healed infarct highlights the fibrosis which is stained green and the viable myocytes red (×200)

Infarct extension is a result of repeated episodes of ischemia to the adjacent myocardial regions which results in a histological picture charcterised by a central zone of infract undergoing repair and a periphery showing various stages in the evolution of ischemia. *Infarct expansion* is an alteration in the ventricular topography due to thinning and lengthening of the infarcted segment, mostly seen in patients with a large, transmural, anterior myocardial infarction. Infarct expansion is acute regional dilatation and thinning of the infarct zone. There are several possibilities for the mechanism of this alteration in cardiac shape: thinning could be caused by cell rupture, stretching of myocytes or slippage of groups of myocytes so that fewer cells are distributed across the wall (15). This process is distinct from extension as there is no further myocyte necrosis.

3.7
Pathological Complications of Myocardial Infarction

The acute and chronic post-infarction complications have changed in the post- reperfusion era, with the decreasing incidence of aneurysm, rupture and Dressler's syndrome.

Myocardial rupture occurs in three forms: rupture of the papillary muscle, rupture of the interventricular septum, and external rupture. Rupture of the papillary muscle is most often associated with an inferior-posterior infarct due to right coronary artery occlusion. Rupture of the interventricular septum, is more common than rupture of the papillary muscle. External rupture increases in incidence with age and is more common in women. It is characterized by sudden loss of arterial pressure with momentary persistence of sinus rhythm and often by signs of cardiac tamponade.

Ventricular septal defects. Transmural infarcts of the interventricular septum may rupture, leading to the acute development of a left to right ventricular shunt.

Right ventricular infarction is seen in patients with ischemic heart disease who have pre-existing right ventricular hypertrophy.

Ventricular aneurysm is common, especially with a large transmural infarct (most commonly anterior) and good residual myocardium. Aneurysms may develop in a few days, weeks, or months. They may be associated with recurrent ventricular arrhythmias and low cardiac output. Another hazard of ventricular aneurysm includes mural thrombus and systemic embolization. The wall of ventricular aneurysms is composed predominantly of collagen but calcification may be seen.

Pseudoaneurysm is a form of rupture of the free LV wall in which an aneurysmal wall containing clot and pericardium prevents exsanguinations.

Post-MI syndrome (Dressler's syndrome) develops in a few patients several days to weeks or even months after acute MI, although the incidence appears to have declined in recent years. It is characterized by fever and pericarditis.

3.8
Chronic Ischemic Heart Disease

Chronic ischemic heart disease is cardiac muscle insufficiency due to scarring from old infarcts, not necessarily large. It results in ischemic cardiomyopathy, characterized by an enlarged, dilated and weakened left ventricle and is a major cause of congestive heart failure. The concept of *myocardial hibernation* [16] is particularly important in understanding the development and progression of ischemic cardiomyopathy. It refers to a state of persistent regional ventricular dysfunction in patients with coronary artery disease that is potentially reversible with early revascularization. The pathophysiology of hibernation seems to be quite complex. It is postulated that despite the reduced coronary blood flow, metabolic activity is sufficient to prevent tissue necrosis and the process most likely involves repetitive post-ischemic dysfunction causing phenotypic changes in myocardial cells leading to the depletion of cardiomyocyte contractile elements, loss of myofilaments and disorganization of cytoskeletal proteins. In addition, the cardiac interstitium exhibits inflammatory changes, leading to fibrotic remodeling. Induction of cytokines and chemokines suggests an active continuous inflammatory process leading to fibrosis and dysfunction. Recovery of the hibernating myocardium has clearly been shown to occur with the establishment of successful and timely revascularization either by coronary bypass surgery or by percutaneous transluminal coronary angioplasty. The differentiation of viable, hibernating myocardium from non-viable myocardium in patients with coronary artery disease and left ventricular dysfunction is a key issue in the current era of myocardial revascularization.

3.9
Pathology of Reperfusion

The restoration of blood flow to regions of evolving infarcts by pharmacological or mechanical thrombolysis alters both the gross and microscopic features of the infarct. Macroscopically, reperfused areas are typically hemorrhagic and do not become pale as early as non-reperfused infarcts. Histologically, these infarcts are characterized by an exaggerated acute inflammatory response, manifested as a very dense and rapid neutrophilic accumulation. One of the hallmarks of reperfusion-induced changes is *contraction band necrosis*. Reperfusion can induce massive myocyte membrane injury and calcium influx as a result of reactive oxygen species production. This triggers a hypercontraction effort in the remaining partly viable myocytes. Ultrastructurally these bands are charcterized by hyper-contracted and disorganized sarcomeres with thickenened Z lines. Under light microscopy, they are visualized as prominent, thick, wavy, densely eosinophilic transverse bands in necrotic myocytes. Other reperfusion induced microscopic changes that have been described include hemorrhagic invasion of the infarct and small blood vessel damage [17].

References

1. Fye WB (2005) A historical perspective on atherosclerosis and coronary artery disease. In Fuster V, Topol EJ, Nabel EG (eds). Atherosclerosis and Coronary Artery Disease, 2nd edn. Lippicott, Williams and Wilkins, Philadelphia, pp. 1–44.
2. Fuster V, Moreno PR, Fayad ZA, Corti R, Badimon JJ (2005) Atherothrombosis and high-risk plaque: part I: evolving concepts. J Am Coll Cardiol 46(6):937–954.
3. Fukuda K, Yuasa S (2006) Stem cells as a source of regenerating cardiomyocytes. Circulation Res 98:1002.
4. Stary HC, Chandler AB, Dinsmore RE et al. (1995) A definition of advanced types of atherosclerotic lesions and a histological classification of atherosclerosis. A report from the Committee on Vascular Lesions of the Council on Arteriosclerosis, American Heart Association Circulation. 92:1355–1374.
5. Virmani R, Kolodgie FD, Burke AP, Farb A, Schwartz SM (2000) Lessons from sudden coronary death: a comprehensive morphological classification scheme for atherosclerotic lesions. Arterioscler Thromb Vasc Biol 20:1262–1275.
6. Lafont A (2003) Basic aspects of plaque vulnerability. Heart 89:1262–1267.
7. Kereiakes DJ (2003) The Emperor's clothes. In search of the vulnerable plaque. Circulation 107:2076.
8. Kolodgie FD, Burke AP, Farb A et al. (2001) The thin-cap fibroatheroma: a type of vulnerable plaque. The major precursor lesion to acute coronary syndromes. Current Opin Cardiol 16:285–292.
9. Libby P (1995) Molecular bases of the acute coronary syndromes. Circulation 91:2844–2850.
10. Schaar JA, Muller JE, Falk E et al. (2004) Terminology for high-risk and vulnerable coronary artery plaques. Report of a Meeting on the Vulnerable Plaque, June 17 and 18, 2003, Santorini, Greece. Eur Heart J 25:1077–1082.
11. Sangiorgi G, Taylor AJ, Farb A et al. (1999) Pathology of postpercutaneous transluminal coronary angioplasty remodeling in human coronary arteries. Am Heart J 138(4):681–687.
12. Farb A, Sangiorgi G, Carter AJ et al. (1999) Pathology of acute and chronic coronary stenting in humans. Circulation 99:44–52.
13. Motwani JG, Topol EJ (1998) Aortocoronary saphenous vein graft disease. pathogenesis, predisposition, and prevention. Circulation 97:916–931.
14. Buja LM (2005) Myocardial ischemia and reperfusion injury. Cardiovasc Pathol 14(4):170–175.
15. Weisman HF, Bush DE, Mannisi JA, Weisfeldt ML, Healy B (1988) Cellular mechanisms of myocardial infarct expansion. Circulation 78:186–201.
16. Brown TA (2001) Hibernating myocardium. Am J Crit Care 10(2):84–91.
17. Reimer KA, Vander Heide RS, Richard VJ (1993) Reperfusion in acute myocardial infarction: effect of timing and modulating factors in experimental models. Am J Cardiol. 72(19):13G–21G.

Chapter 4

Pathophysiology of Diabetic Vascular Complications

Francis Estrada and John R. Buscombe

Contents

4.1	Introduction	45
4.1.1	Diabetes and Cardiovascular Disease: the Complex and Close Association	45
4.2	Pathophysiology of Cardiovascular Complications	46
4.2.1	Macrovascular Complications: Accelerated Atherosclerosis	46
4.2.2	Abnormal Metabolic States in Diabetes	46
4.2.3	Altered Cellular Physiology in Diabetes Mellitus	46
4.2.4	Inflammation in Diabetes and Atherosclerosis	47
4.2.5	Microvascular Complications: Coronary Microcirculation	48
4.3	Molecular Mechanisms	48
4.3.1	The Role of Advanced Glycated End Products and Their Receptors	48
4.3.2	Oxidative Stress	48
4.4	Conclusions	49
	References	49

4.1 Introduction

4.1.1 Diabetes and Cardiovascular Disease: the Complex and Close Association

Diabetes mellitus (DM) is one of the most common chronic diseases in the world. It is classified into type 1 DM, which constitute 10% of cases and type 2 DM, which accounts for 90% of cases. The incidence is increasing and it is estimated that the number of sufferers worldwide will rise from 135 million in 1995 to 300 million in the year 2025 [1].

Cardiovascular complications remain the major cause of morbidity and mortality in people with diabetes [2]. Diabetes is considered an independent risk factor for developing cardiovascular disease in both men and women. Patients with diabetes have increased risks of coronary heart disease (CHD) equivalent to that of non-diabetic patients with a history of stroke.

Patients with type 2 diabetes mellitus have a twofold to threefold increased incidence of diseases related to atheroma [3]. Type 1 diabetes is associated with at least a 10-fold increase in cardiovascular disease compared with an age-matched non-diabetic population [4]. There is also a noted increase in CHD mortality after age 30, particularly in patients with renal complications.

Higher fatality rates from cardiovascular disease is seen in diabetics than in non-diabetic patients. This is for a number of reasons. One of these is the painless presentation of ischemic heart disease in diabetes mellitus, the so-called silent myocardial ischemia. The presence of the co-morbidities of diabetes mellitus, particularly heart failure, is another important factor [5]. Lastly, the development of cardiomyopathy may occur either without or in combination with coronary artery disease (CAD), and hypertension in these patients further increases their morbidity and mortality.

4.2
Pathophysiology of Cardiovascular Complications

4.2.1
Macrovascular Complications: Accelerated Atherosclerosis

Among the multitude of complications, the affect of diabetes on the vascular system accounts for the majority of morbidity and mortality. It promotes accelerated atherogenesis, which leads to the increased incidence and rapid clinical course of coronary artery disease, stroke and peripheral arterial disease [6].

Diabetes is associated with other traditional risk factors for coronary heart disease, which include hypertension and dyslipidemia [7]. Metabolic abnormalities and impairment of normal cellular function are likewise associated with diabetes mellitus, which may hasten the development of atherosclerosis.

4.2.2
Abnormal Metabolic States in Diabetes

Epidemiologic studies have shown that increases in the level of plasma glucose are associated with an increase in cardiovascular events [8]. The UKPDS group demonstrated a commensurate increase in risk of cardiovascular events when the glycosylated hemoglobin is above a level of 6.02%. They also showed that intensive glycemic control reduced the microvascular complications in type 2 DM but it did not decrease the macrovascular events. The DCCT/EDIC trial, a study of intensive glucose control on type 1 DM, documented long-term beneficial effects of such glycemic control on the risk of cardiovascular disease [8]. Hyperglycemia increases the formation of reactive oxygen species, activation of protein kinase C and affects lipid metabolism, which alters endothelial, smooth muscle and platelet function.

Dyslipidemia is another metabolic abnormality associated with diabetes mellitus. Type 1 diabetes mellitus is associated with dyslipidemia which is dependent on good glycemic control, and the most frequent dyslipidemic disorder in poorly controlled patients is low density lipoprotein (LDL)-cholesterol [9]. Type 2 DM should really be considered as a component of a wider metabolic syndrome. Patients with type 2 DM often have a more atherogenic lipid profile characterized by elevated triglycerides, decreased high-density lipoproteins and increased small dense low-density lipoproteins, increased formation of triglyceride-rich LDLs and decreased clearance by lipoprotein lipase leading to the elevated levels of atherogenic triglycerides. The presence of these triglyceride-rich lipoproteins also lowers high density lipoprotein (HDL) by promoting exchanges of cholesterol from HDL to very low density lipoprotein (VLDL) exchange protein [10]. The severity of angiographic CAD is related to the number of triglyceride-rich lipoprotein particles and plasma lipoproteins-a (Lp-a) in type 2 DM. When the LDL apoB of LDL is glycated, its recognition by the LDL receptor on the human fibroblast is decreased. However, it is better recognized by the scavenger receptor on human macrophages, resulting in increased intracellular accumulation of cholesteryl esters within the intimal cells, the so-called foam cells, an important component of the atheroclerotic plaque.

Insulin resistance coexists in about 80% of all type 2 DM. It has also been associated with other traditional risk factors for CHD including central obesity, dyslipidemia, hypertension, hypercoagulability, low-grade inflammation and abnormal vascular reactivity [11]. This is also known as the metabolic syndrome. Haffner et al. showed that metabolic syndrome is common and is associated with an increased risk of CVD and type 2 DM in both sexes [12].

4.2.3
Altered Cellular Physiology in Diabetes Mellitus

Altered cellular function is also noted in diabetic patients. Changes in endothelial function, vascular smooth muscle cell physiology, monocyte–macrophage system, platelet function and coagulation further render diabetic patients susceptible to accelerated atherosclerosis.

The endothelium is the inner layer of the vascular wall, which actively regulates vascular tone and permeability, the balance between coagulation and fibrinolysis, composition of the subendothelial matrix, adhesion and extravastion of leucocytes, and inflammatory activity of vessels. These functions are accomplished through the formation and secretion of extracellular components and regulatory mediators.

Nitric oxide is a key mediator secreted intrinsically by the endothelium [13]. It is a potent vasodilator and possesses anti-platelet, anti-proliferative, permeability-decreasing and anti-inflammatory properties. Nitric oxide formation is noted to be impaired in patients with diabetes mellitus secondary to formation of Advanced Glycation End Products (AGE) and enhanced oxidative stress, which leads to endothelial dysfunction [14].

Endothelial dysfunction has been demonstrated in patients with type 1 and type 2 DM. Type 1 diabetics are documented to have endothelial dysfunction, however, other factors, genetic or environmental, will determine who are likely to develop aggressive angiopathy or who are not. In type 2 diabetes, endothelial cell dysfunction is detectable very early in the course of the disease, even before overt hyperglycemia ensues, and may play a key role in the etiopathology of the vasculopathy associated with this disease. Endothelial dysfunction plays a key role not only in the initiation of atherosclerosis, but also in its progression and clinical consequences. Several molecular mechanisms present in diabetes are known to affect the endothelium, as noted in Table 4.1.

Platelets also play an important role in the development of diabetic vascular complications. Increased platelet aggregation was documented in diabetic patients as early as 1965, with impairment of platelet-mediated vasodilation in NIDDM [15, 16]. Metabolic alterations present in DM are known to affect platelet function. Hyperglycemia causes in vivo platelet activation and nonenzymatic glycation of glycoproteins, causing structural changes and lipid membrane dynamics alterations. Hyperglycemia-induced oxidative stress leads to:
(1) oxidation of arachidonic acid and LDL, resulting in the formation of biologically active isoprotanes;
(2) oxidation of thiols and carbonyl formation, altering structure and function of coagulative proteins; and
(3) activation of transcription factors and redox-sensitive genes which trigger a switch leading to a prothrombotic state.

Enhanced expression of adhesive receptors on the platelet surface of diabetic patients is seen, which increases platelet aggregation [16]. Diabetic patients with clinically apparent atherosclerosis had increased levels of platelet microparticles and P-selectin (markers of platelet activation).

Diabetes mellitus affects vascular smooth muscle function, which influence atherosclerotic plaque formation, plaque instability and clinical events. Increased smooth muscle cell migration is also noted in diabetes mellitus. This results in hyperactive smooth muscle cells in diabetes mellitus secondary to altered subcellular Ca+ distribution [17].

4.2.4 Inflammation in Diabetes and Atherosclerosis

Vascular inflammation is important in the development of atherosclerosis and in determining plaque stability. Acute phase reactants including C-reactive protein (CRP) are increased in patients with diabetes mellitus, and this is related to poorer control as determined by raised HcA1c [18]. CRP may be involved in each of the stages of atherosclerosis by directly influencing processes such as complement activation, apoptosis, vascular cell activation, monocyte recruitment, lipid accumulation and thrombosis. CRP attenuates the survival, differentiation, and function of endothelial progenitor cells,

Table 4.1 Cellular and molecular basis for endothelial dysfunction in diabetes (modified from Calles Escandon J and Cipolla M (2001) Diabetes and endothelial dysfunction: a clinical perspective. Endocrine Reviews 22: 36–52 [16])

Molecular defect	Result
Increased activation of PKC	Increased proliferation of vessels, altered contraction, altered signal transduction
Overexpression of growth factors (endothelin, ANG-II)	Increased growth and phenotypic change of SMC
Nonenzymatic glycation of proteins and Other molecules (DNA)	Change in antigenicity with consequent immune mediated damage
Hyperglycemia induced increase in VSMC	Impaired vasodilation and enhanced proliferation of synthesis of DAG
Impaired insulin activation of PIP-3	Increased growth and proliferation of vessels kinase but normal MAP-kinase response in response to hyperinsulinemia
Increased production of PAI-1	Decreased fibrinolysis, prothrombotic tendency
Oxidative stress	Decreased production of NO, hyperreactivity of SMVC to vasoconstrictive stimuli, increase in proinflammatory, adhesion molecules (ICAM, ELAM, VCAM)

partly by reducing the expression of endothelial nitric oxide synthase. Adverse cardiac outcomes were also associated with elevated CRP and it also predicts future cardiovascular risk [19]. Increased concentrations of soluble adhesion molecules at the atherosclerosis sites are also independently associated with increased coronary risk in NIDDM patients [20].

4.2.5
Microvascular Complications: Coronary Microcirculation

Diabetes also affects the microvessels, particularly those of the eyes, kidneys and nerves, which add to the increased morbidity in diabetes. The effects of the diabetic state on the coronary microcirculation have also been studied.

Several studies, mainly of type 2 DM, have documented reduced coronary flow reserve, i.e., the ratio of myocardial blood flow during near maximal coronary vasodilatation to that of basal myocardial blood flow. Coronary flow reserve is an indirect parameter used to measure coronary circulation by the large epicardial vessels and small resistance vessels. Most of these studies included patients with normal coronary arteries, and were documented angiographically or clinically. Other studies have also shown the presence of coronary flow reserve abnormalities in patients with diabetic nephropathy and retinopathy [21, 22]. The morphologic abnormalities documented in diabetic myocardium include basement membrane thickening, arteriolar thickening, capillary microaneurysms and reduced capillary density. Abnormalities in the vascular smooth muscle cells have also been studied. A study using coronary arterioles from the right atrial appendage of diabetics showed impairment of human coronary dilation to K+ ATP opening leading to reduced dilation to hypoxia [23].

4.3
Molecular Mechanisms

Several biochemical and molecular mechanisms responsible for the microvascular and macrovascular mechanisms of diabetes have been studied and are discussed below.

4.3.1
The Role of Advanced Glycated End Products and Their Receptors

In the milieu of hyperglycemia, a non-enzymatic condensation reaction (Maillard reaction) between glucose and the free amino group of proteins/lipoproteins occurs, which leads to the formation of a heterogeneous group of irreversible adducts called advanced glycation end products (AGE). AGE formation is associated with aging but is accelerated in diabetes mellitus [24].

AGE can promote accelerated atherosclerosis through both non-receptor-mediated and receptor-mediated mechanisms [25], which are listed in Tables 4.2 and 4.3.

4.3.2
Oxidative Stress

DM is associated with oxidative stress. Increased metabolism of hyperglycemia and the elevated levels of free fatty acids in diabetes leads to increased levels of NADH and FADH (electron donors) saturating the electron transport chain with uncoupling of electron transport and oxidative phosphorylation. This results in increased superoxide formation and inefficient ATP synthesis [26]. Increased formation of peroxynitrite is also noted in diabetes mellitus due to oxidation of nitric oxide, which is brought about by increased ROS formation. Peroxynitrite oxidizes BH4 to inactive BH2. It also oxidizes LDL. Oxidized-LDL depletes l-arginine avail-

Table 4.2 Atherosclerosis promoting effects of AGEs: non-receptor. Adapted from Aronson D and Rayfield EJ (2002) How hyperglycemia promotes atherosclerosis: molecular mechanisms. Cardiovascular Diabetology 1:1

Mediated mechanisms
Extra cellular matrix
Collagen cross linking
Enhanced synthesis of extracellular matrix components
Glycosylated subendothelial matrix quenches nitric oxide
Functional alterations of regulatory proteins
bFGF glycosylation reduces its heparin binding capacity and its mitogenic activity on endothelial cells
Inactivation of the complement regulatory protein CD59
Lipoprotein modifications
Glycosylated LDL
Reduced LDL recognition by cellular LDL receptors
Increased susceptibility of LDL to oxidative modification

IGF-I = Insulin-like growth factor I; IL-1 = Interleukin-1; PDGF = Platelet-derived growth factor; TNF-α = Tumor necrosis factor-α.

Table 4.3 Atherosclerosis promoting effects of AGEs: receptor. Adapted from Aronson D and Rayfield EJ (2002) How hyperglycemia promotes atherosclerosis: molecular mechanisms. Cardiovascular Diabetology 1:1

Mediated mechanisms
Promoting inflammation
Secretion of cytokines such as TNF-alpha, IL-Chemotactic stimulus for monocyte-macrophages
Induction of cellular proliferation
Stimulation of PDGF and IGF-I secretion from monocytes and possibly SMC.
Endothelial dysfunction
Increased permeability of EC monolayers
Increased procoagulant activity
Increased expression of adhesion molecules
Increased intracellular oxidative stress (

IGF-I = Insulin-like growth factor I; IL-1 = Interleukin-1; PDGF = Platelet-derived growth factor; TNF-α = Tumor necrosis factor-α.

ability in endothelial cells. The deficiency of l-arginine and BH4 uncouples eNOS resulting in increased superoxide formation instead of nitric oxide [27].

4.3.2.1 Activation of Protein Kinase C

In hyerglycemic patients, there is increased activation of protein kinase C secondary to de novo synthesis of diacylglycerol from the glycolytic intermediates [28]. Protein kinase C is involved in the transcription for growth factors and in the signal transduction in response to growth factors. Protein kinase C increases vascular activation of NADPH leading to increased ROS production, dysfunction of the eNOS system and decreased NO (potent vasodilator) production and increased ET-1 production (potent vasoconstrictor). PKC regulates vascular smooth muscle cell proliferation and apoptosis. It also partly regulates leukocyte adhesion, monocyte transdifferentiation and macrophage growth leading to intimal foam cell formation.

4.3.2.2 Increased Flux to the Polyol Pathway

Glucose freely diffusing into cells is normally reduced to sorbitol through aldose reductase in euglycemic conditions, which is subsequently oxidized to fructose (sorbitol dehydrogenase) [29]. When these cells are exposed to hyperglycemia, there is increased glucose entry into the polyol pathway with subsequent increased production of sorbitol and a concomitant decrease in NADPH. Decreased availability of NADPH decreases endothelial formation of nitric oxide [30]. The potential mechanisms that could promote vascular damage include sorbitol-induced osmotic stress due to accumulated sorbitol, altered or decreased Na/K-ATPase activity, myo-inositol depletion with impaired phosphatidylinositol metabolism, increased prostaglandin production, and alterations in protein kinase C isoform activity.

4.4 Conclusions

The metabolic disorders associated with diabetes result in a multiple stage attack on the coronary arteries, with increased atheroma deposition, resulting coronary artery wall inflammation and increased risk of thrombosis due to increased platelet stickiness and vasospasm caused by factors related to the release of nitric oxide. Understanding these problems allows a more informed assessment of myocardial perfusion to be performed in these patients.

References

1. King H, Aubert RE, Herman WH (1998) Global burden of diabetes, 1995–2025. Diabetes Care 21:1414–1431.
2. Grundy SM, Benjamin IJ, Burke GL, Chait A, Eckel RH, Howard BV et al. (1999) Diabetes and cardiovascular disease. A statement for healthcare professionals from the American Heart Association. Circulation 100:1134–1146.
3. Garcia MJ, McNamara PM, Gordon T, Kannell WB (1974) Morbidity and mortality in diabetics in the Framingham population. Sixteen year followup. Diabetes 23:105–111.
4. Laing SP, Swerdlow AJ, Slater SD et al. (2003) Mortality from heart disease in a cohort of 23,000 patients with insulin-treated diabetes. Diabetologia 46:760–765.
5. The Diabetes Control and Complications Trial/Epidemiology of Diabetes Interventions and Complications (DCCT/EDIC) Study Research Group (2005) Intensive diabetes treatment and cardiovascular disease in patients with Type 1 diabetes. N Engl J Med 353:2643–2653.
6. Kannel WB and McGee DL (1979) Diabetes and cardiovascular disease. The Framingham study. JAMA 241:2035–2038.
7. Soedamah-Muthu SS, Chaturvedi N, Toeller M, Ferriss B, Reboldi P, Michel G, Manes C, Fuller JH (2004) Risk factors for coronary heart disease in Type 1 diabetic patients

in Europe. The EURODIAB Prospective Complications Study. Diabetes Care 27:530–537.
8. Coutinho M, Gerstein HC, Wang Y, Yusuf S (1999) The relationship between glucose and cardiovascular events. Diabetes Care 22:233–240.
9. Perez A, Wagner AM, Cabreras G, Gimenez G et al. (2000) Prevalence and phenotypic distribution of dyslipidemia in Type 1 diabetes mellitus. Effect of glycemic control. Arch Intern Med 160:2756–2762.
10. Kelley DE, Simoneau JA (1994) Impaired free fatty acid utilization by skeletal muscle in non-insulin dependent diabetes mellitus. J Clin Invest 94:2349–2356.
11. F. Xavier Pi-Sunyer (2004) Pathophysiology and long-term management of the metabolic syndrome. Obesity Res 12:Supplement December.
12. Haffner SM (2006) Risk constellations in patients with the metabolic syndrome: epidemiology, diagnosis, and treatment patterns. Am J Med 119(5 Suppl 1):S3–S9.
13. Cohen RA (2005) Role of nitric oxide in diabetic complications. Am J Therapy 12:499–502.
14. Schalkwijk CG and Stehouwer CDA (2005) Vascular complications in diabetes mellitus: the role of endothelial dysfunction. Clinical Sci 109:143–159.
15. Oskarsson HJ, Hofmeyer TG (1997) Diabetic human platelets release a substance that inhibits platelet-mediated vasodilatation. Am J Physiol 273:H371–H379.
16. Tschoepe D, Driesch E, Schwippert B, Nieuwenhuis HK, Gries FA (1995) Exposure of adhesion molecules on activated platelets in patients with newly diagnosed IDDM is not normalized by near-normoglycaemia. Diabetes 44:890–894.
17. Fleischhacker E, Esenabhalu VE, Spitaler M, Holzmann S, Skrabal F, Koidl B, Kostner GM, Graier WF (1999) Human diabetes is associated with hyperreactivity of vascular smooth muscle cells due to altered subcellular Ca2 distribution. Diabetes 48:1323–1330.
18. Ford ES (1999) Body mass index, diabetes, and C-reactive protein among U.S. adults. Diabetes Care 22:1971–1977
19. Koenig W, Sund M, Fröhlich M et al. (1999) C-reactive protein, a sensitive marker of inflammation, predicts future risk of coronary heart disease in initially healthy middle-aged men. Circulation 99:237–242.
20. Jude EB, Douglas JT, Anderson SG, Young MJ, Boulton AJM. (2002) Circulating cellular adhesion molecules ICAM-1, VCAM-1, P- and E-selectin in the prediction of cardiovascular disease in diabetes mellitus. Eur J Int Med May 185–189.
21. Akasaka T, Yoshida K, Hozumi T, Takagi T, Kaji S, Kawamoto T, Orioka S, Yoshikawa J. (1997) Retinopathy identifies marked restriction of coronary flow reserve in patients with diabetes mellitus. J Am Coll Cardiol 30(4):935–941.
22. Ragosta M, Samady H, Isaacs RB, Gimple LW, Sarembock IJ, Powers ER. (2004) Coronary flow reserve abnormalities in patients with diabetes mellitus who have end-stage renal disease and normal epicardial coronary arteries. Am Heart J 147:1017–1023.
23. Bagi Z, Koller A, and Kaley G. Superoxide-NO interaction decreases flow- and agonist-induced dilations of coronary arterioles in Type 2 diabetes mellitus Am J Physiol Heart Circ Physiol 285:H1404–H1410.
24. Bierhaus A, Marion A. Hofmann MA, Reinhard Ziegler R Nawroth PP. (1998) AGEs and their interaction with AGE-receptors in vascular disease and diabetes mellitus. I. The AGE concept. Cardiovasc Res 37.586–600.
25. Mehta JL, Rasouli N, Sinha AK, Molavi A. (2006) Review oxidative stress in diabetes: A mechanistic overview of its effects on atherogenesis and myocardial dysfunction. Int J Biochem Cell Biol 38:794–803.
26. Feron O, Kelly RA. (2001) The caveolar paradox: Suppressing, inducing, and erminating enos signaling. Circulation Res 88:129–131.
27. Inoguchi T, Li P, Umeda F et al. (2000) High glucose level and free fatty acid stimulate reactive oxygen species production through protein kinase C-dependent activation of NAD(P)H oxidase in cultured vascular cells. Diabetes 49:1939–1945.
28. Inoguchi T, Xia P, Kunisaki M, Higashi S, Feener EP, King GL (1994) Insulin's effect on protein kinase C and diacylglycerol induced by diabetes and glucose in vascular tissues. Am J Physiol 267(3 Pt 1):E369–E379.
29. Swidan SZ, Montgomery PA. (1998) Effect of blood glucose concentrations on the development of chronic complications of diabetes mellitus. Pharmacotherapy 18:961–972.
30. Setter SM, Campbell K, Cahoon CJ. (2003) Biochemical pathways for microvascular complications of diabetes mellitus Annals Pharmacotherapy 37(12):1858–1866.

Part II Conventional Investigation of Coronary Artery Disease and Ischaemic Heart Disease

Chapter 5

Clinical Assessment and Evaluation of the Cardiovascular System

Jeanette Sundberg-Cohon,
Nivedita Gauthaman,
Gopinath Gnanasegaran
and Margaret Hall

Contents

5.1	Introduction	53
5.2	Step One: Approach to the Patient and Cardiac History	54
5.3	Step Two: Inspection, Palpation and Auscultation	57
5.3.1	Inspection	57
5.3.2	Palpation	59
5.3.3	Auscultation	60
5.4	Step Three: Conclusion	60
	References	63

5.1 Introduction

"Medicine is an art based on science" – Sir William Osler. Clinical examination was developed and advocated by Hippocrates to understand diseases and patients. Accurate history-taking plays a crucial role in the assessment of patients and clinical examination follows history-taking. Both form a crucial part of good clinical practice.

In spite of phenomenal advancement in diagnostic modalities ranging from excellent biochemical markers to imaging techniques, history and clinical examination is still the first line of assessment. It is still the most important part of investigation and management of a disease. Performing a good examination and obtaining an accurate history takes a certain amount of time, regardless of your level of experience or ability (Figs. 5.1 and 5.2) [1–10]. Initial clinical examination also allows us to identify the severity of symptoms. Astute clinical judgment in the assessment of clinical finding and additional risk factors in the individual patient may alter the diagnostic or therapeutic strategy. A thoughtful examination also lowers the costs of care. The four cardinal principles of good clinical examination involve inspection, palpation, percussion and auscultation. However, in this chapter the discussion is limited to the clinical assessment and evaluation of the cardiovascular system. The physician will concentrate on the cardiac status of patients who present with a history of cardiac disease or who are suspected of having cardiac disease. The time of onset of chest pain, its location, extent, severity, and radiation is vital. Therefore, the attending physician or cardiologist should evaluate the patient's history in detail (cardiac risk factors, family history, and past medical history, etc.) [1–10].

Compared with many bodily systems, the cardiovascular system is an extremely rewarding system to examine, thanks largely to its relative simplicity and accessibility. Many aspects of the function of the heart and vasculature directly follow its structure [1]

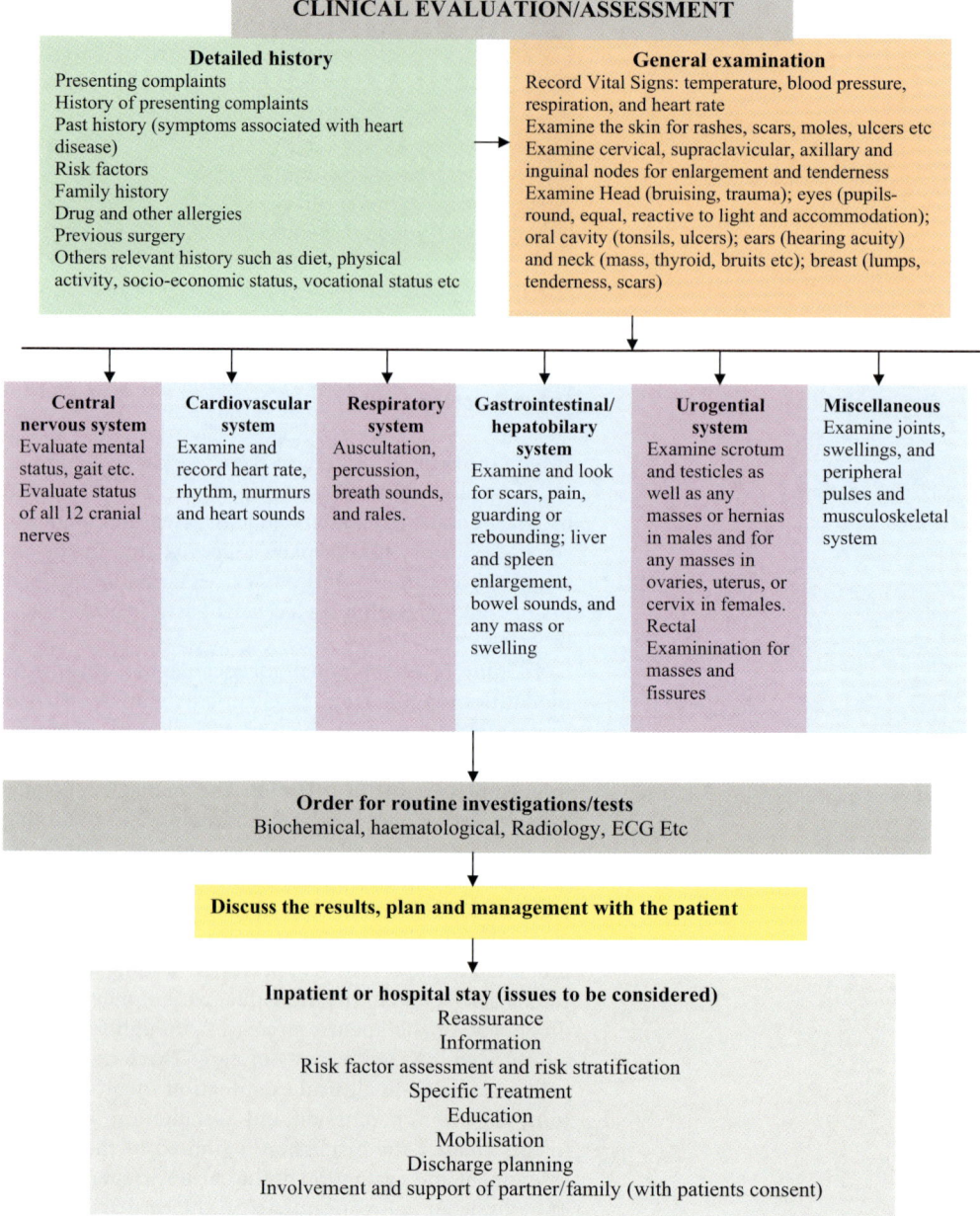

Fig. 5.1 History-taking, general and systemic examination [10]

5.2 Step One: Approach to the Patient and Cardiac History

The importance of that very first impression the patient gains upon meeting the examining doctor cannot be overemphasized. Those first seconds, sometimes starting with the doctor's knock on the door before eye contact has been made can set the tone of the entire interaction. The consequence is that many of us then have a tendency to take comfort in the technical aspects of the examination, and dive directly into the impersonal task of, for instance, staring at the patient's hands. This is directly at the expense of spending just a few invaluable seconds getting to know the patient, and "being there" with them on a human level.

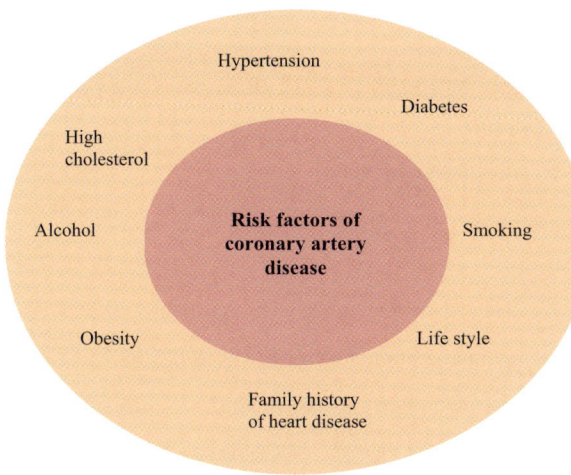

Fig. 5.2 Risk factors for coronary artery disease [1]

became doctors, clinical examinations were a mystery. However, "Good history solves most mysteries".

Establishing a positive vibe or bond with a new patient doesn't take many seconds. Introducing yourself slowly and clearly, confirming their name, introducing yourself to the accompanying relative or friend goes a very long way in your patient's eyes.

In general a good cardiac history should include details of presenting complaints or symptoms (chest pain, fatigue, breathlessness, palpitations, etc.) (Fig. 5.3, Table 5.1) [1–10]. The symptoms, such as chest pain, palpitation, dyspnoea and fatigue, should be recorded in detail with regard to frequency, duration, character, severity, radiation, medication, etc. (Figs. 5.4–5.6, Table 5.2) [5, 11, 12]. Relevant past history or illness (thyroid disease, neoplastic diseases) diabetes, hypertension, and hyperlipidemias should be recorded.

The cardiac history should also make note of the patient's lifestyle and habits (alcohol, smoking) and also any family history of heart disease. The history should also make note of any drug allergies and the patient's current medication, etc.

What can be helpful in ensuring you direct your attention to the individual standing in front of you, rather than to the 'patient with possible heart disease' in front of you is to remind yourself that before we ourselves

Other fundamentals include ensuring that the patient is comfortable, is offered help getting undressed or

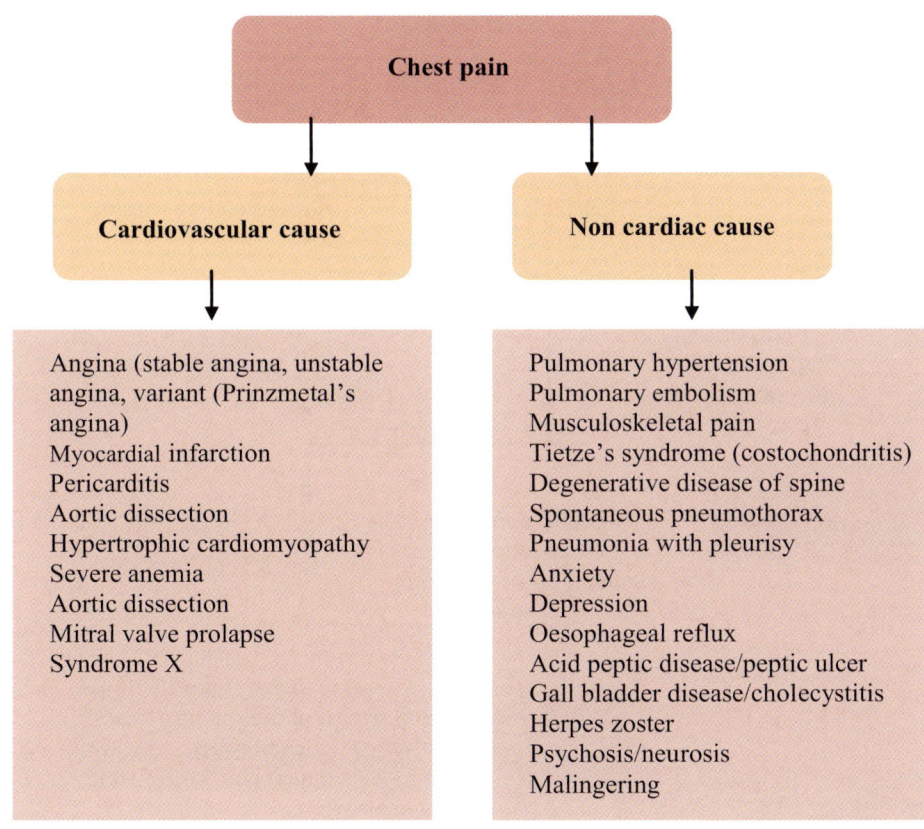

Fig. 5.3 Cardiac and non-cardiac causes of chest pain [5, 11, 12]

Table 5.1 Types of angina and its common features [14–16]

Angina types	Features
Stable angina	The discomfort is due to myocardial ischaemia
Unstable angina	Pain is more severe than stable angina, and it may occur at rest
Prinzmetal or variant	Unpredictable/rest pain
Rest angina	Occurs without precipitating exertion
Spontaneous angina	Occurs due to unexplained sympathetic over activity and unrelated to a particular event
Nocturnal angina	Occurs at night, usually precipitated by nightmares or mild congestive heart failure
Emotional angina	Provoked by autonomic activity during excitement, anger, anxiety, or stress
New onset angina	Occurs in a previously asymptomatic patient due to a change in the coronary dynamics
Refractory angina	Often does not respond to a usually effective medication
Thermal angina	Occurs due to cold weather or cold water
Post-prandial angina	After a meal
Crescendo angina	Rapid increase in the frequency over 2 to 4 weeks
Recrudescent angina	Reappears after a prolonged symptom-free period
Effort angina	Occurs due to exertion

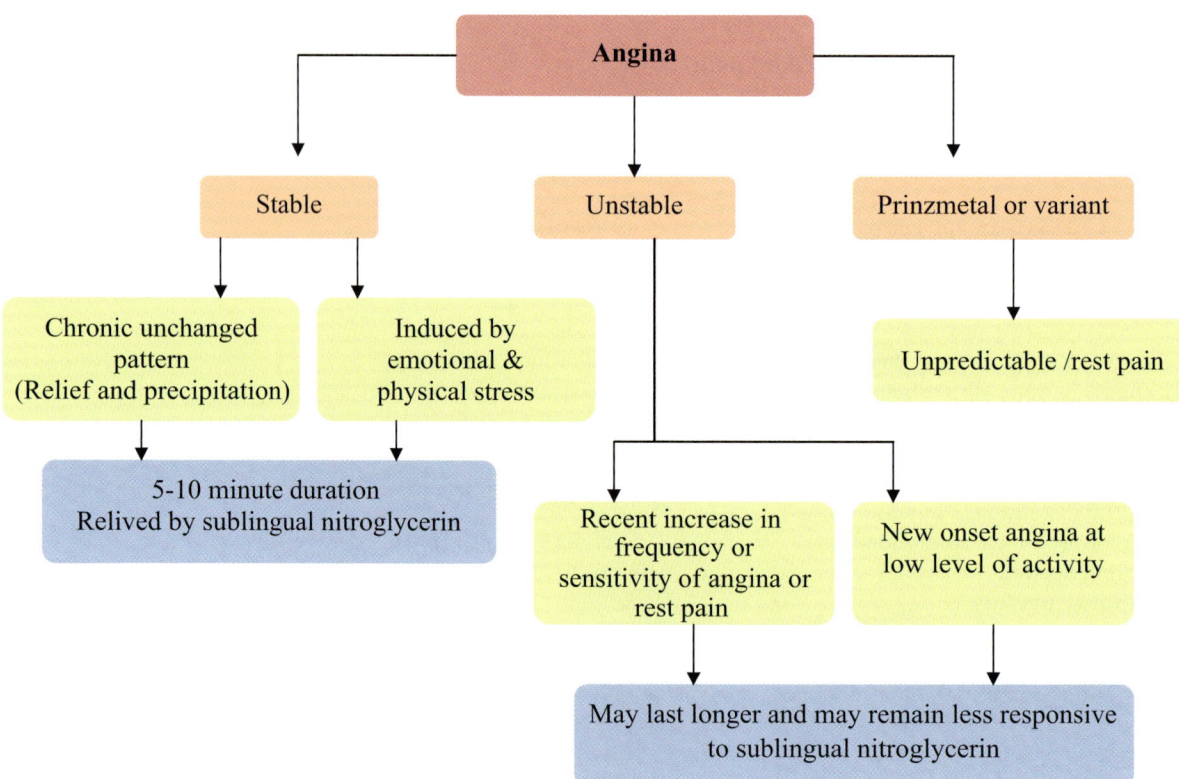

Fig. 5.4 Angina and its patterns [5, 12, 14, 18]

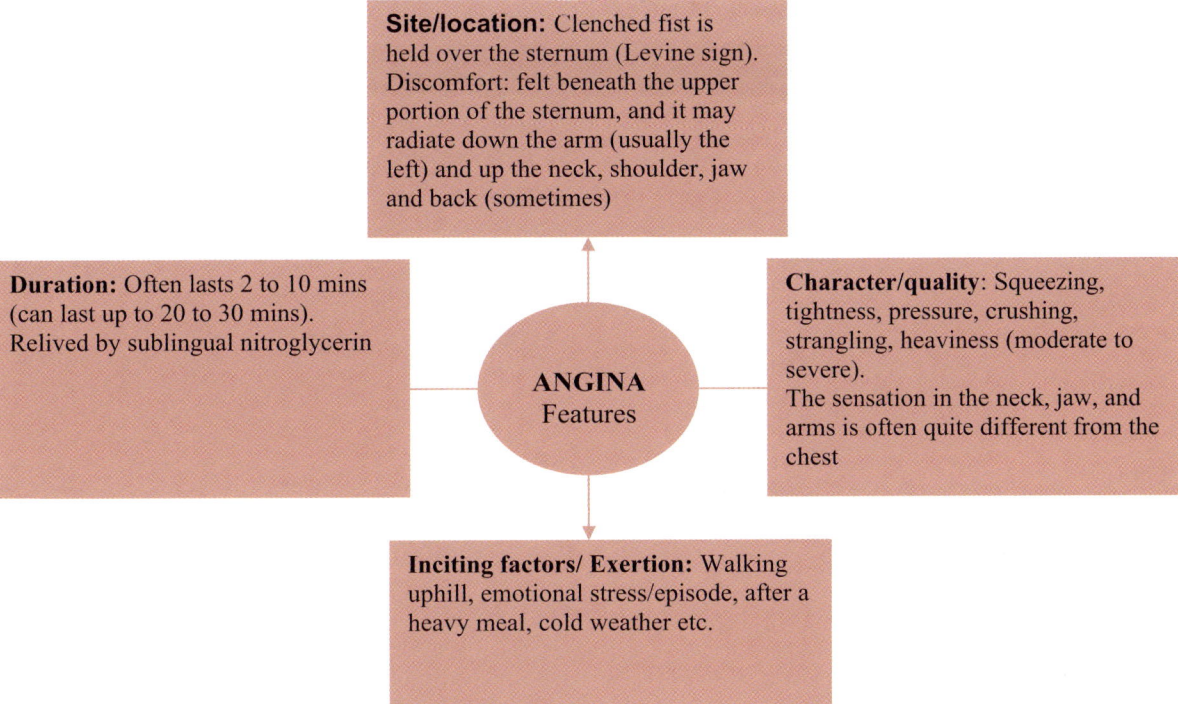

Fig. 5.5 Important features of angina [12]

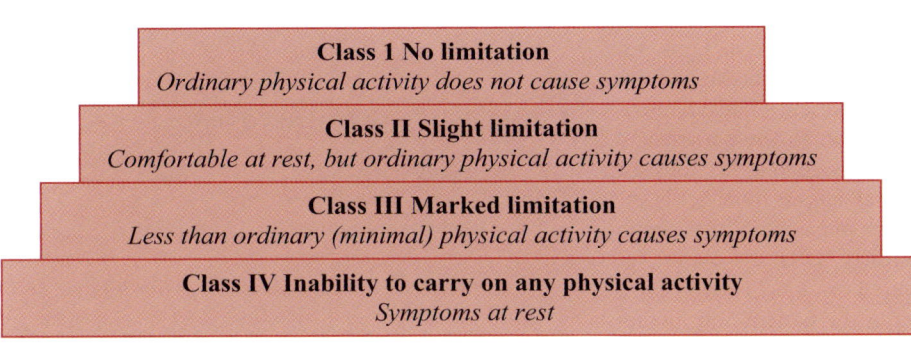

Fig. 5.6 NYHA (New York Heart Association) classification of functional capacity

getting up on the examination table, is not left physically exposed longer than necessary, and has had any preliminary questions answered and has been encouraged to ask questions at any point during the examination. Explaining what you are about to do, what your patient can expect, and what is involved in the clinical examination is essential. Finally, learning a specific sequence in which to examine any system is essential, and although there is no one correct method, most teachers or teaching seems to follow a "route", or path, starting at the foot of the bed, moving up the right arm to face and neck, then down onto the torso.

5.3
Step Two: Inspection, Palpation and Auscultation

5.3.1
Inspection

In general, the patient should be made to feel comfortable and the scenario may be different if the patient is seen as an outpatient in the clinic or as an in-patient (patient who is already admitted to the hospital). First, if the patient is admitted in the ward, the patient's im-

Table 5.2 Common causes and types of dyspnoea [5, 13]

Causes of dyspnoea	Definition and types of dyspnoea
Acute:	Dyspnoea is defined as difficult or unpleasant awareness of ones respiration.
Acute pulmonary oedema	(a) Dyspnoea on effort
Hyperventilation	(b) Orthopnoea
Pneumothorax	(c) Paroxysmal nocturnal dyspnoea
Pulmonary embolism	(d) Cheyne-stokes respiration
Pneumonia	
Airway obstruction	
Chronic:	
Congestive Heart Failure (CHF)	
Pulmonary disease	
Anxiety	
Obesity	
Poor physical fitness	
Pleural effusion	
Bronchial asthma	

mediate surroundings should be observed. Look for medications, a sputum pot, an oxygen mask. Many clues may be gained simply from the patient's bedside environment. Next, turn your attention to the patient and observe for general overall features, such as (a) does she look well? (b) What is her overall appearance? (c) Is she cyanosed? (d) Is there any neck pulsation? (e) Is she in any obvious pain or discomfort? (f) Is she obese? (g) How is the breathing – laboured or quiet? Having completed the overall inspection of the patient and his/her surroundings turn your attention to specific parts such as the hands, nails, eyes, etc. (Figs. 5.7 and 5.8) [1–10]. The findings noted while inspecting these specific organs or organ systems, often give some clue to the final interpretation or diagnosis.

The assessment of the venous pulse is an integral part of the physical examination, since it reflects haemodynamic events in the right atrium. The two main objectives of the bedside examination of the neck veins are the estimation of the CVP and the inspection of the waveform. The maximum pulsation of the internal jugular vein is observed when the trunk is inclined by less than 30° in normal patients. The internal jugular vein is superior for the estimation of venous pressure

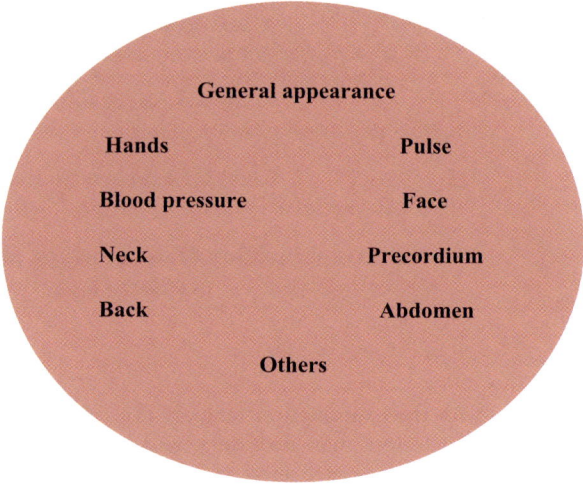

Fig. 5.7 Features to be noted during a cardiovascular examination

and venous waveform because of its more direct route to the right atrium. The most common cause of elevated jugular venous pressure (JVP) is an increased right

Examination of Cardiovascular system

Inspection

Facies: caused by pain, anxiety distress-Angina, MI, PE etc

Skin Color and Texture: Malar flush, brick red color, bronze skin, flushing & telangiectasia, moon face, coarseness /dryness, central cyanosis

Eyes and Lids: Xanthelasma, lid oedema, exophthalmos, corneal arcus, blue sclera, lenses, pupils

Bony developmental Abnormality: Large head, acromegaly, Marfan syndrome, Williams syndrome, Noonan's syndrome

Hands: Tremors, capillary pulsation, Osler's nodes, arachnodactyly

Breathing patterns: use of accessory muscles, breathlessness, stridor, and Cheyne-stokes respiration

Cyanosis: central, peripheral, differential, reverse differential

Palpation

Pulse: rate, rhythm, character, symmetry

Character:
Collapsing pulse: Jerky pulse with full expansion followed by sudden collapse
Pulses alternans: Amplitude varies from beat to beat with regular rate
Pulses bisferiens: 2 strong systolic peaks separated by a mid-systolic dip
Anacrotic pulse: Slow rising pulse
Diacrotic pulse: 2 systolic and diastolic peaks
Paradoxic pulse: Amplitude increases during expiration and decreases with inspiration

Peripheral veins: JVP
Giant "A wave
Cannon "A" wave
Prominent "V" wave
Kussmaul's sign

Apex beat
Left parasternal lift
Abdomen: Abdomen, Liver

Auscultation

Aortic area
Pulmonic area
Tricuspid area
Mitral area:

Heart sounds
S1- closure of mitral and tricuspid valve
S2- Closure of semilunar (AV, PV) valves
S3- passive diastolic filling of the ventricle
S4- vigorous atrial contraction to propel blood into a stiff ventricle

Opening snap: Precedes the mid-diastolic murmur of MS if the valve is not calcified

Ejection clicks: Heard in systole in aortic stenosis and hypertension

Murmurs: Systolic, diastolic & continuous

Fig. 5.8 Examination of cardiovascular system [1–10, 18]

ventricular pressure in conditions such as pulmonary hypertension, pulmonary stenosis, or right ventricular failure (Table 5.3).

5.3.2 Palpation

Examination of pulse and blood pressure is very important and most often it gives valuable information. The radial pulse is considered the best place for assessing the rate and rhythm. A rate faster than 100 beats/minute is considered tachycardia, while less than 60 beats/minute is bradycardia. The normal blood pressure is generally defined as 120/80 mm Hg and this tends to increase with age.

The apex beat is normally located in the 5th intercostal space in the midclavicular line. It is defined as the outermost point of palpation, not the loudest point. If it is displaced laterally, suspect an enlarged heart, especially left ventricular hypertrophy (or pulmonary collapse, a pneumothorax, or spine and rib deformities). In patients with pericardial effusion, pleural effusion, obesity, hyperinflated lungs, or in the case of dextrocardia – the apex often may be difficult to palpate. The apex beat can be normal, sustained, thrusting or tapping depending on the clinical condition. Next, feel for heaves and thrills by laying the hand on the chest. Heaves, where you can feel the heart

Table 5.3 Jugular venous pressure [18]

Normal waves in the JVP	Pathological waves in the JVP
JVP is the vertical height of the pulse in cm above the sternal angle (raised if >3 cm)	**Absent a wave** – Atrial fibrillation
a wave: Atrial contraction	**Large a wave** – Tricuspid stenosis, pulmonary stenosis, pulmonary hypertension
c wave: An invisible flicker in the x descent due to closure of the tricuspid valve, before the start of ventricular systole	**Cannon wave** – Complete heart block, atrial flutter, nodal rhythm, ventricular extra systole and ventricular tachycardia
x descent: Downward movement of the heart causes atrial stretch and drop in pressure	**Raised JVP with normal waveforms** – Bradycardia, right heart failure, fluid overload
v wave: Due to passive filling of blood into atrium against a closed tricuspid valve	**Raised JVP with absent pulsations** – Superior vena cava obstruction
y descent: Opening of tricuspid valve with passive movement of blood from right atrium to right ventricle (causing an S3 when audible)	**Systolic waves** – Tricuspid regurgitation
	Slow y descent –Tricuspid stenosis
	High plateau of JVP with deep x and y descents – constrictive pericarditis, pericardial tamponade

beating (and in extreme cases can see your hand move) indicate hypertrophy, while thrills are palpable murmurs in the mitral and aortic area (Table 5.4) [1–10].

5.3.3
Auscultation

The cardiac contractions are heard through the stethoscope as heart sounds. The low-pitched first heard sound (lub) is associated with closure of the atrioventricular (AV) valves and the second louder sound (dup) is associated with closure of the aortic and pulmonary valves [17]. The first sound marks the onset of systole and the second sound marks the onset of diastole. Murmurs are different types of sounds produced when the blood flow becomes turbulent due to various heart conditions. A knowledge of the physiology behind murmurs facilitates their understanding. Knowing when in the cardiac cycle it occurs, where it's best heard, where it radiates to, what it sounds like, and what happens under special circumstances, such as deep breathing, are all important for diagnosis. Murmurs are commonly graded, or classified by intensity (Table 5.5).

In general, diastolic murmurs can be classified as either early or mid-diastolic and incompetent aortic or pulmonary valves cause an early diastolic murmur. Further, a stenosed mitral or tricuspid valve, or an atrial septal defect (increased flow through these valves) results in a mid-diastolic murmur. Systolic murmurs are due to leakage of mitral/tricuspid valves that should be closed, or narrowed aortic/pulmonary valves that should be open. Mitral or tricuspid incompetence is usually pansystolic. In mitral valve prolapse, however, the valve only leaks halfway through systole after initially functioning well, resulting in a mid- or late systolic murmur. Ejection systolic murmurs occur in stenosed aortic or pulmonary valves that crescendo in mid-systole and are quiet at the start and end [1–10].

5.4
Step Three: Conclusion

"Good education comes with dedication". Once the examination is completed, we should be able to reach a clinical conclusion. However, additional components should be considered, such as fundoscopy for hypertension and diabetes and urine dipstick for glucose, protein and ketones. For completeness, peripheral pulses should be tested, and the abdomen for ascites. Check for an aneurysm, an enlarged and/or pulsatile liver. Finally, listen for bruits at the femoral, renal and umbilical arteries. With the information obtained from taking the history and examining the patient, the physician would have come to a clinical diagnosis or conclusion. Based on his or her observations the patient will be referred for other relevant examinations (Table 5.6).

Table 5.4 Inspection, palpation and auscultation in cardiovascular examination [1–10, 18]

General Considerations:

The patient must be properly dressed/undressed (gown) for the examination. The surroundings and examination room must be pleasant/quiet to perform adequate auscultation.

Arterial Pulses: Rate and Rhythm

Compress the radial artery with your index and middle fingers (check whether the pulse is regular or irregular).

Observe for carotid pulsations (place your fingers behind the patient's neck and compress the carotid artery on one side with your thumb at or below the level of the cricoid cartilage).

Assess the amplitude of the pulse, contour of the pulse wave, variations in amplitude (from beat to beat or with respiration).

Repeat on the opposite side.

Auscultation for Bruits:

Place the bell of the stethoscope over each carotid artery in turn (ask the patient to stop breathing momentarily).

Listen for a blowing or rushing sound (bruit).

Jugular Venous Pressure:

Position the patient supine with the head of the table elevated 30 degrees.

Observe for venous pulsations in the neck (look for a rapid, double wave with each heart beat).

Identify the highest point of pulsation (using a horizontal line from this point, measure vertically from the sternal angle).

In a normal healthy adult it should be less than 3 cm.

Precordial Movement:

Position the patient supine (with the head of the table slightly elevated).

Inspect for precordial movement. Palpate for precordial activity.

Palpate for the point of maximal impulse (or apical pulse).

In general it is normally located in the 4th or 5th intercostal space just medial to the midclavicular line Note the location, size, and quality of the impulse.

Auscultation:

Position the patient supine with the head of the table slightly elevated.

Listen with the diaphragm at:

Aortic area: Right 2nd interspace near the sternum

Pulmonic area: Left 2nd interspace near the sternum

Tricuspid area: Left 3rd, 4th, and 5th interspaces near the sternum

Mitral area: the apex

Table 5.5 Heart sounds in various clinical scenarios [1–10, 18]

Loud S1	Hyperdynamic circulation, high cardiac output (e.g. fever or exercise); mitral stenosis; atrial myxoma
Soft S1	Low cardiac output, tachycardia; severe mitral regurgitation (valve destruction)
Variable S1	AF, complete or third-degree heart block
Wide splitting of S2	RBBB, Pulmonary stenosis, atrial septal defect (ASD)
Reversed splitting of S2	Systemic hypertension, LBBB, aortic stenosis
Loud A2 (Aortic component of S2)	Systemic hypertension; dilated aortic root
Soft A2	Calcific aortic stenosis
Loud P2 (Pulmonary component of S2)	Pulmonary hypertension
Soft P2	Pulmonary stenosis

Table 5.6 Investigations in cardiology

Investigations	Treatment
Biochemical markers	Life style modifications
Resting electrocardiogram (ECG)	Medications
Chest X-ray	Coronary angioplasty ±stent
Exercise stress test (treadmill)	Transmyocardial revascularisation
Holter monitor (ambulatory Electrocardiogram)	Coronary artery bypass graft (CABG)
Echocardiography	Minimal invasive surgery
Stress echocardiography	Cardiac transplantation
Contrast echocardiography	
Dobutamine echocardiography	
Transoesophageal echocardiography (TEE)	
Computed tomography (CT) scan	
Magnetic resonance imaging (MRI)/Magnetic resonance angiography (MRA)	
Coronary angiogram	
Nuclear cardiology: MUGA scan, Thallium MPS, 99mTc-MIBI/Tetrofosmin MPS, and Positron emission tomography (PET)	

References

1. Epstein O, Perkin GD, Cookson J, de Bono DP (2003) Clinical Examination, 3rd edn. Elsevier, Edinburgh.
2. Kumar P, Clark M (2004) Clinical Medicine, 5th edn. Saunders.
3. Brown EM, Collis W, Leng T, Salmon AP (2003) Heart Sounds Made Easy. Churchill Livingstone, London.
4. Souhami RL, Moxham J (1997) Textbook of Medicine, 3rd edn. Churchill Livingstone, London.
5. O'Rourke RA, Shaver JA, Silverman ME (2001) The history, physical examination and cardiac auscultation. In Hurst's The Heart, 10th edn, Fuster V, Alexander RW, O'Rourke RA (eds), pp. 193–280.
6. Tierney LM Jr, McPhee SJ, Papadakis MA (eds) (2001) Current Medical Diagnosis and Treatment, 40th edn. McGraw-Hill, New York.
7. DeGowin RL (ed.) (1994) DeGowin and DeGowin's Diagnostic Examination, 6th edn. McGraw-Hill, New York.
8. Seidel HM, Ball JW, Dains JE, Benedict GW (1999) The history. In Mosby's Physical Examination Handbook, 2nd edn. Mosby, St Louis, pp. 1–8.
9. Chan PD, Winkle PJ (1997) Current Clinical Strategies: History and Physical Examination in Medicine, 2nd edn. CCS Publishing, Laguna Hills, CA, pp. 7–11.
10. Coats AJS, McGee HM, Stokes HC, Thompson DR (1995) BACR Guidelines for Cardiac Rehabilitation. Blackwell Science Ltd.
11. Alexander RW, Pratt CM, Ryan TJ, Roberts R (2001) Diagnosis and management of patients with acute myocardial infarction. In Hurst's The Heart, 10th edn, Fuster V, Alexander RW, O'Rourke RA (eds), pp. 1275–1373.
12. Finnish Medical Society Duodecim (2004) Differential diagnosis of chest pain. In EBM Guidelines. Evidence-based Medicine. Duodecim Medical Publications Ltd., Helsinki, Finland.
13. Hurst JW, Morris DC (1994) The history; symptom and past events related to cardiovascular disease in In Schlant RC et al. (eds), The Heart, 8th edn. McGraw-Hill, New York, pp. 205–216.
14. O'Rourke RA, Schlnt RC, Douglas JS Jr (2001) Diagnosis and management of patients with chronic ischaemic heart disease. In Hurst's The Heart, 10th edn, Fuster V, Alexander RW, O'Rourke RA (eds).
15. Waters DD (2001) Diagnosis and management of patient with unstable angina. In Hurst's The Heart, 10th edn, Fuster V, Alexander RW, O'Rourke RA (eds), pp. 1237–1274.
16. Diamond GA, Staniloff HM, Forrester JS et al. (1983) Computer assisted diagnosis in the non-invasive evaluation of patients with suspected coronary heart disease. J Am Coll Cardiol 1:444–455.
17. Widmaier EP, Raff H, Strang KT (2005) Cardiovascular physiology. In Vanders Human Physiology – The mechanism of Body Function, 10th edn. McGraw-Hill, pp. 387–476.
18. Hope RA, Longmore JM, Hodgetts TJ, Ramrakha PS (1993) Oxford Handbook of Clinical Medicine, 3rd edn. Oxford University Press.

Further Reading

1. Epstein O, Perkin GD, Cookson J, de Bono DP (2003) Clinical Examination, 3rd edn. Elsevier, Edinburgh.
2. Kumar P, Clark M (2004) Clinical Medicine, 5th edn. Saunders.
3. Souhami RL, Moxham J (1997) Textbook of Medicine, 3rd edn. Churchill Livingstone, London.
4. O'Rourke RA, Shaver JA, Silverman ME (2001) The history, physical examination and cardiac auscultation. In Hurst's The Heart, 10th edn, Fuster V, Alexander RW, O'Rourke RA (eds), pp. 193–280.
5. Hope RA, Longmore JM, Hodgetts TJ, Ramrakha PS (1993) Oxford Handbook of Clinical Medicine. Oxford University Press.

Chapter 6

The Plain Chest Radiograph in the Assessment of Cardiac Disease

Nicola Mulholland

Contents

6.1	History and Introduction	65
6.2	Technique	65
6.2.1	Posteroanterior Projection (PA)	65
6.2.2	Anteroposterior Projection (AP)	66
6.2.3	Lateral Projection	66
6.2.4	Assessment of Radiograph Adequacy	66
6.2.5	Pitfalls and Normal Variants	66
6.3	Clinical Applications	68
6.3.1	Assessment of Heart Size	68
6.3.2	Pulmonary Oedema	69
6.3.3	Cardiac Calcifications	70
6.3.4	Radiological Assessment of Pacemakers and Implantable Cardiac Defibrillators (ICD)	71
6.3.5	Pulmonary Arterial Hypertension	72
6.3.6	Congenital Heart Disease	73
6.4	Future Trends in Chest Radiography	74
6.5	Conclusion	75
	References	75

6.1 History and Introduction

Wilhelm Roentgen discovered X-rays on 8 November 1895, and was the first to take a radiograph on 22 December 1895 of his wife's fingers [1]. Roentgen labelled the unknown ray X, and hence the term X-ray was coined. Soon after this the chest radiograph was used and this has become a first line investigation in patients with suspected heart disease. An appreciation of the technique and anatomy, as well as common variants, is vital to the correct interpretation of the chest radiograph. The technique of chest radiography will be described, together with details of the chest radiograph adequacy. Following a description of the normal anatomy and potential pitfalls in interpretation due to normal variants, the clinical applications of the chest radiograph in the assessment of cardiac disease is discussed. Finally, a short discussion on the future trends in chest radiography is given.

6.2 Technique

The traditional chest radiograph is produced using an analogue system, the film-cassette system. Several projections may be used, commonly posteroanterior, anterior and less commonly lateral or lateral decubitus. The patient is encouraged to take a full inspiration, and expiratory films are useful to look for pneumothorax.

6.2.1 Posteroanterior Projection (PA)

The patient stands facing the film cassette/Bucky and grid with the X-ray tube at a distance of 180 cm. The cassette is positioned 5 cm above shoulder height and the stripped patient stands with the shoulders laterally rotated to touch the cassette, the arms forward and the dorsum of the hands on the iliac crests posteriorly. The horizontal central ray is centred at the sternal angle and the exposure is taken on full inspiration. There are two main choices for exposure factors: high and low kilovoltage (kV). A high kV radiograph is taken at 120 kV and has the advantage of demonstrating the mediastinal contours of the lung better than low kV exposures, and increasing the area visualised by decreasing the contrast of the ribs. However, low kV exposures of around 65 kV allow improved lung detail by enhancing the contrast between lung vessels and the surrounding lung, and calcified plaques [2].

6.2.2
Anteroposterior Projection (AP)

The standard practice of obtaining PA radiographs in the erect position during inspiration allows the reproducibility required to enable comparison between radiographs under the same cardiopulmonary physiological conditions. In many cases the patient is too unwell to perform a PA technique and so an AP radiograph is obtained. In this case the semi or fully supine patient lies with his back to the film/cassette and the X-ray tube is anterior to the patient. A low kV exposure is employed to increase contrast and decrease scatter, however the increased exposure time required leads to loss of sharpness due to motion artefact, and the lack of a grid increases scatter. The AP technique causes magnification of the cardiac silhouette so caution is required in its assessment.

6.2.3
Lateral Projection

The lateral projection is no longer routinely obtained in most UK institutions. It may be useful to detect small quantities of free intraperitoneal air or for the early detection of pleural fluid. It is becoming common for cross-sectional imaging with computed tomography to be obtained without a prior lateral radiograph in the investigation of thoracic diseases.

6.2.4
Assessment of Radiograph Adequacy

The initial evaluation of a chest radiograph requires an assessment of the film adequacy. The correct patient name is a simple but essential check. In an ideal projection, the distance between the spinous processes and the clavicles should be equal indicating no rotation. The scapulae should not be projected over the lungs. Penetration is ideal if the T4 vertebral body is visualised and the cardiac and costophrenic angles are well delineated. The degree of inspiration is generally adequate if the lungs project over the anterior ends of the sixth ribs. Great caution must be made in interpreting a radiograph taken with poor inspiratory effort, as the the normal anatomical structures may appear enlarged and the pulmonary vascularity artefactually increased. The patient position should be noted, if the film is not a standard erect PA projection, the position will be marked on the film. In an erect patient, the pulmonary blood flow is influenced by gravity and there is an increase in vessel calibre from cephalad to caudad. Subtle alterations in pulmonary vessel size may be detected in early pulmonary venous hypertension as the upper lobe vessels dilate and the lower lobe vessels constrict. This is lost in a supine patient as the whole lung vasculature is under equal gravity.

6.2.5
Pitfalls and Normal Variants

The chest radiograph provides a two-dimensional image of a three-dimensional object, and interpretation requires a knowledge of the normal anatomy (Fig. 6.1).

Common variants should also be appreciated. Pectus excavatum or funnel chest describes a depressed sternum, usually readily apparent on clinical examination. This causes straightening of the left heart border with shift of the heart to the left, and loss of clarity of the right heart border with increased opacification in the right cardiophrenic angle, simulating right middle lobe collapse (Fig. 6.2a and b). This may be recognised as a variant by the steep downward slope of the anterior ribs and increased penetration of the lower thoracic spine on the PA radiograph. However, it is important to remember that pectus excavatum may be associated with congenital heart disease, e.g., atrial septal defect, and Marfan's syndrome.

Nipple shadows can also cause confusion by simulating lung nodules. They generally have an ill-defined medial margin with a sharp lateral margin [3]. A repeat radiograph with nipple markers usually can resolve the problem. Occasionally a patient may have dextrocardia, only recognisable by correct appreciation of the side marker. Right sided aortic arch may be noted. Right aortic arch with aberrant left subclavian artery has an incidence of 1 in 2500 and is associated with congenital heart disease in 5–12% of patients (Fig. 6.3).

The normal number of ribs seen is 12 pairs. Occasionally seen in normal individuals, the presence of 11 pairs of ribs should alert the physician to the diagnosis of Down's Syndrome or Trisomy 21, which is associated with various congenital heart diseases, e.g., endocardial cushion defect (25%), membranous VSD, ostium primum ASD, AV communis, cleft mitral valve and patent ductus arteriosis.

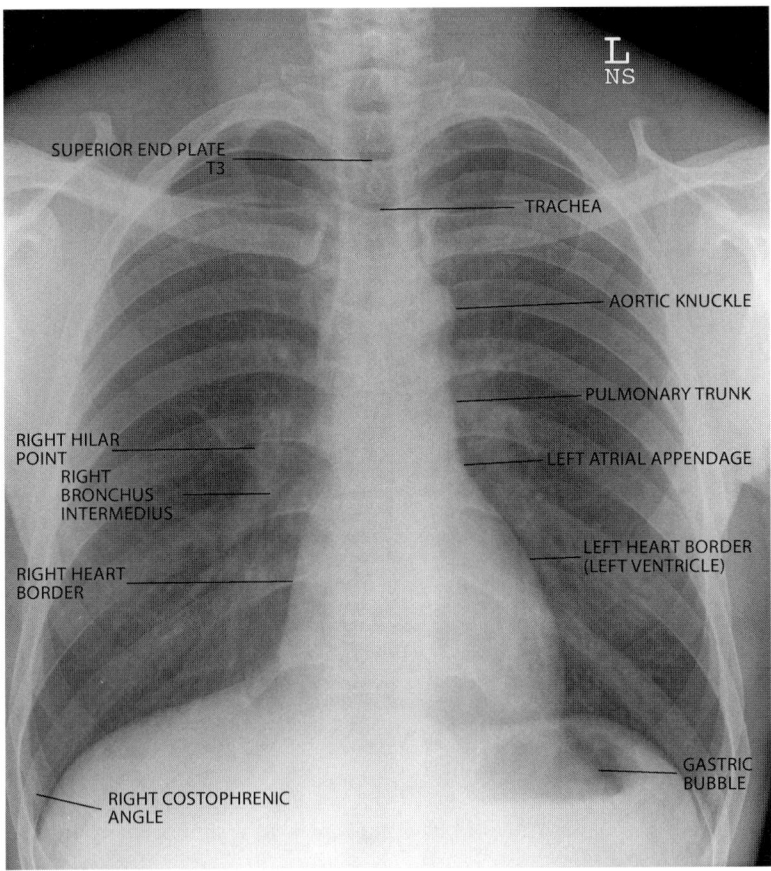

Fig. 6.1 Normal Chest Radiograph

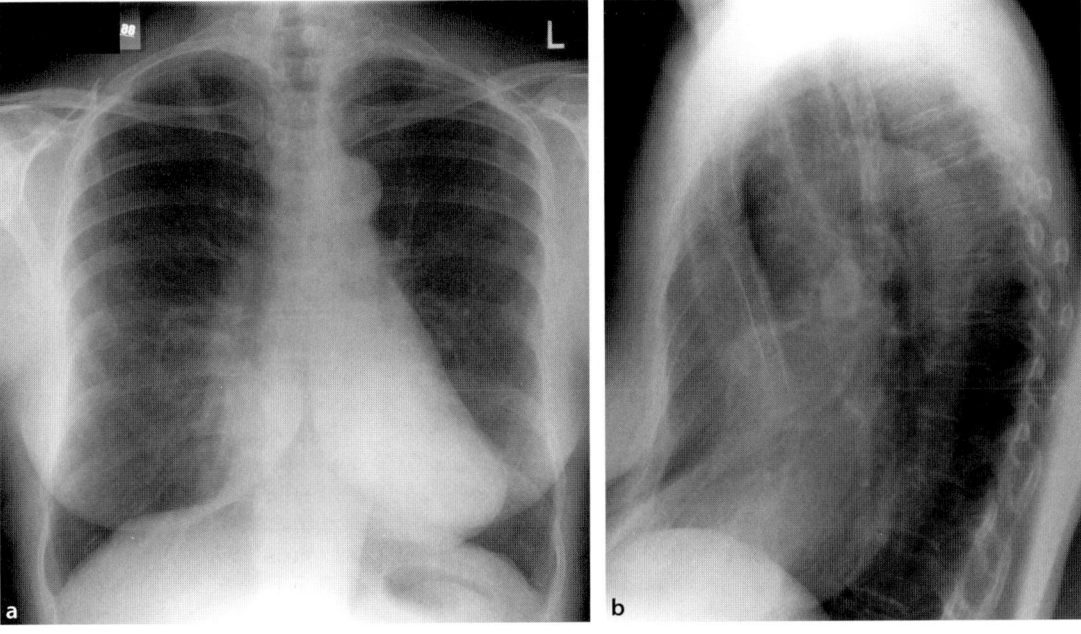

Fig. 6.2 **a** AP Pectus excavatum; **b** lateral radiograph of pectus excavatum. Note the sternal depression

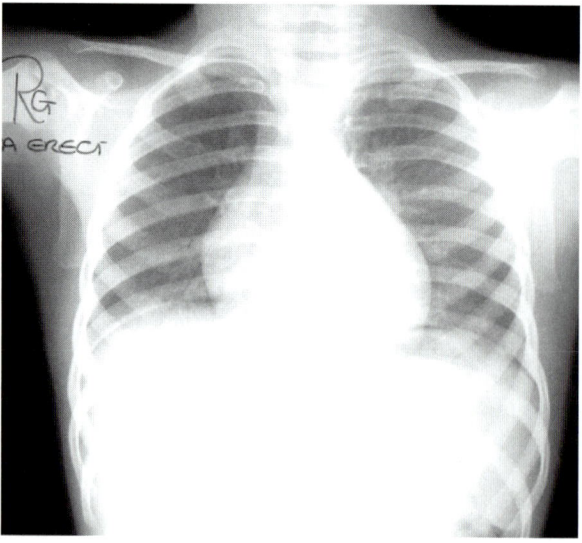

Fig. 6.3 Right sided aortic arch

Table 6.1 General information obtained from a chest X-ray

Heart size

Cardiac silhouette abnormalities

Heart failure

Rib notching

Rib fractures

Pnemothorax

Pneumonia

Placement of tubes and catheters

Atelectasis

Pulmonary parenchymal disease

Pleural and pericardial effusion

6.3
Clinical Applications

The patient with suspected heart disease should undergo a thorough history taking and examination supplemented by an ECG and chest radiograph. The latter is cheap, readily available and carries a low radiation risk; the effective dose equivalent is 0.02 mSv, equivalent to one week's background radiation in the UK. Although the chest radiograph is not the final investigation relied upon for most diagnoses, it provides a useful baseline to allow monitoring of many common disease processes, e.g., heart failure (Table 6.1). Furthermore it allows evaluation of the lungs to ensure no pulmonary lesion is causing the symptoms attributable to the heart.

6.3.1
Assessment of Heart Size

As a general rule, the cardiac silhouette should be no greater than 50% of the maximum width of the thoracic cage on a PA film, the so called cardiothoracic ratio. Accurate measurement is best made with cross-sectional techniques, particularly ultrasound. It is important to note that the cardiac silhouette may appear enlarged not only by cardiac enlargement but by the presence of a pericardial effusion, which can easily be recognised on ultrasound. An increase of the actual heart size by more than 2 cm is likely to represent a significant change in heart size [4].

Selective chamber enlargement can also be recognised. Left atrial enlargement causes elevation of the left main bronchus and eventually splaying of the carina (normal range 55 to 80°) and a double right heart shadow. In rheumatic mitral valve disease particularly there is often enlargement of the left atrial appendage (Fig. 6.4), evident as straightening of the left heart border below the left main bronchus. Left ventricular enlargement can be due to dilatation or hypertrophy. If there is gross enlargement, there will be rounding of the apex of the heart, then elongation of the axis of the left ventricle towards and below the left hemidiaphragm. Right ventricular enlargement may be evident first on the lateral view with an increase in the area of the cardiac shadow in contact with the sternum. On the PA view it is recognised as an increase in the cardiac shadow size, which is triangular in configuration as the enlarged RV makes the left heart border. There is also tilting up of the apex, known as couer en sabot which may be recognised in untreated Fallot's tetralogy (Fig. 6.5). Selective right atrial enlargement is usually due to abnormality of the tricuspid valve, and appears as a bulging right heart border. Ebsteins anomaly is a congenital malformation of the tricuspid valve, which causes gross right atrial enlargement (Fig. 6.6).

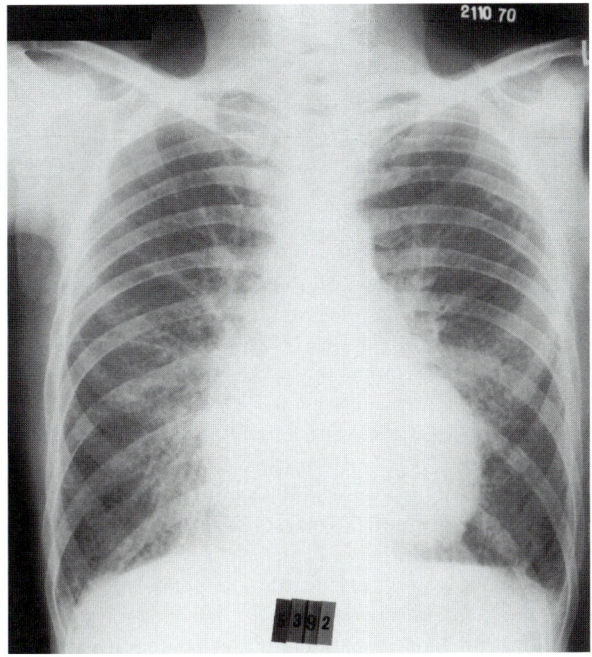

Fig. 6.4 Mitral stenosis due to rheumatic heart disease showing pulmonary haemosiderosis. Note the bulging of the left atrial appendage

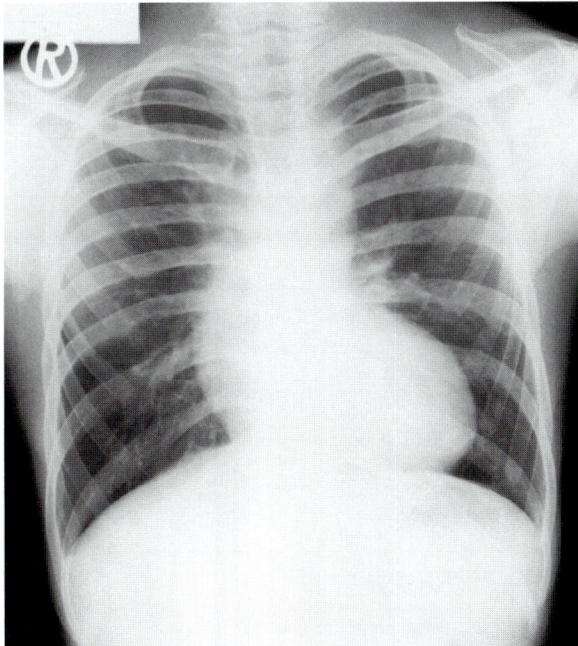

Fig. 6.5 Fallots tetralogy with classic boot shaped heart with enlarged right ventricle and pulmonary oligaemia

6.3.2
Pulmonary Oedema

Pulmonary oedema (Table 6.2) may be cardiogenic, due to left heart failure or non-cardiogenic. The earliest sign of elevated left atrial pressure on the chest radiograph is upper lobe blood diversion. In this instance, the upper lobe vessel size is equal to or greater than the lower lobe vessels, at equal distances from the hilum [5]. This assessment can only be made on erect radiographs, as gravity causes blood redistribution in the supine patient. With increasing pressure (pulmonary capillary wedge pressure PCWP 18–22 mmHg) the signs of interstitial oedema occur: peribronchial cuffing, perihilar haze and septal lines.

s are clearly defined thin septal lines 1–2 mm wide and 3–6 cm long, seen perpendicular to the pleural surface, and represent fluid accumulating in the interlobular septa. As the PCWP exceeds 25 mmHg, fluid passes into the alveoli. This leads to air space opacification, often with sparing of the apices and extreme lung bases (Fig. 6.7). Occasionally, a bat's wing distribution occurs whereby the air space opacification is mainly in the central lung. It is noteworthy that patients with chronic heart failure may tolerate a higher PCWP before signs of pulmonary oedema develop.

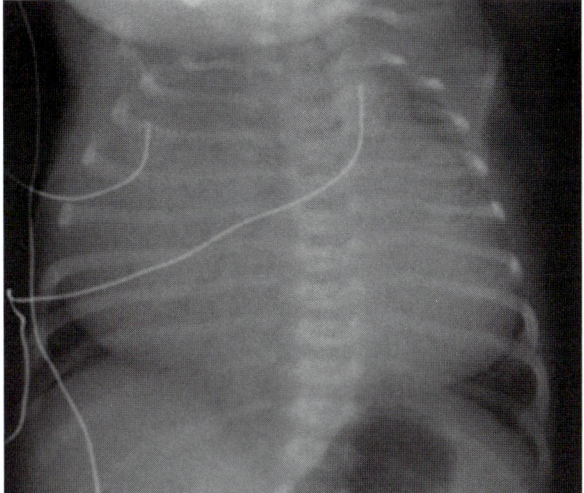

Fig. 6.6 Ebsteins anomaly with dilated right atrium in a neonate

Bilateral pleural effusions are commonly seen together with enlargement of the cardiac silhouette in cardiogenic pulmonary oedema. A meniscus sign of fluid will be seen on an erect radiograph in the presence of pleural fluid (Fig. 6.8); on a supine film, pleural fluid maybe detected as a generally increased greyness of the hemithorax through which lung markings are visible, with or without a lamellar component.

Table 6.2 Causes of pulmonary oedema [12]

Causes of Pulmonary Oedema
Increased hydrostatic pressure
Cardiogenic: left ventricular failure; pulmonary venous disease; pericardial disease; drugs
Non-cardiogenic: fluid overload, neurogenic
Decreased colloid osmotic pressure
Hypoproteinaemia
Increased capillary leakiness
Toxins (inhaled, circulating)
Aspiration (gastric contents, water)
Contusions
Anaphylaxis
Adult respiratory distress syndrome (primarily due to lung pathology or secondary to non-lung causes)

6.3.3
Cardiac Calcifications

Cardiovascular calcification usually occurs in degenerate or dead tissue, and is dystrophic. Myocardial calcification may follow a myocardial infarct (Fig. 6.9), especially with the formation of a left ventricular aneurysm. Other causes such as myocarditis or rheumatic fever may also cause calcifications [6].

Pericardial calcification may occur following resolution of haemorrhage or exudates and may or may not cause constriction (Fig. 6.10a and b). It usually occurs on the visceral layer of the pericardium and predominates over the less pulsatile areas (right atrial and ventricular borders, atrioventricular grooves and pulmonary trunk). CT is more sensitive in the detection of pericardial calcification, and around 50% of patients with constrictive pericarditis show segments of pericardial calcification [7].

Coronary artery calcification appears as a double line, most frequently seen in the left coronary artery. Calcification seen in patients under 50 is suggestive of ischaemic heart disease and was thought to be seen commonly in older asymptomatic patients [8]. However, it is a marker of coronary artery disease and does not reflect ageing; it represents calcification in haemorrhagic areas of atherosclerotic plaques [9]. CT provides more accurate demonstration of this calcification.

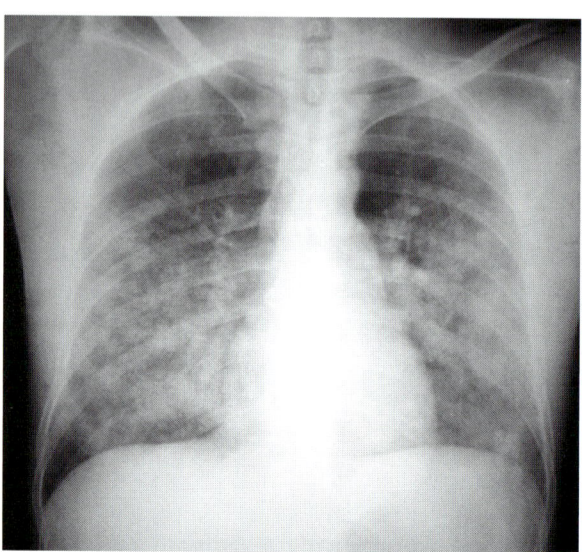

Fig. 6.7 Pulmonary oedema. Note sparing of apices and costophrenic angles

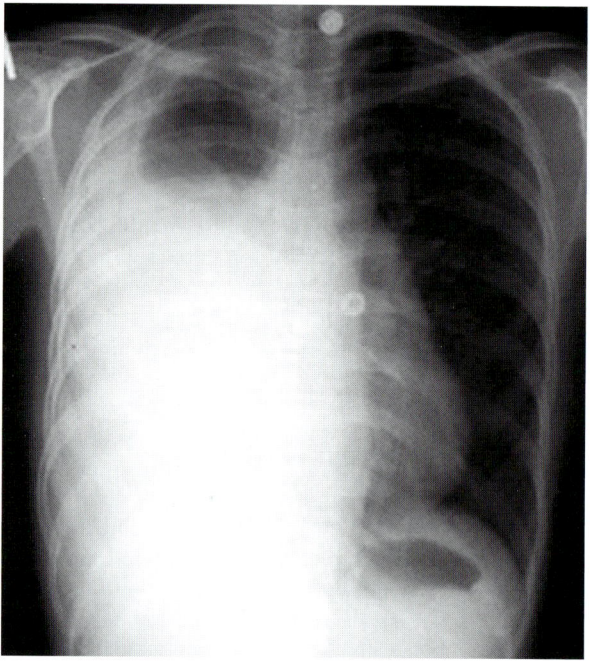

Fig. 6.8 Right pleural effusion. Note meniscus sign

Calcification of the mitral valve annulus is also more common than mitral valve calcification, often seen in elderly patients, particularly female and is usually benign. However, it may be associated with valvular insufficiency and conduction abnormalities. Mitral valve calcification is rare and is secondary to rheumatic heart disease. Aortic valve calcification is not uncommon, detectable using CT in around 30% of people older than 60. The severity of the aortic stenosis correlates with the density of calification but is not usually significant in the absence of left ventricular hypertrophy. The congenital bicuspid valve is usually heavy dense and nodular, and is the commonest cause of aortic calcification in people under 55 [6].

6.3.4
Radiological Assessment of Pacemakers and Implantable Cardiac Defibrillators (ICD)

Pacemakers are becoming more common and the chest radiograph is commonly used to assess for complications. They are commonly inserted for symptomatic bradycardia but may be indicated in other conditions, e.g., heart failure and long QT syndrome [10].

The pacemaker is commonly sited in the left infraclavicular, position, although the right infraclavicular, axillary and submammary positions may be utilised. The percutaneous route is commonly used although pacing leads can also be positioned during surgery. The pacemaker is usually positioned using fluoroscopy. A check CXR is usually performed following this to check for complications. Pneumothorax is a not uncommon complication of lead placement occurring in up to 2.6% of cases [11]. The pneumothorax in the erect film is

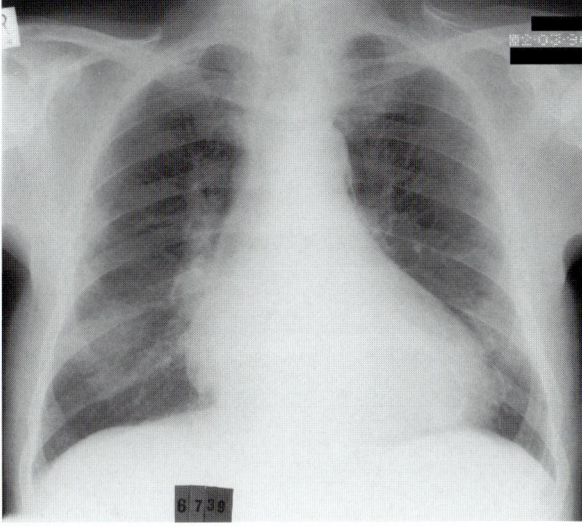

Fig. 6.9 Calcified left ventricle

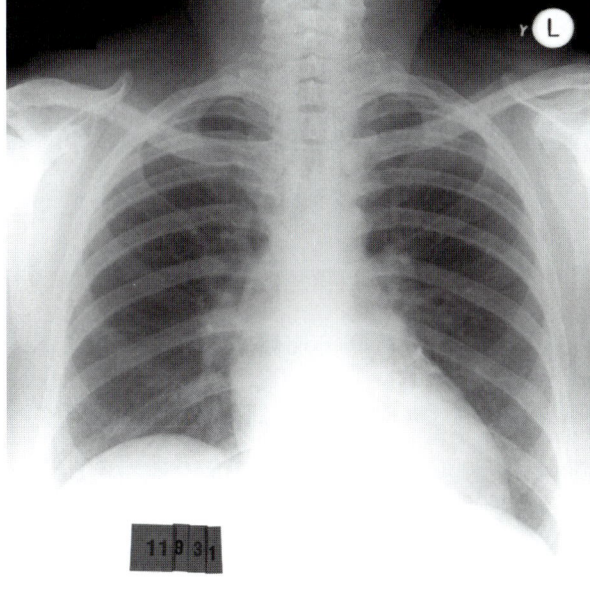 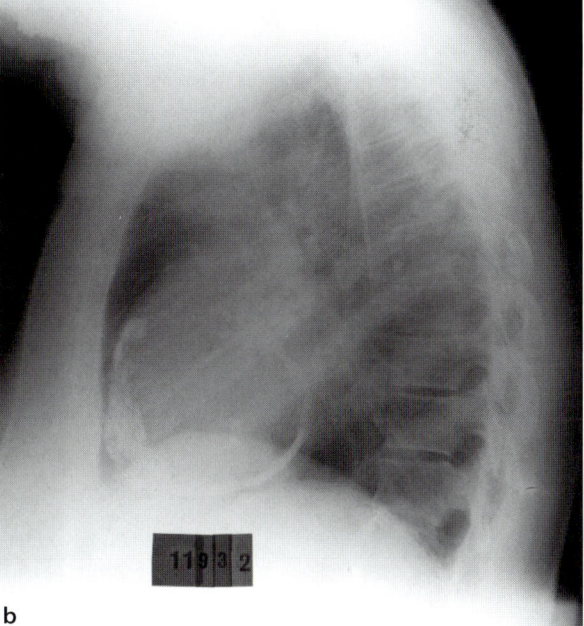

a   b

Fig. 6.10 **a** PA CXR with calcified pericardium; **b** lateral CXR in same patient showing calcified pericardium more clearly

more readily appreciated and a lung edge with no lung markings beyond is characteristically seen (Fig. 6.11). Beware the presence of mediastinal shift – this marks a tension pnemothorax requiring urgent decompression (Fig. 6.12). Pleural air is detected in the supine patient as increased sharpness of the medial mediastinal contour and/or the deep sulcus sign at the bases.

Lead position depends on the type of pacemaker inserted (Table 6.3), and is usually assessed initially at insertion by fluoroscopy and ECG changes. Generic codes are used to describe the operation of different pacemakers. The first letter describes the chamber paced (A for atrium, V for ventricle, D for both), the second letter describes which chamber is sensed, the third letter denotes the response to sensing. This may be inhibition (I), stimulus (T) or both (D).

Late complications include lead fracture, lead displacement and dislodgement, which are all observable on the chest radiograph [10].

6.3.5
Pulmonary Arterial Hypertension

Pulmonary arterial hypertension is present when the pulmonary artery systolic pressure exceeds 30 mmHg.

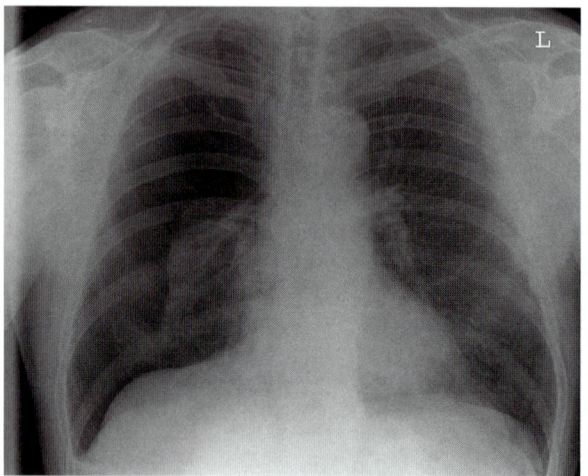

Fig. 6.11 Right-sided pneumothorax. Note the lung edge and lack of lung markings in the periphery

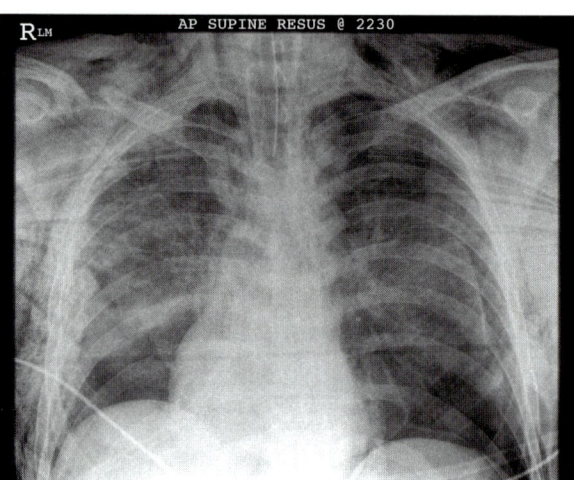

Fig. 6.12 Tension pneumothorax on left. Note the mediastinal shift to the right. There is also extensive subcutaneous emphysema and a fractured right clavicle

Table 6.3 Main indications for pacemaker devices and their lead tip position [10]

Pacemaker type	Indication	Lead tip position
VVIR	Atrial fibrillation with slow ventricular respose	Apex of right ventricle
AAI or AAIR	Sinus node disease	Right atrial appendage
DDD, DDDR	Complete heart block with failure to conduct to ventricles	Right atrium and right ventricle
Biventricular pacing with atrial lead	Heart failure with conduction delay/dyssynchrony of cardiac contractility	Right atrium, right ventricle and coronory sinus lead to pace left ventricle
ICD	Ventricular tachycardia or ventricular fibrillation.	Right ventricle

It may be primary, particularly in young females or secondary to many causes including pulmonary venous hypertension, pulmonary embolism, pulmonary arterial occlusion and respiratory diseases. The radiographic features are dilatation of the proximal elastic pulmonary arteries, and narrowing of the distal pulmonary arteries ("peripheral pruning").

the intercostals arteries enlarge in coarctation of the aorta. In this condition, rib notching is unusual in children under 6. Further signs include a "figure 3" sign, which describes indentation of the lateral margin of the aortic arch at the aortopulmonary window, and left ventricle enlargement (Fig. 6.15).

6.3.6
Congenital Heart Disease

The overall incidence of congenital heart disease (CHD) in liveborn infants is around 8 per 1000 live births. Atrial septal defects (ASD) (Fig. 6.13), patent ductus arteriosus (PDA) and ventricular septal defect (VSD) account for 45% of all CHD.

A chest radiograph is used in the diagnosis and follow-up of CHD. The CXR must be interpreted with some clinical information, importantly the presence of cyanosis. Then the lungs are assessed for degree of pulmonary blood flow, and the heart size is assessed. Table 6.4 outlines diagnostic possibilities. If a left to right shunt is left untreated, eventually the chamber pressures will equalise (balanced shunt) and then a right to left shunt will occur. This is known as Eisenmengher's syndrome and is due to development of high pulmonary vascular resistance. When this occurs, the radiograph will reveal dilated central pulmonary arteries with peripheral pruning and a return to normal size of the left atrium and ventricles (Fig. 6.14).

Rib notching (Table 6.5) may be caused by coarctation of the aorta and in that case is usually bilateral, and spares the first two ribs. It results from dilatation of the components of the neurovascular bundle, for example

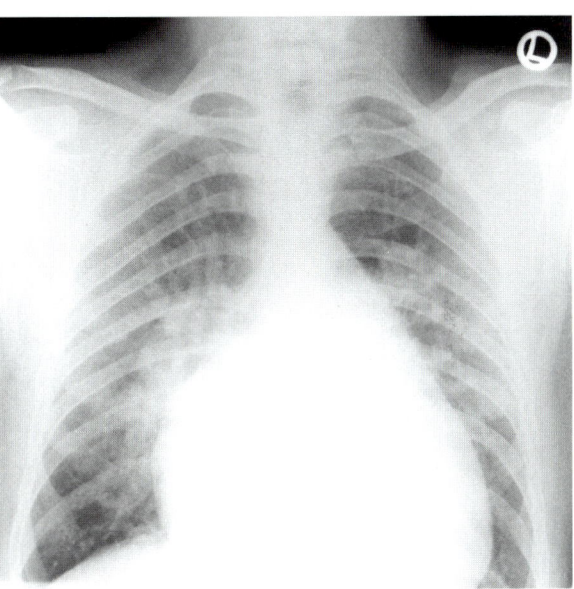

Fig. 6.13 Atrial septal defect showing cardiomegaly and pulmonary plethora

Table 6.4 Classification of congenital heart disease (adapted from [12])

	Cyanotic	Acyanotic
Increased pulmonary blood flow (PBF)	Transposition, Truncus arteriosusm, Single ventricle, Tricuspid atresia, Total anomalous pulmonary venous return	Left to right shunts: VSD, ASD, PDA, Partial anomalous pulmonary venous return
Decreased PBF		Left ventricular outflow obstruction (Aortic stenosis, coarctation, hypoplastic left heart) Left ventricle inflow obstruction (Congenital mitral valve stenosis, Cor triatriatum) Muscle disease (cardiomyopathy)
Decreased PBF	VSD present tetralogy of Fallot, Tricuspid atresia, Pulmonary atresia and VSD	

Table 6.5 Causes of inferior rib notching

Causes of rib notching (inferior margin)
Arterial: Coarctation of the aorta, Pulmonary stenosis, Blalock Taussigh shunt
Venous: SVC obstruction, AV malformation of chest wall
Neurogenic: Intercostals neuroma, Neurofibromatosis, Polio, Paraplegia
Osseous: Hyperparathyroidism, Thalassaemia

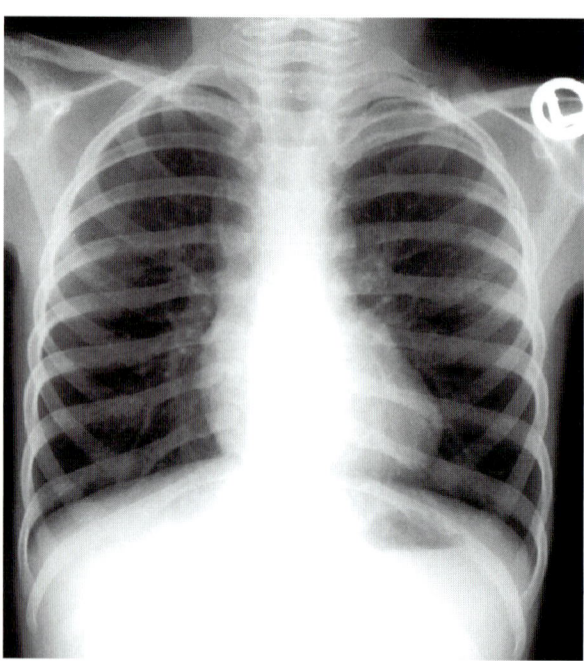

Fig. 6.14 Ventricular septal defect with development of Eisenmenghers syndrome: note return of heart to smaller size, and peripheral pruning of pulmonary vasculature

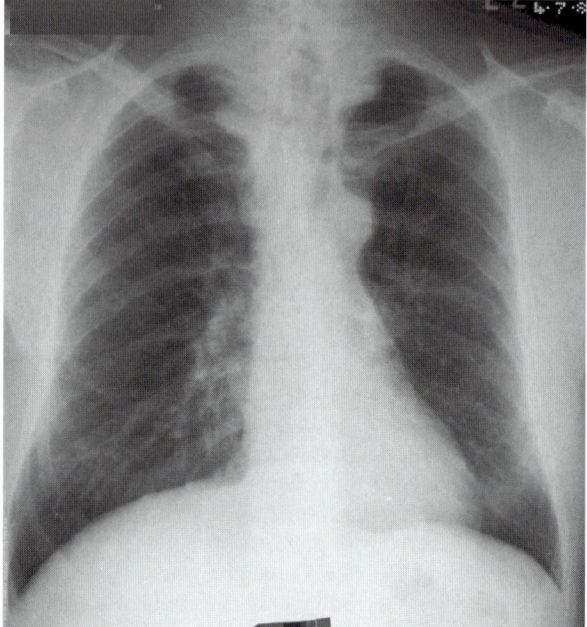

Fig. 6.15 Aortic coarctation showing bilateral rib notching

6.4
Future Trends in Chest Radiography

Computed radiography has replaced traditional analogue systems in many UK hospitals. Photostimulable phosphor plates are used instead of film with conventional X-ray equipment. A scanning laser beam is used to read out the latent image stored on the plate. It has a more forgiving optical density versus radiation exposure response curve than plain film, which allows greater latitude of exposures, resulting in fewer repeat radiographs. It has a lower spatial resolution but a superior contrast resolution. Direct digital radiography uses amorphous silicon with a digital detector. Its spatial resolution is equivalent to traditional film but also has better contrast resolution. It is expensive and is currently used in selected centres only.

Implementation of picture archiving and communication systems (PACS) is a further exciting trend. In this instance, the images are stored on computer and no film needs to be produced. It allows users across the hospital and beyond to see the image, with no more searching for lost old films. It is being used not only for plain chest radiographs, but for images acquired on other modalities, e.g., computed tomography and ultrasound.

6.5
Conclusion

The chest radiograph is the oldest imaging technique available for imaging the heart. It remains a first line and fundamental tool in the evaluation and monitoring of patients with cardiac disease, and its wide availability and low cost help safeguard this position. The technique of chest radiography has been described, with discussion of the assessment of its technical adequacy, together with pitfalls and normal variants. Its application to the assessment of cardiac disease has been described and illustrated.

References

1. Bushberg J, Seibert J, Leidholdt Jr E, Boone J (eds) (2002) Introduction to medical imaging. In The Essential Physics of Medical Imaging. Lippincott Williams and Wilkins, Philadelphia, Ch. 1, p. 4.
2. Hansell DM (2002) Technical considerations. In: Imaging of Diseases of the Chest, 3rd edn, Armstrong P, Wilson A, Dee P, Hansell D (eds). Mosby, London; Ferris R, White A (1976) The round nipple shadow. Radiology 121:293–294.
3. Engeler CE (2001) Interpreting the chest radiograph. In: Grainger and Allison (eds) Diagnostic Radiology. A Textbook of Medical Imaging, 4th edn. Churchill Livingstone, London, pp. 303–314.
4. Simon G (1968) The limitations of the radiograph for detecting early heart enlargement. Br J Radiol 41:862–865.
5. Woodring JH (1991) Pulmonary artery – bronchus ratios in patients with normal lungs, pulmonary vascular plethora and congestive heart failure. Radiology 179:115–122.
6. Mckie SJ, Hardwick DJ, Reid JH, Murchison JT (2005) Features of cardiac disease demonstrated on CT pulmonary angiography. Clin Radiol 60:31–38.
7. Olson MC, PosniakHV, McDonald V, Wisniewski R, Moncada R (1989) Computed tomography and magnetic resonance imaging of the pericardium. Radiographics 9:633–649.
8. McCarthy J, Palmer F (1974) Incidence and significance of coronary artery calcification. Br Heart J 36:499.
9. Yamanaka O, Sawano M, Nakayama R et al. (2002) Clinical significance of coronary calcification. Circulation J 66:473–478.
10. Burney K, Burchard F, Papouchado M, Wilde P (2004) Cardiac pacing systems and implantable cardiac defibrillators: a radiological perspective of equipment, anatomy and complication. Cin Radiol 59:699–708.
11. Grier D, Cook PG, Hartnell GG (1990) Chest radiographs after permanent pacing. Are they really necessary? Clin Radiol 42:244–249.
12. (2000) Heart and great vessels. In Radiology Review Manual, 4th edn, Dahnert W (ed.). Lippincott Williams and Wilkins, Philadelphia, pp. 474–575.

Ischaemic and Inflammatory Biomarkers in Cardiovascular Disease

Gopinath Gnanasegaran, Gregory Shabo and John R. Buscombe

Contents

7.1 Introduction 77
7.2 Current Markers of Myocardial Injury 78
7.2.1 Creatine Kinase (CK) and CK-MB 78
7.2.2 Cardiac Troponins 79
7.2.3 Lactate Dehydrogenase (LDH) 80
7.2.4 Myoglobins 80
7.2.5 C-reactive Protein (CRP) 81
7.3 Clinical Settings and Selection of a Diagnostic Marker 81
7.4 Recent Advances and Future Ischaemic and Inflammatory Markers 83
7.5 Conclusion 83
References 83

7.1 Introduction

Despite major advances in diagnosis and management, coronary artery disease continues to be a major public health problem. Patients with chest pain represent a heterogeneous group with varying presentation or severity of coronary artery disease and cardiac risk. Early prognostic evaluation of future cardiovascular risk is necessary for the application of appropriate treatment and optimal management in patients with chest pain. The role of cardiac markers in the diagnosis and management of patients with chest pain or in patients with suspected acute coronary syndromes (ACS) have improved dramatically with major technological advances. Currently various serum markers such as creatine kinase (CK)-MB, lactate dehydrogenase (LDH), myoglobin and cardiac troponins T (cTnT) and I (cTnI) are readily available and used as plasma diagnostic markers of myocardial necrosis in acute myocardial infarction (AMI) [1–18] (Table 7.1).

Patients with AMI generally present with chest pain with or without radiation to the jaw or arm. In general, patients will have associated electrocardiogram (ECG) changes. In patients presenting with classical symptoms and ECG changes, the role of cardiac markers is generally limited, however, some patients may present atypically. In these circumstances the cardiac markers may assist in the diagnosis of AMI. The cardiac specific diagnostic markers appear and disappear at various stages of myocardial damage.

The time of onset of the symptom is reported to play an important role in the assessment of the importance of these markers. The best marker depends on the time of onset of chest pain or other symptoms. An ideal marker should appear early in the blood and persists for a long time to be measured or detected (Table 7.2) [18].

In the early 1980s creatine kinase (CK)-MB activity and lactate dehydrogenase (LDH) were used as the best markers of myocardial necrosis, and in the 1990s CK-

Table 7.1 Markers of myocardial injury [1, 9–12, 14–17]

Markers of myocardial injury	
Current markers of myocardial injury	**Newer markers for myocardial injury** (Ischaemic and inflammatory markers)
Creatine kinase (CK)	Heart-type fatty acid binding protein
CK-MB	Ischaemia modified albumin
Aspartate amino transferase (AST)	CD40 ligand
Lactate dehydrogenase (LDH)	Myeloperoxidase
Troponin I	Serum amyloid A
Troponin T	Pregnancy-associated plasma protein A
Myoglobin	
B-type natriuretic peptides	
C-reactive protein	

Table 7.2 Criteria for ideal cardiac injury marker [18]

Early appearance in the blood
Persistent elevation in blood
Accurate
Specific
Rapid assay
Cost-effective

Table 7.3 ASNC recommendations in patients with suspected acute ischaemic heart disease [21]

(1) An ECG should be obtained at rest and multilead continuous ST-segment monitoring initiated (or frequent ECGs recorded where monitoring is unavailable).

(2) Troponin T or I should be measured on admission and, if normal, repeated 6 to 12 hours later.

(3) Myoglobin and/or CK-MB mass may be measured in patients with recent (<6 hours) symptoms as an early marker of myocardial infarction and in patients with recurrent ischaemia after recent (<2 weeks) infarction to detect further infarction.

MB was reported to be the gold standard [1, 2, 9]. Currently, in patients early in symptom onset, CK-MB subforms and myoglobin have been reported or proposed to be useful [1, 2, 9]. Cardiac troponins T (cTnT) and I (cTnI) are equally sensitive to CK-MB but more specific for unstable ischaemic syndromes [1, 2, 9]. However, it is important to note that all these markers are not specific for AMI alone. They are also released in non-AMI and non-cardiac conditions. Understanding the release kinetics of these markers is very important in order to apply them logically in an emergency. The final diagnosis of AMI is made from a combination of clinical presentation, serial changes on the electrocardiogram (ECG) and analysis of cardiac enzyme levels, as detailed in the ASNC Recommendations for patients with suspected acute ischaemic heart disease [21] (Table 7.3).

7.2 Current Markers of Myocardial Injury

7.2.1 Creatine Kinase (CK) and CK-MB

CK is a routinely and widely used plasma enzyme to confirm or exclude AMI. CK is commonly found in skeletal, heart, and brain tissues [18]. The use of CK alone without CK-MB has a similar sensitivity, but its specificity is lower: the use of total CK alone in the diagnosis of AMI is discouraged [1]. The molecular weight of CK is 85 kDa and it is comprised of two sub-units, M and B [18], which are coded by different genes [15, 16]. CK contains three main isoenzymes, namely MM, MB and BB, and these are located in the cytoplasm of the cell [1, 13–18].

The CK-MM isoenzyme is found predominantly in the skeletal muscle [1, 13–18] and CK-BB is found predominantly in the brain and internal visceral organs. CK-MB is a hybrid form (formed by one-subunit of M and one of B) of CK found in the heart (smaller amounts could also be detected in normal skeletal muscle) [1, 13, 18]. In the human heart 15% of the CK is in the form of CK-MB [1, 18, 21] and the remainder is in the form of CK-MM. CK-MB is formed of the three isoenzymes and is the most widely used marker today for the diagnosis of AMI. In general, the rise in CK-MB or total CK activity depends on the time and size of infarct. The commonest criteria used in the diagnosis of AMI has been a single result more than twice the upper limit of normal or two serial elevations above the diagnostic cut-off value of CK-MB [21]. CK-MB appears 4–6 hours after the onset of symptoms of AMI and peaks at 24 hours (with a plasma half-life of about 12 hours) [1, 13, 18]. It returns to normal by 48–72 hours [21] (Table 7.4). In general, single sample estimation of CK-MB is of limited value in the diagnosis of AMI [13, 18], and diagnostic sensitivity increases from 50% to approximately 98% when serial sampling is used [13, 18]. CK-MB isoenzyme exists in two isoforms, CK-MB1 and CK-MB2 [21]. The values reported in laboratories represent both these isoforms [21]. CK-MB2 is the tissue form, released initially from the myocardium soon after AMI, and is converted to CK-MB1 peripherally in the serum [21]. The ratio of CK-MB2 to CK-MB1 is calculated and a ratio less than 1 with predominant CK-MB1 is reported as normal, and a ratio more than 1.7 with raised CK-MB2 is reported as a positive test [22–25]. The major limitations of these markers are many and conditions such as skeletal muscle trauma, vigorous exercise, inflammation, and electrical injury, can all elevate CK-MB levels (1–5%) artificially [26–31] (Table 7.5).

7.2.2
Cardiac Troponins

The cardiac troponins are cardio-specific and sensitive markers. Currently, troponin T (TnT), Troponin I (TnI) and Troponin C (TnC) are the three sub-units identified [13]. In general, the genes coding for skeletal and cardiac isoforms of TnT and TnI are different. There are three genes for each of the TnT and TnI that encode for slow and fast skeletal and cardiac muscle [1, 32]. TnT (11 amino acids) and TnI (31 amino acids) have a molecular weight of 38,000 and 23,000, respectively [1, 13]. Cardiac TnI are not present in the skeletal forms [1]. With current assay methods, no cross-reactivity occurs between TnT and TnI [21]. Cardiac troponins appear in the serum 4–8 hours after symptom onset and they remain elevated for approximately 7–10 days post-AMI [21]. An elevated troponin identifies patients at high risk of adverse cardiac outcome up to 6 months after the initial event or presentation [21]. Cardiac troponins are extremely specific for myocardial necrosis. However, they do not discriminate between ischaemic and non-ischaemic etiologies of myocardial injury [1, 13]. High levels of TnT are reported to be found in patients

Table 7.4 Plasma profiles of cardiac markers [1, 9, 14, 21, 23]. (Note: normal values may vary depending on the method/technique, institution/department)

Cardiac markers (normal range)	Reliable sensitivity (>90%)	Max elevation	Normalisation
Total creatine kinase (CK) 24–195 U/L	2–4 hours	24–36 hours	3 days
Creatine kinase isoenzyme (CK-MB) 1-25 U/L (index of CK-MB Per total CK)	12–16 hours	14–36 hours	48–72 hours
LDH 200–450U/mL	8–48 hours	48–72 hours	8–14 days
Troponin-T <0.1 ng/mL	12–16 hours	26–36 hours	10–12 days
Troponin-I <0.5 ng/mL	12–16 hours	26–36 hours	10–12 days
Myoglobin <90 ng/mL	0.5–2 hours	5–12 hours	18–30 hours

Table 7.5 Elevated plasma CK/CK-MB and troponin levels documented in other disease states or clinical settings (1, 7, 14–17, 20, 26, 29–32, 37–41)

CK/CK-MB	Troponins
Polymyositis	Pacing, automated implantable cardioverter-defibrillator
Rhabdomyolysis (trauma, malignant hyper pyrexia)	Tachyarrhythmias
Duchene muscular dystrophy	Hypertension
AMI (acute myocardial infarction)	Myocarditis
Post operative/ surgery/Coronary angiography	Myocardial contusion
Skeletal muscle injury	Acute/chronic congestive heart failure
Severe or excessive exercise	Cardiac surgery
Convulsions	Renal failure
Myositis	Pulmonary embolism
Myocarditis	Subarachnoid haemorrhage
Physiological (Afrocaribbeans)	Sepsis
Hypothyroidism	Hypothyroidism
Drug (statins)	Shock
Electrical injury	

with end-stage renal disease (ESRD) and skeletal muscle injury [33, 34]. Unlike CK-MB and TnT, TnI is highly specific for myocardial tissue and is not detectable in the blood of healthy individuals. Measurement of troponin I clarifies the diagnosis in patients with concomitant myocardial and skeletal muscle injury [33–35].

However, it should be appreciated that a single test for troponins on arrival of the patient in hospital is not sufficient, as in 10 to 15% of patients troponin deviations can be detected in the subsequent hour. In order to demonstrate or to exclude myocardial damage, repeated blood sampling and measurements are required for 6 to 12 hours after admission and after any further episodes of severe chest pain [36]. Further, elevation of cardiac troponins also occurs in the setting of non-ischaemic myocardial injury (Table 7.5) [37–54]. Although current assays have largely overcome these deficiencies, infrequent false-positive results still occur and should be kept in mind. Currently, The European Society of Cardiology [36] consensus committee's recommendations specify a diagnostic cut-off for myocardial infarction using cardiac troponins based on the 99th percentile of levels among healthy controls rather than comparison with CK-MB [36]. The acceptable imprecision (coefficient of variation) at the 99th percentile for each assay should be below 10% [36]. In general, combining troponin with other cardiac biomarkers may offer complimentary information on the underlying pathophysiology and prognosis in an individual patient [13].

7.2.3
Lactate Dehydrogenase (LDH)

Levels generally become elevated 8 to 18 hours after an AMI, peak within 3 days, and return to normal in 6 to 10 days [33, 34]. The levels may also increase with other conditions such as myocarditis, post-cardiac catheterisation, pulmonary infarction, hepatic disease, renal infarction, and leukaemia [33, 34].

7.2.4
Myoglobins

This is a small protein present in the cardiac and skeletal muscles, having a molecular weight of 17,000 [1, 55]. It is not specific to cardiac muscle; it is useful in the detection of myocardial infarction in the absence of skeletal muscle trauma. Myoglobin rises within hours of ischaemic symptoms but it suffers from a lack of specificity. However, obtaining serial myoglobin results can help aid in the earlier identification of an AMI. Reports suggest that myoglobin levels doubling within 1 to 2 hours of presentation were determined to be highly specific for AMI [56]. Elevated levels are observed within a few hours after the onset of chest pain, peak at values up to 5 to 20 times the normal at 5 to 12 hours, and usually return to normal in 18 to 30 hours [57–59]. It is also reported to be more sensitive than CK-MB with an excellent negative predictive value for ruling out acute myocardial infarction in patients with typical or atypical symptoms [42]. The specificity of myoglobin is low since skeletal muscle trauma, intramuscular injections and renal failure all result in elevated levels. There is a short window for detecting elevated levels as myoglobin has rapid renal clearance [57–59].

7.2.5
C-reactive Protein (CRP)

CRP is a serum protein (acute phase protein) synthesized by hepatocytes and it is elevated in infection, inflammation, and tissue injury [60]. The physiological role of CRP is not known and it is moderately elevated in patients with diabetes, hypertension, smokers and in the obese [61]. In general, elevations in CRP levels may predict coronary events, and after acute myocardial infarction CRP values may predict outcome, including death and heart failure [62]. The CRP level increases dramatically in patients with myocardial infarction, starting within 4–6 hours of the onset of symptoms and reaching a peak after ~50 hours [60–64].

7.3
Clinical Settings and Selection of a Diagnostic Marker

Currently there are several cardiac markers available for the diagnosis and management of patients with chest pain. The overall need is use a reliable marker in a cost effective way. Also an ideal marker should be easy and rapid to use and it should have a high and reliable negative predictive value. In an emergency setting the choice is between CK-MB sub-forms and myoglobin (Table 7.6). The most widely used is CK-MB, with myoglobin used as a logical substitute provided the patient has no concomitant muscle trauma or injury [12].

If a patient presents many hours after the onset of chest pain and other related symptoms then the choice would be between CK-MB and troponins. As the troponins TnT and TnI are not normally present in the blood and do not appear to be present in skeletal muscle they appear to be more valuable owing to their higher specificity [1]. If troponins are not available, a single assay for both early and late diagnosis is CK-MB sub-forms, which provide early diagnosis and from which total CK-MB can be derived for the late diagnosis [1]. If both CK-MB and tropinins are available then CK-MB can be used for early diagnosis and TnT or TnI for late diagnosis [1]. Troponin would be ideal in situations where there is concomitant muscle trauma or injury. The choice of markers depends on multiple factors such as onset of pain, baseline ECG changes and availability.

Table 7.6 Clinical settings and selection of a diagnostic marker [1, 2, 21, 22, 36]

Early diagnosis upon admission- CK-MB (first choice) or Myoglobin (concomitant muscle trauma CK-MB preferred)
Presenting 10 hours after the onset of symptoms - CK-MB or TnT, TnI or both (concomitant muscle trauma troponin I preferred)
Presenting/admitted 48–72 hours after the onset of symptoms - LDH (as CK-MB may have returned to normal)
In patients undergoing fibrinolytic therapy or angioplasty - CK-MB, TnT, TnI (4–6 hours, then every 6–8 hours for 36 hours]
Early re infarction (24–48 hours) - CK-MB (secondary rise in CK-MB as initial rise would have reached baseline by 48 hours). Myoglobin though sensitive but non-specific due to venipuncture or minor muscle trauma
Prognostic value in unstable angina - CK-MB, TnT, TnI
Myocardial infarction after non-cardiac surgery - CK-MB, TnT, TnI

Table 7.7 Recent advances and possible future ischaemic and inflammatory markers [10–12, 32, 65 – 70, 74 – 77]

Ischaemic modified albumin [IMA] (albumin cobalt binding)
IMA measures reduction of albumins ability to bind cobalt.
In patients with myocardial ischaemia N-terminus structure is altered and these metals no longer bind.
Detected within minutes and can be used as an early marker of ischaemia at presentation.
96% NPV for a negative troponin 6 hours later [10, 11].
Specificity of IMA is only 69%.
Heart-type fatty acid binding protein [H-FABP]
Low molecular-weight protein, similar to myoglobin.
Released rapidly into the circulation after myocardial damage.
More specific for cardiac muscle than myoglobin.
Reported to be more sensitive and specific than myoglobin (In the early detection of AMI, reinfarction and estimating infarct size) [12, 65, 66].
CD40 ligand
CD40 ligand is distributed on a variety of leukocytes and non-leukocytes cell.
Upon platelet activation, a soluble CD40 ligand is cleaved from the cell membrane [12].
It participates in the plaque destabilization.
May play a role in acute coronary syndrome (found to be elevated) [67].
Based on CD40 levels, it is possible to identify patients who may benefit from antiplatelet and statin therapy [68].
Myeloperoxidase [MPO]
Is a leukocyte enzyme that promotes damage to host tissues at sites of inflammation and modifies intercellular processes that affect plaque stability and thrombogenicity [12].
Plasma MPO levels are significantly elevated in CAD.
Can predict the risk of subsequent cardiovascular events [69, 70].
Appears to rise in the absence of necrosis, unlike troponin and CK-MB.
May be a useful early marker in its ability to detect plaque vulnerability that precedes ACS.
Serum amyloid A (SAA) and pregnancy-associated plasma protein A (PAPP-A)
Currently, SAA &PAPP-A are used as inflammatory markers, especially in troponin negative patients [12].
SAA has been linked to atherosclerosis and can predict the risk of future cardiovascular events [12].
Markers of inflammatory activity
Increased fibrinogen levels and high-sensitivity CRP have been reported as risk markers in ACS, although the data are not consistent [74–77].
Markers of thrombosis
Association between increased thrombin generation and an unfavorable outcome in unstable angina has been found in some although not all trials [78, 79].
Protein C, protein S and antithrombin deficiencies are defects in the anti-coagulant systems associated with the development of venous thromboembolism (so far none of these have been connected to an increased risk of ACS) [32].

7.4 Recent Advances and Future Ischaemic and Inflammatory Markers

Recent advances in biochemistry and molecular medicine have had a tremendous affect on early diagnosis, prediction and management of various pathological conditions. Currently, various types of ischaemic and inflammatory markers are being investigated and some have made their appearance in the clinical world. Some markers that may play an important role in different stages of CAD/IHD are detailed in Table 7.7 [10–12, 32, 65–79]. However, the diagnostic utility of these markers is yet to be established and further studies are awaited.

7.5 Conclusion

Cardiac markers play an important role in the diagnosis and management of patients with chest pain or in patients with suspected acute coronary syndromes. The choice of markers depends on multiple factors such as availability, cost and clinical setting. However, care should be taken as normal values may vary depending on the method/technique, institution/department.

References

1. Alexander RW, Pratt CM, Ryan TJ, Roberts R (2001) Diagnosis and management of patients with acute myocardial infarction In Fuster F, Alexander RW, O'Rourke RA (eds), Hurst's: The Heart, 10th edn. McGraw-Hill, New York, pp. 1275–1360.
2. World Health Organisation (1981) WHO criteria for the diagnosis of acute myocardial infarction. Proposal for the multinational monitoring of trends and determinants of cardiovascular disease. Geneva: Cardiovascular diseases Unit, WHO.
3. Chan PD, Winkle PJ (1997) Current Clinical Strategies: History and Physical Examination in Medicine, 2nd edn. CCS Publishing. Laguna Hills, CA, pp. 7–11.
4. de Winter RJ, Koster RW, Sturk A, Sanders GT (1995) Value of myoglobin, troponin T, and CK-MB mass in ruling out an acute myocardial infarction in the emergency room. Circulation 92:3401–407.
5. Wu AH (1997) Use of cardiac markers as assessed by outcomes analysis. Clin Biochem.30:339–350.
6. Wong SS (1996) Strategic utilization of cardiac markers for the diagnosis of acute myocardial infarction. Ann Clin Lab Sci.26:300–312.
7. Fischbach F (2000) A Manual of Laboratory and Diagnostic Tests, 6th edn. Lippincott Williams & Wilkins, Philadelphia, PA.
8. Morris S, Wu AH, Heller GV (1996) The role of cardiac imaging and biochemical markers in patients with acute chest pain. Curr Opin Cardiol.11:386–393.
9. Schreiber DH (2002) Update on cardiac markers in the emergency department. eMedicine Journal [serial online]; 3(2). www.emedicine.com.
10. Christenson RH, Duh SH, Sanhai WR et al. (2001) Characteristics of an albumin cobalt binding test for assessment of acute coronary syndrome patients: a multicenter study. Clin Chem 47:464–470.
11. Sinha MK, Roy D, Gaze DC, Collinson PO, Kaski JC (2004) Role of ischemia modified albumin, a new biochemical marker of myocardial ischaemia, in the early diagnosis of acute coronary syndromes. Emerg Med J 21:29–34.
12. Melanson SF, Tanasijevic MJ (2005) Innovative Cardiovascular technologies laboratory diagnosis of acute myocardial injury Cardiovasc Pathol 14 156–161.
13. Scirica BM, Morrow DA (2004) Troponins in acute coronary syndromes. Prog Cardiovasc Disease 47:177–188.
14. Marshall WJ, Banget SK (2004) Lipids, lipoproteins, cardiovascular disease. In Clinical Chemistry, 5th edn. Elseiver, pp. 255–271.
15. Walmsley RN, White GH (1994) Plasma Enzymes, 3rd edn. Blackwell Science, pp. 291–320.
16. Laker MF (1996) Enzymes in body fluids. In Clinical Biochemistry for Medical Students. WB Saunders.
17. Kaplan A, Opheim KE Enzymes. In Clinical Chemistry – Interpretation and Techniques. Lippincott Williams & Wilkins, Philadelphia, PA, pp. 277–311.
18. Amsterda EA Deedwania P (2005) Bedside evaluation of cardiac markers, Point-of-care testing can differentiate acute coronary syndromes. Postgrad Med 118:3.
19. Collinson PO (1998) Troponin T or troponin I or CK-MB (or none?). Eur Heart J 19:N16–N24.
20. Fischbach F (2000) A Manual of Laboratory and Diagnostic Tests, 6th edn. Lippincott Williams & Wilkins, Philadelphia, PA.
21. American Heart Association. 2001 Heart and Stroke Statistical Update. Dallas, Tex: American Heart Association; 2000. Available at: http://www.americanheart.org/statistics/index.html.
22. Wong SS (1996) Strategic utilization of cardiac markers for the diagnosis of acute myocardial infarction. Ann Clin Lab Sci 26:301–312.
23. Balk EM, Ioannidis JPA, Salem D, Chew PW, Lau J (2001) Accuracy of biomarkers to diagnose acute cardiac ischemia in the emergency department: a meta-analysis. Ann Emerg Med.37:478–494.
24. Puleo PR, Meyer D, Wathen C et al. (1994) Use of a rapid assay of subforms of creatine kinase-MB to diagnose or rule out acute myocardial infarction. N Engl J Med 1:561–566.
25. Puleo PR, Guadagno PA, Roberts R, Perryman MB (1989) Sensitive, rapid assay of subforms of creatine kinase MB in plasma. Clin Chem 35:1452–1455.

26. Apple FS, Rogers MA, Sherman WM, Costill DL, Hagerman FC, Ivy JL (1984) Profile of creatine kinase isoenzymes in skeletal muscles of marathon runners. Clin Chem 30:413–416.
27. Siegel AJ, Silverman LM, Evans WJ (1983). Elevated skeletal muscle creatine kinase MB isoenzyme levels in marathon runners. JAMA 25 250:2835–2837.
28. Keshgegian AA, Feinberg NV (1984) Serum creatine kinase MB isoenzyme in chronic muscle disease. Clin Chem 30:575–578.
29. Shahangian S, Ash KO, Wahlstrom NO Jr, Warden GD, Saffle JR, Taylor A Jr, Green LS (1984) Creatine kinase and lactate dehydrogenase isoenzymes in serum of patients suffering burns, blunt trauma, or myocardial infarction. Clin Chem 30:1332–1338.
30. McBride JW, Labrosse KR, McCoy HG, Ahrenholz DH, Solem LD, Goldenberg IF (1986) Is serum creatine kinase-MB in electrically injured patients predictive of myocardial injury? JAMA 14:764–768.
31. Tzvetanova E (1971) Aldolase isoenzymes in serum and muscle from patients with progressive muscular dystrophy and from human foetus. J Neurol Sci 14:483–489.
32. Apple FS, Ricchiuti V, Voss EM, Anderson PA, Ney A, Odland M (1998) Expression of cardiac troponin T isoforms in skeletal muscle of renal disease patients will not cause false-positive serum results by the second generation cardiac troponin T assay. Eur Heart J 19:N30–N33.
33. Panteghini M (2006) The new definition of myocardial infarction and the impact of troponin determination on clinical practice International. J Cardiol 106:298–306.
34. Sarko J, Pollack C V Jr (2002) Clinical laboratory in emergency medicine, cardiac troponins. J Emergency Med 23:57–65.
35. Sharma S, Jackson PG, Makan J (2004) Cardiac troponins. J Clin Pathol 57:1025–1026.
36. Bertrand ME, Simoons ML, Fox KA et al. (2002) Management of acute coronary syndromes in patients presenting without persistent ST-segment elevation, Task Force Report, The Task Force on the Management of Acute Coronary Syndromes of the European Society of Cardiology. Eur Heart J 23:1809–1840.
37. Gupta M, Lent RW, Kaplan EL, Zabriskie JB (2002) Serum cardiac troponin I in acute rheumatic fever. Am J Cardiol 89:779–782.
38. Dispenzieri A, Kyle RA, Gertz MA et al. (2003) Survival in patients with primary systemic amyloidosis and raised serum cardiac troponins. Lancet 361:1787–1789.
39. Sybrandy KC, Cramer MJM, Burgersdijk C (2003) Diagnosing cardiac contusion: old wisdom and new insights. Heart 89:458–489.
40. Dworschak M, Franz M, Khazen C, Czerny M, Haisjackl M, Hiesmayr M. (2001) Mechanical trauma as the major cause of troponin T release after transvenous implantation of cardioverter/defibrillators. Cardiology 95:212–214.
41. Cardinale D, Sandri MT, Martinoni A et al. (2000) Left ventricular dysfunction predicted by early troponin I release after high-dose chemotherapy. J Am Coll Cardiol 36:517–522.
42. Sato Y, Yamada T, Taniguchi R et al. (2001) Persistently increased serum concentrations of cardiac troponin T in patients with idiopathic dilated cardiomyopathy are predictive of adverse outcomes. Circulation 103:369–374.
43. Wright RS, Williams BA, Cramner H et al. (2002) Elevations of cardiac troponin I are associated with increased short-term mortality in noncardiac critically ill emergency department patients. Am J Cardiol 90:634–636.
44. Apple FS, Murakami MM, Pearce LA, Herzog CA (2002) Predictive value of cardiac troponin I and T for subsequent death in end-stage renal disease. Circulation 106:2941–2945.
45. Gaze DC, Lawson GJ, Harris A, Collinson PO (2003) Evidence of myocyte necrosis in glycogen storage disease type II. Clin Chem 49:A39
46. Chance JJ, Segal JB, Wallerson G et al. (2001) Cardiac troponin T and Creactive protein as markers of acute cardiac allograft rejection. Clin Chim Acta 312:31–39.
47. Missov E, Mentzer W, Laprade M et al.(2001) Cardiac markers of injury in hemoglobinopathy patients with transfusion hemosiderosis. J Am Coll Cardiol 37:470.
48. Hamwi SM, Sharma AK, Weissman NJ et al.(2003) Troponin-I elevation in patients with increased left ventricular mass. Am J Cardiol 92:88–90.
49. Arlati S, Brenna S, Prencipe L et al. (2000) Myocardial necrosis in ICU patients with acute non-cardiac disease: a prospective study. Intensive Care Med 26:31–37.
50. Mutch WJ, Kulkarmi UV, Croal BL, Simpson WG (2001) Cardiac marker levels in hypothyroidism. Clin Chem 47:A199.
51. Lauer B, Niederau C, Kuhl U et al. (1997) Cardiac troponin T in patients with clinically suspected myocarditis. J Am Coll Cardiol 30:1354–1359.
52. Lopez-Jimenez F, Goldman L, Sacks DB et al. (1997) Prognostic value of cardiac troponin T after noncardiac surgery: 6-month follow-up data. J Am Coll Cardiol 29:1241–1245.
53. Giannitsis E, Muller-Bardorff M, Kurowski V et al. (2000) Independent prognostic value of cardiac troponin T in patients with confirmed pulmonary embolism. Circulation 102:211–217.
54. Spies C, Haude V, Fitzner R et al. (1998) Serum cardiac troponin T as a prognostic marker in early sepsis. Chest 113:1055–1063.
55. Plebani M, Zaninotto M (1998) Diagnostic strategies in myocardial infarction using myoglobin measurement. Eur Heart J 19:N12–N15.

56. Rao M, Jaber, B L, Balakrishnan VS (2006) Inflammatory biomarkers and cardiovascular risk: association or cause and effect? Seminars in Dialysis 19:129–135.
57. Heger JW, Niemann JT, Roth RF, Criley JM (1998) Cardiology, 4th edn. Williams & Wilkins, Baltimore, MD.
58. Wong SS (1996) Strategic utilization of cardiac markers for the diagnosis of acute myocardial infarction. Ann Clin Lab Sci 26:301–312.
59. Conn HF et al. (eds) (2000) Conn's Current Therapy. WB Saunders, Philadelphia, PA, pp. 291–319.
60. Kitsis RN, Jialal I (2006) Limiting myocardial damage during acute myocardial infarction by inhibiting C-reactive protein. New Engl J Med 3(355):513–515.
61. Suleiman M, Khatib R, Agmon Y et al. (2006) Early inflammation and risk of long-term development of heart failure and mortality in survivors of acute myocardial infarction – predictive role of C-reactive protein. J Am Coll Cardiol 47:962–968.
62. Kushner I, Broder ML, Karp D (1978) Control of the acute phase response. Serum C-reactive protein kinetics after acute myocardial infarction. J Clin Invest 61:235–242.
63. de Beer FC, Hind CRK, Fox KM, Allan R, Maseri A, Pepys MB (1982). Measurement of serum C-reactive protein concentration in myocardial ischaemia and infarction. Br Heart J 47:239–243.
64. Griselli M, Herbert J, Hutchinson WL, Taylor KM, Sohail M, Krausz T, Pepys MB (1999) C-reactive protein and complement are important mediators of tissue damage in acute myocardial infarction. J Exp Med 20(190):1733–1740.
65. Seino Y, Ogata K, Takano T, Ishii J, Hishida H, Morita H, Takeshita H, Takagi Y, Sugiyama H, Tanaka T, Kitaura Y (2003) Use of a whole blood rapid panel test for heart-type fatty acid-binding protein in patients with acute chest pain: comparison with rapid troponin T and myoglobin tests. Am J Med 115:185–190.
66. Chan CP, Sanderson JE, Glatz JF, Cheng WS, Hempel A, Renneberg R (2004) A superior early myocardial infarction marker Human heart-type fatty acid-binding protein. Z Kardiol 93:388–397.
67. Garlichs CD, Eskafi S, Raaz D, Schmidt A, Ludwig J, Herrmann M, Klinghammer L, Daniel WG, Schmeisser A (2001) Patients with acute coronary syndromes express enhanced CD40 ligand/CD154 on platelets. Heart 86:649–655.
68. Heeschen C, Dimmeler S, Hamm CW, van den Brand MJ, Boersma E, Zeiher AM, Simoons ML (2003) Soluble CD40 ligand in acute coronary syndromes. New Engl J Med 348:1104–1111.
69. Brennan ML, Penn MS, Van Lente F (2003) Prognostic value of myeloperoxidase in patients with chest pain. New Engl J Med 349:1595–1604.
70. Baldus S, Heeschen C, Meinertz T, Zeiher AM, Eiserich JP, Munzel T, Simoons ML, Hamm CW (2003) Myeloperoxidase serum levels predict risk in patients with acute coronary syndromes. Circulation 108:1440–1445.
71. Klocke FJ, Baird MG, Lorell BH (2003) ACC/AHA/ASNC Guidelines for the clinical use of cardiac radionuclide imaging – executive summary. *Circulation* 108:1404.
72. Johnson BD, Kip KE, Marroquin OC, Ridker PM (2004) Serum amyloid A as a predictor of coronary artery disease and cardiovascular outcome in women: the National Heart, Lung, and Blood Institute-Sponsored Women's Ischemia Syndrome Evaluation (WISE). Circulation 109:726–732.
73. Bayes-Genis A, Conover CA, Overgaard MT (2001) Pregnancy-associated plasma protein A as a marker of acute coronary syndromes. New Engl J Med 345:1022–1029.
74. Lindahl B, Toss H, Siegbahn A, Venge P, Wallentin L (2000) Markers of myocardial damage and inflammation in relation to long-term mortality in unstable coronary artery disease. FRISC Study Group. Fragmin during Instability in Coronary Artery Disease. New Engl J Med 343:1139–1147.
75. Toss H, Lindahl B, Siegbahn A, Wallentin L (1997) Prognostic influence of increased fibrinogen and C-reactive protein levels in unstable coronary artery disease. FRISC Study Group. Fragmin during Instability in Coronary Artery Disease. Circulation 96:4204–4210.
76. Becker RCC, Bovill E et al. (1996) Prognostic value of plasma fibrinogen concentration in patients with unstable angina and non-Q-wave myocardial infarction (TIMI IIIB trial). Am J Cardiol 78:142–147.
77. Pollak H, Fischer M, Fritsch S, Enenkel W (1991) Are admission plasma fibrinogen levels useful in the characterization of risk groups after myocardial infarction treated with fibrinolysis? Thromb Haemost 66:406–409.
78. Ardissino D, Merlini PA, Gamba G et al. (1996) Thrombin activity and early outcome in unstable angina pectoris. Circulation 93:1634–1639.
79. Ernofsson M, Strekerud F, Toss H, Abildgaard U, Wallentin L, Siegbahn A (1998) Low-molecular weight heparin reduces the generation and activity of thrombin in unstable coronary artery disease. Thromb Haemost 79:491–494.

Chapter 8

Electrocardiography and Exercise Stress Test

Humayun Bashir, Gopinath Gnanasegaran and John R. Buscombe

Contents

8.1	Electrocardiography	87
8.1.1	Resting Electrocardiogram	87
8.1.2	Recording ECG	87
8.1.3	ECG and its Major Components	88
8.1.4	ECG Paper	89
8.1.5	Calculation of Rate	90
8.1.6	Analysing an ECG	91
8.1.7	Artefacts in ECG	93
8.1.8	QRS Axis	93
8.1.9	Sinus Rhythm, Sinus Bradycardia and Sinus Tachycardia	94
8.1.10	Sinus Arrhythmias	95
8.1.11	Atrial Arrhythmias	97
8.1.12	Junctional Atrioventricular (AV) Arrhythmias	99
8.1.13	AV Blocks	100
8.1.14	Ventricular Arrhythmias	100
8.1.15	Bundle Branch Block	102
8.1.16	Arial and Ventricular Hypertrophy	104
8.1.17	Computers and ECG	105
8.2	Exercise Stress Testing	105
8.2.1	Types of Exercise	107
8.2.2	Rationale for Testing	107
8.2.3	Indications and Contra-Indications	108
8.2.4	Equipment	108
8.2.5	Stress Protocols	109
8.2.6	Safety	109
8.2.7	Patient Preparation for Exercise Test [21–23]	110
8.2.8	Interpreting Exercise Test Results [21–23]	110
8.3	Conclusion	111
	References	111

8.1 Electrocardiography

8.1.1 Resting Electrocardiogram

In patients with chest pain or suspected heart disease (IHD/CAD), the electrocardiogram (ECG) is one of the principle investigations at the time of presentation. The ECG is a graph obtained when the electrical potentials of an electrical field originating in the heart are recorded at the surface of the body [1–3]. Once the electrical activity is detected it is amplified, displayed on the screen/monitor and finally recorded on a paper chart [1–3]. In general, the ECG records depolarisation (P wave and QRS complex) and repolarisation (ST segment, T wave and U wave) of the heart. The advantages of the ECG are (a) it is an independent marker of myocardial disease, and (b) it detect haemodynamic, anatomical, electrolyte and drug induced abnormalities [1–3]. Although the ECG is useful in the initial stages of chest pain investigation, it has severe limitations.

8.1.2 Recording ECG

The ECG sees the heart in two planes; a vertical/frontal and a horizontal/transverse plane. In general, a routine ECG is recorded using 12 leads to obtain the electrical activity of the heart in 12 views. Each lead records the heart's electrical impulses at different position in relation to the heart. The 12-lead ECG consists of three standard limb leads (I, II, III), three augmented limb leads (aVR, aVL, aVF) and six precordial or chest leads (V1, V2, V3, V4, V5 and V6) [4–7]. The horizontal plane leads are V1 to V6, the vertical plane leads are the standard leads, and augmented vector leads [4–7]. The correct placement of electrodes is important and is described in Table 8.1 and Fig. 8.1. Various artefacts can occur due to conditions such as muscle tremors, incorrect voltages or variations in voltage due to misplacement of leads.

Table 8.1 Position of leads and their significance [1, 5–7] ICS = Intercostal space Leads V5, V6 are in the same horizontal plane as V5

Leads	Recording electrode (+)	Reference electrode (-)
Chest/precordial leads		
V1	4th right ICS (right sternal border)	Limb leads combined
V2	4th left ICS (left sternal border)	Limb leads combined
V3	Half way between V3 & V4 (on the left)	Limb leads combined
V4	Paints apex beat (centered on clavicle)	Limb leads combined
*V5	Anterior axillary line (left of V4)	Limb leads combined
*V6	Mid axillary line	Limb leads combined
Limb leads (standard)		
I	Left arm	Right arm
II	Left leg	Right arm
III	Left leg	Left arm
Limb leads (augmented)		
aVR	Right arm	Left arm and left leg
aVL	Left arm	Right arm and left leg
aVF	Left leg	Right arm and left arm

ICS = Intercostal space
* Leads V5, V6 are in the same horizontal plane as V5

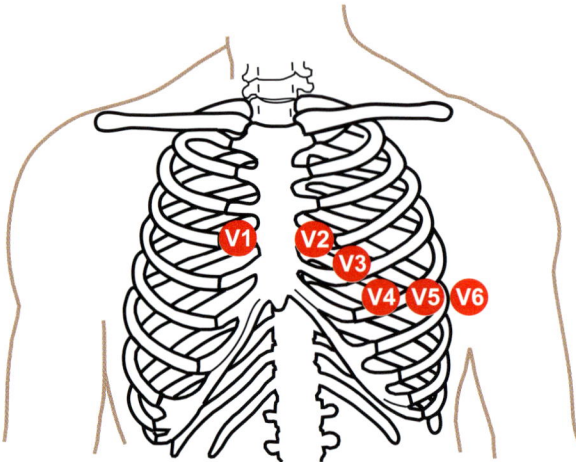

Fig. 8.1 Position of chest and precordial leads

8.1.3
ECG and its Major Components

In general, the ECG detects/displays three major waves (P wave, QRS complex and a T wave), two time intervals (PR interval, QRS duration) and an ST segment [5] (Fig. 8.2).

The P wave represents the electrical activity generated by the right atrium (RA). The P wave is the first deflection recorded on an ECG [5]. The mid-portion of the P wave represents completion of right atrial activation and initiation of left atrial (LA) activation, and the later portion of the P wave is generated by the LA [5–7]. The duration of a normal P wave is 0.12–0.20 seconds. Normal P waves should be upright in I, II, V3–V6, inverted in aVR, usually upright in aVF and V3, and variable in III, aVL, V1 and V2. P waves can be inverted, notched or tall, depending on the clinical scenario (Fig. 8.3).

The PR interval (0.20 second) denotes the time required for the electrical impulse to pass from the atria

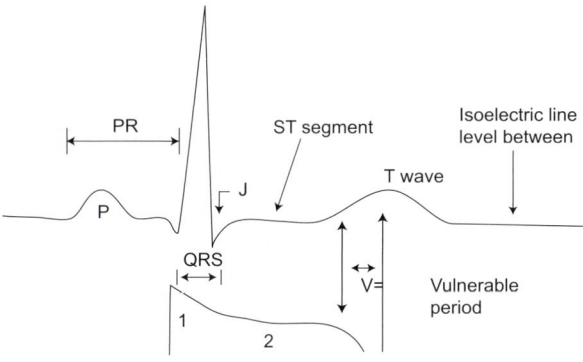

Fig. 8.2 Waves and segments in an ECG

through the AV node, bundle of His, bundle branches and Purkinje fibres [5–7].

The QRS complex represents the time required for the electrical impulse to depolarise the ventricles and is composed of three waves: the Q (negative deflection); R (positive deflection); and S (negative deflection) waves [5–7]. The normal QRS is predominantly positive in lead II with duration of 10 seconds or less. A normal QRS complex indicates depolarisation of ventricles within the normal amount of time [7]. An abnormal QRS complex occurs in such conditions as (a) early arrival of ventricles at the bundle branches, (b) a block in the conduction of impulses through one of the bundle branches, (c) conduction of impulses from the atria to the ventricles through abnormal conduction pathways, (d) electrical impulses from ectopic sites, (e) hyperkalemia, or (f) following administration of drugs such as procanamide, quinidine, etc. [6, 7].

The ST segment occurs between the end of the QRS complex and the beginning of the T wave. The normal duration of the ST segment is 0.08 second [5–7]. During this period, all parts of the ventricle are in a depolarised state. The point at which the ST segment takes off from the QRS complex is called the J point (junctional point) [5, 6].

The QT interval (0.36 second) represents the time between the onset of ventricular depolarisation and the end of ventricular repolarisation [5–7]. The length of the QT interval varies according to gender, age and heart rate. In general, as the heart rate increases, the QT interval decreases and vice versa.

The T wave represents the electrical recovery and repolarisation of the ventricles and is recorded during ventricular systole [5–7].

The U wave follows the T wave and is observed in some individuals only, and its source is uncertain [5, 6].

8.1.4
ECG Paper

The ECG graph paper contains vertical and horizontal lines ruled at 1 mm intervals, with each fifth horizontal and vertical line heavier than the others [5–7]. The vertical axis measures the amplitude of waveforms in millivolts (mV). Each small square represent 0.1 mV vertically and the voltage between two heavy horizontal lines is 0.5 mV [7].

The horizontal axis measures time in seconds and each small horizontal square represents 0.04 second, when the chart paper is moving at 25 mm/second. Each small box equals 40 milliseconds and each large box equals 200 milliseconds [5].

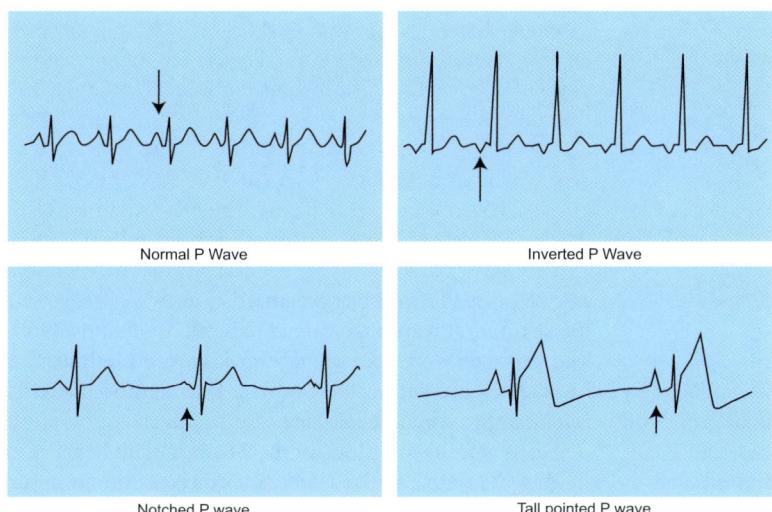

Fig. 8.3 Types of P waves

Table 8.2 Summary of ECG interpretation, artefacts and definition [1–14]

Identification: patient name, date, time	False variations in the voltage,
Explain the procedure to the patient	Overshooting, over-damping
Patient should be lying down in a comfortable position	Hypothermia
Patient and machine should be properly grounded to avoid alternating current interference	Incorrect paper speed
Good contact between the skin and electrodes	**P wave:** Atrial depolarisation. Normally upright in all the leads and inverted in AVR and normal P wave axis is directed toward 40–60 degrees
Quality	
Calibration standardized	**PR interval:** start of atrial depolarisation to start of ventricular depolarisation.
Steps in interpreting ECG	
Rate (atrial, ventricular)	**QRS complex:** QRS complex represents ventricle depolarisation.
Rhythm	
Electrical axis	Initial negative deflection is called a Q wave, positive deflection is called an R wave and a negative deflection which follows an R wave is called a S wave
P wave:	
PR interval (0.12–2.0)	
QRS interval (0.06–1.0)	**T wave:** Ventricular repolaraisation. Normally upright in all the leads except aVR and a normal T wave is asymmetrical (the descending limb is steeper than the ascending limb)
QRS complex, morphology	
ST segment (elevated or depressed)	
T wave: Tall, flat, inverted	**ST segment:** Region between the QRS complex and the T wave
U wave: Prominent or inverted	
QT interval	**QT interval (0.36 s):** Beginning of the QRS complex until the end of the T wave
Compare with previous ECG if any	
Final interpretation: Within normal limits (WNL); Borderline abnormal; Abnormal	**Definition of a sinus rhythm**
	Rhythm – Regular
Artefacts in ECG	Rate – 60–100
Muscle tremor, patient movement and alternate current interference	P waves – normal configuration and direction. P waves precedes each QRS complex
	PR interval – 0.12–0.20 s (normal)
Improper limb-lead positioning or misplacement or Variations in precordial lead placement	QRS – 0.10 s or less (normal)

8.1.5 Calculation of Rate

The heart rate in regular rhythm can be calculated by two common methods: (a) a rapid rate calculation; and (b) a precise rate calculation [7]. In the rapid rate calculation, the number of R waves in a 6-second strip is calculated and then multiplied by 10 (number in 6 seconds × 10 = heart rate/minute) [6, 7]. In the precise rate calculation, the number of small squares between two consecutive R waves are calculated and divided by 1500. The precise rate calculation is an accurate method, the rapid rate calculation method is a fast method, providing an approximate heart rate [7].

However, the simplest method to calculate heart rate in an ECG with regular rhythm is to count the number of large squares between two QRS complexes and divide them into 300, i.e., HR = 300/number of large squares between two QRS complexes [5, 6]. However, in patients with irregular rhythm, we need to count the number of QRS complexes in 30 large squares and multiply by 10 [5, 6].

8.1.6 Analysing an ECG

A 12-lead ECG should be examined systematically for accurate interpretation. The 12 leads provide a number of different views of the heart and provide a comprehensive picture of the electrical activity of the heart. In general, when interpreting ECGs, the following should be observed and measured/calculated: (a) rate, (b) rhythm, (c) P wave, (d) PR interval, (e) QRS interval, (f) QRS complex, (g) ST segment, (h) T wave, (i) electrical axis, (j) U wave, and (k) QT interval [6–13] (Table 8.2). Whatever, the order or methods used, the most important steps include (a) determine regularity of the rhythm; (b) calculate heart rate; (c) assess P waves; (d) measure PR interval; and (e) measure QRS complex [5, 6]. The common causes of ST segment, Q wave, T wave and U wave

Table 8.3 ST segment abnormalities and ECG features [6–13]

ST segment abnormalities
• ST elevation is current injury, ST depression is ischaemia, and Q waves is infarction
• Abnormal elevation (>1 mm in two or more contagious limb leads): acute MI, coronary artery spasm, acute pericarditis, LBBB, LVH, LV aneurysm
• Subendocardial infarction: Infarct affecting a part of the thickness.
• Transmural infarction: infarct affecting the entire thickness of myocardium
Abnormal elevation (probable Q wave infarction)
• Elevation in I, aVL, V5 and V6 is anterolateral infarction
• Elevation in I, II, III and aVF is inferior infarction
• Elevation in2 or more contagious leads indicates anterior infarction
• Elevation in V1-V3 indicates anteroseptal or anteroapical
• Elevation in V3-V6 indicates anterior infarction
• Elevation in V3R, V4R with inferior infarction indicates added RV infarction
• Elevation in II, III, aVF, or V4 associated with tall R waves in V1, V2 may indicates added posterior infarction
• Elevation in aVR greater than elevation in V1 is a marker of left main coronary artery occlusion
Condition mimicking ST elevation infarction
Normal variants in some healthy ethnic groups
Acute pericarditis
Coronary artery spasm,
LBBB, LVH, LV aneurysm
Cocaine abuse
Pulmonary embolism
Hypertrophic cardiomyopathy, Acute myocarditis
Conditions causing ST depression
Ischaemia
Hypokalemia
Tachycardia
Subendocardial infarct
LVH , Bundle branch block
Digitalis, Hypothermia
Non specific ST –T changes (<1 mm)
Ischaemia
Improper electrode contact
Electrolyte abnormalities
Arrhythmias
Pericarditis
Cardiomyopathy
Pulmonary embolism
Hyperventilation ethanol abuse
Digoxin subarachnoid hemorrhage
Interventricular conduction defects

Table 8.4 Q wave facts and ECG abnormalities [6–13]

Q wave facts	Condition mimicking Q wave MI or pseudinfarction
During the assessment of Q waves, the following should be noted (a) depth (b) width (c) leads in which observed and (d) age of the patient	• Hyperthropic cardiomyopathy
	• Myocarditis
Normal:	• Wolff–Parkinson–White syndrome
Q wave wider than 0.03 second is abnormal (except in III, aVR, V1 where it is considered normal)	• Chagas' disease,
	• Acquired immunodeficiency syndrome
Q waves of acute infarction are always associated with ST elevation	• LVH, LBBB
	• Dextrocardia
Q wave myocardial infarction (MI)	• Emphysema
• Extensive anterior MI: Q, QS or QR in V2–V4/V5 or V1–V6	• Non-penetrating chest trauma, chest deformity
• Anteroseptal/apicoanterior MI: Q, QS in V1–V3	• Massive pulmonary embolism
• Apical MI: Q in I, II, III	• Left sided pnemothorax
• Anterolateral MI: Q in I, aVL, V5, V6 with ST segment abnormality	• Sarcoidosis, amyloidosis, acute pancreatitis, scleroderma
• Inferior wall MI: Q in II, III, aVF with some nonspecific ST–T changes	• Hyperkalemia
• Infero-lateral MI: Q in II, III, aVF, V4–V6	• Cardiac tumours
• Right ventricular MI: Inferior wall MI + ST elevation in V3R and V4R	• Friedreich's ataxia
	Transient Q waves
• Posterior (MI Infero-posterior): Inferior wall MI + tall R in V1, V2	• Hyperkalaemia
• True posterior: V1 (tall R wave)	• Cardiac contusion
	• Hypothermia
	• Coronary spasm, Hypoxia

Table 8.5 T wave facts and ECG abnormalities [6–13]

T wave facts:	In some patients with partial thickness ischaemia the T waves show a biphasic pattern
Represents repolarisation	
Abnormal T waves: Inverted, flat and tall T waves	**Normal/variants:**
Tall T waves are one of the earliest changes seen in acute myocardial infarction	Always upright in I, II, V4–V6, (b) Usually upright in aVF, (c) Variable in III, aVL (d) inverted in aVR (e) often inverted in V1 (33% males, 50% females)
Isolated tall T waves in leads V1 to V3 may also be due to ischaemia of the posterior wall of the left ventricle	**T wave abnormalities:**
T waves that are deep and symmetrically inverted strongly suggest myocardial ischaemia.	Inverted T waves (in absence of ST elevation)
	Ischaemia
T wave inversion can be normal – It occurs in leads III, aVR, and V1 (and in V2, but only in association with T wave inversion in lead V1)	LVH
	Post MI (evolutionary changes)

Table 8.5 (continued) T wave facts and ECG abnormalities [6–13]

Myocarditis, pericarditis	**Tall T waves:**
Cardiomyopathies	Hyperkalemia,
Pulmonary embolism	Acute myocardial infarction
Alcohol and cocaine abuse	**Small T waves:**
Post SVT or VT	Hypokalemia
Electrolyte imbalance	Hypothyroidism
Pancraetitis, subarachnoid haemorrhage	Pericardial effusion
Cardiac tumours, pheochromocytoma	**Suggested criteria for size of T wave**
Minor T wave changes – hyperventilation, postprandial, mitral valve prolapse, pneumothorax, LVH	1/8 size of the R wave
	< 2/3 size of the R wave
	Height <10 mm

Table 8.6 Causes of U wave abnormalities [6–14]

U waves
Prominent:
Hypokalaemia
Hypercalcaemia
Digitalis toxicity
Exercise
Congenital long QT interval
Antiarrythmic agents Class IA & 3
Thyrotoxicosis
Intracranial haemorrhage
Inverted U:
IHD
Left ventricular volume overload

abnormalities are discussed in Tables 8.3, 8.4, 8.5 and 8.6, and Figs. 8.4 and 8.5 [3, 5–7, 11, 12].

Finally, interpretation should conclude with the designation (a) normal ECG, (b) border line ECG, or (c) abnormal ECG.

Regularity of the rhythm can be assessed by measuring the R–R interval using either an index card or calipers [7]. If the rhythm varies by 0.12 second or more between the shortest and longest R wave (on the index card), the rhythm is reported to be irregular; if it varies by less than 0.12 second, the rhythm is regular [7].

8.1.7
Artefacts in ECG

Incorrect placement of ECG chest electrodes (leads) is a major source of error, introducing short-term variations in amplitude and waveform of chest lead ECGs [15]. However, artefacts can also be due to hypothermia, electric interference, etc.

8.1.8
QRS Axis

In general, the cardiac axis indicates the direction that the depolarisation wave takes as it flows through the ventricle. The ventricular depolarisation axis is determined by the QRS complex axis [6–14] (Fig. 8.6). In general, the QRS axis may shift due to physical change in the position of the heart, chamber hypertrophy, or conduction blockage [6–14]. The normal QRS axis is from around −30° to +90°, less than −30° is termed left axis deviation and greater than +90° is termed right axis deviation. When more electrical forces move to the right than normal, a right axis deviation is noted on the ECG [6–14]. When the electrical forces take longer (prolonged) time to the ventricle, or electrical forces move to the left, a left axis deviation is noted on the ECG [6–14]. Common causes of these deviations are detailed in Table 8.7. The QRS axis can be assessed by various methods such as:

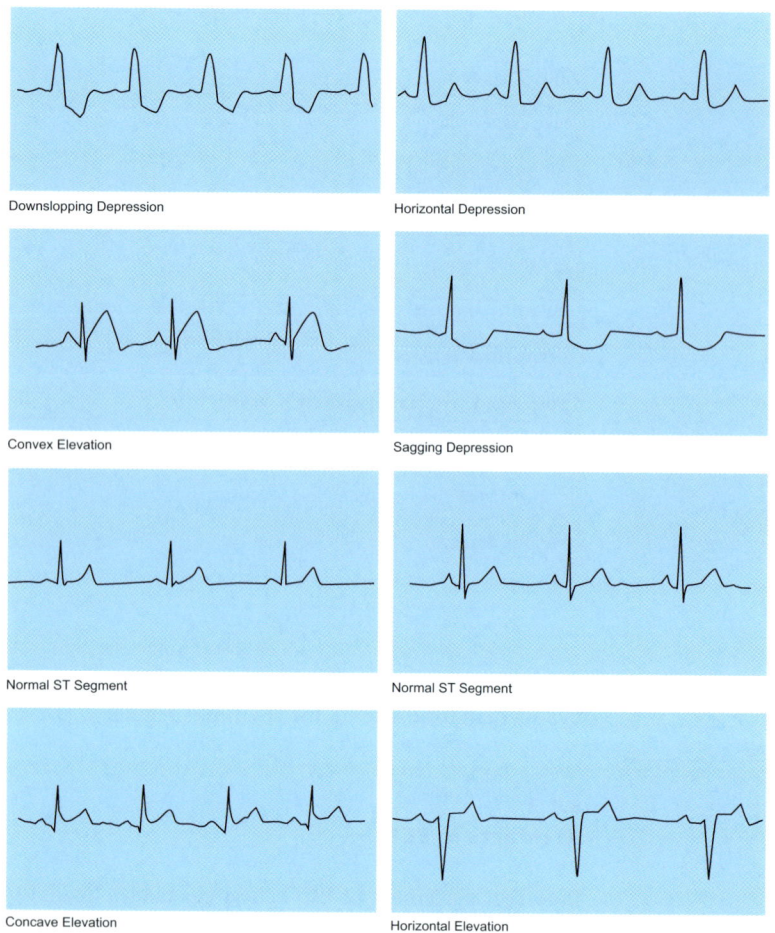

Fig. 8.4 Examples of types of ST segment

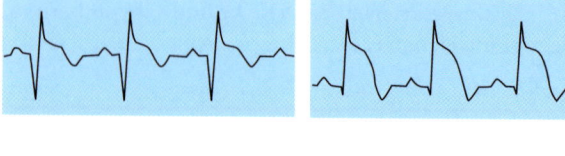

Fig. 8.5 ST elevation inverted T

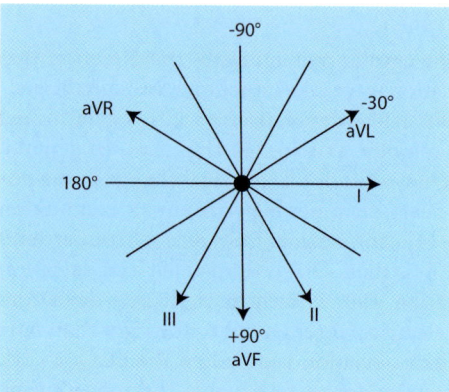

Fig. 8.6 Hexial reference system

(a) a vector method; (b) inspection; and (c) an equiphasic lead method. QRS axis assessment using the inspection method is faster than using the vector method, and is done by checking QRS orientation [6–14].

8.1.9
Sinus Rhythm, Sinus Bradycardia and Sinus Tachycardia

In a normal sinus rhythm, impulses are formed in the sinoatrial node (SA) and these are discharged at a regular rate 60–100 times/minute [5] (Fig. 8.7a). The normal sinus rhythm of the heart has no clinical significance. Sinus bradycardia originates in the SA node and discharges the impulses regularly at ta rate between 40 and

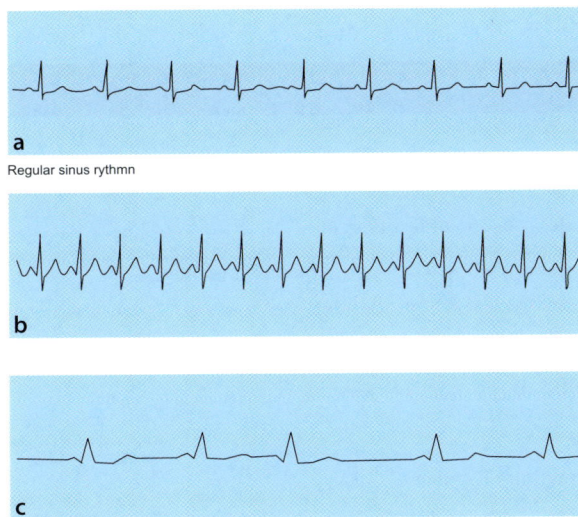

Fig. 8.7 **a** Normal sinus rhythm; **b** sinus tachycardia; **c** sinus arrhythmia

Table 8.7 Common causes of QRS axis deviation and ECG features [6–14]

Common causes of right axis deviation
Left posterior hemi block
Normally found in children
Normally found in thin and tall adults
Anterior lateral MI
Right ventricular hypertrophy (RVH)
Left ventricular disease
Chronic obstructive lung disease (without pulmonary hypertension)
Pulmonary embolism
Atrial septal detect (ASD)
Ventricular septal detect (VSD)
Common causes of left axis deviation
Left ventricular hypertrophy (less than −30°)
Left anterior hemi block
WPW syndrome
Inferior wall MI (Q waves)
Tricuspid atresia
Hyperkalaemia
Emphysema
Ostium primum ASD
Artificial cardiac pacing
Axis:
−30° to +90°: normal
−30° to −90°: left axis
+90° to +180°: right axis
−90° to −180°: indeterminate.
OR
Normal cardiac axis: Lead I-positive QRS and Lead II-positive QRS
Left axis deviation: Lead I- positive QRS and Lead II-Negative QRS
Right axis deviation: Lead I -negative QRS and Lead II-positive QRS

and 60/minute [5]. In general, conditions increasing the parasympathetic tone and decreasing the sympathetic tone causes sinus bradycardia (Table 8.8) [6–14].

Sinus tachycardia originates in the SA node and discharges impulses at a regular rate between 100 and 160 beats/minute [5]. In general, conditions decreasing the parasympathetic tone and increasing the sympathetic tone causes sinus tachycardia.

8.1.10 Sinus Arrhythmias

These arise from disturbances in the impulse discharge or impulse conduction from the sinus node [7]. The heart rate may be normal and may result from variation in the autonomic tone. The heart rate gradually increases during inspiration and decreases during expiration. The distinguishing feature of this rhythm is the sinus origin and irregular rhythm [7]. Sinus arrest is caused by a failure of the SA node to produce a discharge impulse and the underlying rhythm will not resume on time after the pause [7]. In sinus exit block, the impulses are generated by the SA node but are blocked as they exit the sinus node, thus preventing conduction of the impulse to the atria [7]. The pause associated with both sinus arrest and sinus exit block may be short or transient producing no or some symptoms such as hypotention, dizziness or syncope [7]. However, sometimes it may produce longer pauses and then lose pacemaker control. The common causes and ECG patterns of sinus arrhythmias are discussed in Table 8.8 and Fig. 8.7b and 8.7c [6–14].

Table 8.8 Causes and ECG features of sinus arrhythmias [6–14]

Common causes	ECG findings
Sinus arrhythmia	
Normal phenomenon	**Rhythm** – irregular
Variations in autonomic tone	**Rate** – 60–100 or less than 60
Associated with phases of respiration	**P waves** – normal configuration and direction. P waves precedes each QRS complex
Common among children and elderly	**PR interval** – 0.12–0.20 seconds
	QRS – 0.10 seconds or less
Sinus tachycardia	
Exercise	**Rhythm** – Regular
Hypertension	**Rate** – 100–160
Hypoxia	**P waves** – normal configuration and direction. P waves precedes each QRS complex
Cardiac failure	PR interval – 0.12-0.20 seconds
Anaemia	**QRS** – 0.10 seconds or less
Pulmonary embolism	
Acute pericarditis	
Sinus node dysfunction	
Drugs (adrenaline, noradrenaline, dobutamine, dopamine, atropine, tricyclic antidepressants)	
Pregnancy	
Thyrotoxicosis	
Anxiety/excitement /fever	
Sinus bradycardia	
Normal in athletes	**Rhythm** – Regular
Beta-blockers, Calcium channel blockers	**Rate** – 40–60
Sleep	**P waves** – normal configuration and direction. P waves precedes each QRS complex
Hypothyroidism	**PR interval** – 0.12–0.20 seconds
Obstructive jaundice	**QRS** – 0.10 seconds or less
Uremia	
Sinus node dysfunction	
Glaucoma	
Raised intra cranial pressure	
Vasovagal syncope	

Table 8.8 *(continued)* Causes and ECG features of sinus arrhythmias [6–14]

Common causes	ECG findings
Sinus arrest and sinus exit block	
Nausea, vomiting, valsalva maneuver, carotid sinus massage	**Rhythm** – usually regular and irregular during pause
SA node damage or dysfunction, sick sinus syndrome	**Rate** – normal (60–100) or less (<60)
Hyperkalemia and hypoxia	**P waves** – P waves present with underlying rhythm and absent during pause
Digitalis, beta blockers and calcium channel blockers	**PR interval** – normal during underlying rhythm and absent during pause
Differentiating features:	**QRS** – normal during underlying rhythm and absent during pause
Sinus block: underlying rhythm resumes on time after pause	
Sinus arrest: underlying rhythm does not resumes on time after pause	

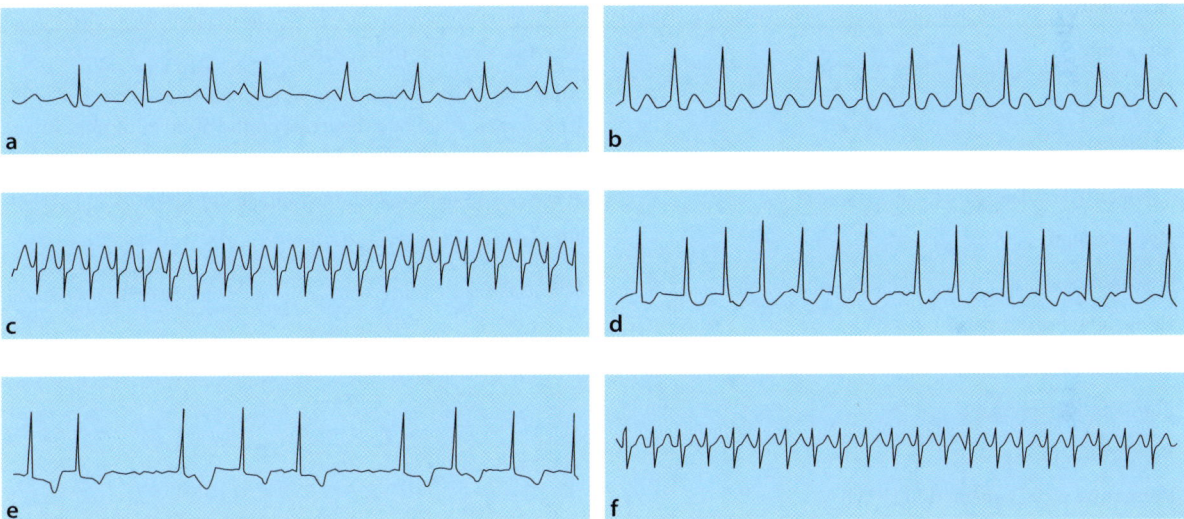

Fig. 8.8 **a** Premature atrial contractions; **b** atrial flutter; **c** paroxysmal atrial tachycardia; **d** atrial fibrillation (controlled rate) **e** controlled rate; **f** atrial tachycardia

8.1.11
Atrial Arrhythmias

In general, atrial arrhythmias originate from ectopic sites in the atria and the P waves will have different configurations. In fast atrial rhythms, the abnormal P wave is either superimposed on the preceding T wave or may have a sawtooth or wavy pattern [7–11]. In slow atrial arrhythmias, the P wave is often small, upright or invisible and if it originates from the lower atrium, it may be inverted. Various atrial arrhythmias such as paroxysmal atrial tachycardia (PAT), atrial flutter, premature atrial contraction (PAC), atrial fibrillation and wandering trail pacemaker can occur [7–11] (Table 8.9, Fig. 8.8a–e). The basic mechanism often responsible for atrial arrhythmias is altered automaticity and re-entry [7].

PAC originates from an ectopic pacemaker in the atria and is caused by enhanced automaticity in the atrial tis-

Table 8.9 Causes and ECG features of atrial arrhythmias [6–14]

Common causes	ECG findings
Atrial fibrillation	
Idiopathic	**Rhythm** – grossly irregular
Hypertension (HTN)	**Rate** – atrial rate is 400 or more; ventricular rate varies with number of impulses conducted through AV node to ventricles
Mitral valve prolapse	
Thyrotoxicosis	**P waves** – irregular wavy deflections (f waves)
Cardiomyopathy	**PR interval** – not measurable
Hypothyroidism	**QRS** – normal
Hyperkalemia	
Sepsis	
Sick sinus syndrome	
Cardiac surgery	
Alcohol	
Atrial flutter	
Idiopathic	**Rhythm** – regular or irregular
IHD	**Rate** – atrial rate is 250–400; ventricular rates varies and will be less than atrial rate (depends on the number of impulses conducted through AV node)
Cardiomyopathy	
Valvular heart disease	**P waves** – V-shaped with sawtoothed appearances
Hypertension	**PR interval** – not measurable
Cor pulmonale	**QRS** – normal
Congenital heart disease	
Thyrotoxicosis	
Pulmonary embolism	
Pericarditis, myocarditis	
Premature atrial contraction (PAC)	
Emotional stress	**Rhythm** – underlying rhythm is regular and the becomes irregular with PACs
Alcohol, coffee/nicotine	**Rate** – underlying rhythm
Electrolyte imbalances (low potassium or magnesium)	**P waves** – associated with PACs is premature and abnormal in size, shape or direction
Hypoxia	**PR interval** – prolonged or normal
Myocardial ischaemia, coronary artery disease	**QRS** – normal
Chronic lung disease	
Digitalis toxicity	
Hyperthyroidism	
Dilated/hypertrophied atria	
Adrenaline, Isoproteronol, Theophylline	

Table 8.9 *(continued)* Causes and ECG features of atrial arrhythmias [6–14]

Common causes	ECG findings
Wandering atrial pacemaker (WAP)	
Increased vagal tone	**Rhythm** – regular or irregular
Chronic lung disease	**Rate** – normal or may be slower
Mitral and tricuspid valvular disease	**P waves** – vary in shape, size and direction
Digitalis	**PR interval** – vary depending on the changing pacemaker location
	QRS – normal
Paroxysmal atrial tachycardia (PAT)	
Exercise	**Rhythm** – regular (with exception of PAC)
Drugs	**Rate** – normal (may vary)
Hypoxia, Hypovolemia	**P waves** – normal and precedes QRS complex
Fever	**PR interval** – PR associated with early beat is longer than normal
Anxiety	
AMI	**QRS** – normal
Congestive heart failure	

sue [7]. It may originate from a single ectopic or multiple sites in the atria. The P wave is abnormal and its location depends on the location of the ectopic pacemaker site. A non-conducted PAC results from an ectopic atrial focus so early that it finds the AV node refractory and the impulses are not conducted to the ventricles [7].

PAT originates from an ectopic pacemaker in the atria and is caused by rapid firing from an ectopic atrial site from accelerated automaticity or a re-entry circuit [7–11]. It starts and ends abruptly and is often initiated by PAC. The rate is between 140 and 250/minute [7]. The P waves may be difficult to identify because they are often hidden in the preceding T waves. In general, the causes of PAT are similar to PACs. PACs may appear as a single beat, every other beat (bigeminal), every third beat (trigeminal), every fourth beat (quadrigeminal) in pairs (couplets) or in runs. Frequent PACs may trigger more serious arrhythmias such as PAT, atrial tarchycardia, atrial flutter and fibrillation [7–11].

Atrial flutter results from rapid accelerated automaticity or due to a rapid re-entry circuit in the atria [7–11]. The atria are depolarised at rates of 250–400/minute by producing wave deflection called flutter waves (F waves). A typical atrial flutter consists of an initial negative component followed by a positive component producing a sawtooth appearance [7].

Atrial fibrillation is an arrhythmia arising from multiple ectopic pacemakers or sites of rapid re-entry circuits [7–11]. The atrial are depolarised at rates of 400/minute or more. These waves are called fibrillatory waves (f waves) and if the waves are large, they are called coarse fibrillatory waves. The wave deflection in both atrial flutter and fibrillation affects the whole baseline and are sometimes seen mixed. In general, atrial fibrillation is recognised by a wavy baseline and a grossly irregular ventricular rhythm [7–11]. The clinical significance of atrial fibrillation and flutter is similar and their causes are described in Table 8.9. Finally, a wandering atrial pacemaker occurs when the pacemaker site shifts back and forth between the sinus node, other atrial sites and occasionally the AV node [7]. In general, it is thought to occur because of multiple pacemaker sites competing with each other for control of the heart [7].

8.1.12
Junctional Atrioventricular (AV) Arrhythmias

Junctional AV arrhythmias originate from an area around the AV node [6, 7] The AV node can function as a secondary pacemaker site if the SA node fails to function Because it contains specialised pacemaker cells. The inherent firing rate of the functional pacemaker is around 40–60/minute and the rhythm occurring at this rate is called the junctional rhythm [6, 7]. Occasionally the firing may exceed its inherent rate resulting in arrhythmias such as premature junctional contractions (PJC), accelerated junctional rhythm and junctional tachycardia

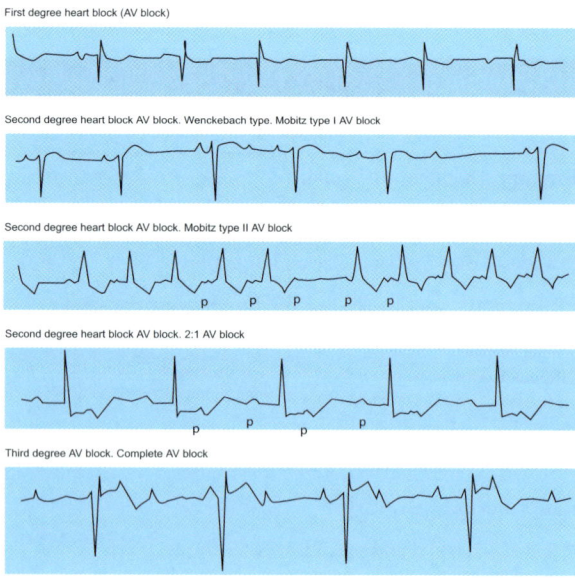

Fig. 8.9 Examples of types of conduction or heart blocks

[6, 7]. The PJC is caused by the enhanced automaticity of the junctional tissue that originates from a beat from the ectopic pacemaker site in the AV junction. The PJC is characterised by an abnormal P wave and they occur in similar patterns to the PACs (single/pairs; bigeminy/trigeminy, etc.). However, PACs are more common than PJCs [6, 7]. Occasionally the ectopic junctional beats will occur late instead of early and these are called juctional escape beats [6, 7].

Junctional rhythm is an arrhythmia originating in the AV junction with a rate of 40–60 beats/minute [7] and is often called a junctional escape rhythm. Junctional rhythm is the normal response of the AV junction when the rate of the dominant pacemaker (SA node) becomes less than the rate of the AV node or when the impulses from SA node fail to reach the AV node [7]. Accelerated junctional rhythm can be seen in a number of clinical situations and is usually transient. The accelerated junctional rhythm also originates from the AV junction with a rate between 60 and 100 (accelerated) and is caused by enhanced automaticity of the AV Junctional tissue [6–13]. Accelerated junctional rhythm is a continuous rhythm, which is usually transient in nature and commonly seen because of digitalis toxicity [6–13].

8.1.13
AV Blocks

AV blocks occur when there is delayed or failed conduction of supraventricular impulses through the AV node into the ventricles. These conduction disturbances could be transient or permanent and the site of pathology could be at the level of the AV node or just below the AV node in the bundle of His or in its branches [6, 7]. AV heart blocks are classified into first degree, second degree (type I and type II) and third degree (Fig. 8.9). This classification is based on the site of the block and severity of the conduction disturbances, and the ability to diagnose them accurately needs careful scrutiny [6, 7].

The sinus impulse is conducted to the AV node normally there is then a delay at the AV node to conduct the impulses to the ventricles. This delay results in the first-degree AV block, which is an abnormal sinus rhythm with prolonged PR interval [6, 7]. The first degree AV block requires no treatment, but needs to be monitored as it may progress to higher blocks [6, 7].

The second-degree AV block is of two types, the type I (Mobitz I or Wenckebach) and type II (Mobitz II) [6, 7]. The type I second-degree AV block is due to the failure of some sinus impulses to be conducted to the ventricles. The impulses are conducted normally to the AV node and thereafter each impulse has more and more difficulty passing through the AV node, until an impulse does not pads through. The common location of conduction disturbances is at the level of the AV node. Although the mechanism of type II AV block is similar to that of type I, there are a few differences, such as the location (below the AV node in the bundle of His or its bundle branches), severity of conduction disturbances and ECG features [6–13]. The QRS complex may be narrow (if located in the bundle of His) and wide (if located in the bundle branches). However, the most common location is the bundle of His. In general, Mobitz II is less common and more serious than Mobitz type I because of its anatomical location (lower in the conducting system) [6–13].

The third-degree AV block, also called the complete heart block, represents complete absence of conduction between atria and ventricles. In this condition, the atria and ventricles beat independently and there is no relationship between atrial and ventricular activity. The common causes and ECG patterns of AV blocks are discussed in Table 8.10 [6–14].

8.1.14
Ventricular Arrhythmias

Ventricular arrhythmias originate below the bundle of His in the right or left ventricle [6, 7]. The electrical impulses arise from the ventricular tissue and spread to the ventricle in an abnormal fashion. The resultant QRS complexes are abnormal and ventricular arrhythmias include ventricular tachycardia, premature ventricular contractions (PVCs), ventricular fibrillations, idioven-

Table 8.10 Causes and ECG features of AV junctional arrhythmias and AV blocks [6–14]

Common causes	ECG findings
First degree AV block	
Increased vagal tone	**Rhythm** – Regular
Idiopathic	**Rate** – Heart rate is that of underlying rhythm; atrial and ventricular
IHD	**P waves** – Sinus; P waves precedes each QRS complex
Rheumatic carditis	**PR interval** – Prolonged (> 0.2 second)
Digoxin toxicity	**QRS** – Normal
Betablockers	
Electrolyte disturbances – hyperkalemia	
Calcium channel blockers	
Degeneration of conduction pathways	
Second degree AV block type I (Wenkeback/Mobitz I)	
Inferior MI	**Rhythm** – Atrial is regular, ventricular is irregular
Digoxin toxicity	**Rate** – Atrial is that of underlying rhythm (sinus); ventricular rate will depend on number of impulses conducted through the AV node (will be less than atrial)
Beta blockers	
Calcium channel blockers intoxication	**P waves** – Sinus
Increased vagal tone	**PR interval** – Varies and progressively lengthens until a P wave occurs without a QRS
	QRS – Normal
Second degree AV block type II (Mobitz II)	
Degenerative disease of the conducting system	**Rhythm** – Atrial is regular. Ventricular is regular (unless the AV conduction ratio varies)
Anteroseptal MI	**Rate** – Atrial is that of underlying rhythm (sinus); ventricular rate will depend on number of impulses conducted through the AV node (will be less than atrial)
	P waves – Sinus; two or three P waves before each QRS
	PR interval – Normal or prolonged
	QRS – Normal if located in bundle of His and is wide if located in bundle branches
Third degree heart block	
Infranodal degenerative fibrosis	**Rhythm** – Atrial is regular. Ventricular is regular
MI (anteroseptal-permanent; inferior-transient)	**Rate** – Atrial is that of underlying rhythm (sinus); ventricular rate will be between 40 and 60 (if paced by AV node) and between 30 and 40 (if paced by ventricles)
Digitalis toxicity	
Beta blockers	**P waves** – Sinus P waves
Congenital	**PR interval** – Varies
After cardiac surgery	**QRS** – Normal if located at the level of AV node or bundle of His and is wide if blocked at the level bundle branches
Acute myocarditis	

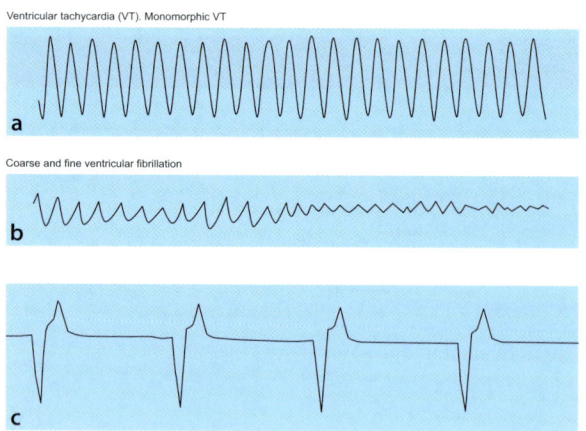

Fig. 8.10 **a** Ventricular tachycardia; **b** coarse and fine ventricular fibrillation; **c** idioventricular rhythm

tricular rhythm, accelerated idioventricular rhythm and ventricular standstill [6–14].

PVC is an ectopic impulse originating in one of the ventricles (right or left) and is caused by increased automaticity. The PVCs may appear as a single beat, every other beat (bigeminal), every third beat (trigeminal), every fourth beat (quadrigeminal) in pairs (couplets) or in runs. PVCs are termed ventricular tachycardia (VT) if there is a run of three or more consecutive PVCs [6–13].

In general PVCs can be classified as unifocal (arising from a single or the same focus, identical in shape, size and direction) and multifocal (arising from different foci with different shape, size and direction) [6–13]. A PVC is called interpolated when it is sandwiched between two normally conducted sinus beats, without greatly disturbing the rhythm [6, 7] and R on T phenomenon is a term used to indicate a PVC that occurs during the vulnerable period of ventricular repolarisation. If the ventricular beat occurs late instead of early, it is called ventricular escape beats and is more likely as a result of increased vagal effects on the SA node [6–13].

Ventricular tachycardia (VT) originates from an ectopic focus in the ventricles, discharging at a rate of 140–250/minute [6, 7] (Fig. 8.10a). The rhythm is associated with re-entry or increased automataticity. The rhythm on the ECG appears as a series of wide QRS complexes, usually with the absence of P waves (occasionally hidden in the QRS complexes) [6–13]. VPCs may occur at rates greater than 250/minute and the QRS complexes may appear as a sawtooth (ventricular flutter). In general, VT is often preceded by frequent and repetitive ventricular ectopy. VT may occur as a sustained (lasting more than 30 seconds) or as a non-sustained (lasting less than 30 seconds) rhythm [6–13]. In general non-sustained VT is rare and does not cause any haemo-dynamic compromise. But it can progress to sustained VT, which is life threatening. VT can be monomorphic (stable or unstable) with a pulse or polymorphic. Finally, a special type of polymorphic VT called Torsedes de pointes (twisting of the points) occurs [6, 7]. This classically occurs in a setting of delayed ventricular repolarisation. Recognition of torsedes de pointes is vital, as the treatment differs from monomorphic VT [6, 7].

Ventricular fibrillation is a chaotic, disorganised electrical focus in the ventricle and the ventricle beats ineffectively and asynchronously similar to the atria in atrial fibrillation [7]. The P and QRS complexes are absent as organised depolarisation from the atria and ventricle is absent. The fibrillatory waves may be large (coarse ventricular fibrillation) or small (fine ventricular fibrillations) (Fig. 8.10b). Clinically these may be important because coarse ventricular fibrillations indicate a more recent onset (reversed by defibrillations alone) and in contrast, fine fibrillations indicate arrhythmias present over a period and may require drug treatment to start before defibrillation [6–9].

Idioventricular rhythm (IVR) or ventricular escape rhythm originates in a subsidiary pacemaker site in the ventricles, with a heart rate between 30 and 40/minute (Fig. 8.10c) [6–9]. It occurs when the rate of impulse in the dominant pacemaker (SA node) and the backup pacemaker in the AV node is less than the ventricular pacemakers or when the impulses from the SA node, atria or AV node fail to reach the ventricles due to sinus arrest, sinus block or third degree AV block [6, 7]. Ventricular escape rhythm may be transient or continuous. IVR is termed accelerated IVR (AVIR) (50–100/minute), when the rate exceeds the inherent IVR rate (30–40/minute) [6, 7]. AVIR is a transient phenomenon and usually seen after an inferior wall myocardial infarction [6, 7]. Finally, ventricular standstill/ventricular aystole occurs in the absence of all electrical activities in the ventricles [6, 7]. The ECG tracing may show a straight line or P waves without complexes. During ventricular standstill the patient becomes unconscious (no cardiac output, peripheral pulses and blood pressure) and death is imminent unless the arrhythmia is treated. The common causes and ECG patterns of ventricular arrhythmias are discussed in Table 8.11 [6–14].

8.1.15
Bundle Branch Block

In general, bundle branch block (BBB) refers to an obstruction in the transmission of electrical impulses though one of its branches (left or right) [5–9]. The electrical impulse normally travel through the right bundle branch and the left bundle branch and their fascicles simultaneously, thereby leading to synchronous depo-

Table 8.11 Causes and ECG features of ventricular arrhythmias [6-14]

Common causes	ECG findings
Ventricular premature beats (VPC)	
Normal individuals	**Rhythm** – Regular
IHD	**Rate** – Normal (usually)
Left ventricular dysfunction	**P waves** – Normal and precedes QRS complex (except with premature beat, when there is no P)
Digoxin toxicity	**PR interval**
Every other beat-bigeminy	**QRS** – Normal (except with premature beat, when there is wide and bizarre QRS)
Every third beat-trigeminy	
One in a row is isolated VPC	
Two in a row couplet/pair	
Three in a row is VT	
Ventricular tachycardia[VT] (polymorhic)	
IHD	**Rhythm** – Regular or slightly irregular
Left ventricular dysfunction	**Rate** – 140–250
Electrolyte imbalance	**P waves** – Often obscured by ORS and may be inverted
Long QT interval	**PR interval** – Cannot be measured or difficult to determine
Acute myocardial infarction	**QRS** – Wide and beyond 0.12 second
Catecholamine sensitivity	
Normal individuals	
Torse de pointes	
AV block	**Rhythm** – Regular
Long QT interval	**Rate** – 250
Congenital long QT interval	**P waves** – None identified
IHD	**PR interval** – Cannot be measured or difficult to determine
Amiodarone, Sotolol, Anti-arrhythmic agents (class IA), Tricyclic anti-depressants	**QRS** – Wide, 0.12–0.22 second
Subarachnoid haemorrhage	
Myxoedema	
Hypokalemia, Hypomagnesaemia	
Ventricular fibrillation	
IHD	**Rhythm** – chaotic (irregular)
Cardiomyopathy	**Rate** – 0 (P & QRS complexes are absent)
Mitral valve prolapse	**P waves** – Absent
Cardiac trauma	**PR interval** – Not measurable
Hypoxia	**QRS** – Absent

Table 8.11 (continued) Causes and ECG features of ventricular arrhythmias [6-14]

Common causes	ECG findings
Cocaine toxicity	
Electrolyte imbalances	
Drug toxicity (digitalis, proarrhythmic agents)	
Ventricular standstill/asystole	
Terminal arrhythmia after VT/VF	Rhythm – None/no QRS complexes
Metabolic acidosis	Rate – 0 (QRS complexes are absent)
Hypoxia, Hyperkalemia, Hypokalemia	P waves – Straight line or P waves without QRS complexes
Hypothermia	PR interval – Not measurable
	QRS – Absent
Idioventricular Rhythm	
MI	Rhythm – Usually regular
Electrolyte/metabolic imbalances	Rate – 30–40
Digitalis toxicity	P waves – Absent
Post-resuscitation rhythm	PR interval – Not measurable
	QRS – wide (0.12 second or more)

larisation of both ventricles [6–13]. BBB can be recognised by the presence of bizarre and wide QRS complexes on the ECG. The presence of left bundle branch block (LBBB) is a sign of organic heart disease in most cases. However, in contrast, right bundle branch block (RBBB) may be present in normal patients or in patients with organic heart disease [7–9]. BBB by itself is not significant and usually requires no treatment. The common causes and ECG patterns of bundle branch block are discussed in Table 8.12 (Fig. 8.11a and b) [2, 6–14, 16].

8.1.16
Arial and Ventricular Hypertrophy

The initial part of the P wave is due to right atrial depolarisation and enlargement of the right atrium produces a P wave prominence [5–9]. In left atrial enlargement the P wave duration is of 120 milliseconds or more, with definite

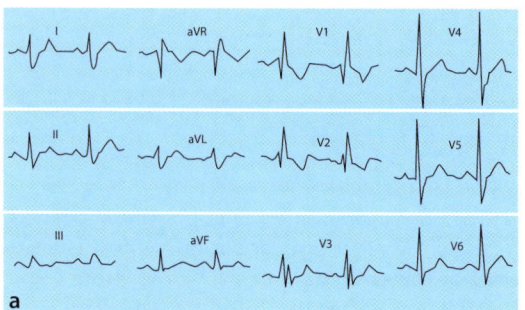
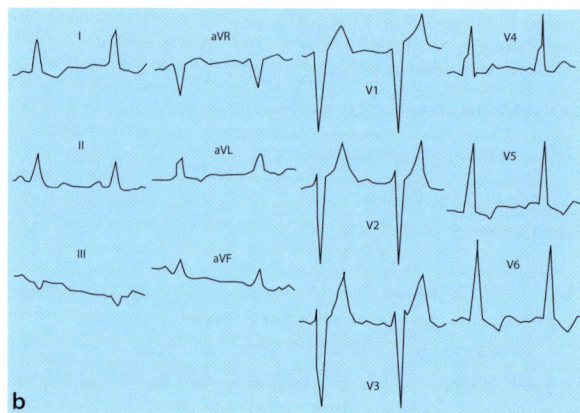

Fig. 8.11 a RBB; b LBBB

Table 8.12 Causes and ECG features of bundle branch blocks [6–14]

Common causes	ECG changes
LBBB	
IHD, HTN	Wide QRS > 0.12 second
Fibrotic degeneration	QRS negative in V1, V2
Congestive cardiomyopathy	QRS positive in V5, V6 (often notched)
Hypertrophic cardiomyopathy	Monophasic R wave, often notched or slurred in lead (absence on normal Q waves) I, aVL, V5, V6
Calcific aortic stenosis	V1, V2 reveal QS or rS pattern with poor R wave progression in V2, V3
Post-cardiac surgery	
Congenital heart disease	
RBBB	
IHD, HTN	Wide QRS (>0.12 second)
Fibrotic degeneration	Secondary R wave in V1 or V2 (rSR', rsR', or rsr' complex often is M shaped)
Atrial septal detect (ASD)	Wide, slurred S wave in leads V5, V6 and I
Cardiomyopathy	Axis may be (a) normal, (b) left axis-consider left anterior fasicular block (hemiblock)
Fallot's tetrology	
Pulmonary embolism	

notching and prominence of the terminal portion of the P wave, or prominent negativity of the terminal portion of the P wave in V1 [17]. Left ventricular hypertrophy (LVH) is an enlargement of the left pumping chamber of the heart and the most common cause is hypertension. Right ventricular hypertrophy is commonly associated with any form of right ventricular outflow obstruction or pulmonary hypertension. The causes and ECG findings are summarised in Table 8.13 [11, 13, 17].

8.1.17
Computers and ECG

Use of computers for the interpretation for ECGs is popular. The computer is programmed to measure ECG parameters such as (a) automatic wavefront recognition section, set valves and control, (b) identification of various rhythms, both normal and abnormal (c) interpretation of previously acquired information, and to recognise changes [18]. These have added advantages, when used properly. Currently the majority of them use some type of automated system to record an ECG [18–20] (Table 8.14). However, it should be emphasised that all these tracings should be checked by qualified personnel to make the final diagnosis. Management of patients based only on a computerised interpretation may lead to medico legal implications due to improper diagnosis and patient care. The ACC/AHA Task force guidelines for electrocardiography clearly states, "There is no computer program that can replace the skilled physician" [2, 18].

8.2
Exercise Stress Testing

An exercise stress test is a screening tool used to test the effect of physiological stress on the heart. It is an inexpensive noninvasive tool that provides cardiopulmonary information in healthy and diseased populations and elicits cardiovascular abnormalities that are not present at rest [21, 22]. During exercise coronary blood

Table 8.13 Causes and ECG features of atrial and ventricular hypertrophy [6–14]

Common causes	ECG changes
Left atrial hypertrophy	
Left ventricular failure	Broad notched P waves
Mitral stenosis	P wave duration >0.12 seconds in II,III,or aVF
Mitral regurgitation	Negative notched P waves in V1
Left ventricular hypertrophy	Depth of negative deflection is V1 >1 mm
Aortic valve disease	
Right atrial hypertrophy	
Congenital heart disease	Tall (>2.5 mm) peaked waves in II (often III and aVF)
Cor pulmonale	Positive component of P wave in lead V1, V2, V3 is tall and peaked (1.5 mm)
Pulmonary stenosis	
Pulmonary hypertension	P frontal axis is greater than 75°
Tricuspid stenosis	
Tricuspid regurgitation	
Right ventricular hypertrophy	
Left ventricular hypertrophy	
Hypertension	Deep S waves in V1, V2
Aortic stenosis	Tall R waves in V5, V6
Coarctation of aorta	ST–T changes (ST depression)
Hypertrophic cardiomyopathy	T wave inversion
Aortic incompetence	Wide QRS-T angle
Mitral imcompetance	**Sokolow–Lyon Voltage Criteria:**
	R wave in lead I + S wave in lead III >25 mm (2.5 mV)
	R wave in V6 > 26 mm (2.6 mV)
	R wave in aVL > 11 mm (1.1 mV)
	R wave in V6 + S wave in V1 > 35 mm (3.5 mV)
	Cornell Voltage Criteria
	S wave in V3 + R wave in aVL > 28 mm in men or > 20 mm in women
Right ventricular hypertrophy	
Pulmonary hypertension	QRS negative in lead I
Fallot tetralogy	QRS positive in lead V1
Pulmonary valve stenosis	ST–T changes
Ventricular septal defect (VSD)	Right axis deviation
Tricuspid incompetence	
Over-transfusion, acute nephritis	

Table 8.14 Possible advantages of using computerised ECG tracing and reporting methods [18]

Faster reports
Optimal utilization of emergency ECG services
Measurements are reproducible
Possible reduction in physicians' reading times
Can handle large throughput
Retrieval with better comparison with previous tracings
Good quality control

Table 8.15 Interpretation and conclusion of exercise stress test [23]

Interpretation of the results
Basic ECG interpretation
Symptoms during stress testing
Reasons for ending exercise
Estimatation of exercise capacity in METS
Blood pressure and heat rate response
Presence and frequency of arrhythmias
Presence and frequency of ectopics
ECG changes during stress and recovery
Final conclusions/interpretation
Positive test
Negative test
Equivocal test
Uninterruptible

flow increases to meet the higher metabolic demands of the myocardium and any factor limiting the coronary blood flow may result in electrocardiographic changes that can be recorded. Exercise stress testing is an important diagnostic and prognostic tool for assessing patients with suspected or known ischaemic heart disease [21, 22]. Exercise stress is commonly performed using a treadmill or a bicycle ergometer.

The stressing team or personnel must be adequately trained and should be aware of all emergency procedures. Regardless of the stress modality used, an appropriate exercise protocol should be used.

The history, physical examination and laboratory studies necessary to evaluate the patient's suitability for performing an exercise stress test should be performed prior to the test. The patient should receive the proper preparatory instructions for the exercise stress test as required [21].

Once the test is completed, the results should be interpreted and this includes reviewing the test results while considering the patient's history, medications and indication for the test. Further, intensity, modality of exercise, frequency and duration should be taken into account (Table 8.15) [21, 23].

8.2.1
Types of Exercise

Three types of muscular contraction or exercise can be applied as a stress to the cardiovascular system:

Isotonic (dynamic or locomotory): Exercise defined as a muscular contraction resulting in movement (e.g. treadmill, ergometer). Isotonic exercise provides a volume load to the left ventricle and response is proportional to the size of working muscle mass and the intensity of exercise [21, 22].

Isometric (static): Exercise defined as a muscular contraction without movement (e.g hand grip). Cardiac output is not increased as much as in isotonic exercise because increased resistance in active muscle group limits blood flow [21, 24].

Resistance (a combination of isometric and isotonic): Exercise that combines both isometric and isotonic exercise (e.g weight lifting).

8.2.2
Rationale for Testing

Exercise testing has been reported to have variable diagnostic accuracy depending on the characteristics of the study population. Meta-analysis studies report a sensitivity of 50–68% and a specificity of 74–90% for detecting coronary artery disease [24]. The clinical utility of the test is its high specificity. Sensitivity will be higher in patients with triple-vessel disease and lower in patients with single-vessel disease. Improvements in sensitivity for single-vessel disease have recently been reported with the use of three right precordial leads in addition to the conventional 12-lead during stress ECG [25]. The exercise ECG results should always be interpreted in the light of the pre-test probability of coronary artery disease [21–23].

Table 8.16 Common indications and contra-indications in exercise stress testing [21–23]

Indications	Contraindications
• Assessment of chest pain	**Absolute**
• Assessment of symptoms like syncope	• Acute myocardial infarction (within 2 days)
• Severity of ischaemic heart disease	• Unstable angina (rest pain in previous 48 hours)
• Prognosis of ischaemic heart disease	• Uncontrolled cardiac arrhythmias causing symptoms or hemodynamic compromise
• Risk stratification after myocardial infarction	• Symptomatic severe aortic stenosis
• Evaluation of medical, revascularization and surgical therapy for ischaemic heart disease	• Uncontrolled symptomatic heart failure
• Screening for latent coronary heart disease	• Acute pulmonary embolus and pulmonary infarction
• Detection of labile hypertension	• Acute myocarditis or pericarditis
• Evaluation of congestive heart failure	• Acute aortic dissection
• Evaluation of arrhythmias	• Severe pulmonary hypertension
• Evaluation of functional capacity	**Relative**
• Evaluation of congenital heart disease and cardiomyopathies	• Left main coronary stenosis
	• Moderate stenotic valvular heart disease
	• Electrolyte abnormalities
	• Severe arterial hypertension (systolic > 200 mmHg, diastolic > 110 mmHg) [3]
	• Tachyarrythmias
	• Bradyarrythmias
	• Severe hypertrophic obstructive cardiomyopathy or other outflow tract obstructions
	• Mental or physical impairment leading to inability to exercise adequately
	• High degree atrioventricular block

8.2.3 Indications and Contra-Indications

Table 8.16 summarises the currently accepted indications and contra-indications for exercise stress testing. In general, contraindication is classified as absolute and relative. Exercise stress test may often worsen the clinical scenario in high-risk patients such as unstable angina, sustained uncontrolled arrhythmia, cardiac failure, high-grade heart blocks. In such patients extra vigilance during the test is important.

8.2.4 Equipment

Treadmills and cycle ergometers are used for exercise testing. Cycle ergometers are generally less expensive than treadmills, occupy less space and produce less motion of the upper body, which makes monitoring convenient. However, the easy fatigue of the quadriceps muscles in patients who are not experienced cyclists is a major limitation. In contrast, treadmills are easy to use by all age groups. It has been observed that patients can

Table 8.17 Bruce protocol (modified from M.H. Ellestead (2003) Stress Testing Principles and Practice, 5th edn, Stress Testing Protocol. Oxford University Press [22])

Stage	Speed	Grade	Time	Cumulative time
1	1.7	10	3 min	3 min
2	2.5	12	3	6
3	3.4	14	3	9
4	4.2	16	3	12
5	5	18	3+	15+

Table 8.18 Submaximal protocol (modified from modified from M.H. Ellestead (2003) Stress Testing Principles and Practice, 5th edn, Stress Testing Protocol. Oxford University Press [22])

Stage	Speed	Grade	Time	Cumulative time
1	1.5	0	3 min	3 min
2	1.5	4	3	6
3	1.5	8	3	9
4	1.7	10	3	12
5	2	12	3+	15+

be reluctant to push on because of fatigue on an ergometer. It is easier to obtain their cooperation on a treadmill, as it is difficult for them to stop voluntarily on a moving treadmill.

8.2.5 Stress Protocols

Exercise testing is commonly performed using a treadmill or a bicycle ergometer. The treadmill has been shown to have greater diagnostic sensitivity than the bicycle ergometer. The bicycle ergometer is more appropriate for those individuals with limitations such as obesity or difficulty in walking. In general, the Bruce protocol is the most common.

8.2.5.1 Treadmill

The protocols for exercise testing include an initial warm-up (low load), progressive uninterrupted exercise with increasing loads and an adequate time interval at each level, and a recovery period. The Bruce protocol starts at 4.6 METS of work, a speed of 1.7 mph and a gradient of 10°. Each 3 minutes the workload is increased by a combination of increasing the speed and the gradient of the treadmill [21, 22, 24].

The Bruce protocol (Table 8.17) is the most widely adopted protocol and has been extensively validated [21, 22]. The protocol has seven stages, each lasting 3 minutes, resulting in a 21 minutes exercise for a complete test. In stage 1 the patient walks at 1.7 mph (2.7 km) up a 10% incline. Energy expenditure is estimated to be 4.8 METs (metabolic equivalents) during this stage. One MET is the amount of oxygen consumed at rest. It is equivalent to 3.5 mL of oxygen/kg/min. Workload is increased by a combination of increasing the speed and the gradient of the treadmill each 3 minutes [22, 23].

The modified Bruce protocol starts at 2.9 METS of work and its third stage corresponds to the first stage of the Bruce protocol [21–23]. Thus the person who does 9 minutes on the modified Bruce protocol does 3 minutes on Bruce. The optimum protocol for any test should last 6 to 12 minutes and should be adjusted to the subject's needs [21, 22].

A modified sub-maximal protocol (Table 8.18) starts at a lower workload than the Bruce protocol and is used for exercise testing in patients (a) within 2 to 3 weeks of myocardial infarction, (b) with a history of symptoms at a low workload, (c) for those with sedentary habits, and (d) the elderly who are unable to keep up with the pace of the Bruce protocol [21, 22].

8.2.5.2 Cycle

The cycle ergometer is usually less expensive, and it is easy to obtain blood pressure measurements and to record the ECG. However, a major limitation to cycle ergometer testing is discomfort and fatigue in the quadriceps muscles. In this test, the initial power output is usually 10 or 25 W (150 kpm/min), usually followed by increases of 25 W every 2 or 3 minutes until end points are reached [21, 22].

8.2.6 Safety

The exercise stress test has been in use for several decades now and the number of studies performed is continuously on the rise. It is generally considered a safe procedure, however there are reported complication rates of 3.5 infarctions, 48 serious arrhythmias and 0.5–1 deaths per 10,000 [26, 27]. Full cardiopulmonary resuscitation facilities must be available, and test supervisors must be trained in cardiopulmonary resuscitation [21–23] (Table 8.19).

Table 8.19 Essential resuscitation equipment in the stress test room [23]

Defibrillator: regularly charged (with electrode pads)
Suction
Airway and self-inflating ventilation bag
Oxygen
Appropriate oxygen masks
Intravenous cannulas
Drugs/medications: atropine, lignocaine, adrenaline, and sotalol or amiodarone, salbutamol inhaler
Short-acting nitrates: sublingual glyceryl trinitrate/GTN spray

8.2.7
Patient Preparation for Exercise Test [21–23]

Clinical history should be taken, which includes indication, risk factors, medication and prior diagnostic and therapeutic procedures.

(a) The patient should instructed not to eat or smoke for at least 2 or 3 hours before the test.
(b) Patients should come dressed appropriately for exercise.
(c) Nitrates, beta-blockers, calcium antagonists, Dipyridamole (Persantin), Digoxin should be discontinued for the test after consultation with the referring physician.

8.2.8
Interpreting Exercise Test Results [21–23]

(a) An exercise test should end when diagnostic criteria have been reached or when the patient's symptoms and signs dictate termination of the test (Table 8.20).
(b) In clinical practice patients rarely exercise for the full duration (21 minutes) of the Bruce protocol.

Table 8.20 Indications for terminating an exercise test, and measurements available from the exercise stress test [21–23]

Electrocardiographic criteria	**Electrocardiographic**
• Severe ST segment depression (>3 mm) • ST segment elevation >1 mm in non-Q wave lead • Frequent ventricular extrasystoles • Sustained ventricular tachycardia • New atrial fibrillation or supraventricular tachycardia • Development of new bundle branch block • New second or third degree heart block • Cardiac arrest	• Maximum ST depression • Maximum ST elevation • ST depression slope (down, horizontal, up) • Number of leads showing ST changes • Duration of ST deviation in recovery • ST/HR (heart rate) indexes • Exercise induced ventricular arrhythmias • Time to onset of deviation
Symptoms and signs criteria	**Haemodynamic**
• Patient requests stopping because of severe fatigue (most common cause of stopping) • Moderate to severe angina • Decrease in systolic blood pressure >10 mm Hg from baseline, despite an increase in workload, with evidence of ischaemia • Hypertensive response (systolic >250 mm Hg, diastolic >115 mm Hg) (3) • Increasing nervous system symptoms (e.g ataxia, dizziness, near syncope) • Fatigue, dyspnea, leg cramps or claudication	• Maximum exercise heart rate • Maximum exercise blood pressure (BP) • Maximum exercise double product (HR × BP) • Total exercise duration • Exertional hypotension • Chronotropic incompetence
	Symptomatic
	• Exercise induced angina • Exercise limiting symptoms • Time to onset of angina

(c) Reaching 85% of the maximum predicted changes in heart rate is usually satisfactory and can be achieved on completion of 9–12 minutes of exercise.
(d) Maximum predicted heart rate, by convention, is calculated as 220 minus the patient's age.
(e) Attainment of maximum heart rate is a good prognostic sign.
(f) ST segment changes (or arrhythmias) may occur during the recovery period that are not apparent during exercise. Such changes generally carry the same significance as those occurring during exercise.
(g) ECG changes must be interpreted in the light of the probability of coronary artery disease and physiological response to exercise.
(h) A normal test result or a result that indicates a low probability of coronary artery disease is one in which 85% of the maximum predicted heart rate is achieved with a physiological response in blood pressure and no associated ST segment depression (Table 8.21).
(i) A test that indicates a high probability of coronary artery disease is one in which there is substantial ST depression at low work rate associated with typical angina-like pain and a drop in blood pressure (Table 8.22).

Table 8.21 Normal electrocardiographic changes during exercise [21–23]

- P wave increases in height
- R wave decreases in height
- J point becomes depressed
- ST segment becomes sharply up sloping
- Q–T interval shortens
- T wave decreases in height

Table 8.22 Findings suggesting high probability of coronary artery disease [21–23]

- Horizontal ST segment depression >2 mm
- Downsloping ST segment depression
- Early positive response within 6 minutes
- Persistent ST depression for more than 6 minutes into recovery
- ST segment depression in five or more leads
- Exertional hypotension

8.3 Conclusion

ECG is an important investigation preformed routinely in patients presenting with chest pain and it is vital to understand the patterns, variants and limitations of ECG. Exercise testing with a treadmill remains an important part of cardiovascular evaluation and provides valuable information. The exercise treadmill test plays an important role in the diagnosis and management of cardiovascular diseases.

References

1. Macfarlane PW, Lawrie TDV (eds) (1989) Comprehensive Electrocardiography; Theory and Practice in Health and Disease. Pergamon Press, New York.
2. Task Force Report of the American College of Cardiology and the American Heart Association (1992). ACC/AHA Guidelines for Electrocardiography. Circulation 19:473–481.
3. Castellanos A, Interian A, Myerburg RJ (2001) The resting electrocardiogram. In Hurst's The Heart, Fuster V, Alexander RW, O'Rourke RA (eds), pp. 281–314.
4. Taback L, Marden E, Mason HL et al (1959) Digital recording of electrocardiographic data for analysis by a digital computer. IRE Trans Med Electron 6:167–171.
5. Boyle J III (2001) Cardiovascular physiology. In Physiology, 2nd edn, Bullock J et al. (eds). The National Medical Series for Independent Study, pp. 93–148.
6. Khan GM (2003) Rapid ECG Interpretation, 2nd edn. Saunders.
7. Huff J (2002) ECG Workout. Exercises in Arrhythmia Interpretation, 4th edn. Lippincott Williams & Wilkins.
8. Houghton AR, Gray D (2003) Making Sense of the ECG, 2nd edn. Arnold Publishers.
9. Goldschlager N, Goldman MJ (1984) Electrocardiography – Essentials of Interpretation. Lange Medical Publications.
10. Hampton JR (2003) The ECG in Practice. Churchill Livingstone.
11. Chung EK (2001) Pocket Guide to ECG Diagnosis, 2nd edn. Blackwell Science, Malden, MA.
12. Aehlert B (2002) ECGs Made Easy, 2nd edn. Mosby, Inc, St Louis, MO.
13. Jenkins RD, Gerred SJ (2005) ECG by Example Elsevier/Churchill Livingstone.
14. Swanton RH (2003) Cardiac Investigations in Cardiology, 5th edn. Blackwell Publishing
15. Rautaharju PM, Park L, Rautaharju FS, Crow RA (1998) Standardized procedure for locating and documenting ECG chest electrode positions: consideration of the effect

of breast tissue on ECG amplitudes in women. J Electrocardiol 31:17–29.
16. Huszar RJ (2002) Basic Dysrhythmias: Interpretation & Management, 3rd edn. Mosby, St Louis, MO.
17. Atrial and Ventricular Depolarization Changes. www.americanheart.org
18. Brailer DJ, Kroch E, Pauly MV (1997) The impact of computer-assisted test interpretation on physician decision making: the case of electrocardiograms. Med Decision Making 17:80–86.
19. Massel D (2003) Observer variability in ECG interpretation for thrombolysis eligibility: experience and context matter. J Thromb Thrombolysis 15:131–140.
20. Rodger M, Makropoulos D, Turek M et al. (2000) Diagnostic value of the electrocardiogram in suspected pulmonary embolism. Am J Cardiol 86:807–809.
21. Gibbons RJ, Balady GJ, Bricker JT et al. (2002) ACC/AHA (2002) guideline update for exercise testing: a report of the American College of Cardiology/American Heart Association Task force on Practice Guidelines (Committee on Exercise Testing). 2002. American College of Cardiology website. Available at: www.acc.org/clinical/guideline/exercise/dirIndex.htm
22. Ellestad MH (2003) Stress testing protocol. In Stress Testing Principles and Practice, 5th edn. Oxford University Press, Chapter 8.
23. Morise AP, Diamond GA (1995) Comparison of the sensitivity and specificity of exercise electrocardiography in biased and unbiased populations of men and women. Am Heart J 130:741–747.
24. Hill J, Timmis A (2002) Exercise tolerance testing. BMJ 324:1084–1087.
25. Michaelides AP, Psomadaki ZD, Dilaveris PE et al. (1999) Improved detection of coronary artery disease by exercise electrocardiography with the use of right precordial leads. New Eng J Med 340:340–345.
26. Stuart RJ, Ellestad MH (1980). National survey of exercise stress testing fascilities. Chest 77:94.
27. Rochimis P, Blackburn H (1971) Exercise test (1971). A survey of procedures, safety, and litigation experience in approximately 170,000 tests. JAMA 217:1061.

Ambulatory Electrocardiography, Transient Event Monitors, and Continuous Loop Recorders

R. Wayne Kreeger, John Brooks and Assad Movahed

Contents

9.1 Introduction 113
9.2 Summary 114
9.3 Synopsis of ACC/AHA/NASPE Guidelines for Ambulatory EcG Monitoring [12] 115
References 116

9.1 Introduction

Palpitations are sensations of an irregular or rapid heartbeat [1]. Although usually benign, palpitations may be related to dangerous cardiac arrhythmias or portend the likelihood of syncope or near-syncope [2]. If their etiology cannot be discerned from the clinical history, physical examination, or resting electrocardiogram, ambulatory electrocardiographic (AECG) monitoring is recommended [3, 4]. Various modalities exist and their selection depends upon the duration of monitoring likely to capture or record the electrocardiogram during symptoms, whether daily palpitations or sensations separated by days, weeks or even months. The gold standard for diagnosing an arrhythmia is obviously symptom–rhythm correlation. AECG monitoring permits monitoring synchronous with normal daily activity. A standard electrocardiogram is a focal record of 9–10 seconds of the heart's rhythm and rate. The ECG is limited in its dynamic ability since it is a "snapshot" of the heart rhythm. The AECG provides a mechanism to effectively capture the presence and features of an arrhythmia (if one exists) simultaneous with symptoms. True arrhythmogenic symptoms should have corresponding electrocardiographic abnormalities.

Ambulatory electrocardiographic monitoring encompasses continuously recording monitors or Holter monitors as well as patient- or auto-activated event recorders (loop recorders). The latter are either worn by skin-patch leads or application of electrode contact points to the skin synchronous with symptoms. Other types of devices are subcutaneously implanted for longer duration monitoring. Ambulatory ECG monitoring is frequently used for patients with symptoms suspected to be caused by an arrhythmia, such as palpitations, dizziness, or syncope. Holter monitors are worn continuously to record data for several ECG leads while the

the patient keeps a diary of any symptoms and time of occurrence. Named after Dr Norman Holter, these devices are lightweight, battery-operated, and portable. The monitor may be utilized for 24 hours or longer, recording continuous multi-lead electrocardiographic signals by digital or tape format, attempting to simultaneously capture an event to see whether arrhythmogenic or not. The recorded data is converted to digital format for analysis. The Holter monitor's efficacy is limited by the patient's having and capturing the symptoms while the device is on and recording. Its optimal use is for frequent, especially daily, symptoms suspicious for an arrhythmia, such as flutters or palpitations.

Patients with infrequent symptoms have a higher diagnostic yield with either a patient-activated or an auto-activated event recorder set to record synchronous with preset bradycardia and tachycardia threshold criteria [5, 6]. Loop recorders or event monitors are devices similar to Holter monitors but are worn or carried for a longer period of time for post-symptom recording. Implantable loop recorders are pre-symptom recorders with the capability of patient-triggering or activation with symptoms or auto-triggering to record based upon bradycardia or tachycardia parameters. Patient-activated or auto-recording occurs with antegrade and retrograde memory for sandwiching the onset and offset of a brady- or tachyarrythmia. Intermittent recorders, either those transcutaneously applied (and wearable for days to weeks) or those implantable loop recorders that have the capability of capturing events for over a year's time, are especially beneficial for infrequent or widely separated suspected arrhythmic symptoms. Transtelephonic monitors can download recordings to a central monitoring station for analysis; however, different from Holters, they save data for only a couple of minutes at the time of activation. Multiple time-separated events can be stored then retrieved, downloaded, and analyzed either transtelephonically or in the physician's office. The key benefits of implantable recorders (called ILRs or implantable loop recorders) are for infrequent or fleeting episodes separated by days, weeks, or even months. Implantable loop recorders weigh less than 20 grams and are about the size of two French-fries side by side. They have surface electrodes for electrocardiographic single lead monitoring. They are inserted in the left pectoral subcutaneous tissue. ILRs are particularly useful in recurrent unexplained syncope. They store information either automatically, based on programmable rate criteria parameters set at the time of implant, or are externally activated to record by a transcutaneous signaling device to start recording [7]. With any analysis of captured events, the physician's obligation is to assess whether a corresponding arrhythmia is present, whether it is a threat to the patient's well-being or survival, and to formulate a treatment plan. The plan may include simple reassurance, pharmacologic intervention, or a mechanical interventional such as ablation or an implantable cardiac rhythm control device such as a pacemaker or defibrillator.

Syncope and presyncope account for up to 3–6% of emergency room visits as well as 0.5–2% of hospitalizations. Fleeting arrhythmias may have serious consequences such as syncope or presyncope but are often difficult to assess because they may be brief in duration and may not be present at the time of ER or office visit. Misdiagnoses have been made attributing true arrhythmias to anxiety or panic disorders [8]. The utility of any of the monitoring modalities hinges on symptom–rhythm correlation. Short-term cardiac monitoring in a hospital setting is preferred for high risk patients, such as those with obvious electrocardiographic conduction abnormalities at presentation such as rapid tachycardias, profound bradycardias, bundle branch or AV blocks, malfunctioning pacemakers or defibrillators, and especially if symptoms were associated with significant bodily trauma or injury. Yet, in the setting of normal presenting electrocardiograms, short-term monitoring is often unfruitful in making a diagnosis, while longer periods of monitoring enhance the likelihood of capturing events. Some studies have noted that the incidence of detected symptomatic events increases with longer periods of monitoring [9]. Zimetbaum et al. [5] cited six studies comparing 48 hour Holter monitoring versus transtelephonic event monitors. The diagnostic yield was superior with the event monitors, which captured from 66–83% events compared with 33–35% by the Holters [10–12].

9.2
Summary

AECG has utilized computer technology for data retrieval, comparison, quantitation, and analysis for over 20 years. The primary use of AECG is in determining the association of a patient's transient symptoms with any cardiac arrhythmia. Symptom–rhythm correlation occurs with the crucial recording of an ECG during the precise time of symptom onset or occurrence. Yield in syncope is low unless a syncopal episode is captured while the monitor is recording. Holter monitoring sensitivity is low since its usefulness is when symptoms occur daily. Externally worn or applied or implantable recorders enhance the sensitivity of capturing an event. Implantable devices requiring short duration surgical implantation are reserved for highly symptomatic palpitations that are elusive or when other diagnostic modalities for recurrent syncope are inconclusive [7]. Symptom–rhythm correlations occurred most frequently in syncopal and near-syncopal patients in up to 56% of loop recorder patients versus 22% of Holter monitor patients [12]. Ambulatory ECG monitoring is suitable for patients with suspected arrhythmogenic symptoms such as palpitations, light-headedness, "flutters", or syncope. The ability to recognize timing and record symptoms in a diary or have the symptoms logged by another person is important to arrive at a symptom–rhythm correlation. Those patients with daily and frequent symptoms may be evaluated by a 24 or 48 hour Holter monitor. When symptoms occur infrequently, separated by days, weeks, or even months, a patient-activated or implantable device is preferred. Holter monitors are simple and require little interaction by the patient. Patient-activated devices allow capture of symptomatic and asymptomatic arrhythmias but their strengths are extended period of monitoring as well as enhanced sensitivity and specificity by activation at the time of perceived symptoms or preset heart rate criteria.

Guidelines as to when AECG and event monitors are indicated have been developed by the American College of Cardiology (ACC), American Heart Association (AHA), and the Heart Rhythm Society, and were published in 1999 [13]. The guidelines reflect the ever-evolving technology changes and appropriate application of Holter monitors and patient-activated or auto-activated event or loop recorders.

9.3
Synopsis of ACC/AHA/NASPE Guidelines for Ambulatory EcG Monitoring [12]

Recommendations are classed based on their level of evidence as described below.
Class I – Conditions for which there is evidence and/or agreement a procedure or treatment is useful or effective.

Class II – Conditions for which there is conflicting evidence or divergence of opinion about a treatment procedure.
IIa – weight of evidence in favor of usefulness/efficacy
IIb – weight of evidence is less well established

Class III – Conditions for which there is evidence that procedure/treatment is NOT useful/effective

1. The indication to utilize AECG in patients with symptoms of arrhythmia:
   Class I – patients with unexplained syncope, near syncope, or dizziness without identifiable cause
   Class IIb – patients with shortness of breath, chest pain of fatigue which is ill defined; patients with paroxysms of atrial fibrillation/flutter
   Class III – patients with stroke without evidence of arrhythmia; patients with synope/near syncope with an identified cause

2. The indication for ACEG in patients with arrhythmic risks:
   Class I – none
   Class IIb – post-myocardial infarction with LV dysfunction (ef<40%); congestive heart failure; idiopathic hypertrophic cardiomyopathy
   Class III – sustained myocardial contusion, hypertension with LVH, post-myocardial infarction with normal ejection fraction, pre-operative arrhythmia assessment for non-cardiac surgery, sleep apnea, valvular heart disease

3. The indication for AECG in patients after anti-arrythmic therapy:
   Class I – to assess drug response in patients whose rhythm has been recurrent enough to permit analysis.
   Class II – to detect proarrythmic responses to therapy in high risk patients
   Class IIb – to assess rate control in patients with atrial fibrillation; to document recurrent or asymptomatic non-sustained arrhythmia during outpatient therapy

4. Indications for AECG to assess pacemaker and implantable cardioverter defibrillator function:
   Class I – evaluate frequent symptoms of palpitations, syncope or near syncope to assure no pacemaker-induced tachycardia and to assist in enhanced features as rate responsivity and mode switching; evaluation of component failure when device interrogation is not definitive; evaluation of pharmacologic therapy in patients receive therapies from a device
   Class IIb – evaluation of immediate postoperative function of a device; evaluation of supraventricular arrythmias in patients with implantable defibrillators
   Class III – Assessment of device malfunction when device interrogation, ECG or other data are sufficient in elucidating an etiology; routine follow-up in an asymptomatic patient

5. Indication for AECG in monitoring for myocardial ischemia:
   Class I – none
   Class IIa – patients with variant angina
   Class IIb – evaluation of patients with chest pain who cannot exercise; pre-operative evaluation for vascu-

lar surgery who cannot exercise; patients with known coronary artery disease and atypical chest pain syndrome

Class III – initial evaluation of patients with chest pain who are able to exercise; routine screening of asymptomatic patients

References

1. Barsky AJ (2001) Palpitations, arrhythmias, and awareness of cardiac activity. Ann Internal Med 134 (9pt2):832–837.
2. Weber BE, Kapoor WN (1996) Evaluation and outcomes of patients with palpitations. Am J Med 100:138–148.
3. Abbott AV (2005) Diagnostic approach to palpitations. Am Family Physician 71(4):743–750, 755–756.
4. Zimetbaum P, Josephson ME (1998) Evaluation of patients with palpitations. New Eng J Med 338:369–1373.
5. Zimetbaum PJ, Josephson ME (1999) The evolving role of ambulatory arrhythmia monitoring in generally clinical practice. Ann Internal Med 130(10):848–856.
6. Zimetbaum PJ, Kim KY, Josephson ME, Goldberger AL, Cohen DJ (1998) Diagnostic yield and optimal duration of continuous-loop event monitoring for the diagnosis of palpitations. A cost-effective analysis. Ann Internal Med 128(11):890–895.
7. Farwell DJ, Freemantle N, Sulke AN (2004) Use of implantable loop recorders in the diagnosis and management of syncope. Eur Heart J 25(14):1257–1263.
8. Lessmeier TJ, Gamperling D, Johnson-Liddon V, Fromm BS, Steinman RT, Meissner MD et al. (1997) Unrecognized paroxysmal supraventricular tachycardia. Potential for misdiagnosis as panic disorder. Arch Internal Med 157:537–543.
9. Kinlay S, Leitch JW, Neil A, Chapman BL, Hardy DB, Fletcher PJ et al. (1996) Cardiac event recorders yield more diagnoses and are more cost-effective than 48-hour Holter monitoring in patients with palpitations. A controlled clinical trial. Ann Internal Med 124(1pt1):16–20.
10. Fogel RI, Evans JJ, Prystowsky EN (1997) Utility and cost of event recorders in the diagnosis of palpitations, presyncope, and syncope. Am J Cardiol 79:207–208.
11. Zimetbaum PJ, Kim KY, Ho KK, Zebede J, Josephson ME, Goldberger AL (1997) Utility of patient-activated cardiac event recorders in general clinical practice. Am J Cardiol 79:371–372.
12. Morey S (2000) ACC/AHA Guidelines for Ambulatory ECG. American Family Physician, Practice Guidelines, Feb 1.
13. Sivakumaran S, Krahn, AD, Klein GJ, Finan J, Yee R, Renner S, Skanes AC (2003) A prospective randomized comparison of loop recorders versus Holter monitors in patients with syncope or presyncope. Am J Med 115(1):1–5.
14. Crawford MH, Bernstein SJ, Deedwania PC, DiMarco JP, Ferrick KJ, Garson A Jr et al. (1999) ACC/AHA guidelines for ambulatory electrocardiography: executive summary and recommendations. A report of the American College of Cardiology/American Heart Association task force on practice guidelines. Circulation 100(8):886–893.

Chapter 10

Echocardiography and Contrast Echocardiography

Firas A Ghanem, Jaffar Ali Raza, Ishtiaque H. Mohiuddin and Assad Movahed

Contents

10.1	Introduction	117
10.2	Principles of Ultrasound	118
10.3	Imaging Modalities	118
10.4	Doppler Echocardiography	120
10.5	Contrast Echocardiography	120
10.6	Clinical Application of Echocardiography (Table 10.2) [14]	122
10.6.1	Murmurs and Valvular Heart Disease	122
10.6.2	Chest Pain and Ischemic Heart Disease	122
10.6.3	Heart Failure and Assessment of Left Ventricular Function	122
10.6.4	Pericardial Disease	122
10.6.5	Cardiac Masses and Tumors	122
10.6.6	Diseases of the Great Vessels	123
10.6.7	Systemic Hypertension	123
10.6.8	Neurological Disease and other Cardioembolic Disease	123
10.6.9	Arrhythmias and Palpitations	123
10.6.10	Congenital Heart Disease	123
10.7	Newer Devices and Strategies in Echocardiography	123
10.7.1	3D Echocardiography	123
10.7.2	Intracardiac Echocardiography (ICE)	123
10.7.3	Tissue Doppler Echocardiography	124
10.7.4	Strain Doppler Echocardiography (Strain Rate Imaging)	124
10.8	Limitations of Echocardiography (Table 10.3)	124
	References	125

10.1
Introduction

In 1953, Dr. Helmut Hertz of Sweden together with Dr. Inge Edler began to use a commercial ultrasonoscope to examine the heart, thus starting the era of clinical echocardiography [1].

Echocardiography has become an integral part of clinical cardiology. It is used widely in addition to history and physical examination to make the initial diagnosis, management, treatment decision and follow-up of various cardiovascular diseases. It uses the principle of ultrasound reflection off cardiac structures to produce real-time images of the heart. The main purpose of the echocardiogram is to study the structure of the cardiac chambers, valves, septa and the great vessels (the aorta and pulmonary vessels). The M-mode examination obtains a one-dimensional view of the heart whereby distance is plotted against time. Two-dimensional (2D) echocardiography plots distance against distance, and more accurately recreates a spatially oriented heart on either videotape or digital video disc [2]. Doppler technology offers the possibility to demonstrate the intracardiac flow as well as the flow across valves and is particularly useful for the quantitative assessment of valvular stenosis. The use of color flow mapping enables the qualitative assessment of valvular regurgitation [3]. Using various Doppler equations, valve areas, regurgitant fractions, pressure gradients and flow velocities can be calculated. Contrast echocardiography utilizes the interaction of microscopic gas bubbles with ultrasound to augment recognition of blood pool and/or the blood/tissue interface. This can help identify cardiac and extracardiac shunts and a patent foramen ovale (PFO) [4]. The major advantage of echocardiography over other diagnostic modalities is its noninvasiveness and portability, offering the ability to be used in emergency, intraoperative and critical care settings.

10.2
Principles of Ultrasound

Echocardiography uses ultrasound transducers, which have piezoelectric crystals that both generate and receive ultrasound waves. Ultrasound waves between the frequencies 1,000,000 and 20,000,000 Hz (1.0 to 20 MHz) are used in current echocardiogram machines. The velocity of the ultrasound beam within the tissue is related to the frequency and wavelength of the sound wave. It is approximately 1,540,000 mm/s in human tissue. The formula is velocity (m/s) = wavelength (m) × frequency (Hz). The ability to distinguish between two objects that are spatially close together (resolution) varies directly with frequency and inversely with wavelength. Increasing the frequency causes attenuation and decreases the depth of tissue penetration. The distance traveled by the ultrasound wave is directly related to the wavelength and inversely related to the frequency. Hence, transducers with higher frequencies have an increased spatial resolution with a reduction in tissue penetration, and the opposite applies for transducers with increased wavelength.

The ultrasound beam travels in a straight line through a homogeneous medium. When the beam travels through a medium that is not homogeneous or through a medium with two or more interfaces, its path is altered. This relationship between ultrasound waves and tissues is described by the terms reflection, scattering, refraction, and attenuation. Reflection occurs when the ultrasound wave hits a tissue boundary/interface and is reflected back to the transducer, like a mirror. Scattering, refraction and attenuation, all act to decrease the magnitude of the ultrasound wave. Refraction and scattering result in loss of the sound wave and they do not return to the transducer. Attenuation refers to the loss of ultrasound power as it traverses tissue leading to poorer image quality. Attenuation is dependent on the acoustic impedance of the tissue structures. Air has a very high acoustic impedance, resulting in significant signal attenuation, while fluid has low acoustic impedance and generally enhances ultrasound imaging.

As mentioned above, ultrasound transducers use piezoelectric crystals to generate and receive ultrasound waves. These crystals, made of either quartz or titanate ceramic, alternately compress and expand when alternating electric current is applied to generate the ultrasound waves. At a time 1–6 ms after transmission, the same piezoelectric crystal receives the reflected ultrasound waves and generates an electric current. This produces an image based on the distance traveled and the amplitude of the received signal.

There are various kinds of transducers: mechanical transducers physically move the crystal in the transducer while phased-array transducers have a series of crystals arranged so that they can be electronically steered. Currently, phased-array transducers are the most common type used in clinical echocardiography.

Harmonic imaging takes advantage of the sound wave becoming more distorted as it travels further through tissue [5]. This generates additional sound frequencies that are harmonics of the original frequency. Harmonic imaging uses broadband transducers that receive at double the transmitted frequency. As a result, the transducer receives only the additional generated harmonics and filters the fundamental signal; this effectively boosts the signal from deeper structures, acting as a form of depth compensation, enhancing the quality of the images from deeper tissues.

10.3
Imaging Modalities

A comprehensive echocardiographic examination in clinical practice currently involves utilizing both M-mode and 2D recordings to provide adequate information about cardiac anatomy and physiology. M-mode echocardiography has been in use since the 1950s to evaluate the heart. This technique uses a single crystal that rapidly alternates between transmitting and receiving ultrasound waves. Due to their high temporal resolution (>1000 Hz), rapidly moving structures (e. g. valve leaflets) cause reflection of the sound waves resulting in characteristic motion that can be recorded. The ultrasound waves are propagated along the same axis; hence different parts of the heart are studied by changing the direction of the beam manually (Fig. 10.1)

2D guidance is used to ensure proper alignment with the chamber or area of interest. It is very useful in evaluating subtle abnormalities such as fluttering of the anterior mitral leaflet due to aortic insufficiency or movement of vegetations. Although chamber measurements were made in the past by using M-mode, currently they are also made during the 2D examinations. The main drawback of using M-mode echocardiography is that it yields a one-dimensional ("ice-pick") view of the cardiac structures moving over time.

Two-dimensional echocardiography allows the heart to be imaged in real time, giving the operator a sense of both depth and width of the tissue imaged. Hence, it is easier to appreciate the anatomical relationships between various structures. Although various imaging planes through the heart are possible, standard views are used to evaluate the intra and extracardiac struc-

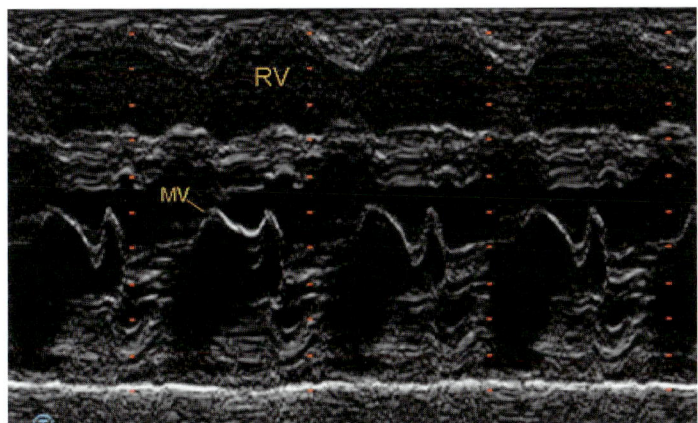

Fig. 10.1 Normal M-mode echocardiogram. MV = mitral valve; RV = right ventricle

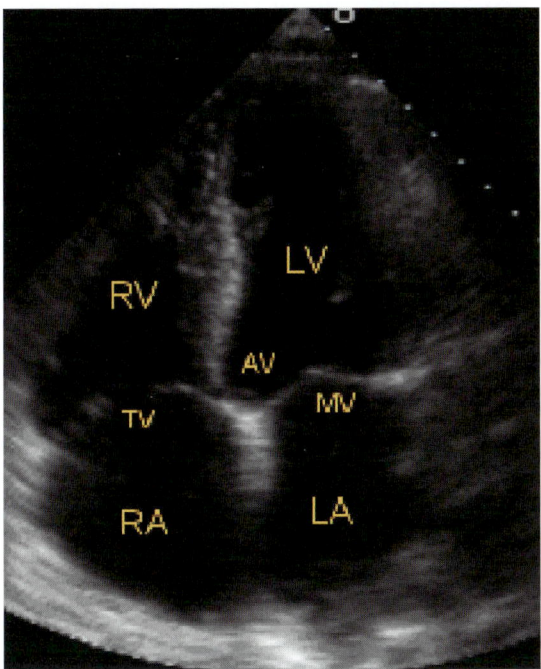

Fig. 10.2 Apical four chamber view. AV = aortic valve, LA = left atrium; LV = left ventricle; MV = mitral valve ; RA = right atrium; RV = right ventricle; TV = tricuspid valve

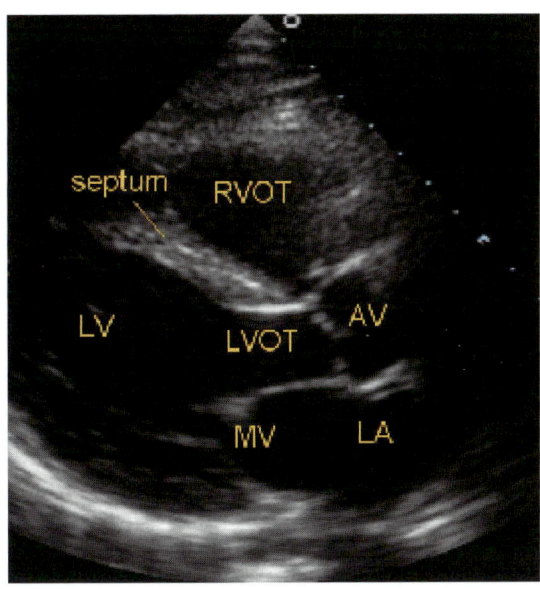

Fig. 10.3 Long axis view (shown from parasternal position). AV = aortic valve, LA = left atrium; LV = left ventricle; LVOT = left ventricular outflow tract MV = mitral valve ; RA = right atrium; RVOT = right ventricular outflow tract

tures. 2D echocardiographic images should be obtained in three orthogonal planes; the long-axis plane transects the heart from the aortic root to the left ventricular apex, the short axis corresponds to the plane of the atrioventricular junction, and the four-chamber plane that is at right angles to both the long and short axes runs from the apex to the base of the heart and is perpendicular to both the interventricular septum and interatrial septum (Figs. 10.2 and 10.3).

10.4
Doppler Echocardiography

$$\Delta F = \frac{V \times 2F_0 \times \cos\theta}{C}$$

where ΔF = change in frequency, V = velocity of RBC, F_0 = transducer frequency, C = velocity of sound in tissue (C = 1540 m/s), θ is the intercept angle between the ultrasound beam and the lines of flow.

The angle θ is of crucial importance in the calculation of blood flow velocities. When the ultrasound beam is directed parallel to the blood flow, the measured velocity will be maximal (angle θ = 0° and the cosine of 0° = 1). On the other hand, when the ultrasound beam is perpendicular to the blood flow, no Doppler shift will be recorded (angle θ = 90° and the cosine of 90° = 0). Hence, every effort should be made to measure the true velocity by having the angle as parallel as possible to the blood flow. Color Doppler can be used to help place the Doppler signal parallel to the blood flow.

There are two main types of Doppler measurements used in clinical practice today, i.e. continuous wave (CW) and pulsed wave (PW). CW Doppler is the older and electronically simpler of the two kinds. It involves a two-crystal transducer that continuously generates ultrasound waves using one crystal and continuously receives using the other. Doppler shift data is obtained from the reflected ultrasound waves off every red blood cell along the course of the ultrasound beam. The main advantage of CW Doppler is its ability to measure high blood velocities accurately. The disadvantage of using CW is that it lacks the sensitivity to differentiate between the depths of returning signals.

PW Doppler uses a transducer that alternates transmission and reception of ultrasound signals. The main advantage of PW Doppler is its ability to provide data selectively from a small segment along the ultrasound beam where the operator places the sample volume.

Since PW Doppler repeatedly samples the returning signal, there is a maximum limit to the frequency shift that can be measured. Accurate identification of the frequency of an ultrasound requires sampling at least twice per wavelength. Thus the maximum detectable frequency shift, also known as the "Nyquist limit" is one-half the pulse repetition frequency (PRF). When the velocity exceeds the Nyquist limit, "wraparound" of the signal occurs and this is known as aliasing. It is seen as a cut-off of the velocity tracing with the cut section seen in the opposite side of the spectral tracing. The main disadvantage of PW Doppler is "aliasing". Aliasing happens when PW Doppler is unable to accurately measure high blood flow velocities (above 1.5 to 2 m/s) that are seen in some valvular heart disease. Limitations of Doppler echocardiography are listed in Table 10.1.

Color Doppler is a form of PW Doppler that uses various sample volumes along many tracer lines to record the doppler shift. It uses the PRF principle to transmit and receive the signals. The signals are obtained from the sampling sites and the mean velocity is analyzed. These velocities are displayed in color scale showing the flow toward the transducer as red and flow away as blue. Usually about eight sampling sites are used. Turbulence in the flow caused by regurgitant lesions or nonlaminar flow is displayed as variance in the color scheme. Color Doppler echocardiography is a sensitive and useful modality for diagnosis and quantitation of regurgitant lesions. It is more sensitive in recognizing minor degrees of valvular regurgitation than clinical examination [6]. Because of their higher sensitivity, there is a potential risk of over diagnosis of regurgitation. Trivial regurgitation seen on color Doppler may be normal in some adults [7].

10.5
Contrast Echocardiography

Contrast echocardiography utilizes the interaction of microscopic gas bubbles with ultrasound to enhance recognition of the blood pool and/or the blood/tissue interface. Blood appears black on conventional 2D

Table 10.1 Limitations of Doppler

PW and CW
Inability to obtain parallel angle
Flow velocity exceeding Nyquist limit (aliasing)
Mirror imaging
Overlap of adjacent flows (beamwidth artefact)
Electronic interference from other sources
Color Doppler
Inability to obtain parallel angle
Aliasing
Shadowing from strong reflectors
Color flow not corresponding with normal flow pattern (ghosting)
Loss of flow signal due to low gain
Electronic interference from other sources

PW, pulsed wave; CW, continuous wave

echocardiography because of the weakness of the ultrasound scattered by red blood cells. Contrast bubbles oscillating in an ultrasound beam are much more effective at scattering sound than red blood cells and as a result greatly increase the blood pool signal strength.

Traditionally, contrast echocardiography has been performed using agitated saline solution. The large size and fragility of these microbubbles limited their passage to the pulmonary circulation, and they became visibile only on the right side of the heart. Newer agents, characterized by both smaller mean size and prolonged persistence, can pass through the pulmonary circulation intact and achieve left heart opacification following intravenous injection [8]. Technological advances such as harmonic and pulse inversion imagings are able to exploit the interactions that occur between microbubbles and the ultrasound to give high quality images.

Hand agitated saline produces large air bubbles that are predominantly confined to the right heart. The presence of air bubbles in the left side of the heart is likely to be the result of an intracardiac shunt. In clinical practice, this is used for detection of shunts, especially PFO in patients with suspected paradoxical embolism [9].

One of the limitations of echocardiography is the suboptimal visualization of the entire endocardium in a significant number of patients. The use of the newer transpulmonary contrast agents has enabled opacification of the left heart structures and enhanced endocardial border definition. This has improved the ability to assess left ventricle (LV) anatomy and systolic function, identify regional wall motion abnormalities and confirm/

Table 10.2 Indications for echocardiogram

Assess LV function and wall motion abnormalities
Identify cause of a cardiac murmur
Estimate severity of valve disease
In atrial fibrillation – LAA clots
In stroke patients – cardiac source of emboli
Post MI patients – LV thrombus
Aortic root assessment
Pericardial effusion
Infective endocarditis
Congenital heart disease
Septal defects or PFO
Cardiac tumors

LV, left ventricular; LAA, left atrial appendage; PFO, patent foramen ovale.

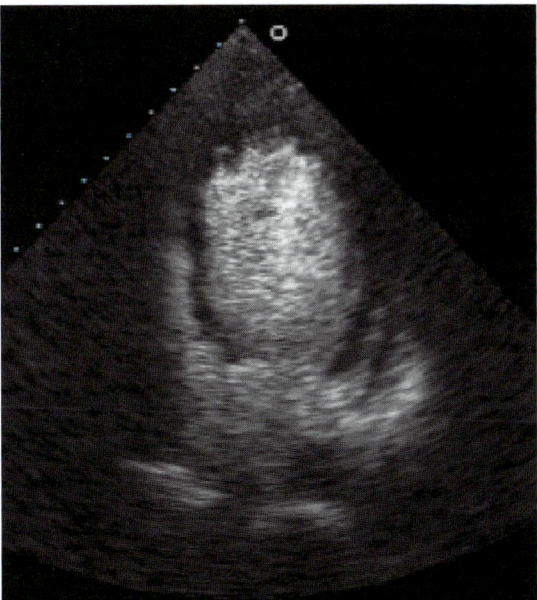

Fig. 10.4 Left ventricular opacification. Apical 2 chamber view showing the contrast filling the left ventricle in a difficult to image patient showing clear demarcation of the endocardium

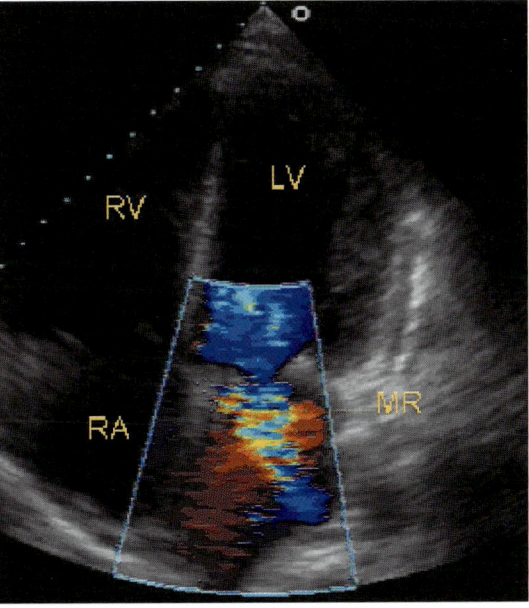

Fig. 10.5 Apical four-chamber transthoracic view showing moderate to severe mitral regurgitation. LV = left ventricle; MR = mitral regurgitation; RA = right atrium; RV = right ventricle

exclude LV thrombus [10, 11] (Fig. 10.4). In addition, the use of second-generation contrast agents in stress echocardiography has further optimized LV opacification and completeness of wall segment visualization [12].

Newer applications include coronary artery flow detection and flow reserve measurement (i.e., myocardial contrast echocardiography). Using the latest-generation contrast agents as blood flow tracers, non-invasive images of the myocardium can be obtained to reflect myocardial perfusion during rest or stress [13].

10.6
Clinical Application of Echocardiography (Table 10.2) [14]

10.6.1
Murmurs and Valvular Heart Disease

Heart murmurs are produced by turbulent blood flow and often represent valvular or structural heart disease. A Doppler echocardiogram can define the primary lesion and its etiology, severity and hemodynamics as well as evaluate cardiac size and function and establish a reference point for future observations. Doppler echocardiography allows measurement of peak flow velocity through a stenotic valve and allows accurate prediction of the pressure gradient across the valve. It is also valuable in detecting and semi-quantitating valvular regurgitation [15] (Fig. 10.5). In patients with mitral valve prolapse an echocardiogram is useful for diagnosis and risk stratification, particularly by identifying leaflet thickening and LV dilation. Echocardiographic findings in infective endocarditis include an oscillating intracardiac mass or vegetation, an annular abscess or new valvular regurgitation, or a prosthetic valve partial dehiscence.

10.6.2
Chest Pain and Ischemic Heart Disease

Echocardiography can be performed when possible during chest pain in the emergency room. The absence of regional wall motion abnormalities indicates the unlikelihood of having either an acute infarction or ischemia with a weighted mean negative predictive accuracy of approximately 98%. Segmental LV wall motion abnormalities are characteristic of myocardial infarction and their location correlates well with the distribution of CAD. These can also be seen with transient myocardial ischemia, chronic ischemia (hibernating myocardium), or a myocardial scar. Echocardiography can be used to evaluate any complication of acute myocardial infarction such as acute mitral regurgitation, infarct expansion and LV remodeling, ventricular septum and free wall rupture, intracardiac thrombus, RV infarction and pericardial effusion.

10.6.3
Heart Failure and Assessment of Left Ventricular Function

The most commonly used index of LV ejection phase is ejection fraction (LVEF). It is derived using algorithms developed for volume determination from M-mode linear dimensions, visual estimation or quantitative analysis from two-dimensional images. Assessment of RV size and systolic function, on the other hand, remains mostly qualitative. In clinical scenarios like edema and dyspnea, echocardiography can help distinguish cardiac causes if the history and physical examination are not diagnostic. Echocardiography is invaluable in the evaluation of heart failure, as it furnishes comprehensive assessment of morphology and function and often allows assessment of hemodynamic status. In the presence of normal ejection fraction, indices of diastolic dysfunction can be obtained based on information from M-mode and two-dimensional Doppler mitral and pulmonary vein flow profiles. The most commonly used Doppler indices are the early E wave and late A wave and their ratio, the deceleration time of the E wave, and the isovolumic relaxation time.

10.6.4
Pericardial Disease

Echocardiography provides a semi-quantitative assessment of pericardial effusion, a qualitative description of its distribution and helps guide pericardiocentesis. Echocardiographic evidence of right atrial collapse at onset of systole and RV collapse in diastole are signs of hemodynamic compromise that can be seen in cardiac tamponade.

10.6.5
Cardiac Masses and Tumors

When clinically indicated, echocardiography can identify primary tumors of the heart, such as atrial myxoma, metastatic disease from extracardiac primary sites, thrombi within any of the four chambers, and vegetations (infectious or noninfectious) on any of the four cardiac valves.

10.6.6
Diseases of the Great Vessels

Echocardiography is well suited to diagnose aortic dissection, aortic aneurysm, aortic root dilation in Marfan syndrome, or aortic rupture. It is also useful to diagnose pulmonary hypertension and detect the effects of pulmonary embolism by the presence of RV dilatation and dysfunction.

10.6.7
Systemic Hypertension

Echocardiography is the preferred procedure in evaluating the cardiac effects of systemic hypertension which is the most common cause of LV hypertrophy and congestive heart failure in adults. It can aid in selecting patients for aggressive treatment and follow-up on LV remodeling.

10.6.8
Neurological Disease and other Cardioembolic Disease

The available data suggests a high prevalence of potential cardiac sources of embolus in subjects with neurological embolic events. Two-dimensional echocardiography is easily applied for detection of a potential cardioembolic source. The intravenous injection of agitated saline can be used to evaluate for a right-to-left shunting across a PFO.

10.6.9
Arrhythmias and Palpitations

Echocardiography can be used in the setting of arrhythmias with clinical suspicion of structural heart disease or in a patient with a family history of a genetically transmitted cardiac lesion associated with arrhythmias. Also, it can be used in a patient presenting with syncope and clinically suspected heart disease or periexertional syncope.

10.6.10
Congenital Heart Disease

Echocardiography is extremely useful in evaluating and monitoring clinically suspected congenital heart disease. It can be used to guide therapy as well as periodic evaluation of those with repaired lesions and those who require follow-up on pulmonary artery pressure, LV function and atrioventricular valve regurgitation.

10.7
Newer Devices and Strategies in Echocardiography

10.7.1
3D Echocardiography

Three-dimensional (3D) echocardiography has the potential for a better understanding of the cardiac morphology under normal and pathological conditions. Various techniques have been described that permit integration of information from multiple 2D imaging planes to generate a 3D reconstruction of the LV. 3D echocardiography appears to produce LVEF values similar to radionuclide ventriculography (RVG) and offers incremental benefit over 2D techniques and improved accuracy and reproducibility [16–20]. One study, for example, compared LVEF measurements obtained by 3D echocardiography, quantitative and qualitative 2D echocardiography, and RVG in 51 patients with heart disease; there was excellent correlation between 3D echocardiography and RVG (r = 0.94 to 0.97) without significant overestimation or underestimation [16]. 3D echocardiography was superior to both quantitative and qualitative 2D echocardiographic techniques. In other studies, 3D echocardiography has also been shown to correlate well with measurements made using cardiac magnetic resonance imaging [18–20]. 3D echocardiography has also been investigated as a tool to quantify LV dyssynchrony in patients being considered for biventricular pacing, also referred to as cardiac resynchronization therapy. It has been evaluated for its utility in assessing mitral stenosis. Recently matrix-array real-time (RT) 3D technology has been a significant breakthrough technology that allows instant visualization of cardiac anatomic details that could not be well delineated by 2D imaging [21].

10.7.2
Intracardiac Echocardiography (ICE)

ICE uses an intracardiac catheter that provides online 2D, color Doppler, pulsed wave and continuous wave Doppler images and was first reported in 2002. Since then the scope of ICE has widened. ICE has been used in transseptal puncture [22], ablation of RA flutter [23], isolation and ablation of pulmonary veins [24], ablation of accessory pathways [25], and closure of atrial septal defect or PFO. More recent studies have demonstrated successful use of ICE in balloon valvuloplasty [26] and mitral valve apparatus repair [27].

10.7.3
Tissue Doppler Echocardiography

Tissue Doppler echocardiography (TDE) is a relatively recent addition to the diagnostic ultrasound examination; it permits an assessment of myocardial motion using ultrasound imaging with color coding. The technique uses frequency shifts of ultrasound waves to calculate myocardial velocity. This is similar to the use of routine Doppler ultrasound to assess blood flow, but its technological features focus on lower velocity frequency shifts. Although Doppler ultrasound has been in widespread clinical use to assess intracardiac blood flow and noninvasive hemodynamics for many years, interest in TDE increased significantly when the color-coded TDE method was introduced [13–18]. Routine echocardiographic assessment of regional LV wall motion is subjective because it is determined by visual determination of endocardial excursion and wall thickening. TDE offers the promise of an objective measure to quantify regional and global LV function through the assessment of myocardial velocity data.

10.7.4
Strain Doppler Echocardiography (Strain Rate Imaging)

An important refinement of tissue Doppler imaging used in the assessment of regional left ventricular function has been the calculation of the myocardial velocity gradient, or strain rate imaging. Strain, which is a change in length corrected for the original length, or the fractional or percentage change from the original or unstressed dimension, reflects deformation of a structure and therefore directly describes the contraction/relaxation pattern of the myocardium. Strain rate is the rate of this deformation and is a strong index of left ventricular contractility [28–31]. Strain rate imaging involves mathematical subtraction of the whole heart or translational motion from regional thickening velocity using a transmural data set from color-coded TDE [32–34]. The results are less subjective than with wall motion scoring with traditional dobutamine echocardiography. This quantification of the spatial distribution of intramural velocities across the myocardium has improved the ability of TDE to reflect directional and incremental alterations in regional and global left ventricular contractility in patients with cardiovascular disease [32, 35]. The technique can also identify regional diastolic asynchrony due to post-systolic shortening during ischemia, thereby defining the extent of ischemic myocardium [36]. When used with low dose dobutamine, it is also a useful method for assessing the degree of myocardial viability [37].

10.8
Limitations of Echocardiography (Table 10.3)

The main limitation of transthoracic echocardiography lies in its dependency on operator skills and the ability to image from satisfactory examining windows. For patients with chronic obstructive pulmonary disease the interposition of air-filled lung between the body surface and the heart severely limits access, and may prevent complete examination. Moreover, the diagnosis of prosthetic valve endocarditis by the transthoracic technique is more difficult than diagnosis of endocarditis of native valves because of image artefacts related to both mechanical and bioprosthetic valves [14]. Echocardiographic studies tend to be of poorer quality in obese patients with decrease ability to obtain pulmonary artery systolic pressure or to differentiate between subepicardial adipose tissue and pericardial effusion [38]. Other potential limitations include decreased ability to image the left atrial appendage, superior vena cava and the majority of aorta and pulmonary arteries above valve/root level necessitating the use of transoesophageal echocardiogram.

Table 10.3 Limitations of echocardiogram

Poor image quality, e.g., body habitus, COPD, post-cardiac surgery
Sidelobe artefacts
Reverberations from two strong reflectors like prosthetic valves and calcifications
Shadowing from prosthetic valves
Near field cluttering
Refraction
Range ambiguity
Electronic processing artifacts
Technologist dependent
Reader dependent

References

1. Feigenbaum H. History of Echocardiography. http://www.asecho.org/freepdf/FeigenbaumChapter.pdf. Accessed 06/10/2006.
2. Feigenbaum H (1977) Principles of echocardiography. Am J Med 62(6):805–812.
3. Lee RT, Bhatia SJ, St John Sutton MG (1989) Assessment of valvular heart disease with Doppler echocardiography. J Am Med Assoc 262(15):2131–2135.
4. Stewart MJ (2003) Contrast echocardiography. Heart 89(3):342–348.
5. Caidahl K, Kazzam E, Lidberg J et al. (1998) New concept in echocardiography: harmonic imaging of tissue without use of contrast agent. Lancet 352(9136):1264–1270.
6. Jaffe WM, Roche AH, Coverdale HA, McAlister HF, Ormiston JA, Greene ER (1988) Clinical evluation versus Doppler echocardiography in the quantitative assessment of valvular heart idsease. Circulation 78:267–275.
7. Sahn DJ, Maciel BC (1994) Physiological valvular regurgitation. Doppler echocardiography and the potential for iatrogenic heart disease. Circulation 78:1075–1077.
8. Goldberg BB, Liu JB, Forsberg F (1994) Ultrasound contrast agents: a review. Ultrasound Med Biol 20:319.
9. Kerut EK, Norfleet WT, Plotnick GD, Giles TD (2001) Patent foramen ovale: a review of associated conditions and the impact of physiological size. J Am Coll Cardiol 38(3):613–623.
10. Senior R (1999) Role of contrast echocardiography for the assessment of left ventricular function. Echocardiography 16:747–752.
11. Takeuchi M, Ogunyankin K, Pandian NG et al. (1999) Enhanced visualization of intravascular and intracardiac left atrial thrombus with the use of a thrombus-targeting ultrasonographic contrast agent: in vivo experimental echocardiographic studies. J Am Soc Echocardiogr 12:1015–1021.
12. Rainbird AJ, Mulvagh SL, Oh JK et al. (2001) Contrast dobutamine stress echocardiography: clinical practice assessment in 300 consecutive patients. J Am Soc Echocardiogr 14:378–385.
13. Caiati C, Montaldo C, Zedda N, Bina A, Iliceto S (1999) New noninvasive method for coronary flow reserve assessment: contrast-enhanced transthoracic second harmonic echo Doppler. Circulation 99(6):771–778.
14. Cheitlin MD, Armstrong WF, Aurigemma GP, Beller GA, Bierman FZ, Davis JL et al. (2003) ACC/AHA/ASE 2003 guideline update for the clinical application of echocardiography: a report of the American College of Cardiology/American Heart Association Task Force on Practice Guidelines (ACC/AHA/ASE Committee to Update the 1997 Guidelines for the Clinical Application of Echocardiography). 2003. Accessed at http://www.acc.org/clinical/guidelines/echo/index.pdf on June 11, 2006.
15. Missri JC (1986) Doppler echocardiography in the evaluation of valvular heart disease. Can J Cardiol 2(1):16–23.
16. Gopal AS, Shen Z, Sapin PM et al. (1995) Assessment of cardiac function by three-dimensional echocardiography compared with conventional noninvasive methods. Circulation 92:842.
17. Nosir YF, Fioretti PM, Vletter WB et al. (1996) Accurate measurement of left ventricular ejection fraction by three-dimensional echocardiography. A comparison with radionuclide angiography. Circulation 94:460.
18. Danias PG, Chuang ML, Parker RA et al. (1998) Relations between the number of image planes and the accuracy of three-dimensional echocardiography for measuring left ventricular volumes and ejection fraction. Am J Cardiol 82:1431.
19. Nosir YF, Lequin MH, Kasprzak JD et al. (1998) Measurements of day-to-day variables of left ventricular volumes and ejection fraction by three-dimensional echocardiography and comparison with magnetic resonance imaging. Am J Cardiol 82:209.
20. Kuhl HP Schreckenberg M, Rulands D et al. (2004) High-resolution transthoracic real-time three-dimensional echocardiography: quantitation of cardiac volumes and function using semi-automatic border detection and comparison with cardiac magnetic resonance imaging. J Am Coll Cardiol 43:2083.
21. Seliem MA, Fedec A, Cohen MS et al. (2006) Real-time 3-dimensional echocardiographic imaging of congenital heart disease using matrix-array technology: freehand real-time scanning adds instant morphologic details not well delineated by conventional dimensional imaging. J Am Soc Echocardiogr 19:121–129.
22. Ren JF, Marchlinski FE, Callans DJ, Herrmann HC (2002) Clinical use of AcuNav diagnostic ultrasound catheter imaging during left heart radiofrequency ablation and transcatheter closure procedures. J Am Soc Echocardiogr 15:1301–1308.
23. Okishige K, Kawabata M, Yamashiro K et al. (2005) Clinical study regarding the anatomical structures of the right atrial isthmus using intra-cardiac echocardiography: implication for catheter ablation of common atrial flutter. J Intervent Card Electrophysiol. 12(1):9–12.
24. Verma A, Marrouche NF, Natale A (2004) Pulmonary vein antrum isolation: intracardiac echocardiography-guided technique. J Cardiovasc Electrophysiol 15(11):1335–1340.
25. Citro R, Ducceschi V, Salustri A et al. (2004) Intracardiac echocardiography to guide transseptal catheterization for radiofrequency catheter ablation of left-sided accessory pathways: two case reports. Cardiovasc Ultrasound 2(1):20.
26. Green NE, Hansgen AR, Carroll JD (2004) Initial clinical experience with intracardiac echocardiography in guiding balloon mitral valvuloplasty: technique, safety,

27. Naqvi TZ, Zarbatany D, Molloy MD et al. (2006) Intracardiac echocardiography for percutaneous mitral valve repair in a swine model. J Am Soc Echocardiogr 19(2):147–153.
28. Mirsky I, Parmley WW (1973) Assessment of passive elastic stiffness for isolated heart muscle and the intact heart. Circ Res 33(2):233–243.
29. Abraham TP, Nishimura RA (2001) Myocardial strain: can we finally measure contractility? J Am Coll Cardiol 37(3):731–734.
30. Greenberg NL, Firstenberg MS, Castro PL et al. (2002) Doppler-derived myocardial systolic strain rate is a strong index of left ventricular contractility. Circulation 105(1):99–105.
31. Sutherland GR, Di Salvo G, Claus P et al. (2004) Strain and strain rate imaging: a new clinical approach to quantifying regional myocardial function. J Am Soc Echocardiogr 17(7):788–802.
32. Sutherland GR, Stewart MJ, Groundstroem KW et al. (1994) Color Doppler myocardial imaging: a new technique for the assessment of myocardial function. J Am Soc Echocardiogr 7(5):441–458.
33. Uematsu M, Miyatake K, Tanaka N et al. (1995) Myocardial velocity gradient as a new indicator of regional left ventricular contraction: detection by a two-dimensional tissue Doppler imaging technique. J Am Coll Cardiol 26(1):217–223.
34. Uematsu M, Nakatani S, Yamagishi M et al. (1997) Usefulness of myocardial velocity gradient derived from two-dimensional tissue Doppler imaging as an indicator of regional myocardial contraction independent of translational motion assessed in atrial septal defect. Am J Cardiol 79(2):237–241.
35. Edvardsen T, Skulstad H, Aakhus S et al. (2001) Regional myocardial systolic function during acute myocardial ischemia assessed by strain Doppler echocardiography. J Am Coll Cardiol 37(3):726–730.
36. Pislaru C, Belohlavek M, Bae RY et al. (2001) Regional asynchrony during acute myocardial ischemia quantified by ultrasound strain rate imaging. J Am Coll Cardiol 37(4):1141–1148.
37. Hoffmann R, Altiok E, Nowak B et al. (2002) Strain rate measurement by doppler echocardiography allows improved assessment of myocardial viability inpatients with depressed left ventricular function. J Am Coll Cardiol 39(3):443–449.
38. Ansari A, Rholl AO (1986) Pseudopericardial effusion: echocardiographic and computed tomographic correlations. Clin Cardiol 9:551–555.

utility, and limitations. Catheter Cardiovasc Intervent 63(3):385–394.

Dobutamine Stress Echocardiography

Satish C. Govind and S. S. Ramesh

Contents

11.1	Introduction	127
11.2	Clinical Application	127
11.3	Technique	129
11.3.1	Protocol	129
11.3.2	Analysis	129
11.4	Feasibility and Safety	131
11.5	Discussion	132
11.6	Comparison with Other Stress Modalities	133
11.6.1	Exercise ECG	133
11.6.2	Exercise Echocardiography	133
11.6.3	Dipyridamole Echocardiography	133
11.6.4	Radionuclide Imaging	134
11.7	Viable Myocardium	134
11.8	Use of Dobutamine Stress Echo in Non-ischemic Heart Disease	134
11.9	Future Trends	135
11.10	Conclusion	135
	References	135

11.1 Introduction

Dobutamine stress echocardiography (DSE) has developed over the years into a widely accepted routine, non invasive clinical diagnostic test for evaluating patients with suspected or established coronary artery disease (CAD). This technique was initially reported in the late 1980s [1]. When the myocardium is subjected to stress by the use of a pharmacological agent like dobutamine, it induces ischemia in patients with significant coronary artery stenosis and the detection of the ischemia is reflected by wall motion abnormalities (WMA) in regional segments of the left ventricle (LV), as elaborated by the American Society of Echocardiography (ASE) [2]. DSE has gradually evolved over the last three decades into an established application; it has faced many technical challenges, culminating in a refined and accurate test. Although the exercise electrocardiogram (ECG) continues to be the primary initial test for CAD, DSE has proved to be an excellent alternative for those patients for whom the exercise ECG has low diagnostic power, and for patients who are unable to exercise. DSE is a relatively demanding technique with a steep learning curve, but recent advances in echocardiography have made this an easier and more sophisticated test, with better predictive accuracy. This chapter describes the increasing use of DSE as a comprehensive, non-invasive tool in the diagnosis and monitoring of CAD.

11.2 Clinical Application

DSE, as a test to diagnose CAD is more efficient than the exercise ECG and is comparable with myocardial perfusion studies, however, for logistical reasons in performing the test, it is confined to certain patient categories. The indications are summarised in Table 11.1.

Exercise testing is generally the initial step taken when looking for the presence or absence of CAD. In the ACC/AHA guidelines for exercise testing [3], the combined results of a meta-analysis were 68% sensitivity and 77% specificity. This modest level of accuracy

Table 11.1 Indications for Dobutamine stress echo

1. Non-diagnostic exercise ECG
2. Unable to do exercise ECG – severely deconditioned
3. Orthopaedic or neurological limitations
4. Peripheral vascular disease (PVD)
5. LV hypertrophy with strain
6. Women with high probability of CAD
7. Risk stratification before major surgery
8. Left bundle branch block and WPW syndrome
9. Digitalis therapy
10. Post myocardial infarction risk stratification
11. Post myocardial revascularisation follow-up
12. Dilated cardiomyopathy

reflects the limitations of exercise ECG. Thus patients with an inconclusive or negative exercise ECG, but with a high pretest probability would require further testing. In one study [4], about 35% of patients were unable to perform exercise ECG because of orthopaedic, neurological or vascular diseases, or failed to reach the required target level. These subsets of patients are ideal for DSE testing. The diagnosis of CAD in patients with left ventricular hypertrophy (LVH) is often a clinical challenge since the coexistence of these conditions is frequently seen. The resting ECG itself is a poor marker for LVH and of limited value, although by itself it is well validated for the definition of LVH. The issue of LVH and DSE was discussed in a study [5] that showed that increased LV mass index alone did not affect the accuracy of DSE. Sensitivity of exercise testing was reduced to 36% in concentric LVH. In those patients without ECG evidence of LVH, DSE sensitivity was 93% and specificity was 100%, and the corresponding results for exercise ECG were 72% and 29%. This emphasizes that DSE is better than exercise ECG.

Another separate group that deserves special attention is women. The accuracy of exercise ECG in women is even lower. This is compounded by the fact that, other than in elderly women, CAD has a lower prevalence in women than in men of the same age. In addition mitral valve prolapse and altered vascular reactivity in women cause ST segment response not related to CAD. DSE has a sensitivity of 87% and 89% in women [6]. As a practical test for women, the accuracy of the test results are not compromised, and although as an initial test it is more expensive, it is cost effective in the long run because it avoids unnecessary coronary angiograms [7]. For the preoperative assessment of perioperative cardiac risk in non-cardiac surgery, DSE is an invaluable tool in patients unable to undergo exercise ECG. Literature results [8] show that preoperatively, patients who undergo DSE and who show new WMA have a higher perioperative risk for cardiac events than those with a negative test result.

Another dilemma concerns patients with left bundle branch block (LBBB), where the utility of the exercise ECG is poor. The prognostic value of myocardial ischemia in patients with this conduction abnormality was defined in a major study [9] in which a positive echocardiographic result (evidence of ischemia) was detected in 28% of patients. The 5-year survival was 77% in the ischemic group and 92% in the nonischemic group. The 5-year infarction-free survival was 60% in the ischemic group and 87% in the nonischemic group. Stress echocardiography significantly improved risk stratification in patients with LBBB, but without previous myocardial infarction, and not in those with previous myocardial infarction. In particular, it provided additional value over clinical and resting echocardiographic findings in predicting cardiac events among patients without previous infarction. The conclusion is that myocardial ischemia during pharmacologic stress echocardiography is a strong prognostic predictor in patients with LBBB, particularly in those without previous myocardial infarction. DSE has excellent diagnostic specificity in LBBB patients with suspected coronary artery disease.

In patients with abnormal resting septal thickening, however, DSE may lack good sensitivity for detection of coronary artery disease in the anterior circulation. Routine exercise ECG testing has variable sensitivity in patients following cardiac bypass surgery. DSE is an accurate method for the diagnosis and localization of vascular compromise in patients evaluated after coronary artery bypass graft surgery. The test provides useful data for selection of patients for whom coronary angiography may be indicated [10]. Although similar conclusions are drawn from other studies, data pertaining to the efficacy of DSE and prognosis of late detection of recurrent CAD are limited [11]. DSE has a low sensitivity but high specificity for detecting restenosis after coronary angioplasty in a patient population with high prevalence of single vessel disease. At late post revascularization follow-up, results have been shown to correlate well with those of perfusion scintigraphy. Whether or not screening for restenosis is better than using the test to investigate for new symptoms is still not clear [11, 12]. Dobutamine stress echo provides potentially useful information on idiopathic dilated cardiomyopathy, and in these patients an extensive contractile reserve identified by high-dose dobutamine stress echocardiography is associated with better survival [13].

Contraindications to DSE include severe aortic stenosis, hypertrophic obstructive cardiomyopathy, uncontrolled hypertension, uncontrolled atrial fibrillation, known severe ventricular arrhythmias and electrolyte abnormalities (mainly hypokalaemia).

11.3
Technique

11.3.1
Protocol

The protocol varies from centre to centre with regard to dobutamine dose (range 5 to 50 µg/kg per min), atropine addition (up to 2 mg) and stage duration (range 2 to 8 min). To date, the most widely adopted protocol uses dobutamine up to 40 µg/kg per min, with the addition of atropine up to 1 mg [14]. Dobutamine is a synthetic catecholamine with a relatively short plasma half-life of 2–3 min due to rapid metabolisation to inactive metabolites in the liver. It has a strong $beta_1$ receptor and mild $alpha_1$ and $beta_2$ receptor agonist activity. When used at low doses up to 10 to 20 µg/kg body weight per min, marked inotropic effects ($alpha_1$- and $beta_1$-receptor stimulation) are encountered. When used at higher doses, heart rate is progressively increased ($beta_1$-receptor stimulation). Systemic blood pressure increases only minimally, since an increase in cardiac output due to the peripheral vasoconstrictive effects ($alpha_1$-receptor stimulation) is offset by a decrease in systemic vascular resistance due to the predominance of the vasodilative effects ($beta_2$-receptor stimulation). In patients without an adequate increase in heart rate, the addition of atropine helps to further increase the heart rate. The protocol starts with a resting ECG being taken, intravenous access is secured and 2-D images are acquired. Dobutamine is then infused intravenously by an infusion pump, starting at 5 or 10 µg/kg per min for 3 min, increasing by 10 µg/kg per min every 3 min up to a maximum of 40 µg/kg per min. In patients not achieving 85% of their maximal heart rate (220 beats/min minus age in males, 210 beats/min minus age in females) and without symptoms or signs of myocardial ischemia, atropine is additionally injected with maximal dose of dobutamine, starting with 0.25 mg intravenously and repeated up to a maximum of 1.0 mg within 4 min, with dobutamine infusion being continued. Throughout dobutamine infusion, a 12-lead ECG is continuously monitored and recorded at 3-min intervals. Blood pressure is measured and recorded every 3 min. The patient is continuously imaged and images are recorded on video or quad screen during the final minute of each dobutamine stage and recovery. Reasons for terminating the test are new wall motion abnormalities; ECG showing horizontal or downsloping ST segment depression more than 2 mm in two or more contiguous leads at an interval of 80 ms after the J point compared with baseline, ST segment elevation more than 1 mm in two or more contiguous leads in patients without a previous MI; severe angina; a symptomatic reduction in systolic blood pressure more than 40 mm Hg from baseline; blood pressure more than 240/120 mm Hg; significant tachyarrhythmias; or any serious side effect regarded as due to dobutamine. A beta-blocker that can be injected intravenously must be available to reverse the effects of dobutamine if they do not revert spontaneously and quickly. The addition of atropine is contraindicated in patients with narrow-angle glaucoma, myasthenia gravis, obstructive uropathy or obstructive gastrointestinal disorders.

11.3.2
Analysis

In the analysis of the images, the LV is divided into the 16-segment model as recommended by the ASE [14]. The quad screen format (with rest, low and high dose and recovery images next to each other in one screen) facilitates better analysis and is more helpful (Fig. 11.1). Wall motion or thickening is reported according to an accepted numerical classification: 1 = normal, characterized by a uniform increase in wall excursion and thickening; 2 = hypokinesia, denoted by reduced inward systolic wall motion; 3 = akinesia, marked by an absence of inward motion and thickening; 4 = dyskinesia, indicated by systolic thinning and outward systolic wall motion. As a result of the hemodynamic changes during DSE there is an increase in oxygen demand. But, in myocardial regions supplied by a coronary artery with a critical stenosis, the increase in oxygen demand cannot be met by an adequate increase in blood flow. Hence, regional ischemia develops and causes regional WMA that can be detected by two-dimensional echocardiography. A normal stress echocardiogram is defined by a uniform increase in wall motion and systolic wall thickening, with a reduction in end systolic cavity area and end systolic volume. A positive test is denoted by development of new WMA or by worsening of regional WMA in one or more segments (Fig. 11.2). In patients with rest WMA, a "biphasic" response (i.e., initial improvement of WMA at low dose followed by worsening of WMA at high dose) has improved detection of CAD. Isolated mild wall motion deterioration in mid- or basal inferoposterior segments needs to be interpreted with caution because these segments are known to be less specific for CAD. Several investigators have reported that the inclusion of rest WMA in addition to new or worsening WMA as the criterion for a positive test result in a gain in sensitivity without a loss in specificity

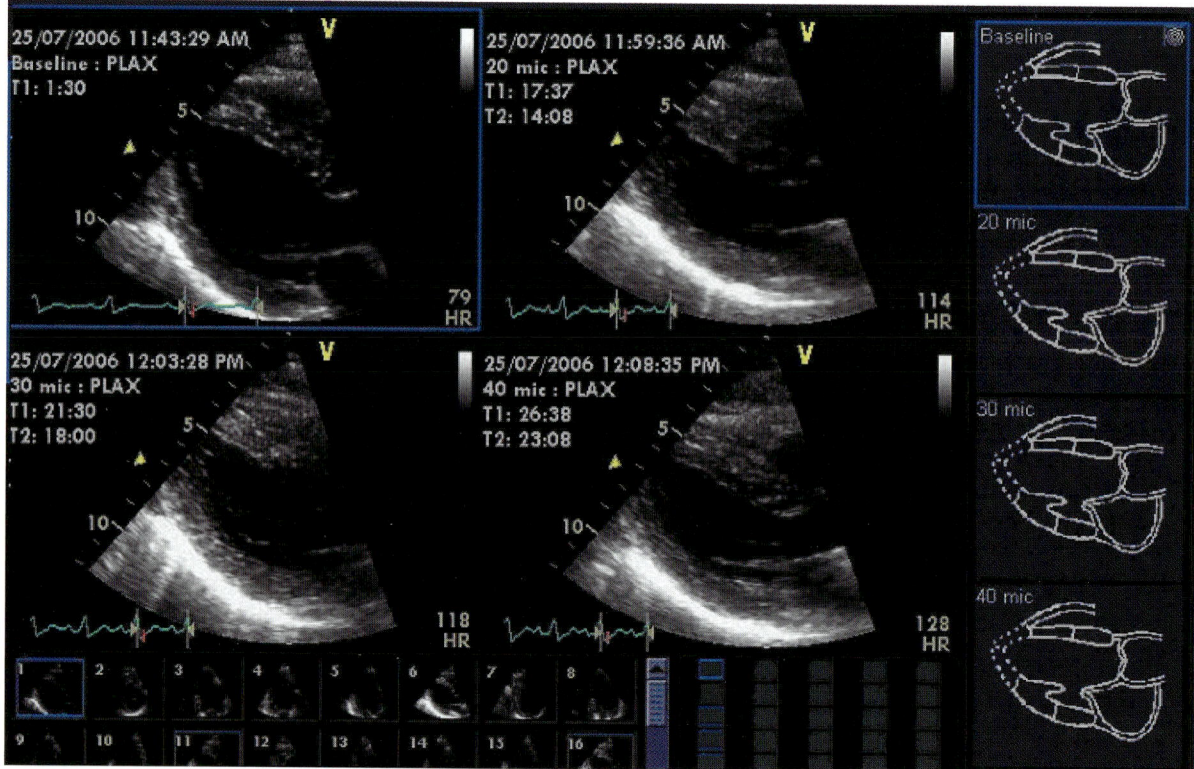

Fig. 11.1 Quad image of Dobutamine stress echo showing the left ventricle in the parasternal long axis view at different stages of the test

for the detection of CAD. However, the inclusion of rest WMA as a criterion for CAD is appropriate only in patients without a previous MI because in patients with a previous MI, this diagnosis is nearly certain and does not require further testing for this purpose.

Generally, dobutamine stress causes an increase in cardiac output and a small reduction in systemic vascular resistance with a small increase in systolic blood pressure as a net result. Although the pathophysiology of dobutamine stress-induced hypotension has not been completely defined, theoretically, it could be from an inadequate increase in cardiac output to compensate for an expected decrease in systemic vascular resistance, or a disproportionate decrease in systemic vascular resistance in the presence of a normal increase in cardiac output. An inadequate increase in cardiac output may be due to inadequate contractile reserve, severe ischemic left ventricular dysfunction or left-sided obstructive heart disease. Dynamic left ventricular cavity obliteration due to strong inotropic stimulation was proposed as an important cause for reduced cardiac output and hypotension, especially in patients with dehydration. Later studies could not confirm this mechanism, and the proposed bolus of saline before dobutamine did not prevent cavity obliteration in a canine model. The second mechanism, a disproportionate decrease in systemic vascular resistance, may be due to excessive sensitivity of the peripheral circulation to beta$_2$-receptor stimulation, increased beta$_2$-receptor density (deconditioned patients) or a neurally mediated mechanism in which vigorous myocardial contraction stimulates the intramyocardial mechanoreceptors, resulting in sympathetic withdrawal and enhanced parasympathetic activity (the Bezold–Jarisch reflex). In contrast to exercise stress-induced hypotension, all presently available data indicate that there is no relation between ischemic left ventricular systolic dysfunction or angiographically detected CAD and dobutamine stress-induced hypotension.

With regard to ECG changes, ST segment changes are the hallmark of ischemia in exercise tests but they seem to have less value during dobutamine stress. In an early study in patients with mainly unstable angina and severe coronary lesions, dobutamine stress-induced ST segment depression was described as a highly accurate diagnostic test. However, subsequent reports in stable patients with less severe lesions could never confirm

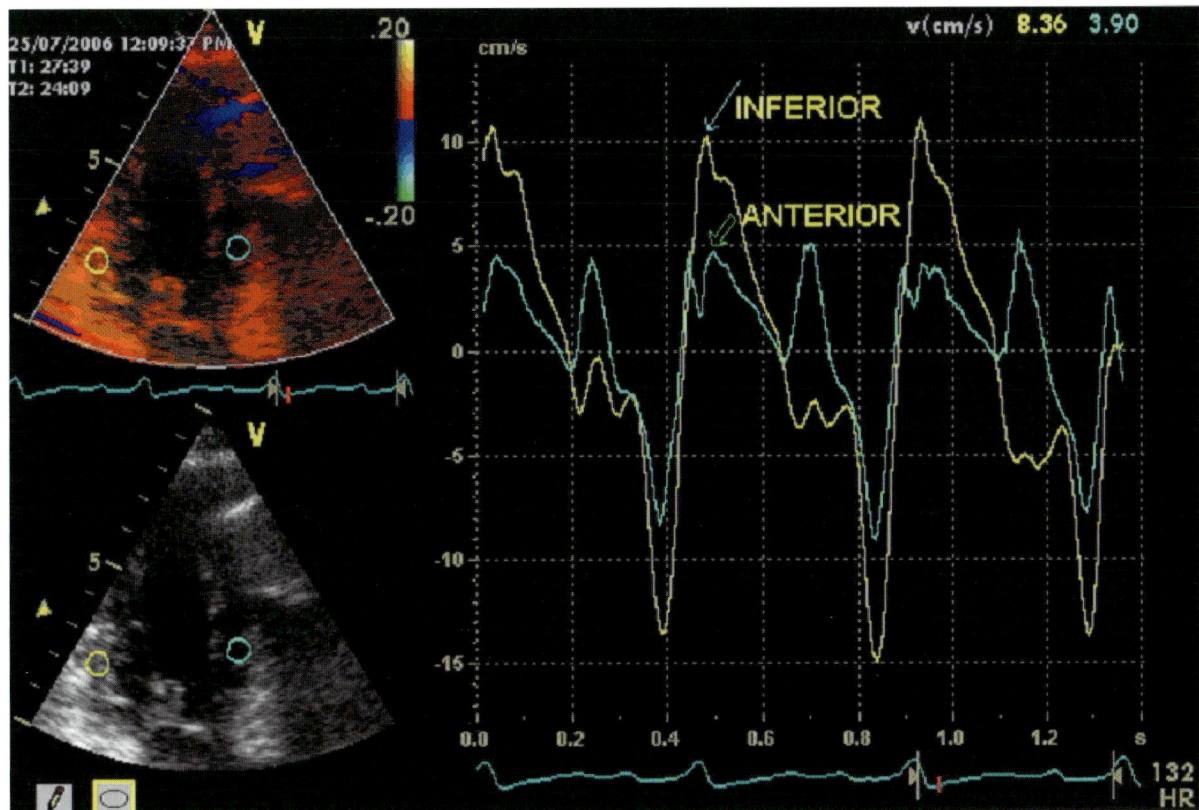

Fig. 11.2 Tissue Doppler image of Dobutamine stress echo showing the velocity curves in apical two-chamber view at peak stress. Inferior wall shows a normal velocity response, while the anterior wall shows a decreased and abnormal velocity response. Subsequent coronary angiogram showed a significant stenosis of the left anterior descending artery

these data. Whether this is due to altered placement of electrodes (because of the requirement for a good apical acoustic window), less stress (lower rate – pressure product than for exercise tests) or other factors still needs to be established. In contrast, as in exercise testing, dobutamine stress-induced ST segment elevation in patients without a previous MI was consistently reported to be associated with significant coronary artery disease.

11.4
Feasibility and Safety

In about 5% of patients, an inadequate acoustic window precludes the performance of successful DSE, although this proportion may underestimate the actual number of patients with an inadequate acoustic window in an unselected population. Furthermore, in 10% of tests, absent ischemic markers in submaximal tests result in nondiagnostic tests because of an insufficient hemodynamic response to dobutamine–atropine administration or limiting side effects. Noncardiac side effects like nausea, headache, chills, urgency and anxiety are usually well tolerated, without the need for test termination. The most common cardiovascular side effects are angina, hypotension and cardiac arrhythmias. Although angina occurs in about 20% of patients, severe angina as a test end point without accompanying new or worsening wall motion abnormalities is rare. Dobutamine stress-induced hypotension occurs, in 5% to 37% of patients. A more than 20 mm Hg decrease in systolic blood pressure occurs in about 20%. Severe, symptomatic hypotension necessitating test termination occurs only rarely. The test may have to be terminated when symptomatic hypotension occurs. Arrhythmias are not uncommon, with frequent premature atrial or ventricular contractions occurring in about 10% of patients and supraventricular or ventricular tachycardias each occurring in about 4% of patients. Ventricular tachycardias are usually nonsustained and have been attributed to beta$_1$-receptor stimulation and dobutamine-induced reduction in plasma potassium concentrations. These arrhythmias are more frequently encountered in patients with a history of previous ventricular arrhythmias or baseline WMA. On the basis of combined diagnostic and safety reports on DSE, it can be roughly estimated that ventricular fibrillation or MI occurs in 1 of 2000 studies. These severe complications can occur up to 20 min after dobutamine withdrawal, and it has been suggested that in these patients, alpha$_1$-mediated coronary and systemic vasoconstriction might be paradoxically exacerbated, not reversed, by beta-blocker administration. Atropine intoxication, although generally requiring a dose of atropine of at least 5 mg, has been reported in a few patients receiving less than 1 mg of atropine.

Intraobserver and interobserver agreement for ischemia within institutions as reported in individual studies ranged from 95% to 98% and from 92% to 96%, respectively. Agreement was clearly higher in patients without CAD or with extensive CAD and was lower in patients with limited echocardiographic image quality.

DSE has its strengths and limitations. The advantages are: it is real time, low cost of the test and supporting equipment, easy availability and portability, no radiation, immediate availability of results, and other information such as intracardiac thrombus, aneurysm, pericardial effusion and abnormal valve anatomy can be detected with the test. In addition, echo has excellent spatial resolution and when this is combined with Doppler techniques, it can offer information on chamber volumes, dimensions, wall thickness, assessment of systolic and diastolic function and various gradients. The limitations are that it is operator dependent, DSE is more a functional assessment than perfusion, and it largely relies on adequate echo windows with appropriate endocardial definition. Use of anti-ischemic drugs decreases the sensitivity of the test.

11.5
Discussion

As with other tests for the detection of CAD, the diagnostic accuracy of DSE is expressed by its sensitivity, specificity and accuracy. These indexes depend on several technical factors, such as describing a positive test and the threshold for defining significant CAD. Also, several characteristics of the patients studied may affect these indexes, such as the presence or absence of myocardial infarction, patient gender, referral bias, the level of stress induced, the stenosis severity and extent of diseased vessels.

The overall sensitivity, specificity and accuracy of DSE in detecting CAD for a total of 2246 patients in 28 studies were 80%, 84%, and 81%, respectively. The number of diseased coronary arteries assessed in 15 studies and 897 patients showed that mean sensitivity increased significantly from 74% for single-vessel disease to 86% for double-vessel disease and to 92% for triple-vessel disease. One of the most important avoidable factors influencing test sensitivity is the use of beta-blockers. These medications lower peak cardiac workload and inotropic response during DSE and thus have the potential to lower the sensitivity of the test, especially when atropine is not added to dobutamine. It has been found consistently that sensitivity was lower in patients with beta-blocker therapy despite the finding that patients taking beta-blockers generally have a higher prevalence of significant CAD.

The coronary arteries and their branches supply different regions of the LV myocardium. Based on the known anatomic relations between coronary arteries and various myocardial regions, it is possible to infer disease of a given coronary artery by noting the location of a WMA on echocardiography. For the left anterior descending, left circumflex and right coronary arteries, the mean reported sensitivities are 72%, 55% and 76%, respectively, and the mean specificities were 88%, 93% and 89%, respectively. The lower sensitivity for detection of disease in the left circumflex artery can be explained by the variation in coronary anatomy (with a small circumflex territory in some patients) and problems with resolution of the lateral wall endocardium.

Although values for sensitivity and specificity have a useful role, the use of DSE in diagnostic practice is to assist in the clinical recognition of CAD [14]. In this sense, tests are used to reclassify the initial clinical impression of the probability of CAD into high, low and intermediate risk subgroups. According to the Bayes theorem, the likelihood of a positive test result is determined by the pretest probability of CAD in the patient studied, as well as the accuracy of the test. Multicentre trials provide the necessary information for an unrestricted acceptance of any new diagnostic procedure. This was the scenario for Dobutamine stress echo in the early 1990s. A large multicentric multicentre study [15] made a credible case for routine use of DSE. Results were obtained in 24 experienced echocardiography laboratories where 2949 DSEs were carried out on 2799 patients. In 341 DSEs (12% of the overall population, 21% of the negative tests) the test could not be completed because of complex ventricular tachyarrhythmia's (134, 38% of all submaximal studies); nausea and/or headache (71, 20%); hypotension and/or bradycardia (62, 17%); supraventricular tachyarrhythmia's (44, 12%); hypertension (24, 7%); and others (20, 6%). Dangerous events (life-threatening complications or side-effects requiring specific treatment and lasting more than 3 hours, or new hospital admission) occurred in 14 cases (1 every 210 tests) – nine cardiac (three ventricular tachycardias; two ventricular fibrillations;

two myocardial infarctions; one prolonged antidote-resistant myocardial ischaemia; one severe, persistent hypotension) and five extra cardiac (atropine poisoning with hallucinations lasting several hours in the absence of either myocardial ischaemia or hypotension). The test is generally well tolerated, although it may be interrupted by minor, self-limiting side effects. Rarely, life-threatening complications may occur during dobutamine/atropine stress echocardiography.

The advent of tissue Doppler imaging (TDI) gave a boost to myocardial quantification. It has been developed from a pulsed Doppler acquisition tool towards a method where extraction of velocities can be performed from colour-coded images [16]. This has introduced further development into different forms of parametric images describing different myocardial functions as colour-coded information, such as deformation imaging, motion imaging and phase imaging. The technical requirements have been established with temporal requirements of frame rates in acquisition exceeding 100 frames/s. The most powerful application of the tissue Doppler technique today is perhaps to quantify the myocardial functional reserve, during stress echocardiography, and making the method applicable to diagnose the presence of coronary disease with an accuracy exceeding that of nuclear and other non-invasive techniques. The method also has great potential for future developments with the introduction of more regional measuring variables. Off-line post-processing of colour tissue Doppler images from digital loops may allow objective quantification of dobutamine stress echocardiography. Quantification of myocardial functional reserve by off-line analysis of colour tissue Doppler acquired during dobutamine stress is feasible [17] and reproducible in 11 segments of the left ventricle. The most reliable measurements are systolic velocities of longitudinal motion in basal segments. Data suggest [18] that a fully quantitative interpretation of DSE using site-specific normal ranges of tissue Doppler, which account for regional variations of base-apex function, is feasible and equivalent in accuracy to expert wall motion scoring. Furthermore TDI improved the accuracy of wall motion scoring by novices and an experienced group [19].

11.6
Comparison with Other Stress Modalities

11.6.1
Exercise ECG

Apart from the special issues discussed in a previous section, several studies directly compared DSE with exercise ECG in a more heterogeneous patient group. Pooled data from eight studies directly comparing DSE and exercise electrocardiography in 560 patients show that the sensitivity (76% vs. 63%, $p < 0.0001$), specificity (88% vs. 64%, $p < 0.0001$) and accuracy (79% vs. 63%, $p < 0.0001$) of DSE was clearly superior. However, since most studies did not specify how many patients were able to exercise adequately, were using digoxin or had abnormal rest ECG results, these results do not indicate that the routine exercise test should be replaced by DSE. In particular, in patients with a low pretest likelihood of CAD and in men with normal results on the rest ECG it can be anticipated that DSE will provide little incremental diagnostic information in a cost-effective manner.

11.6.2
Exercise Echocardiography

Exercise echocardiography can be performed in the same set of DSE patients. Directly comparing DSE and exercise echocardiography in four studies involving 334 patients shows that the sensitivity (75% vs. 85%, $p < 0.01$) and accuracy (79% vs. 86%, $p < 0.05$) of exercise echocardiography were significantly higher. It should be emphasized that these differences were caused by one particular study in which DSE showed low accuracy. In that study a large number of DSE tests were submaximal because a modest decline in systolic blood pressure was used as a not uncommon end point, and a substantial number of the study patients were using beta-blockers while atropine was not added to dobutamine. It seems likely that in this patient cohort, the previously described dobutamine–atropine protocol would have resulted in better diagnostic accuracy, probably comparable with that of exercise echocardiography. However, the choice for the latter in patients who are expected to exercise adequately can be justified by better patient acceptance, fewer unpleasant side effects and the complementary functional information provided by exercise, such as duration of exercise, increase in heart rate, blood pressure response and reproducibility of symptoms.

11.6.3
Dipyridamole Echocardiography

In patients unable to perform adequate exercise, echocardiographic imaging can also be performed with dipyridamole as a pharmacologic stressor. In normal arteries dipyridamole, an indirect coronary vasodilator, causes a three- to five-fold increase in both subendocardial and subepicardial coronary flow. However, in stenosed arteries this augmentation is limited depending on stenosis severity, creating flow heterogeneity.

Echocardiographically detected functional evidence of ischemia is caused by coronary steal – either "subendocardium to subepicardium" or "stenotic vessel to nonstenotic". Directly comparing DSE and dipyridamole echocardiography in 422 patients, DSE is more sensitive for the detection of CAD (73% vs. 65%). This is mainly because of higher sensitivity in patients with single-vessel disease. The specificity (82% vs. 89%) and accuracy (76% vs. 72%) of the respective tests were not significantly different. These results are not surprising because dipyridamole creates primarily, blood flow heterogeneity, which is not detected by echocardiography and "real" ischemia is seen only in a limited number of patients. Moreover, the detection of ischemia with dobutamine stress is facilitated by the improved thickening of normal segments as opposed to decreased thickening of ischemic segments, whereas dipyridamole has less effect on normal segments. However, recent reports have suggested that the addition of atropine to dipyridamole increases the sensitivity of the dipyridamole test for the detection of CAD to a level comparable with DSE.

11.6.4
Radionuclide Imaging

During DSE, coronary blood flow to the vascular bed of a normal artery increases dramatically, whereas through a stenosed artery it may be altered. On the basis of this regional flow heterogeneity, DSE can also be performed in conjunction with radionuclide perfusion imaging. Comparing DSE with dobutamine technetium-99m (Tc-99m) imaging in 318 patients, sensitivity was 76% versus 81%, specificity 85% versus 71% and accuracy 80% versus 78%. The finding that DSE is more specific but may be less sensitive, especially in patients with single-vessel disease, is in line with the "ischemic cascade" theory, which states that perfusion abnormalities due to limited coronary flow reserve precede echocardiographic and ECG changes. Two studies with available angiographic data reported the diagnostic accuracy of DSE versus vasodilator perfusion imaging. In one study comparing DSE with adenosine Tc-99m imaging in 97 patients, sensitivity was 85% versus 86%, specificity 82% versus 71% and accuracy 84% versus 80%. In another study comparing DSE with dipyridamole thallium-201 imaging in 54 patients, sensitivity was 93% versus 98%, specificity 73% versus 73% and accuracy 89% versus 93%. Therefore, DSE and radionuclide perfusion imaging seem to have almost comparable diagnostic accuracy, and the choice of one test over the other can be based on patient characteristics and the availability of the laboratory performing the test.

11.7
Viable Myocardium

Pulsed wave TDI at rest and during low-dose dobutamine has been used to differentiate stunned, hibernating, and scarred myocardium using perfusion metabolism patterns on single-photon emission computed tomography (SPECT) imaging as the standard [20, 22, 23]. In a study of 70 patients with left ventricular dysfunction, there was a gradual decline in the systolic wall motion velocities between stunned, hibernating, and scarred myocardium. These differences became more pronounced during low-dose dobutamine infusion. The same investigators extended these observations to assess not only systolic, but also diastolic function of viable and nonviable myocardium. Early diastolic velocities were increased at rest compared with nonviable regions. However, with low-dose dobutamine there was no difference in early diastolic velocities in viable versus nonviable regions. Detection of post-systolic shortening, a potential marker of viability, can be readily recognized with TDI. Myocardium that is thin (non-preserved, i.e., less than 6 mm) has a very low likelihood of viability and recovery of function after revascularization (negative predictive value of 93%). A combination of increased contractile reserve during DSE and preserved myocardial thickness yields the best diagnostic accuracy for echocardiography in predicting recovery of function. Studies that have compared determination of viability with DSE and radionuclide studies have shown slightly higher sensitivity and lower specificity for radionuclide techniques.

11.8
Use of Dobutamine Stress Echo in Non-ischemic Heart Disease

Stress imaging techniques allow a unique application of DSE in valvular heart disease [23]. The majority of patients with valvular stenosis have a conclusive evaluation based on a resting echocardiogram and Doppler examination. In patients with unexplained symptoms and what appears to be moderate mitral stenosis at rest, a hemodynamic re-evaluation with DSE would be helpful. DSE can provide re-evaluation of valvular gradients during stress and simultaneous determination of pulmonary artery pressure from the tricuspid regurgitation jet. In patients with mitral regurgitation (MR), dobutamine protocols assess for the change in severity of regurgitation and the pulmonary artery pressure in response to stress, and also to detect underlying LV dysfunction. It also helps in the prognostic assessment of patients with mitral valve prolapse to provoke new MR to identify a group of high-risk individuals with normal resting echocardiographic parameters. In patients with apparent severe aortic stenosis and significant LV dysfunction, the reduction in blood flow may exaggerate the reduction in orifice area of the stenotic valve. In these instances, DSE plays a significant role in re-evaluating valvular hemodynamics and contractile reserve and confirming the presence or absence of significant aortic stenosis. The same methodology can also be applied to hypertrophic cardiomyopathy to elicit an obstructive gradient during stress.

11.9
Future Trends

Strain represents relative myocardial deformation and strain rate represents the speed of deformation. Strain and strain rate are derivatives from tissue Doppler velocities. These are relatively homogeneous throughout the myocardium, and compared with tissue velocity imaging, are less influenced by cardiac motion. Hence, myocardial function can be more accurately assessed with strain and strain rate imaging. However, the strain and strain rate signals generally have more background noise and require high frame rates. Strain rate imaging is Doppler based and sensitive to improper alignment between the cardiac axis and the ultrasound beam. Preferably, the smallest possible sector should be used and a single wall recorded at a time to get a good signal. Myocardial strain rates reflect rapidity of regional myocardial shortening or lengthening; they are calculated from TDI velocities measured at two locations separated by a given distance. Strain rate equals the instantaneous spatial velocity gradient and has units of l/s. When the two velocities being measured are different, there is deformation of the tissue in-between. Strain is calculated as the time integral of strain rate and is a dimensionless quantity expressed as a percentage. In the long axis it represents shortening fraction, and in the short axis, thickening fraction.

It is also suggested [21] that with appropriate data collection and post-processing methodologies, strain rate and strain imaging can be applied to the quantification of DSE. However, appropriate post-processing algorithms must be introduced to reduce data analysis time in order to make this a practical clinical technique. Presently, the feasibility of strain rate imaging is less than that of conventional wall motion assessment and tissue Doppler velocity imaging. Strain rate imaging offers great promise for the accurate and reproducible quantification of regional myocardial function. Further studies are indicated to prove their accuracy, efficiency, and superiority over existing methods.

Contrast imaging is another application that has tremendous potential. A standardized imaging and contrast injection protocol for contrast-enhanced DSE has been assessed [22] and power modulation contrast imaging can be applied with a completely standardized protocol for DSE in the majority of patients with excellent endocardial border definition. Similar to two-dimensional echocardiography, contrast echocardiography can be used for enhancement of endocardial border definition and possibly for myocardial perfusion.

Technological advances in transducer and computer technology have allowed the recent introduction of real-time 3D echocardiography [23]. A real-time 3D volume set can be acquired within one to four cardiac cycles. Subsequent analysis allows multiple tomographic interrogations off-line, thus avoiding foreshortening of the ventricle and possibly improving accuracy. Initial studies with 3D echocardiography during pharmacologic stress have been encouraging.

11.10
Conclusion

DSE is a feasible, safe and useful exercise-independent stress modality for assessing the presence, localization and extent of CAD. The diagnostic accuracy of DSE seems at least comparable with other, competitive non-invasive stress modalities used in patients with limited exercise capacity. Tissue Doppler and strain rate imaging will play an increasing role in stress echocardiography and offer great promise for more accurate quantification of cardiac function at rest and with stress. Further studies are needed to document the accuracy, efficiency, and effectiveness of these over existing methods. New technical developments are expected to further increase its strengths and should make the interpretation of stress echocardiograms more uniform and less subjective. Further developments in myocardial contrast echocardiography would allow the simultaneous assessment of myocardial regional function and perfusion, which would then establish it as the ultimate test.

References

1. Berthe C, Pierard LA, Hiernaux M, Trotteur G, Lempereur P, Carlier J et. al. (1986) Predicting the extent and location of coronary artery disease in acute myocardial infarction by echocardiography during dobutamine infusion. Am J Cardiol 58(13):1167–1172.

2. Schiller NB, Shah PM, Crawford M, DeMaria A, Devereux R, Feigenbaum H et al. (1989) Recommendations for quantitation of the left ventricle by two-dimensional echocardiography. American Society of Echocardiography Committee on Standards, Subcommittee on Quantitation of Two-Dimensional Echocardiograms. J Am Soc Echocardiogr 2(5):358–367. Review.
3. Gibbons RJ, Balady GJ, Beasley JW, Bricker JT, Duvernoy WF, Froelicher VF et.al. (1997) ACC/AHA Guidelines for Exercise Testing. A report of the American College of Cardiology/American Heart Association Task Force on Practice Guidelines (Committee on Exercise Testing). J Am Coll Cardiol 30(1):260–311.
4. Zoghbi WA (1991) Use of adenosine echocardiography for diagnosis of coronary artery disease. Am Heart J 122:285–292.
5. Smart SC, Knickelbine T, Malik F, Sagar KB (2000) Dobutamine-atropine stress echocardiography for the detection of coronary artery disease in patients with left ventricular hypertrophy. Importance of chamber size and systolic wall stress. Circulation 101(3):258–263.
6. Dionisopoulos PN, Collins JD, Smart SC, Knickelbine TA, Sagar KB (1997) The value of dobutamine stress echocardiography for the detection of coronary artery disease in women. J Am Soc Echocardiogr 0(8):811–817.
7. Marwick TH, Anderson T, Williams MJ, Haluska B, Melin JA, Pashkow F et al. (1995) Exercise echocardiography is an accurate and cost-efficient technique for detection of coronary artery disease in women. J Am Coll Cardiol 26(2):335–341.
8. Krahwinkel W, Ketteler T, Godke J, Wolfertz J, Ulbricht LJ, Krakau I et al. (1997) Dobutamine stress echocardiography. Eur Heart J Suppl D:D9–D15.
9. Cortigiani L, Picano E, Vigna C, Lattanzi F, Coletta C, Mariotti E et al. (2001) EPIC (Echo Persantine International Cooperative) and EDIC (Echo Dobutamine International Cooperative) Study Groups. Prognostic value of pharmacologic stress echocardiography in patients with left bundle branch block. Am J Med 110(5):361–369.
10. Elhendy A, Geleijnse ML, Roelandt JR, Cornel JH, van Domburg RT, El-Refaee M et al. (1996) Assessment of patients after coronary artery bypass grafting by dobutamine stress echocardiography. Am J Cardiol 77(14):1234–1236.
11. Marwick TH (2003) Stress Echocardiography - Its Role in the Diagnosis and Evaluation of Coronary Artery Disease, 2nd edn. Kluwer Academic Publishers, Boston, MA.
12. Heinle SK, Lieberman EB, Ancukiewicz M, Waugh RA, Bashore TM, Kisslo J (1993) Usefulness of dobutamine echocardiography for detecting restenosis after percutaneous transluminal coronary angioplasty. Am J Cardiol 72(17):1220–1225.
13. Pratali L, Picano E, Otasevic P, Vigna C, Palinkas A, Cortigiani L et al. (1997) Prognostic significance of the dobutamine echocardiography test in idiopathic dilated cardiomyopathy. Am J Cardiol 88(12):1374–1378.
14. Geleijnse ML, Fioretti PM, Roelandt JR (1997) Methodology, feasibility, safety and diagnostic accuracy of dobutamine stress echocardiography. J Am Coll Cardiol 30(3):595–606.
15. Picano E, Mathias W Jr, Pingitore A, Bigi R, Previtali M (1994) Safety and tolerability of dobutamine-atropine stress echocardiography: a prospective, multicentre study. Echo Dobutamine International Cooperative Study Group. Lancet 344(8931):1190–1192.
16. Brodin LA (2004) Tissue Doppler, a fundamental tool for parametric imaging. Clin Physiol Funct Imaging 24(3):147–155.
17. Fraser AG, Payne N, Madler CF, Janerot-Sjoberg B, Lind B, Grocott-Mason RM, Ionescu AA, Florescu N, Wilkenshoff U, Lancellotti P, Wutte M, Brodin LA, MYDISE Investigators (2003). Feasibility and reproducibility of off-line tissue Doppler measurement of regional myocardial function during dobutamine stress echocardiography. Eur J Echocardiogr 4(1):43–53.
18. Cain P, Baglin T, Case C, Spicer D, Short L, Marwick TH (2001) Application of tissue Doppler to interpretation of dobutamine echocardiography and comparison with quantitative coronary angiography. Am J Cardiol 87(5):525–531.
19. Fathi R, Cain P, Nakatani S, Yu HC, Marwick TH (2001) Effect of tissue Doppler on the accuracy of novice and expert interpreters of dobutamine echocardiography. Am J Cardiol 88(4):400–405.
20. Pellikka PA (2005) Stress echocardiography for the diagnosis of coronary artery disease: progress towards quantification. Curr Opin Cardiol 20(5):395–398.
21. Kowalski M, Herregods MC, Herbots L, Weidemann F, Simmons L, Strotmann J, Dommke C, D'hooge J, Claus P, Bijnens B, Hatle L, Sutherland GR (2003) The feasibility of ultrasonic regional strain and strain rate imaging in quantifying dobutamine stress echocardiography. Eur J Echocardiogr 4(2):81–91.
22. Thibault H, Timperley J, Ehlgen A, Pariente A, Dawson D, Becher H (2005) Can contrast dobutamine stress echocardiography be performed with standardized imaging settings for everybody? J Am Soc Echocardiogr 18(11):1194–1202.
23. Armstrong WF, Zoghbi WA (2005) Stress echocardiography: current methodology and clinical applications. Review. J Am Coll Cardiol 45(11):1739–1747.

Chapter 12

Transesophageal echocardiography

Satish C. Govind and S. S. Ramesh

Contents

12.1	Introduction	137
12.2	Technique	138
12.3	Clinical Application	138
12.3.1	Endocarditis	139
12.3.2	Atrial Fibrillation	139
12.3.3	Valvular Evaluation	140
12.3.4	Aorta	141
12.3.5	Intraoperative Monitoring	142
12.3.6	Congenital Heart Disease	142
12.3.7	Catheter-Based Procedures	142
12.4	Discussion	142
12.5	Future Trends	143
	References	143

12.1 Introduction

Transesophageal echocardiography (TOE) is a specialised echo application that is frequently utilised by cardiologists and also by surgeons, anaesthesiologists and intensivists for quick decision making, monitoring and guiding operative procedures, interventions, and managing critically ill patients. It is the term used to describe the study of the heart from the oesophagus using two-dimensional, three-dimensional, M-mode or Doppler echocardiography. The clinical application of TOE continues to grow, and the indications, diagnostic utility and related issues of this application are discussed briefly here.

Imaging through the gastro-oesophageal tract provides unobstructed ultrasound signals and allows use of high frequency ultrasound, thereby providing excellent spatial resolution. There is a steep learning curve for the interpretation of structural and haemodynamic information. The technique, which has wide applicability, can be readily utilised in day to day clinical practice.

Transesophageal Doppler echocardiography was first reported by Side and Gosling in 1971. They used a dual element construction mounted on a standard gastroscope to obtain continuous wave Doppler information about the velocity of cardiac blood flow [1].

Over the next few decades technological developments facilitated the transition of TOE to its present clinical status. This included the introduction of the flexible endoscope, miniaturisation, and improvements in transducer design, improvement from monoplane, biplane to multiplane imaging, and the addition of spectral and colour Doppler imaging. Newer applications such as tissue Doppler imaging and multi-dimensional echo have also made their entry. TOE is currently used in approximately 5–10% of patients being evaluated in the Echo lab. It is a low risk procedure that yields an enormous amount of clinically relevant information when used appropriately. Although it is semi-invasive, TOE is generally very safe.

12.2
Technique

The oesophagus is a muscular tube with an average diameter of 20 mm extending approximately 25 cm from the pharynx to the stomach [2]. As it descends inferiorly into the thorax, the oesophagus courses behind the trachea, left mainstem bronchus, left atrium (LA), and left ventricle (LV) before it passes through the diaphragm. Because of the close proximity of the oesophagus to the posterior surface of the heart, the ultrasound beam needs to penetrate only the muscular oesophageal wall before reaching the pericardium, making the oesophagus an ideal echocardiographic window for cardiac examination.

Medical history is taken to look for contraindications such as, haematemesis, dysphagia and cervical spine disease. Absolute contraindications to TOE include oesophageal stricture, diverticulum, tumour, and recent oesophageal or gastric surgery. The patient must be fasting for at least 4–6 hours before the procedure. Blood pressure and heart rate are measured. Dentures and oral prostheses should be removed. Airway, oxygen delivery system, bite guard, suction, and standard crash cart should be immediately available. An intravenous access should be established.

Awake patients are premedicated with topical anesthesia of oropharynx and hard and soft palates, which diminishes the gag reflex. This is induced by an aerosol local anesthetic lidocaine solution that should ideally be applied with the patient in the sitting position to reduce the risk of aspiration. Other agents used include viscous lidocaine. Sedation may be required to decrease anxiety and discomfort, with administration of an intravenous sedative belonging to the benzodiazepines group like diazepam or midazolam. Drying agents that are optional lessen salivary and gastrointestinal secretions, reducing the risk of aspiration. The anticholinergic agent glycopyrrolate is used to control secretions effectively. Antibiotics help prevent infective endocarditis in selected high-risk patients. The issue of endocarditis prophylaxis during TOE remains controversial. Since the procedure is similar to that of endoscopic examinations, there may be some merit to administering infective endocarditis prophylaxis in patients with previous endocarditis, prosthetic valves and those with multivalvar disease. Patients receiving long-term anticoagulation therapy should have their dosing appropriately adjusted to reduce the risk of bleeding prior to the procedure.

Being semi-invasive, appropriate training requirements are needed and have been laid down by the American Society of Echocardiography (ASE) [3] and European Society of Cardiology (ESC) [4]. Though procedural risks are low in trained hands they need to be explained clearly to the patient. These include throat pain, minor throat bleeding, nausea, laryngospasm, bronchospasm, aspiration, hypotension, hypertension, tachycardia, mucosal bleeding, oesophageal rupture, angina, heart failure, and rarely, risk of death.

After obtaining informed consent and anesthetizing, the patient is placed in the left lateral position and the neck slightly flexed to allow for better oropharyngeal positioning. Dentures and oral prostheses must be removed before the examination. Intubation can also be performed with the patient in the supine position and if necessary the upright sitting position. A bite guard is essential to allow manipulation and protection of the TOE probe. The distal portion of the transducer is coated with lubricating jelly. The examiner passes the probe tip through the bite guard and over the tongue, all along maintaining it in the midline. The tip is slowly advanced until resistance is encountered, then the patient is asked to swallow and with gentle forward pressure the transducer is advanced until loss of resistance is felt then the transducer is passed into the oesophagus. There is no standardized protocol for obtaining the necessary views in the TOE examination, but a general rule of thumb would be to obtain the most clinically relevant views first, based on the reason for the procedure, then methodically move on to complete the rest of the imaging. When the procedure is over, the precautions that should be taken by the patient include not to drink any liquid until oropharyngeal anesthesia has worn off (1 hour), not to eat until gag reflex returns (1–4 hours) and not to drive for 12 hours (if a sedative was given). The incidence of unsuccessful probe introductions is about 1.9%, whereas 0.9% of examinations maybe interrupted before completion because of patient intolerance A small proportion of patients cannot tolerate the study and, either gag so much that the probe can not be inserted, or remove the probe forcibly before the study is completed

12.3
Clinical Application

The indications for a TOE study have continued to grow over the last few years. Now TOE is indicated in almost any condition in which routine transthoracic echocardiography fails to provide definitive diagnostic information (e.g., the presence of an atrial septal defect is unclear on TTE) or during surgery. Also, it is indicated whenever it is expected to add important information beyond that obtained by routine echo and whenever the clinical question is important enough to take the small risk and discomfort associated with the procedure. The principal indications for a TOE study are published in the Guidelines from the Working Group on Echocardiography of the ESC [4].

The most common indications [2] for TOE are evaluation for infective endocarditis (IE), assessment of embolic risk prior to cardioversion for atrial fibrillation (AF), and evaluating the heart and aorta as a source for systemic emboli. Other clinical situations would include aortic dissection, intraoperative and perioperative cardiac monitoring, and instances in which the transthoracic echocardiogram (TTE) is diagnostically inadequate due to poor quality or limited echocardiographic windows. Despite technical advances and better image resolution, TOE continues to be superior to transthoracic echocardiography for better visualisation of the shape, size of vegetations and ensuing sequelae, which may affect surrounding structures [6].

12.3.1
Endocarditis

The diagnosis of infective endocarditis is straightforward in some patients with bacteremia, active valvulitis and immunologic vascular phenomena, while in others, classical features could be few or even absent. This may occur during acute courses of IE, particularly among intravenous drug users in whom IE is often due to Staphylococcus aureus infection of right-sided heart valves, or in patients with IE caused by other microorganisms such as haemophilus parainfluenza, Actinobacillus, Cardiobacterium hominis, Eikenella and Kingella species. Acute IE evolves too quickly for the development of immunologic vascular phenomena, which are more characteristic of subacute IE. In addition, acute right-sided IE valve lesions do not create the peripheral emboli and immunologic vascular phenomena that can result from left-sided valvular involvement [7]. The variability in the clinical presentation of IE requires a diagnostic strategy that will be both sensitive for disease detection and specific for its exclusion across all forms of the disease. Duke's criteria, which forms the basis of current guidelines, incorporate echocardiographic documentation of vegetations in establishing a diagnosis of infective endocarditis (IE). Transthoracic echocardiography has excellent specificity for vegetations (98%) but the overall sensitivity for vegetations, however, is <60%. TOE provides a significant improvement in sensitivity, primarily at detecting small vegetations (<5 mm), which are difficult to visualise by TTE. Obesity, poor echo window, prosthetic valves also preclude optimal visualisation. In these situations TOE is the ideal investigation to detect vegetations. TOE is also important for assessing the structural complications such as myocardial abscess, fistulas, mycotic aneurysms, valvar valvular aneurysms or perforations, flail leaflets, or prosthetic valve dehiscence which are indicators for surgical intervention. TOE in experienced hands has high sensitivity of detection of vegetations. It has a substantially higher sensitivity (76% to 100%) and specificity (94%) than TTE for perivalvular extension of infection. It also enhances visualization of prosthetic valves, with 86% to 94% sensitivity and 88% to 100% specificity for vegetations and additionally could be very useful in detecting and quantitating regurgitation. Suspicion of IE may persist after an initially negative TOE. While a negative TOE does not have enough diagnostic accuracy to rule out IE, potential sources of false-negative TOE studies include vegetations that are smaller than the limits of resolution, previous embolization of vegetation, or inadequate views to detect small abscesses. Multiple TOE and TTE planes are absolutely essential before a negative conclusion is drawn. When both TOE and TTE studies are negative, there is a 95% negative predictive value. When clinical suspicion of IE is high and the TOE results are negative, a repeat study is necessary within 7 to 10 days, which may demonstrate previously undetected vegetations. False positive findings for vegetations in TOE, however, may occur due to misinterpretation of artefacts, sewing ring suture, surgically severed or retained chordae tendinae, fibrin strands, or periprosthetic material.

12.3.2
Atrial Fibrillation

Atrial fibrillation has a predilection towards emboli formation. Atrial stunning, whether brief or prolonged after cardioversion results in inadequate emptying and dilatation of the left atrium and left atrial appendage, which subsequently predisposes to stasis of blood and thrombus formation. Paroxysmal atrial fibrillation may lead to thrombus formation in the left atrium. Left atrial thrombus may be detected in the presence of sinus rhythm. In the absence of thrombus, spontaneous echo contrast has been shown to be a strong predictor of ischaemic strokes. An annual thromboembolic event rate of 12% has been observed in patients with spontaneous echo contrast compared with 3% in patients without it [6]. Among patients presenting with new-onset atrial fibrillation, TOE studies have demonstrated an incidence of atrial thrombi in 12–15% of patients and an incidence of 27% in patients with chronic atrial fibrillation. The frequency increases to 50% among patients presenting with atrial fibrillation in the clinical background of acute thromboembolism [5]. Combining pulsed wave Doppler and 2-D imaging by TOE has further augmented risk stratifying the thromboembolic risk of patients with atrial fibrillation. An enlarged left atrium, spontaneous echo contrast and a reduced flow rate (<25 cm/s) within the enlarged left atrial appendage are associated with an increased thromboembolic risk even in the absence of a left atrial thrombus and are also associated with a high recurrence rate of atrial fibrillation after successful cardioversion. Thus the prevailing use of TOE in patients with AF is primarily twofold: (1) risk stratification for the likelihood or cause of embolic events and the need for anticoagulation; and (2) detection of thrombi in left atrium or left atrial appendage prior to DC cardioversion [8].

For potential cardiac sources of emboli, TOE has been shown to have high accuracy in identifying abnormal lesions in patients with cardioembolic strokes which may include abnormalities of the left and right atrium and their appendages, aortic atheromas, patent foramen ovale (PFO), atrial septal aneurysm (ASA), vegetations, spontaneous contrast, left ventricular clots, and various cardiac masses. The diagnostic yield of TOE for a cardiac source of emboli in patients presenting with unexplained stroke or transient ischaemic attacks is high, with potential lesions identified in over 50% of the studies. A common part of the evaluation for cryptogenic stroke is the demonstration of a possible PFO, for which TOE is currently considered to be the reference standard for its detection. During the TOE examination for PFO, it is necessary to evaluate for the presence of ASA as well as a Chiari network because these conditions are associated with a significant number of PFOs. M-mode TOE of the IAS helps to facilitate the measurement of septal excursion, where an excursion >15 mm yields the diagnosis ASA [2].

12.3.3
Valvular Evaluation

Compared with transthoracic echocardiography, TOE provides improved signal-to-noise ratio and improved spatial resolution using high frequency transducers, and with this unique advantage there is improved acoustic penetration through mechanical valves thus making TOE the first-choice modality for the investigation of patients with prosthetic valves, especially those with mechanical mitral valve replacement. TOE is used routinely to evaluate prosthetic valves, both at the time of implantation as well as well as later when complications associated with these valves are suspected (Figs. 12.1 and 12.2). Prosthetic valves are classified either as biological (tissue) or mechanical. Biological valves are subsequently subdivided into homografts (allografts) or heterografts (xenografts). Mechanical heart valves are subdivided into ball-in-cage, single leaflet tilting disc, or double leaflet tilting disc types. A single tilting disc valve will have two orifices, one larger than the other, within a symmetric flow profile. The bileaflet tilting disc valve will have two large valve orifices with a small narrow central orifice. Flow through the central orifice will result in relatively high velocities with localized gradients often higher than the overall gradient across the entire valve. Additional findings such as thrombi in the left atrium and left atrial appendage as well as valvular or paravalvular leakages can easily be detected by TOE. These findings are nearly always missed by TTE, especially in mechanical prostheses, because of shadowing. TOE is the procedure of choice for detecting other abnormalities of mitral valve prostheses, such as cusp abnormalities in tissue prosthesis, embolic events, patient–prosthesis mismatch, and malfunction of repaired

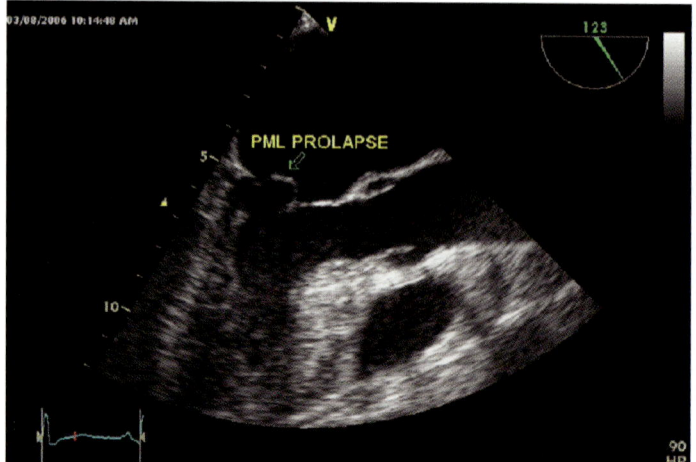

Fig. 12.1 Lower oesophageal view showing clear delineation of the mitral and aortic leaflets with marked prolapse of the posterior mitral leaflet (PML) (*arrow*)

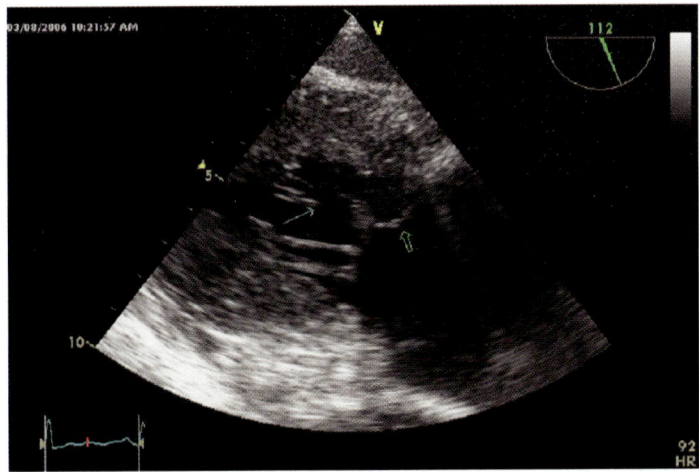

Fig. 12.2 Transgastric view showing the mitral leaflets and chordae (*thin arrow*) with a prolapsed posterior mitral leaflet (*thick arrow*)

valves and implanted rings. TOE is also useful in diagnosing prosthetic valve thrombosis and for deciding whether thrombolytic treatment is required. TOE allows close examination of the sewing ring and the occluder, thus helping differentiate pannus from a thrombus, and for establishing the mechanism of a choked valve. The aortic valve lies in a plane perpendicular with the oesophagus, with a flow that has an asymmetric profile, therefore assessment of a prosthetic aortic valve by TOE may be more challenging while it is useful in providing a high resolution assessment of valves in tricuspid and pulmonic positions. Another indication for TOE in valvular assessment is evaluation of the patient prior to possible balloon mitral valvuloplasty (BMV). The TOE must include a thorough assessment of the LA and LA appendage for the presence of thrombus, as well as the quantification of mitral regurgitation (MR), since the presence of either a thrombus or moderate MR is a relative contraindication for BMV. The mitral valve itself should be carefully evaluated (mitral scoring) for mobility, thickening, calcification and with a characterization of the subvalvular apparatus. The mitral valve-echo scoring system is used to determine a patient's suitability for BMV. Thus TOE allows assessment of prosthetic valve anatomy and function and paraprosthetic anatomy, and serves as the diagnostic imaging modality of choice for patients with suspected prosthesis dysfunction or endocarditis [9]. TOE also plays a major role in the determination of MR aetiology, mechanism and severity when mitral valve repair is being planned [10]. A thorough anatomical examination of the mitral apparatus via multiplane TOE, delineating where the pathology is and the type of pathology being detected, becomes a necessity. It is also extremely sensitive in detecting aortic leaflet morphology and also minute amounts of aortic regurgitation, although it has a very limited role to play in aortic stenosis.

12.3.4
Aorta

TOE is now commonly used to evaluate the thoracic aorta. This would include acute and chronic aortic diseases, such as aortic dissection, aneurysm, atherosclerosis and aortic trauma. When compared with other technologies that are used to evaluate the thoracic aorta, TOE has the unique advantages of portability and the ability to obtain high-resolution images of the normal and pathologic anatomy of the three layers of the aortic wall and the aortic lumen [11, 12]. Aortic dissection is a catastrophic illness with a dangerously high mortality rate during the first 48 h of presentation. Mortality can be improved upon by early diagnosis and prompt initiation of aggressive medical/surgical therapy. In comparative imaging of multiplane TOE with spiral computed tomography (CT) and magnetic resonance imaging (MRI), the sensitivity and specificity of TOE for diagnosing aortic dissections has been reported as 98% and 95%, respectively [6]. The chief advantage of TOE in imaging aortic dissections is that it provides diagnostic information faster than other modalities, and it is the only modality that can be used intraoperatively during surgery. Based on TOE findings, intramural haematoma and penetrating atherosclerotic ulcers are now believed to be major precursors of aortic wall dissection. These conditions may lead to perforation of the intima and initiate dissection. The most important diagnostic finding of aortic dissection that can be seen on TOE is the presence of an undulating intimal flap within the aortic lumen that differentiates a false (usually larger) lumen from a true (usually smaller) lumen. What has to be kept in mind is that small dissections could lead to false negative assumptions while artefacts can result in false positive findings. TOE has also been used to assess atheroma features such as atheroma protrusion, ulceration and flow dynamics. The high-risk patients for embolic events are those with mobile plaques, ulcerated plaques, and plaques that protrude into the aorta by >4–5 mm. As such, these plaque characteristics should be specifically reported in any patient undergoing TOE. Other conditions of the aorta where TOE is of help are the penetrating aortic ulcers which occur when an ulceration of an atherosclerotic plaque erodes through the internal elastic lamina into the aortic wall media, and aortic intramural hematoma which is a localized separation of the layers of the aortic wall by partially or totally clotted blood in the absence of an intimal tear.

12.3.5
Intraoperative Monitoring

TOE is an important intraoperative diagnostic adjunct during cardiac surgery, where it is used to evaluate a hypotension/low-cardiac output state and to discern valve-related problems, particularly during aortic valve replacement and mitral valve repair. Three important and often remedial reasons for hypotension/low cardiac output in this setting include the following: left ventricular (LV) or right ventricular (RV) systolic dysfunction; hypovolemia; and outflow tract obstruction [2]. During myocardial revascularization TOE allows for the non-invasive evaluation of global and regional left ventricular function. The myocardium is observed for all three coronary distributions. In this setting, the transgastric short-axis images are particularly valuable since they tend to avoid the foreshortening of the apex that is inherent in images obtained from the oesophageal images. Hypovolaemia could be a cause of hypotension in the early post-operative setting, in which the pulmonary capillary wedge pressure may provide misleading data due to changes in LV compliance resulting from cardiopulmonary bypass. In this setting, TOE images reveal diminished cavity size and hyper dynamic LV, thereby requiring fluid resuscitation. TOE has become an integral part in the evaluation of patients for mitral valve repair. A quality echocardiographic examination of the mitral valve apparatus is necessary to determine the anatomic pathology of the mitral apparatus as well as the abnormal flow characteristics across it. Knowledge of the anatomic structure aids the surgeon in deciding which of the surgical procedures to perform. TOE is the best imaging modality for imaging the heart at immediate postoperative state, as there is immediate availability of the haemodynamic and anatomical information, thus permitting rapid and adequate therapeutic intervention.

12.3.6
Congenital Heart Disease

TOE is superior to trans-thoracic echocardiography for the evaluation of specific defects, such as atrial septal defects, anomalous pulmonary venous connections, and complex cardiac malformations. Sinus venosus defects and anomalous pulmonary vein drainage are detected more easily by TOE than by trans-thoracic echocardiography because of the proximity of these structures to the transducer. TOE is recommended in any patient with an unexplained right heart dilatation for ruling out a sinus venosus atrial septal defect and associated pulmonary venous abnormalities. TOE is also useful for visualising the margins of an atrial septal defect for identifying patients who may benefit from non-surgical device closure of the defect.

12.3.7
Catheter-Based Procedures

TOE also plays a role in the interventional laboratory for percutaneous interventions such as transcatheter closure of atrial septal defects and ventricular septal defects. It is used before the procedure for identifying the defect, excluding multiple defects, measuring the adequacy of the rim of the interatrial septum and its relation to the adjoining structures.

It also has an important role to play in balloon valvuloplasties of the mitral, aortic and pulmonary valves, septal ablation in hypertrophic obstructive cardiomyopathy, atrial septostomy, radiofrequency ablation of cardiac arrhythmias, implantation of the left atrial appendage occluder, closure of PFO and also plays an important role in patients with heart failure undergoing implantation of left ventricular assist devices for selecting the type of assist device necessary (right versus left or biventricular) [6].

12.4
Discussion

In the world of emerging sophisticated technologies to image the heart and the great vessels within the chest, such as multi-slice computed tomography and cardiovascular magnetic resonance imaging, TOE has achieved a firm place in the diagnostic armamentarium of the cardiologist. TOE is remarkable in its capability to scan the heart at bedside from perspectives that cannot be easily attained by any other modality, and is especially suited to visualize small and rapidly moving structures thus enhancing its diagnostic yield [5]. The wide acceptability, its easy utilisation, its portability, and the relatively low cost of the procedure has resulted in increased usage in clinical applications for the evaluation of patients with cardiovascular disease. This is particularly so with respect to intensivists, surgeons, anesthesiologists, as well as specialists in cardiovascular diseases, for the evaluation and treatment of all types of patients. CT scanning and MRI, although providing enhanced images, are not performed in real time. Thus TOE is an integral part of present-day practice of cardiology, with a broad range of utilities providing a unique combination of anatomical and haemodynamic information at bedside, and looks set to grow further with the emergence and development of newer applications. Despite its value in many clinical scenarios, several limitations and pitfalls need to be borne in mind.

12.5
Future Trends

A promising new application may be TOE guided cardioversion using the same probe. This would allow for exclusion of atrial thrombi and electrical cardioversion via the oesophagus within the same session. This technique would not only contribute to save time and costs but also to reduce discomfort for the patient, who can be safely treated in only one session needing only one sedation. A probe assembly for simultaneous transesophageal echocardiography and transesophageal cardioversion has been developed. This probe allows cardioversion with the delivery of much lower energy than the standard external approach. The use of a combined probe may be the technique of choice for patients who require both cardioversion and transesophageal echocardiography [13]. Future miniaturisation of the TOE transducer would help minimise discomfort from longer monitoring of cardiovascular haemodynamics and treatment. Tissue Doppler and strain rate imaging applications in TOE are gaining increasing recognition because of their quantitative ability. Three-dimensional transesophageal echocardiography (3D-TOE) provides unique "en face" views of intracardiac structures. One study showed that 3D-TOE and transcatheter methods are two complementary techniques for the success of transcatheter ASDs closure [14]. Real-time 3D-TOE, which is still evolving, would further refine TOE and make it a comprehensive procedure.

References

1. Side CD, Gosling RG (1971) Non-surgical assessment of cardiac function.Nature 232(5309):335–336.
2. Milani RV, Lavie CJ, Gilliland YE, Cassidy MM, Bernal JA (2002) Overview of transesophageal echocardiography for the chest physician. Chest 124(3):1081–1089. Review.
3. Shanewise JS, Cheung AT, Aronson S, Stewart WJ, Weiss RL, Mark JB et al. (1999) ASE/SCA guidelines for performing a comprehensive intraoperative multiplane transoesophageal echocardiography examination: recommendations of the American Society of Echocardiography Council for Intraoperative Echocardiography and the Society of Cardiovascular Anesthesiologists Task Force for Certification in Perioperative Transesophageal Echocardiography. J Am Soc Echocardiogr 12(10):884–900.
4. Flachskampf FA, Decoodt P, Fraser AG, Daniel WG, Roelandt JR (2001) Subgroup on Transesophageal Echocardiography and Valvular Heart Disease; Working Group on Echocardiography of the European Society of Cardiology. Guidelines from the Working Group. Recommendations for performing transesophageal echocardiography. Eur J Echocardiogr 2(1):8–21.
5. Kuhl HP, Hanrath P (2004) The impact of transesophageal echocardiography on daily clinical practice. Eur J Echocardiogr 5(6):455–468. Review.
6. Sengupta PP, Khandheria BK (2005) Transoesophageal echocardiography.Heart 91(4):541–547. Review.
7. Bayer AS, Bolger AF, Taubert KA, Wilson W, Steckelberg J, Karchmer AW et al. (1998) Diagnosis and management of infective endocarditis and its complications. Circulation 98(25):2936–2948.
8. Asher CR, Klein AL (2003) Transesophageal echocardiography in patients with atrial fibrillation. Pacing Clin Electrophysiol 26(7 Pt 2):1597–1603. Review.
9. Bach DS (2000) Transesophageal echocardiographic (TEE) evaluation of prosthetic valves. Cardiol Clin 18(4):751–771. Review.
10. Perrino AC Jr, Scott T, Reeves A (2003) Practical Approach to Transesophageal Echocardiography. Lippincott Williams & Wilkins, Philadelphia, PA.
11. Willens HJ, Kessler KM (1999) Transesophageal echocardiography in the diagnosis of diseases of the thoracic aorta: part I – Aortic dissection, aortic intramural hematoma, and penetrating atherosclerotic ulcer of the aorta. Chest 116(6):1772–1779. Review.
12. Willens HJ, Kessler KM (2000) Transesophageal echocardiography in the diagnosis of diseases of the thoracic

aorta: part II-atherosclerotic and traumatic diseases of the aorta. Chest 117(1):233–243. Review.
13. Kronzon I, Tunick PA, Scholten MF, Kerber RE, Roelandt JR (2005) Combined transesophageal echocardiography and transesophageal cardioversion probe: technical aspects. J Am Soc Echocardiogr 18(3):213–215.
14. Abdel-Massih T, Dulac Y, Taktak A, Aggoun Y, Massabuau P, Elbaz M et al. (2005) Assessment of atrial septal defect size with 3D-transesophageal echocardiography: comparison with balloon method. Echocardiography 22(2):121–127.

Chapter 13

Clinical Cardiac Electrophysiology – An Overview

Senthil Thenappan, Jaffar Ali Raza, R. Wayne Kreeger and Assad Movahed

Contents

13.1	Introduction	145
13.2	Basic Electrophysiologic Principles	145
13.3	The Electrical Conduction System of the Heart	145
13.4	Mechanism of Arrhythmias	146
13.4.1	Disorders of Impulse Formation	146
13.5	Differential Diagnosis of Arrhythmias	147
13.6	Diagnostic Cardiac Electrophysiological Study	147
13.7	Genetics of Cardiac Arrhythmias	148
13.8	Pharmacological Treatment of Cardiac Arrhythmias	149
13.9	Implantable Cardioverter–Defibrillator Therapy	149
13.9.1	Clinical Indications [35]	150
13.9.2	Contraindications [35]	150
13.10	Catheter Ablation Therapy	151
13.11	Pacing Therapy	151
13.12	Cardiac Resynchronization Therapy	152
	References	152

13.1 Introduction

Clinical cardiac electrophysiology is a subspecialty of cardiology dealing with the evaluation and management of patients with complex rhythm or conduction abnormalities. In the last four decades, clinical cardiac electrophysiology has evolved into an established discipline credited with improving and saving hundreds of thousands of lives. We briefly review the basic electrophysiologic principles, anatomy of the electric system of the heart, mechanism of arrhythmias, genetical predisposition to arrhythmias, types of arrhythmias, diagnostic electrophysiologic studies, and pharmacologic and device therapies available for the treatment of different types of arrhythmias.

13.2 Basic Electrophysiologic Principles

Most cardiac cells have a resting membrane potential of –80 to –90 mV except the sinuatrial and atrioventricular nodes, and the potassium gradient across the cell membrane determines it. Movement of ions across the cell membrane produces a transient depolarization called action potential, which results in activation of the cardiac cell. The configuration of the action potential depends on the type of ion movement, and it varies from one cardiac cell to the other. The action potential of the Purkinje fibers consists of five phases (phase 0–4). Phase 0 is the rapid depolarization caused by the influx of sodium ions into the cardiac cell followed by a slow depolarization caused by calcium ion influx. Phases 1, 2, and 3 are repolarization phases caused by outflow of potassium ions. Phase 4 is the resting membrane potential.

13.3 The Electrical Conduction System of the Heart

The conducting system of the heart consists of specialized cardiac muscle present in the sinuatrial node

(SAN), the atrioventricular node (AVN), the atrioventricular bundle, its right and left terminal branches, and the subendocardial plexus of Purkinje fibers (specialized cardiac muscle fibers that form the conducting system of the heart). The SAN is located in the wall of the right atrium just to the right of the opening of the superior vena cava. The AVN lies at the lower part of the atrial septum just above the attachment of the septal cusp of the tricuspid valve. The atrioventricular bundle (bundle of His) emerges from the AVN, descends through the fibrous skeleton of the heart, and passes anteriorly across the membranous interventricular septum. Usually, the bundle of His is the only pathway of cardiac muscle that connects the myocardium of the atria and the ventricles. At the upper part of the muscular part of the septum, the bundle of His divides into the right and left bundle branches. The bundle branches eventually become continuous with the fibers of the Purkinje system, which ultimately extends through the endocardium of the right and left ventricles.

Under normal conditions, electrical impulses originate from the SAN, spread in all directions through the cardiac muscle of the atria, and cause the atrial muscle to contract. The impulses from the SAN reach the AVN rapidly through three special pathways namely, the anterior, the middle, and the posterior internodal pathways. The rate of conduction of the impulses through the AVN is slow, resulting in the PR interval. From the AVN, the impulses travel down through the bundle of His, the bundle branches, and the Purkinjee fibers to reach the ventricular myocardium. The autonomic nervous system regulates the activities of the conduction system; parasympathetic stimulation slows the rate of conduction of the impulse while sympathetic stimulation increases it.

13.4
Mechanism of Arrhythmias

Cardiac arrhythmias result from either disorders of impulse formation or disorders of impulse conduction (Fig. 13.1) [1]. The clinical examination and current diagnostic modalities do not precisely determine the electrophysiologic mechanisms of many arrhythmias, especially ventricular arrhythmias. In addition, some arrhythmias have more than one mechanism.

13.4.1
Disorders of Impulse Formation

13.4.1.1 Automaticity

Automaticity is the ability of cardiac cells to spontaneously initiate an impulse and depolarize repeatedly without any stimulation. A period of electrical dormancy does not exist, and this results from spontaneous phase 4 depolarization (Fig. 13.2).

Under normal conditions, only specialized cardiac cells, the pacemaker cells, have the property of automaticity. The SAN is the dominant pacemaker of the heart. The cells in the specialized fibers in the atria, the coronary sinus, the pulmonary veins, the AV valves, the AV junction, the bundle of His, the ventricles, and the right and left ventricular outflow tracts are also capable of manifesting automaticity. These are called ectopic or latent or subsidiary pacemakers, and are normally prevented from reaching the threshold potential level by overdrive suppression from the rapidly firing SAN. The other cardiac cells do not normally possess automaticity. Enhancement of the normal automaticity of the pacemaker cells or development of abnormal automaticity (resulting from a decrease in the membrane potential), either in the pacemaker cells or the normal cardiac cells, initiates an arrhythmia.

13.4.1.2 Triggered Activity

After-depolarizations generate triggered arrhythmias. After-depolarizations are oscillations in membrane voltage during the recovery or repolarization phase, induced by one or more preceding action potentials. An after-depolarization of sufficient magnitude may reach "threshold" and trigger an early action potential. There are two types of after-depolarizations, early and delayed.

Early after-depolarizations (EAD) occur during phase 2 or 3 of the cardiac action potential and prolong the QT interval [2]. Increased intracellular positivity causes EADs. The L-type calcium channel may have a role [3]. EAD appears to be responsible for acquired and congenital long QT syndromes and torsades de pointes [4–6]. Magnesium and increased heart rate suppress EAD.

Delayed after-depolarizations (DAD) occur after phase 3 when the action potential is fully repolarized. The mechanism is unclear; however, it is associated with high intracellular Ca^{++} concentrations. DAD is the underlying mechanism in digitalis-induced tachyarrythmias, accelerated idioventricular rhythm in acute infarction, and exercise induced ventricular tachycardia.

13.4.1.3 Re-Entry

Re-entry is the most common mechanism for arrhythmia, and is associated with repetitive excitation of a region of the heart. Re-entry results from conduction of an electrical impulse around a fixed obstacle in a defined circuit referred to as re-entrant tachycardia. The initiation and maintenance of re-entry requires electro-

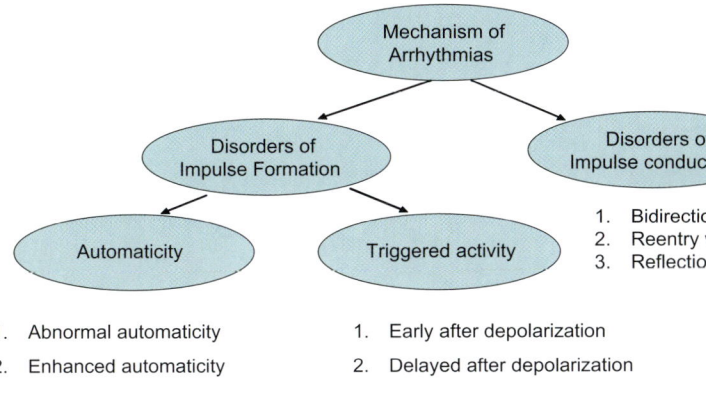

Fig. 13.1 Mechanism of cardiac arrhythmias (from Zipes DP. Mechanisms of clinical arrhythmias. J Cardiovasc Electrophysiol. 2003;14(8):902–912)

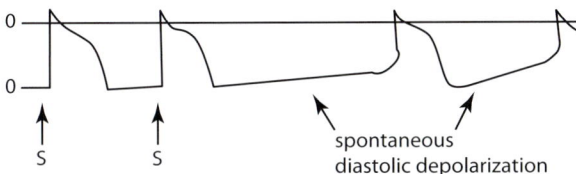

Fig. 13.2 Action potential of the sinoatrial node with spontaneous phase 4 depolarization

physiologic inhomogeneity in two or more regions of the heart connected with each other to form a closed loop, unidirectional block in one pathway, slow conduction over an alternative pathway, allowing time for the initially blocked pathway to recover excitability, and re-excitability of the initially blocked pathway to complete a loop of activation. Repetitive circulation of the impulse over this loop results in tachyarrhythmias. Re-entry can occur over an anatomically established pathway (AVN and an accessory pathway to produce AV re-entry tachycardia), or it can be functional in nature (ventricular ischemia) [7]. Interrupting the re-entry pathways by catheter ablation or by anti-arrhythmic drugs terminates re-entrant tachycardias. Clinical arrhythmias resulting from re-entry include AV nodal re-entrant tachycardia (AVNRT), atrioventricular reentrant tachycardia (AVRT), pre-excitation syndromes (e.g., WPW), ventricular tachycardias, ventricular fibrillation, the Brugada syndrome, atrial fibrillation, atrial flutter, and atrial tachycardias.

13.5
Differential Diagnosis of Arrhythmias

Tachyarrhythmias are characterized as narrow complex (QRS duration <120 milliseconds) and wide complex (QRS duration >120 milliseconds) tachycardias, based on the QRS morphology. Figure 13.3 lists the causes of narrow and wide complex tachyarrythmias. Narrow complex tachycardias are usually supraventricular (SVT) in origin. However, wide complex tachycardias could be either SVT with aberrant conduction or ventricular tachycardia (VT). Differentiating SVT and VT is crucial, since anti-arrhythmic agents used to treat SVT, particularly verapamil or diltiazem, may precipitate hemodynamic collapse in a patient with VT. If it is unclear whether an arrhythmia is SVT or VT, one should treat it as VT unless proved otherwise.

A bradyarrhythmia is any rhythm that results in a ventricular rate less than 60. The differential diagnoses include sinus arrest or sinus pause, sinus bradycardia, first-degree AV block, second-degree AV block (Mobitz type I and Mobitz type II block) and third-degree AV (complete) AV block.

13.6
Diagnostic Cardiac Electrophysiological Study

Electrophysiological (EP) study involves programmed electrical stimulation in the electrophysiology (EP) laboratory to assess the detailed mechanisms of arrhythmias. In addition, it evaluates the efficacy of anti-arrhythmic medications and identifies patients who are prone to develop life-threatening arrhythmias. EP study is a relatively safe procedure when performed under the carefully controlled conditions of the EP laboratory [8]. Typically, a number of catheters (wires) are placed in the heart under x-ray fluoroscopic guidance, and electrograms are recorded from various sites, most frequently the high right atrium, His bundle (i.e., AV junction), coronary sinus, and right ventricle. This setup provides the ability to assess the conduction properties of the heart, as well as the ability to induce and terminate cardiac arrhythmias

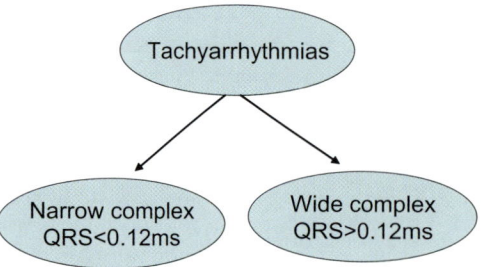

Fig. 13.3 Differential diagnosis of tachyarrhythmias

Narrow complex QRS<0.12ms
1. Atrial tachycardia,
2. Atrial flutter,
3. Atrial fibrillation,
4. Atrioventricular reciprocating tachycardia (AVRT),
5. Atrioventricular nodal reciprocating tachycardia (AVNRT)
6. Permanent form of junctional reciprocating tachycardia (PJRT)

Wide complex QRS>0.12ms
1. Supraventricular tachycardia with bundle-branch block,
2. Supraventricular tachycardia with atrioventricular conduction over an accessory pathway,
3. Accelerated idioventricular rhythm (AIVR),
4. Ventricular tachycardia (VT)
5. Ventricular fibrillation (VF)

using various pacing protocols. Analysis of the electrogram patterns and the patient's response to pacing interventions and drugs provides accurate diagnosis of the mechanisms and circuits for most arrhythmias [8, 9].

Indications for programmed electrical stimulation include risk stratification (regarding ventricular arrhythmias) in patients with structural heart disease, risk assessment in patients with Wolff–Parkinson–White (WPW) syndrome, evaluation of patients with syncope, characterization of AV conduction, determination of mechanism and treatment of supraventricular tachycardia, and assessment of efficacy of catheter ablation [8].

13.7
Genetics of Cardiac Arrhythmias

In recent years, several types of inherited defects in genes encoding cardiac ion channel proteins have been identified that can cause cardiac arrhythmias. These abnormalities have been explored in greatest depth in the long QT syndromes (LQTS) [10], which is characterized by prolongation of the QT interval resulting in recurrent syncope and sudden death in patients with a structurally normal heart. Currently, at least eight LQTS genes (variants of the LQTS) have been discovered and more than 300 mutations have been identified that account for approximately 70% of affected patients [11]. Most mutations are missense mutations, leading to a single amino acid substitution. LQTS1 and LQTS2 are the most commonly affected genes. The ionic abnormalities cause a reduction in the repolarizing currents provided by K^+ channels or an increase in the inward plateau Na^+ current [12]. These ionic alterations increase intracellular positivity, which results in a prolongation of atrial and ventricular repolarization thus creating a milieu for development of EAD-induced ventricular and possibly atrial tachyarrhythmias. Identical genetic abnormalities can have different clinical expressions, and therefore, the type of gene mutation may not necessarily predict the clinical phenotype.

The other inherited causes of arrhythmia and sudden death include the Brugada syndrome, arrhythmogenic right ventricular dysplasia, and hypertrophic cardiomyopathy. The Brugada syndrome is a primary electrical disease [13], characterized by right bundle branch block on ECG with persistent ST segment elevation in V1–V3, a normal appearing heart and sudden death secondary to VT [14]. It is often familial with an autosomal dominant inheritance, and it is related to ion channel gene mutation (SCN5A)[15].

Arrhythmogenic right ventricular dysplasia is a heart muscle disorder characterized pathologically by fatty or fibrofatty replacement and electrical instability of the right ventricular myocardium [16]. Hypertrophic cardiomyopathy, characterized by an asymmetrically hypertrophied and non-dilated left ventricle, is a relatively common genetic cardiac disease with heterogeneous clinical, morphologic, and genetic expression [17].

13.8
Pharmacological Treatment of Cardiac Arrhythmias

The development of catheter ablation therapies and implantable cardioverter defibrillators (ICD), paralleled by the recognition that anti-arrhythmic drugs may increase mortality despite suppressing cardiac arrhythmias, has changed the approach to the treatment of arrhythmias remarkably. The chronic use of anti-arrhythmic drugs has been increasingly limited and is now marked by uncertainty and apprehension.

Anti-arrhythmic agents are classified based on their mechanism of action. The Vaughan Williams classification is the most commonly used, and is based on the predominant electrophysiological effects of a drug on the action potential (Table 13.1). Class I drugs block the sodium channels responsible for the fast response in atrial, ventricular, and Purkinje fibers, thus depressing conduction velocity. Class II drugs are beta blocking agents. Class III drugs prolong cardiac repolarization by blocking potassium channels during phase 2 and 3 of the action potential and thereby increase the refractory period. Class IV drugs block calcium channels, depressing the slow response in the SA node and AV node. The usefulness of this classification system in predicting anti-arrhythmic drug efficacy is limited. Not all drugs in the same class have identical effects, and some drugs in different classes have overlapping actions. The Sicilian Gambit classification proposed by the European arrhythmia society requires in-depth knowledge regarding cellular and molecular targets of anti-arrhythmic agents, which may make it cumbersome for regular clinical use.

The most commonly used anti-arrhythmic agents are amiodarone, sotalol, dofetilide, procainamide, propafenone, lidocaine, flecainide and mexiletine. Among the class I and III anti-arrhythmic drugs, only amiodarone has been shown to reduce arrhythmic deaths in patients after myocardial infarction and to be the most effective anti-arrhythmic drug in maintaining sinus rhythm in patients with atrial fibrillation.

All anti-arrhythmic drugs are proarrhythmics (precipitation of life threatening ventricular fibrillation/tachycardia by prolonging the QT interval) and must be used with caution. Using anti-arrhythmic agents to suppress premature ventricular contractions and non-sustained VT in patients with myocardial infarction and decreased left ventricular function resulted in increased mortality [18]. Hence, specific guidelines have been given for the use of anti-arrhythmic medications, especially those that prolong the QT interval and increase proarrhythmia [19]. Type IC agents are contraindicated in patients with coronary artery disease and ischemia, but are relatively safe when used in patients with a normal heart. Type IA and type III agents are generally initiated in hospital with telemetry monitoring.

13.9
Implantable Cardioverter–Defibrillator Therapy

Sudden death from cardiac arrest remains a major public health problem [20, 21]. Most of these deaths are related to either ventricular fibrillation or ventricular tachycardia. Mirowski et al., motivated by the death

Table 13.1 The Vaughan Williams classification of anti-arrhythmic drugs

Class	Action	Drugs
I	Sodium channel blockade	
IA	Prolong repolarization	Quinidine, procainamide, disopyramide
IB	Shorten repolarization	Lidocaine, mexiletine, tocainide, phenytoin
IC	No or little effect on repolarization	Encainide, flecainide, propafenone
II	Beta-adrenergic blockade	Propanolol, esmolol, acebutolol, l-sotalol
III	Prolong repolarization Potassium channel blockade	Ibutilide, dofetilide, sotalol (d,l), amiodarone, bretylium
IV	Calcium channel blockade	Verapamil, diltiazem, bepridil
Miscellaneous	Miscellaneous actions	Adenosine, digitalis, magnesium

of a colleague, developed the concept of an implantable device that could automatically monitor and analyze cardiac rhythm and deliver defibrillating shocks when it detected ventricular arrhythmias [22, 23]. Subsequently, the implantable cardioverter–defibrillator (ICD) therapy has been identified as an effective method of preventing sudden cardiac death.

The ICD consists of a pulse generator and one or more leads for pacing and defibrillation electrodes [24]. The pulse generator is implanted subcutaneously on the anterior chest wall, and it contains the electronic circuitry, power source, memory and microprocessor. The leads from the pulse generator are positioned transvenously in the right ventricle by active-fixation (screw-in) or passive-fixation. The defibrillation lead contains a coil for delivering a shock and also bipolar electrodes for ventricular pacing and sensing. Dual-chamber and biventricular devices also have ports for atrial or left ventricular electrodes, which are used for pacing and sensing.

The function of ICD involves two major steps: sensing and detection of arrhythmia and therapy for the arrhythmia [24]. ICD devices identify the cardiac rhythm based on the rate of R waves detected by the ventricular sensing circuit and deliver therapy when the rate exceeds the programmed rate cutoff. One or more tachycardia-detection zones may be programmed. The fastest rate, or ventricular-fibrillation zone, is treated by delivery of a high-energy shock. Zones with lower rate boundaries may be treated with antitachycardia pacing or low-energy synchronized shocks or, in some cases, just observed. Antitachycardia pacing is not always effective, and it can accelerate ventricular tachycardia. Hence, delivery of a high-energy shock is always included in the prescription for therapy when antitachycardia pacing is ineffective. The sensing circuit filters the incoming signal to eliminate unwanted low-frequency components (e.g., T waves and baseline drift) and high-frequency components (e.g., skeletal-muscle electrical activity). In addition, they have a sensitivity-gain adjustment for detecting low-amplitude signals during episodes of ventricular fibrillation [25].

ICD was initially used only in patients surviving sudden cardiac deaths, but now it has emerged as a standard treatment for prevention of a first fatal arrhythmia (primary prevention) and for prevention of a recurrence of life threatening arrhythmia or cardiac arrest (secondary prevention). Few other interventions have been shown to consistently provide equivalent absolute and relative effects on survival among high-risk patients. Several studies have documented the superiority of ICD over anti-arrhythmic agents in patients with serious ventricular arrhythmias, both as primary prevention [26–30] and secondary prevention [31–34]. ICD should be the initial treatment of choice for patients with a high risk for ventricular tachyarrhythmias.

13.9.1
Clinical Indications [35]

Primary prevention
1. Chronic coronary artery disease with LVEF < 30%.
2. Coronary artery disease with LV dysfunction and inducible VT.
3. Non-ischemic dilated cardiomyopathy with moderate to severe LV dysfunction.
4. Hypertrophied cardiomyopathy.
5. Brugada syndrome,
6. Long QT syndrome.

Secondary prevention
1. Cardiac arrest due to VT or VF.
2. Sustained VT with structural heart disease.
3. Unexplained syncope with inducible sustained VT or VF or advanced structural heart disease and no other identifiable cause.

13.9.2
Contraindications [35]

1. Syncope of undetermined cause in a patient without inducible ventricular tachyarrhythmias and without structural heart disease.
2. Incessant VT or VF.
3. VF or VT resulting from arrhythmias amenable to surgical or catheter ablation.
4. Ventricular tachyarrhythmias due to a transient or reversible disorder.
5. Significant psychiatric illnesses that may be aggravated by device implantation or may preclude systematic follow-up.
6. Terminal illnesses with projected life expectancy less than 6 months.
7. Patients with coronary artery disease with LV dysfunction, prolonged QRS duration in the absence of spontaneous or inducible sustained or non-sustained VT, and who are undergoing coronary bypass surgery.
8. Patients with NYHA Class IV symptoms and drug-resistant congestive heart failure, who do not qualify for cardiac transplantation.

The complications associated with ICD can be grouped into device-related or therapy- related. The device related complications include infection, hematoma, pneumothorax, lead dislodgement, lead malfunction or fracture, inadequate defibrillation threshold, connection problems and electromagnetic interference. The therapy-related complications are frequent shocks, either appropriate or inappropriate, acceleration of ventricular tachycardia into fibrillation, prolonged hospital stay and psychological reactions.

13.10
Catheter Ablation Therapy

Percutaneous radio-frequency (RF) catheter ablation has revolutionized the field of electrophysiology. It has replaced anti-arrhythmic drug therapy and open-heart surgery for the treatment of many arrhythmias.

Catheter ablation procedures are performed in an electrophysiology laboratory. Usually both the diagnosis and ablation can be accomplished in a single session [36]. Three or four electrode catheters are inserted percutaneously into the femoral, internal jugular or subclavian vein and positioned within the heart to allow pacing and recording at key sites [13]. The efficacy of catheter ablation depends on the accurate identification of the site of origin of the arrhythmia (mapping). Once this site has been identified, an electrode catheter is positioned in direct contact with it and RF energy is delivered through the catheter to destroy it [37–39]. The RF energy coagulates the abnormal tissue that is in immediate contact with the electrode and creates a well-demarcated lesion [40]. A small scar develops at this site, and the effect is usually permanent.

Through targeting the specific site of origin of the arrhythmia, as with atrial tachycardia, or through interruption of a critical pathway needed for the maintenance of a re-entrant arrhythmia, such as an accessory pathway, arrhythmias due to various mechanisms can be eliminated. In experienced laboratories, RF ablation is curative in 95% of patients with SVT and 90% of patients with VT and no structural heart disease. However, in patients with structural heart disease (for example, prior heart attack), the complete cure rate is 40 to 50% [41, 42].

RF ablation has become the technique of choice to cure patients with recurrent paroxysmal SVT due to AVRT using an accessory pathway, AVNRT, atrial tachycardia, and atrial flutter [36]. It is also used for AVN ablation followed by pacemaker insertion or AVN modification in patients with poorly controlled atrial fibrillation. Patients with idiopathic non-ischemic VT arising from the left ventricle or right ventricular outflow tract can also similarly be cured. RF ablation offers curative therapy, thus eliminating recurrent symptoms, life-threatening events, tachycardia induced cardiomyopathy, and the need for life-long drug therapy. However, atrial fibrillation and ventricular tachyarrhythmias are difficult to ablate especially in patients with structural heart disease.

Although the incidence of complications is low, serious complications such as valvular disruption, coronary occlusion, cerebrovascular accident, and death can occur. Procedural deaths occur in 0.2% of patients who undergo AVN ablation and 0.1% of patients with accessory pathways [41, 42]. The most common complication in AVN modification has been the development of heart block through the inadvertent ablation of both the fast and slow AVN pathways [43]. Despite these complications, studies have clearly shown that symptomatic patients can have significant improvement in the quality of life with catheter ablation. The benefits gained with catheter ablation are superior to those achieved through medical therapy, and the cost of catheter ablation is less over time than the cost of alternatives such as medical therapy or surgical interventions.

13.11
Pacing Therapy

Permanent pacemakers (PPM) are life saving in patients with symptomatic bradyarrhythmias. A PPM is a mechanical device that consists of a pulse generator and pacemaker leads [44]. The most commonly used device is a dual chamber pacemaker, in which one lead is placed into the right atrium and another lead is positioned in the right ventricle. The leads are connected to the pulse generator placed subcutaneously in the anterior chest wall. The generator consists of circuitry and a lithium-iodine battery. The circuit and battery generate an electrical impulse, which passes through the leads and excites the endocardial cells, resulting in a wave of depolarization in the myocardium. The electronic circuitry can modulate the frequency and the amount of current flow, and in addition, sense spontaneous electrical activity in the heart through the leads. The pacemaker functions using a complicated time sequence that senses atrial and ventricular activity. Modern pacemakers are extremely sophisticated, capable of treating tachyarrhythmias as well as bradyarrhythmias, and incorporate extensive recording capabilities and a variety of physiological sensors to match the pacing rate and mode with physiological needs [45]. The pacing mode is determined by a four-digit code. The first letter of the code describes the pacing site, the second letter describes the sensing site, and the third letter describes the sensing modality.

The fourth letter is used if rate responsiveness is programmed on. For example, in DDDR pacing, D stands for dual-chamber pacing, sensing, and modality and R for rate responsiveness.

The standard indications for pacing include complete heart block, Mobitz type II second-degree heart block, irreversible symptomatic bradycardia, bradycardia requiring essential medications, severe symptomatic carotid hypersensitivity, and cardio inhibitory type neurocardiogenic syncope [35]. Recent applications of pacemakers include biventricular pacing to treat heart failure and biatrial pacing to prevent atrial fibrillation [45].

13.12
Cardiac Resynchronization Therapy

Cardiac resynchronization is a recently developed technique in which biventricular pacing is used to improve ventricular function. In patients with depressed ejection fractions, interventricular conduction delay, and advanced heart failure (New York Heart Association (NYHA) functional class III or IV symptoms), cardiac resynchronization improves hemodynamic function, increases exercise tolerance, and lowers the NYHA functional class [46, 47]. Several randomized trials indicate that combining cardiac resynchronization with defibrillator therapy may improve functional status and lower mortality [48–52].

References

1. Hoffman BF (1999) Cardiac arrhythmias: what do we need to know about basic mechanisms? J Cardiovasc Electrophysiol 10(3):414–416.
2. Satoh T, Zipes DP (1998) Cesium-induced atrial tachycardia degenerating into atrial fibrillation in dogs: atrial torsades de pointes? J Cardiovasc Electrophysiol 9(9):970–975.
3. Anderson ME (2002) Calmodulin and the philosopher's stone: Changing Ca2+ into arrhythmias. J Cardiovasc Electrophysiol 13(2):195–197.
4. Coumel P, Leclercq JF, Lucet V (1985) Possible mechanisms of the arrhythmias in the long QT syndrome. Eur Heart J 6Suppl D: 115–129.
5. El-Sherif N (2001) Mechanism of ventricular arrhythmias in the long QT syndrome: On hermeneutics. J Cardiovasc Electrophysiol 12:973–976.
6. El-Sherif N, Caref EB, Yin H, Restivo M (1996) The electrophysiological mechanism of ventricular arrhythmias in the long QT syndrome. Tridimensional mapping of activation and recovery patterns. Circ Res 79(3):474–492.
7. Zipes DP (2003) Mechanisms of clinical arrhythmias. J Cardiovasc Electrophysiol 14(8):902–9012.
8. Zipes DP, DiMarco JP, Gillette PC et al. (1995) Guidelines for clinical intracardiac electrophysiological and catheter ablation procedures: a report of the American College of Cardiology/American Heart Association Task Force on Practice Guidelines (Committee on Clinical Intracardiac Electrophysiologic and Catheter Ablation Procedures), developed in collaboration with the North American Society of Pacing and Electrophysiology. J Am Coll Cardiol 26:555–573.
9. Tracy et al. (2000) Clinical competence statement on invasive electrophysiology. J Am Coll Cardiol 36: 1725–1736.
10. Chiang CE (2004) Congenital and acquired long QT syndrome. Current concepts and management. Cardiol Rev 12(4):222–234.
11. Roden DM, Viswanathan PC (2005) Genetics of acquired long QT syndrome. J Clin Invest 115(8):2025–2032.
12. Moss AJ, Kass RS (2005) Long QT syndrome: from channels to cardiac arrhythmias. J Clin Invest 115(8):2018–2024.
13. Alings M, Wilde A (1999) Brugada syndrome: clinical data and suggested pathophysiological mechanism. Circulation 99:666–673.
14. Gussak I, Antzelevitch C, Bjerregaard P et al. (1999) The Brugada syndrome: clinical, electrophysiological and genetic aspects. J Am Coll Cardiol 33:5–15.
15. Chen Q, Kirsch GE, Zhang D et al. (1998) Genetic basis and molecular mechanism for idiopathic ventricular fibrillation. Nature 19:293–296.
16. Kies P, Bootsma M, Bax J, Schalij MJ, van der Wall EE (2006) Arrhythmogenic right ventricular dysplasia/cardiomyopathy: Screening, diagnosis, and treatment. Heart Rhythm 3(2):225–234.
17. Nishimura RA, Holmes DR Jr (2004) Hypertrophic obstructive **cardiomyopathy**. N Engl J Med 350:1320–1327.
18. The Cardiac Arrhythmia Suppression Trial (CAST) (1989) Investigators. Preliminary report: effect of encainide and flecainide on mortality in a randomized trial of arrhythmia suppression after myocardial infarction. N Engl J Med 321:406–412.
19. Chaudhry GM, Haffajee CI (2000) Anti-arrhythmic agents and proarrhythmia [review]. Crit Care Med 28:N158–N164.
20. Zipes DP, Wellens HJJ (1998) Sudden cardiac death. Circulation 98:2334–2351.
21. Huikuri HV, Castellanos A, Myerburg RJ (2001) Sudden death due to cardiac arrhythmias. N Engl J Med 345:1473–1482.
22. Mirowski M, Mower MM (1973) Transvenous automatic defibrillator as an approach to prevention of sudden death from ventricular fibrillation. Heart Lung 2:867–869.

23. Mirowski M, Mower MM, Langer A, Heilman MS, Schreibmen J (1978) A chronically implanted system for automatic defibrillation in active conscious dogs: experimental model for treatment of sudden death from ventricular fibrillation. Circulation 58:90–94.
24. DiMarco JP (2003) Implantable cardioverter-defibrillators. N Engl J Med 349:1836–1847.
25. Swerdlow CD, Chen PS, Kass RM, Allard JR, Peter CT (1994) Discrimination of ventricular tachycardia from sinus tachycardia and atrial fibrillation in a tiered-therapy cardioverter-defibrillator. J Am Coll Cardiol 23:1342–1355.
26. Moss AJ, Hall WJ, Cannom DS et al. (1996) Improved survival with an implantable defibrillator in patients with coronary disease at high risk for ventricular arrhythmia. N Engl J Med 335:1933–940.
27. Moss AJ, Zareba W, Hall WJ et al. (2002) Prophylactic implantation of a defibrillator in patients with myocardial infarction and reduced ejection fraction. N Engl J Med 346:877–883.
28. Bardy GH, Lee KL, Mark DB et al. (2005) Amiodarone or an implantable cardioverter-defibrillator for congestive heart failure. N Engl J Med 352:225–237.
29. Bigger JT Jr, Whang W, Rottman JN et al. (1999) Mechanisms of death in the CABG Patch trial: a randomized trial of implantable cardiac defibrillator prophylaxis in patients at high risk of death after coronary artery bypass graft surgery. Circulation 99:1416–1421.
30. Bänsch D, Antz M, Boczor S et al. (2002) Primary prevention of sudden death in idiopathic dilated cardiomyopathy: the Cardiomyopathy Trial (CAT). Circulation 105:1453–1458.
31. The Anti-arrhythmic versus Implantable Defibrillators (AVID) Investigators (1997) A comparison of anti-arrhythmic-drug therapy with implantable defibrillators in patients resuscitated from near-fatal ventricular arrhythmias. N Engl J Med 337:1576–1583.
32. Connolly SJ, Gent M, Roberts RS et al. (2000) Canadian Implantable Defibrillator Study (CIDS): a randomized trial of the implantable cardioverter defibrillator against amiodarone. Circulation 101:1297–1302.
33. Kuck KH, Cappato R, Siebels J, Ruppel R (2000) Randomized comparison of anti-arrhythmic drug therapy with implantable defibrillators in patients resuscitated from cardiac arrest: the Cardiac Arrest Study Hamburg (CASH). Circulation 102:748–754.
34. Connolly SJ, Hallstrom AP, Cappato R et al. (2000) Meta-analysis of the implantable cardioverter defibrillator secondary prevention trials: AVID, CASH and CIDS studies. Eur Heart J 21:2071–2078.
35. Gregoratos et al. (2002) ACC/AHA/NASPE 2002 Guideline Update for Implantation of Cardiac Pacemakers and Antiarrhythmia Devices.
36. Morady F (1999) Radiofrequency ablation as treatment for cardiac arrhythmias. N Engl J Med 340: 534–544.
37. Scheinman MM, Morady F, Hess DS, Gonzalez R (1982) Catheter-induced ablation of the atrioventricular junction to control refractory supraventricular arrhythmias. J Am Med Assoc 248:851–855.
38. Morady F, Calkins H, Langberg JJ et al. (1993) A prospective randomized comparison of direct current and radiofrequency ablation of the atrioventricular junction. J Am Coll Cardiol 21:102–109.
39. Olgin JE, Scheinman MM (1993) Comparison of high energy direct current and radiofrequency catheter ablation of the atrioventricular junction. J Am Coll Cardiol 21:557–564.
40. Huang SK, Graham AR, Wharton K (1988) Radiofrequency catheter ablation of the left and right ventricles: anatomic and electrophysiologic observations. Pacing Clin Electrophysiol 11:449–459.
41. Evans GTJ, Scheinman MM, Zipes DP et al. (1988) The Percutaneous Cardiac Mapping and Ablation Registry: final summary of results. Pacing Clin Electrophysiol 11:1621–1626.
42. Scheinman MM (1995) NASPE survey on catheter ablation. Pacing Clin Electrophysiol 18:1474–1478.
43. Hindricks G (1996) Incidence of complete atrioventricular block following attempted radiofrequency catheter modification of the atrioventricular node in 880 patients: results of the Multicenter European Radiofrequency Survey (MERFS): the Working Group on Arrhythmias of the European Society of Cardiology. Eur Heart J 17:82–88.
44. Kusumoto FM, Goldschlager N (1996) Cardiac pacing. N Engl J Med 334:89–97.
45. Hayes DL, Furman S (2004) Cardiac pacing: how it started, where we are, where we are going. J Cardiovasc Electrophysiol 15(5):619–627.
46. Abraham WT, Hayes DL (2003) Cardiac resynchronization therapy for heart failure. Circulation 108(21):2596–2603.
47. Abraham WT, Fisher WG, Smith AL et al. (2002) Cardiac resynchronization in chronic heart failure. N Engl J Med 346:1902–1905.
48. Auricchio A, Stellbrink C, Sack S (2002) Long-term clinical effect of hemodynamically optimized cardiac resynchronization therapy in patients with heart failure and ventricular conduction delay. J Am Coll Cardiol 39:2026–2033.
49. Cazeau S, Leclercq C, Lavergne T et al. (2001) Effects of multisite biventricular pacing in patients with heart failure and intraventricular conduction delay. N Engl J Med 344: 873–880.
50. Bristow MR, Feldman AM, Saxon LA (2000) Heart failure management using implantable devices for ventricular resynchronization: Comparison of Medical Therapy, Pacing and Defibrillation in Chronic Heart Failure (COMPAN-

ION) trial. COMPANION Steering Committee and COMPANION Clinical Investigators. J Card Fail 6:276–285.
51. Kühlkamp V (2002) Initial experience with an implantable cardioverter-defibrillator incorporating cardiac resynchronization therapy. J Am Coll Cardiol 39:790–797.
52. Lozano I, Bocchiardo M, Achtelik M et al. (2000) Impact of biventricular pacing on mortality in a randomized crossover study of patients with heart failure and ventricular arrhythmias. Pacing Clin Electrophysiol 23:1711–1712.

Chapter 14

Cardiac Catheterization and Selective Coronary Angiography: Current Status and Limitations

Matt Cummings, Aravinda Nanjundappa and Assad Movahed

Contents

14.1	History/Introduction	155
14.2	Clinical Application/Indications for Cardiac Catheterization	156
14.3	Contraindications	157
14.4	Principle/Purpose/Technique/Types/Equipment/Contrast	158
14.5	Vascular Access	158
14.6	Injection Techniques	158
14.7	Views	158
14.8	Lesion Classification	159
14.9	Complications	159
14.10	Post-catheterization Care	160
	References	160

14.1 History/Introduction

Cardiac catheterization and selective coronary angiography has revolutionized the evaluation of cardiac anatomy and physiology over the past three decades. In an age of advanced noninvasive cardiac imaging, selective coronary angiography remains the gold standard for defining cardiac anatomy. In addition to defining the site, severity, and morphology of coronary lesions, cardiac catheterization provides the most accurate quantitative assessment of cardiac structure and hemodynamics.

The first catheterization of a living human heart was performed in 1929 by Dr Werner Forssman in Eberswald, Germany [1]. Remarkably, Dr Forssman performed the procedure on himself, utilizing the left antecubital vein to access the venous system and the right atrium [1, 2]. In the early 1940s, Drs. Cournand and Richards pioneered the use of right heart catheterization to evaluate cardiac function and intracardiac pressures, and established right heart catheterization as the gold standard for evaluation of cardiac hemodynamics. This established cardiac catheterization as the gold standard for the evaluation of cardiovascular hemodynamics [1]. The first attempts to visualize coronary arteries in human subjects involved non-selective injection of a bolus of radiopaque contrast directly into the sinuses of Valsalva. A bolus of radiopaque contrast was injected directly into the sinus of valsava with subsequent visualization of the coronary arteries [2]. While coronary artery opacification was successful, visualization of the distal coronary tree was suboptimal, and the overlying opacified aortic root obscured a detailed coronary examination. The first selective coronary artery catheterization was done by Dr Mason Sones at the Cleveland Clinic in 1958. Dr Sones inadvertently cannulated the right coronary ostium while attempting to inject contrast medium into the aortic root in a patient with aortic regurgitation [3]. Dr Sones' subsequent work in 1959 eventually led to selective coronary angiography via the retrograde brachial approach and established the selective technique of coronary angiography. Selective catheterization allows for use of smaller amounts of radiopaque contrast agent, thereby minimizing the toxic effects. Use of the Seldinger technique allowed Ricketts and Adams to use preformed catheters to perform the first selective coronary arteriography via a percutaneous transfemoral approach in 1961 [4]. Modifying the techniques, Judkins and Amplatz further developed catheters and described techniques still used today for selective coronary angiography [3, 4].

14.2
Clinical Application/Indications for Cardiac Catheterization

By far the most common indication for coronary angiography is the evaluation of coronary anatomy in patients with clinical evidence of myocardial dysfunction or ischemia. Until recently, cardiac catheterization was prerequisite for all cardiac surgery patients. Currently, various noninvasive imaging techniques provide adequate data to direct surgical correction of many cardiac abnormalities such as valvular and congenital heart disease.

Selective coronary angiography remains the most accurate method to assess coronary anatomy and the extent of obstruction, providing sufficient information to guide coronary revascularization and is generally recommended to establish the presence or absence of suspected cardiac abnormalities that cannot be adequately evaluated by noninvasive cardiac imaging techniques [7]. Guidelines published by the ACC/AHA in 1999 outline the indications for coronary angiography in detail (Table 14.1). Coronary angiography is performed to define coronary anatomy in patients with typical symptoms of coronary ischemia. Coronary angiography is advised in patients with known coronary artery disease who continue to have symptoms of angina despite adequate medical therapy, or who have evidence of worsening ischemia by noninvasive testing. In the setting of atypical chest pain, coronary angiography is advised only when noninvasive testing is suggestive of ischemia.

For example, Patients with chest pain and nuclear stress tests showing scintographic evidence of reversible ischemia would warrant evaluation with angiography. Coronary angiography is clearly indicated in patients presenting with unstable angina. For patients with unstable angina whose symptoms do not improve within one hour of aggressive medical therapy, cardiac catheterization should be done on an urgent basis. In patients with unstable angina who respond to initial medical therapy, current guidelines indicate that two approaches to catheterization may be appropriate: either an "early invasive" or "early conservative" strategy [8]. In the early invasive approach, all patients with unstable angina are referred for cardiac catheterization within 48 hours of presentation. With the early conservative approach, only patients with high-risk indications such as recurrent ischemia, high-risk findings on non-invasive stress testing or ischemic ECG changes, are referred for catheterization. In the setting of acute ST segment elevation myocardial infarction, cardiac catheterization is the standard of care when available, and ideally should be performed within 90 minutes of presentation. In patients with failure to reperfuse, despite thrombolytics therapy, cardiac catheterization should be performed. Coronary angiography is also recommended in patients

Table 14.1 Indications for coronary angiography

- Stable angina with noninvasive testing showing high risk findings.
- Stable angina non responsive to medical therapy
- Unstable angina despite optimal medical treatment
- Acute ST segment elevation myocardial infarction
- Non-ST segment elevation myocardial infarction
- Angina post-coronary revascularization
- Preoperative evaluation showing high risk features on non invasive testing
- Congestive heart failure patients who have not undergone previous coronary angiogram
- Valvular heart disease evaluation and patients with need to evaluate concomitant coronary artery disease
- Congenital heart disease

who have survived a cardiac arrest and a non-cardiac cause for the arrest cannot be identified.

Coronary angiography may also be indicated for preoperative cardiac evaluation. Catheterization is performed for patients with coronary artery disease undergoing non-cardiac surgeries who continue to have angina despite optimized medical therapy or have high-risk noninvasive cardiac tests. Cardiac catheterization and coronary angiography is useful in the evaluation of valvular diseases as well. It is often advised to define coronary anatomy in patients with valvular disease prior to valve surgery, since the presence of coronary artery disease can worsen the prognosis. Cardiac catheterization plays an important role in evaluating patients with congenital heart disease for concomitant congenital coronary anomalies.

Cardiac catheterization plays a pivotal role in evaluation of congestive heart failure. Cardiac catheterization may be advised to evaluate the possibility of ischemic ventricular dysfunction, unexplained acute episodes of pulmonary edema and in patients with scintigraphic evidence of reversible myocardial ischemia. Finally, coronary angiography may be occasionally indicated to evaluate coronary anatomy in the setting of aortic abnormalities such as aortic dissection.

14.3
Contraindications

While there are no absolute contraindications to cardiac catheterization, there are several conditions widely accepted as relative contraindications. The most common include renal failure, active gastrointestinal bleeding, active infection, coagulaopathy, uncontrolled hypertension, severe anemia, digitalis toxicity, decompensated heart failure, and a history of contrast allergy without pre-medication prior to catheterization [7, 9] (Table 14.2). Since the majority of these are self-limited or reversible, if possible, it may be beneficial to delay catheterization to reduce risk related to these relative contraindications. Furthermore, the clinician must carefully assess the risk-benefit ratio when such situations arise, since rarely do the risks associated with catheterization outweigh the risks associated with these conditions.

Of the relative contraindications to cardiac catheterization, contrast nephropathy is by far the most studied as it occurs in a significant number of patients undergoing cardiac catheterization [7]. The most reliable predictor of procedure related contrast nephropathy is the presence of underlying renal insufficiency, and diabetes mellitus. It is estimated that 10–40% of patients with pre-existing renal insufficiency will develop worsening renal function, while only 0–0.5% of patients with normal renal function will develop a significant reduction in renal function following catheterization. Patients with renal insufficiency in the setting of diabetes mellitus, are at greatest risk of developing contrast nephropathy. Most patients recover completely, but up to 10% will require dialysis [8].

Several steps can be taken to reduce the risk of contrast nephropathy in high risk patients. Adequate hydration with intravenous normal saline prior to catheterization has been shown to reduce the incidence of contrast nephropathy. Minimizing the dose of contrast media is imperative with the recommended doses for diagnostics studies and interventional procedures are ≤ 30ml and ≤ 100ml respectively. Delaying interventional procedures for 48 hours following a diagnostic catheterization provides added benefit as well [10]. Use of nonionic low-osmolar contrast medium has been shown to significantly reduce nephrotoxicity in patients with com-

Table 14.2 Relative contraindications for coronary angiogram

- Patients who are unable to consent to the procedure
- Active bleeding
- Coagulopathy
- Severe Stage 3 hypertensions (B.P >160/90)
- Severe electrolyte imbalance such as hypokalemia or hyperkalemia
- Digitalis toxicity
- Severe anemia and thrombocytopenia
- Decompensated congestive heart failure
- Patients with anaphylactic contrast allergy
- Active infection

promised renal function, although no benefit has been demonstrated in patients with normal renal function. Periprocedural oral administration of acetylcysteine may also reduce the risk of contrast nephropathy, although this benefit is controversial [11–14]. Discontinuing nephrotoxic drugs, such as anti-inflammatory agents and metformin reduces risk further.

14.4
Principle/Purpose/Technique/Types/Equipment/Contrast

Prior to cardiac catheterization, informed consent must be obtained from all patients or responsible parties. The physician should explain the catheterization procedure in detail along with the indications for the procedure. The risks and benefits of the procedure, are explained and any concerns or questions that may arise. A thorough pre-catheterization evaluation should include a detailed history and physical examination, baseline ECG, CXR, and thorough laboratory evaluation. Important aspects of the history include a history of diabetes mellitus, hypertension, chronic kidney disease, peripheral vascular disease, bleeding diatheses, as well as a history of contrast medium and latex allergy. Laboratory evaluation should include a complete blood count, basic metabolic panel, and coagulation studies, with close attention to renal function, platelet count, and hematocrit values. In general, all patients are given pre- and post-catheterization intravenous hydration. In patients with elevated serum creatinine, N acetyl acetylcysteine administration prior to catheterization has been shown to reduce the incidence of contrast nephropathy [11]. Oral anticoagulants are stopped prior to catheterization with an International Standardized ratio goal of less than 1.8, and oral antihistamines are frequently given to prevent allergic reactions to contrast medium and or latex. Metformin should be discontinued on the day of the procedure and withhold until the creatinine is stable for at least 48 hours following the procedure. Patients with documented contrast medium allergy should receive either oral or intravenous corticosteroid prophylaxis prior to the procedure. Several steroid regiments have been described.

14.5
Vascular Access

Several techniques and access sites are commonly used including:
- Retrograde brachial approach: Cut down utilizing Sones technique and percutaneous Seldinger technique
- Retrograde femoral: Seldinger technique
- Retrograde radial approach
- Ante grade percutaneous trans-myocardial left ventricular puncture.

14.6
Injection Techniques

Hand injection utilizing a multi-channel manifold system.
  Automatic injector:
- ASCIST © Bracco Diagnostics, Inc. Princeton, New Jersey, USA
- MEDRAD Avanta® Fluid Management Injection System, Medrad, Inc. Indianola, PA, USA

14.7
Views

A diagnostic angiogram is performed with 5 French or 6 French Judkins left, right and pigtail catheters over a 0.035-inch guide wire for selective cannulation of the coronary arteries under continuous hemodynamic monitoring. All catheters should be exchanged over a 0.035-inch guide wire to avoid vascular trauma and catheter whipping, and to reduce atheroembolism. The left main coronary artery is cannulated in the left anterior 30° view. Several angulations [17] for coronary angiograms have been proposed; the key is to perform imaging with adequate coronary visualizations and minimal vessel overlap. The initial imaging is done in the 20° right anterior oblique and 20° caudal views. The left main coronary artery (LMCA) in its entirety, proximal left anterior descending artery (LAD), proximal left circumflex coronary artery (LCX) and the collaterals to the right coronary artery (RCA) if it is occluded are visualized. The next image is preferable in the anterior posterior 5° and a cranial 30° view. The proximal, mid and distal LAD can be seen. The third imaging view should be set up in the left anterior oblique 35° and cranial 30°. The course of the LAD and its relation to diagonal arteries will be visualized. The fourth image is acquired in the left anterior 40° and caudal 30°. This so called "spider view", will illustrate the proximal LAD, ramus intermedius artery if present and the LCX artery in its entirety. The left coronary system can be safely imaged with 4 cm³/s for a total of 6 to 8 cm³ of contrast material with hand injection, or an automated pressurized injector delivering a pressure of 500 psi. The RCA is cannulated in the left anterior oblique 30° and the first imaging study of the RCA is performed in the same view. The proximal, mid and distal RCA vasculature can be seen. The next image is obtained in the anterior-posterior 5° and 30° cranial view, which will delineate the distal bifurcation of RCA into posterior lateral ventricular branch and posterior descending artery. The right coronary system is usually injected with 3 cm³/s for a total of 5 to 6 cm³ injected at 400 psi.

The left ventricular cavity is crossed in the right anterior oblique 30° with a pigtail catheter. Once the pigtail catheter has crossed the aortic valve into the mid portion of the left ventricle, the catheter is connected to hemodynamic monitoring. Care must be taken to observe for ventricular arrhythmias and flushing the catheter with heparinized saline is essential to obtain accurate left ventricular end diastolic pressure readings. The left ventriculogram is obtained in RAO 30° unless lateral wall motion abnormality or possible ventricular septal defect is suspected. These special situations warrant left anterior oblique 30° with 30° cranial tilt. The left ventriculogram is performed with 15 cm³/s for a total of 45 cm³ of radiocontrast material at 600 psi.

14.8
Lesion Classification

The joint task force from ACC/AHA have proposed coronary lesion classification as Type A, B and C. Several characteristics are incorporated to define lesions, which include lesion length, tortuosity, calcification, location, severity, native coronary or bypass grafts, duration of occlusion, side branch involvement and thrombus. The type of lesion will predict success rate and degree of risk involved with the procedure (Table 14.3).

14.9
Complications

While cardiac catheterization is generally considered a relatively safe procedure, it does carry serious risks of morbidity and mortality, as is the case with most interventional procedures. In general, the condition of the patient prior to catheterization determines the overall outcome, with patients in a poor state of health undergoing catheterization in an emergency setting obviously being at greatest risk for complications. The total risk of all major complications from coronary angiography is 1.7%, based on a 1990 registry data study from the Society for Cardiac Angiography and Interventions (SCAI). These include death, myocardial infarction, stroke, arrhythmia, vascular complications, contrast reaction, hemodynamic complications, and ventricular perforation.

Table 14.3 Characteristics of American College of Cardiogy/American Heart Association Type A, B and C lesions

TYPE A LESIONS (High success, > 85%; low risk)	
Discrete (< 10mm length)	Little or no calcification
Concentric	Less than totally occlusive
Readily accessible	Notostial in location
Nonangulated segment < 45 degree	No major branch involvement
Smooth contour	Absence of thrombus
TYPE B LESIONS (Moderate success, 60 to 85%; moderate risk)	
Tubular (10–20 mm length)	Ostial in location
Eccentric	Bifurcation lesions requiring
Moderate tortuosity of prox. segment	Double guidewire
Moderately angulated, 45–90°	Some thrombus present
Irregular contour	Total occlusion < 3 months old
Moderate to be avy calcification	
TYE C LESIONs (Low success, < 60%; high risk)	
Diffuse (> 2cm length)	Degeneration vein grafts with friable lesions
Extremely angulated > 90 degree	Total occlusion > 3 months old
Inability to protect major side branch	

Several large trials have identified patients at risk for complications related to cardiac catheterization [15–17]. Additional registry data from the SCAI database has identified patients at greatest risk for complications related to catheterization. Patients at highest risk include those with a moribund status, shock, or an acute myocardial infarction within the previous 24 hours. The risk of complications is also higher in those with symptomatic heart failure, hypertension, aortic or mitral valve disease, cardiomyopathy, unstable angina, and renal insufficiency. The major predictors of complications are obesity, elderly females, patients with shock, renal failure, heart failure, valvular heart disease, unstable angina and cardiomyopathy.

14.10
Post-catheterization Care

All patients who undergo coronary angiography are evaluated for hemodynamic stability prior to discharge from the catheterization laboratory. Vascular access is managed by manual compression or use of closure devices. Manual pressure is held above and medial to the access site for a minimum of 15 minutes depending on the size of the sheath used. The simple rule of "3" is 3 minutes for each size of sheath, e.g., 6 French requires 18 minutes of compression, 7 French will need 21 minutes of compression. Several vascular closure devices utilizing mechanical compression devices, collagen vascular plugs and suture devices are available. There is minimal benefit of vascular closure devices in terms of reduced time of bed rest compared with manual compression. However, closure devices carry a higher risk of bleeding, hematoma and blood transfusions. A minimum of 4 to 6 hours of bed rest is mandatory prior to ambulation. The majority of patients can be safely discharged home the same day, with the few exceptions being vascular complications, volume overload and renal insufficiency patients. Prior-to-discharge, patients must be evaluated for signs of CVA/TIA, heart failure, limb ischemia, access site hematoma and atheroembolism. Patients who require anticoagulation can be given anticoagulants 8 hours post-sheath removal. Metformin use in diabetics should be held for 48 hours and patients must have normal serum creatinine prior to resuming metformin use. All patients will have a physician check within one week.

References

1. Braunwald E (2003) Cardiology: the past, the present, and the future. J Am Coll Cardiol 42:2031–2041.
2. Conti RC (1977) Coronary arteriography. Circulation 55(2):227.
3. Ryan TJ (2002) The coronary angiogram and its seminal contributions to cardiovascular medicine over five decades. Circulation 106:752–756.
4. Abrams HL (1996) History of Cardiac Radiology. Am J Radiol 167(2):431–438.
5. Fischman DL, Leon MB, Baim DS, Schatz RA, Savage MP, Penn I (1994) A randomized comparison of coronary-stent placement and balloon angioplasty in the treatment of coronary artery disease. N Engl J Med 331:496–501.
6. Scanlon PJ, Faxon DP, Audet AM, Carabello B, Dehmer GJ, Eagle KA (1999) ACC/AHA guidelines for coronary angiography: a report of the American College of Cardiology/American Heart Association Task Force on Practice Guidelines (Committee on Coronary Angiography). J Am Coll Cardiol 33:1756–1824.
7. ACC/AHA (2002) Guideline Update for the Management of Patients with Unstable Angina and Non-ST-Segment Myocardial Infarction – Summary Article: J. Am. Coll. Cardiol 40:1366–1374.
8. Parfrey PS, Griffiths SM, Barrett BJ, Paul MD, Genge M, Withers J et al. (1989) Contrast material-induced renal failure in patients with diabetes mellitus, renal insufficiency, or both. A prospective controlled study. 320(3):143–149.
9. Braunwald E (2004) Braunwald's Heart Disease: A Textbook of Cardiovascular Medicine, 7th edn. WB Saunders, Philadelphia.
10. Sos TA, Baltaxe HA (1977) Cranial and caudal augulation for coronary angiography revisited. Circulation 56:119–123.
11. Tepel M, Von Der Giet M, Schwarzfeld C et al. (2000) Prevention of radiographic contrast agent induced reactions in renal function by acetylcysteine. N Engl J Med 343:180.
12. Kay J, Chow W, Chan TM et al. (2003) Acetylcysteine for prevention of acute deterioration of renal function following elective coronary angiography and intervention. J Am Med Assoc 289:553.
13. Briguori C, Maganelli F, Scarpato P et al. (2002) Acetylcysteine and contrast agent-associated nephrotoxicity. J Am Coll Cardiol 40:298.
14. Durham JD, Caputo C, Dokko J et al. (2002) A randomized controlled trial of N-acetylcysteine to prevent contrast nephropathy in cardiac angiography. Kidney Int 62:2202.

15. Davidson CJ, Mark DB, Pieper KS et al. (1990) Thrombotic and cardiovascular complications related to non-ionic contrast media during cardiac catheterization. Analysis of 8517 patients. Am J Cardiol 65:1481.
16. Laskey W, Boyle J, Johnson LW and the Registry Committee of the Society for Cardiac Angiography and Interventions (1993) Multivariable model for prediction of risk of significant complication during diagnostic cardiac catheterization. Cathet Cardiovasc Diagn 30:185.
17. Clark VL, Khaja F (1994) Risk of cardiac catheterization in patients aged >80 years without previous cardiac surgery. Am J Cardiol 74:1076.

Emerging Role of Multi-detector CT Imaging

Shahid Mahmood and John Hoe

Contents

15.1	Introduction	163
15.2	Clinical Applications in CAD	164
15.2.1	Diagnosis	164
15.2.2	Acute Chest Pain	166
15.2.3	Revascularization	167
15.2.4	Prognosis and Plaque Imaging	171
15.3	Role in Congenital Heart Diseases	171
15.4	Hybrid Imaging	172
15.5	Conclusion	173
	References	174

15.1 Introduction

The innovative advances in imaging technologies during the last decade have profoundly helped medicine and research. The recent enhancements in radionuclide imaging, echocardiography, computed tomography (CT) and magnetic resonance imaging (MRI) have broadened the horizons of non-invasive cardiac imaging for various cardiovascular diseases [1]. However, among all these, the introduction of multi-detector/multi-slice computed tomography (MDCT/MSCT), has been the most significant contribution, permitting increased imaging speed with reduced examination time and high resolution images [2, 3]. This has helped CT to enter the arena of cardiac imaging, however, its exact role under various clinical scenarios will be established in the near future.

The basic principles of data acquisition, image reconstruction, post-processing and display in CT are very similar to those in Single Photon Emission Computerised Tomography (SPECT). Based on the similar principles, Godfrey Hounsfield developed the first CT or CAT (Computerized Axial Tomography) scanner [4]. There followed successive generations of CT scanners, with progressive improvements in speed and resolution [5]. CT density units are expressed in Hounsfield Units (HU) and range from −1024 to +3071. The density value of water is predefined as 0 HU, while that of non-enhanced soft tissues and blood is between −100 HU and +200 HU.

The first generation CT scanners used a pencil-beam X-ray source and xenon detectors, with poor temporal resolution. With advancement in technology, ceramic scintillators replaced xenon detectors. One-second scanners were introduced in 1985. However, until 1990 all scanners were sequential scanners. In these scanners, the table moved to the next slice position only after complete acquisition of one slice. The introduction of spiral imaging in 1989 was a major technical breakthrough in CT technology [6]. In spiral CT scanners, the table moves at a constant speed, with simultaneous data acquisition by a number of detectors.

The small diameters and continuous motion of coronary arteries demand the highest temporal and spatial resolutions. ECG gating helps to acquire images during diastole, when motion is least. Despite the capability of ECG triggered imaging in this previous generation of scanners, the temporal and z-resolutions remained limited for meaningful clinical coronary imaging [7].

The restricted speed of rotation of the tube has been one of the major factors in limiting temporal resolution and cardiac imaging in previous CT scanners. To overcome this shortcoming, electron-beam CT (EBCT) was developed and until recently, was the only way to achieve adequate cardiac CT imaging [8]. There are no moving parts in EBCT, rather a beam of electrons is accelerated through a vacuum and is precisely reflected onto a tungsten anode, under the patient table. This generates a fan-shaped X-ray beam, which is collected by two 240° detector rows above the patient. EBCT was initially pioneered to measure coronary calcifications, and to a lesser extent for coronary angiography [9, 10]. EBCT did not gain wide clinical acceptance due to its higher costs and controversies regarding the prognostic value of coronary calcifications.

In 1995, subsecond scanners were introduced and were enhanced to multi-slice/multi-detector scanners (4-slice) in 1998 [11]. The term multi-slice implies that for each gantry rotation more than one image slice or image section is created, whereas multi-detector row indicates that the detector is composed of several rows of detectors. The terms "multi-slice" and "multi-detector" CT are generally used interchangeably for this new technology. The current generation of MSCT/MDCT were launched in 2002, with 16 rows of detectors, with faster gantry rotation times of 400–500 ms and a resolution of $0.5 \times 0.5 \times 0.6$ mm. The arrays of detectors used in new systems have variable geometry (isotropic arrays, adaptive arrays). The latest 64-slice MDCTs have a temporal resolution of approximately 165 ms (using half scan reconstruction techniques), a nearly isotropic voxel resolution of 0.4 mm, and a gantry rotation time of only 0.33 s. Recently introduced dual X-ray tube MDCT scanners, with a temporal resolution of 83 ms and using single segment reconstruction, appear to be independent of heart rate, with the ability to scan two different energy windows [12]. Theoretically, different energies may translate into characterization of different tissues in one study. The newer generation of all-purpose MDCT scanners have made non-invasive coronary imaging economically viable and have almost replaced expensive EBCT. A detailed discussion regarding different acquisition protocols, processing and artefacts is beyond the scope of this book.

Relatively higher radiation doses of 11.0 ± 4.1 mSv for cardiac 64-MDCT and 6.4 ± 1.9 mSv for 16-MDCT versus 1.1 mSv for electron beam CT have been a recent topic of discussion [13]. This is primarily due to the use of continuous overlap scanning and the increased number of detectors used. The new systems have variable tube output to decrease total radiation exposure during the CT examination by up to 50%, but a heart rate of less than 60 bpm is mandatory for accurate use of this technique. The dual source CT also appears to be associated with similar or higher radiation doses compared qwith 64-slice MDCT [14]. There is now use of prospective ECG gating for cardiac CT scanning, which significantly reduces dose (by about 70%), and the effective dose received is similar to the background radiation dose [15]. Similarly, recently launched 256- and 320-slice CT scanners also appear to promise a reduction in radiation exposure.

15.2
Clinical Applications in CAD

15.2.1
Diagnosis

The incidence of coronary artery disease will continue to escalate, with more disease prevalence in younger people and in developing countries. In order to reduce the mortality from CAD, early detection and intervention prior to adverse events would be most helpful. This however necessitates reliable detection of early disease processes in intermediate and high-risk subject groups.

The gold standard for the diagnosis of CAD has been coronary angiography, but this is an invasive and costly procedure. The ideal screening and diagnostic test must be non-invasive, cheaper and easily available.

The ECG stress test is still the most widely used diagnostic test, but suffers from a poor sensitivity of 68% and specificity of 77% [16]. In combination with radionuclide myocardial perfusion imaging, besides improved sensitivity and specificity, excellent prognostic information is also gained [17]. However, this does not provide any anatomical/morphological details, which may be necessary in certain cases for management decisions.

Coronary calcifications represent coronary atherosclerosis in proportion to the atheromatous burden. Both EBCT and MDCT have the ability to detect the presence, severity, and location of coronary calcifications, generating an index, known as the Agaston coronary calcium score, in asymptomatic subjects (Fig. 15.1) [18, 19]. A high calcium score suggests only the presence of underlying CAD, as the sites of the greatest calcium deposits are not usually sites of stenosis (Fig. 15.2). Due to controversies regarding the use of calcium scoring alone for prognosis, and the higher costs associated with EBCT, it has gained only limited acceptance

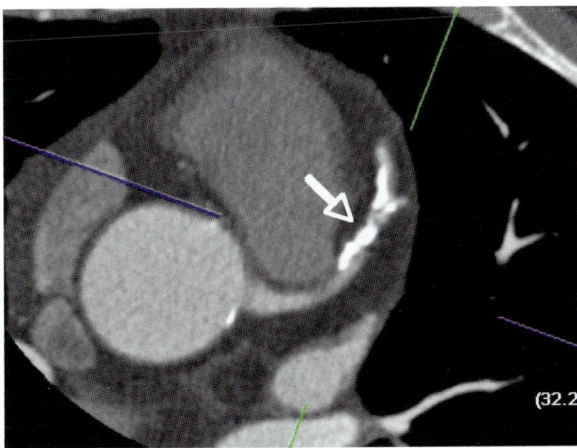 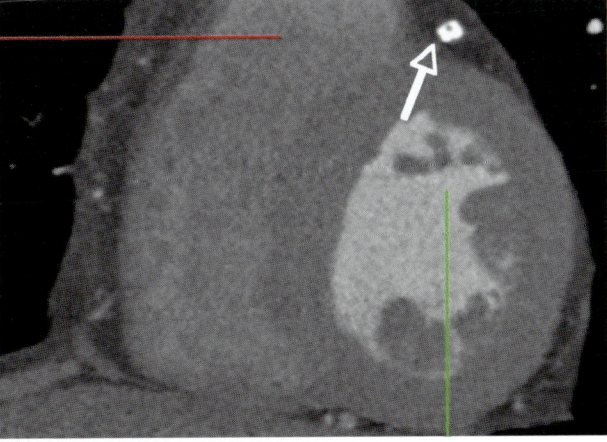

Fig. 15.1 Heavily calcified coronary artery in an asymptomatic 52-year-old male with risk factors of DM, hypertension and hyperlipidaemia. Coronary CT revealed that Calcium score was 1796 Agatston (90–100th percentile). The lumen of LAD was not assessable due to large calcified plaques. A coronary calcium score of 1–10 is considered minimal, 11–100 as mild, 100–400 as moderate and more than 400 is considered as severe disease

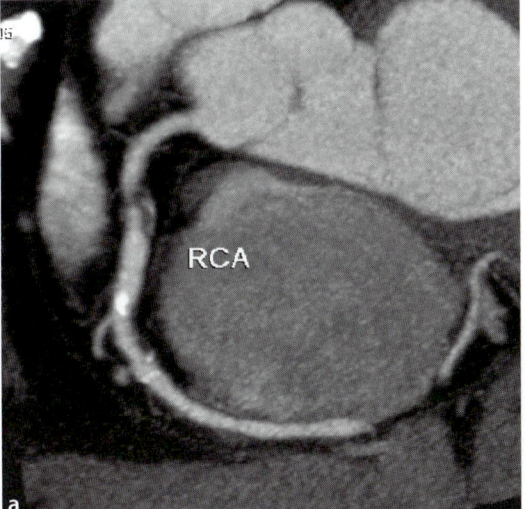 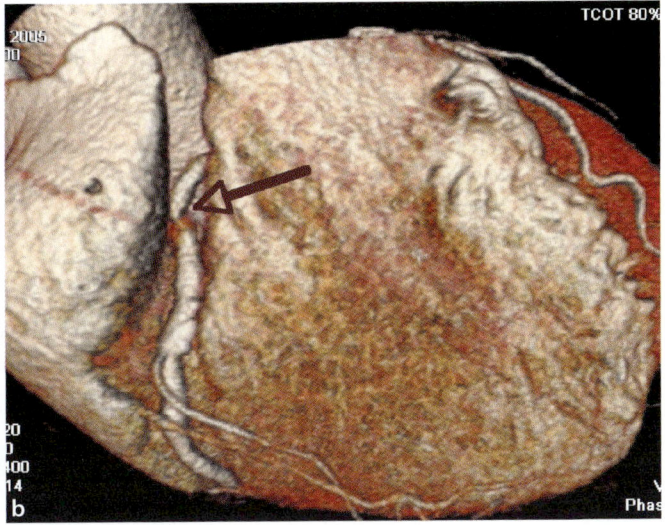

Fig. 15.2a,b CT coronary angiogram of a 58-year-old male, demonstrating a large plaque (mainly non-calcified) at the junction of proximal and mid-RCA causing significant obstruction (*arrow*). 3D volume rendered image also shows significant short segment of stenosis (b). The patient had a calcium score of 274. Soft plaques are normally the sites of significant stenoses and rupture and are responsible for major coronary events

clinically. However, recent studies confirm the complementary role of calcium scoring in risk stratification, in conjunction with the Framingham score [20].

The recent iteration of MSCT/MDCT scanners has enabled not only better estimation of coronary calcium scoring, but also non-invasive visualization of coronary anatomy and luminal obstruction with high negative predictive values of 99% (Fig. 15.3) [21–26]. The basic principle of coronary CT angiography is tomographic visualization of contrast material in the vessel lumen, which is similar to catheter-based coronary angiography. Although more major systematic trials are required, it is likely to transform the practice of cardiovascular medicine [27–29]. MDCT coronary angiography may find an important role in screening and early diagnosis of CAD in intermediate-risk group patients, if, with the newer

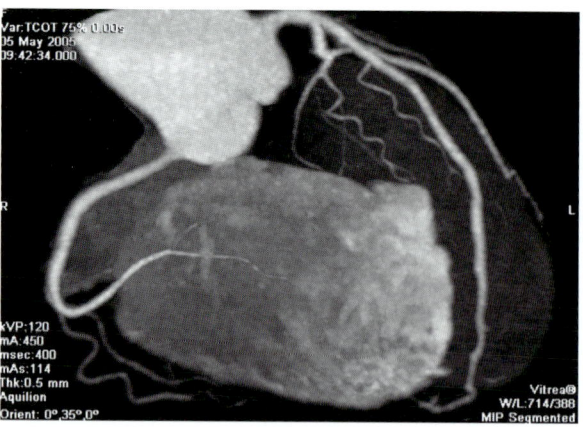

Fig. 15.3 CT coronary angiogram demonstrating high resolution 3-D MIP images

scanning techniques, the radiation dose is reduced to that of background radiation (Figs. 15.4a, 15.4b, 15.5a, 15.5b, 15.5c).

The incidence of occult CAD in asymptomatic diabetics ranges from 20% to more than 50% and is a major cause of silent ischaemia [30, 31]. Hyperglycaemia is not only responsible for impaired endothelial function, but also contributes to the worsening of other coronary risk factors such as obesity, dyslipidaemia and hypertension. Due to a low probability of significant obstructive CAD in uncomplicated diabetics, most physicians tend to screen diabetic patients only in the presence of complications or ECG abnormalities. However, due to the high risk of cardiac and non-cardiac complications, all patients with type-2 diabetes should be screened for CAD at the time of diagnosis and thereafter (Fig. 15.6a and 15.6b) [32–34].

Syndrome X or non-obstructive (spasmodic) atherosclerotic coronary disease occurs in approximately 10% of women and 6% of men with ST-segment elevation, representing with chest pain, myocardial ischemia or myocardial infarction [35, 36, 37]. Since, both obstructive and spasmodic lesions have similar perfusion abnormalities on myocardial perfusion SPECT imaging, CT coronary angiography at the time of chest pain could be of help in depicting coronary artery spasm (Fig. 15.7).

The number of unnecessary invasive procedures can be reduced substantially by inclusion of non-invasive approaches like myocardial perfusion SPECT and coronary CT angiography. Patients, with atypical symptoms and/or normal or equivocal stress test results for CAD, could be evaluated by non-invasive CT coronary angiography establishing a definitive diagnosis [38]. It is likely, based on the present trend, that CT coronary angiography will gradually become an integral component of many screening programmes. However, the long-term clinical benefits of such an approach can only be determined in the future.

15.2.2 Acute Chest Pain

Acute coronary occlusion is a sudden manifestation of the atherosclerotic process, with higher risk. A non-invasive imaging test with high negative predictive value would be of great help to a clinician, with the prospect to missing 3–5% of myocardial insults in an emergency department [39]. Radionuclide myocardial

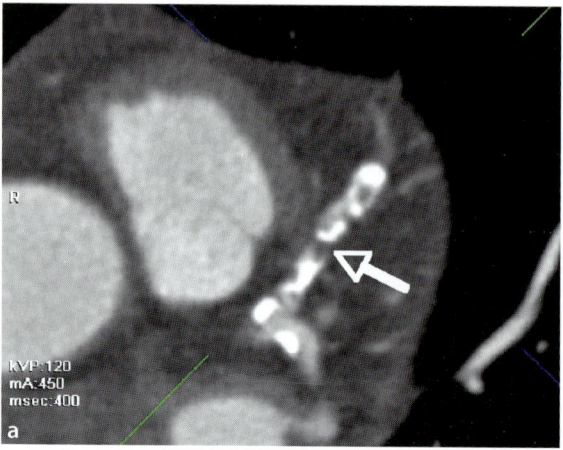
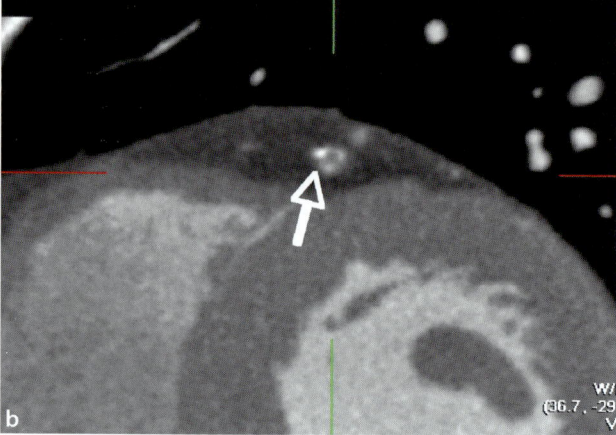

Fig. 15.4 CT coronary angiogram demonstrating extensive calcified plaques in proximal LAD (calcium score of 1515), in a 51-year-old male with risk factors of hyperlipidaemia and smoking. A significant stenosis caused by non-calcified plaque (*arrow*) can be visualized despite high calcifications, due to the improved resolution of the 64-slice scanner

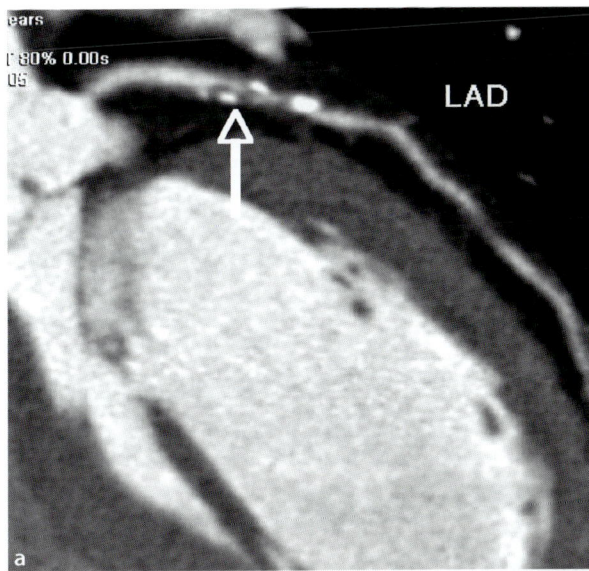
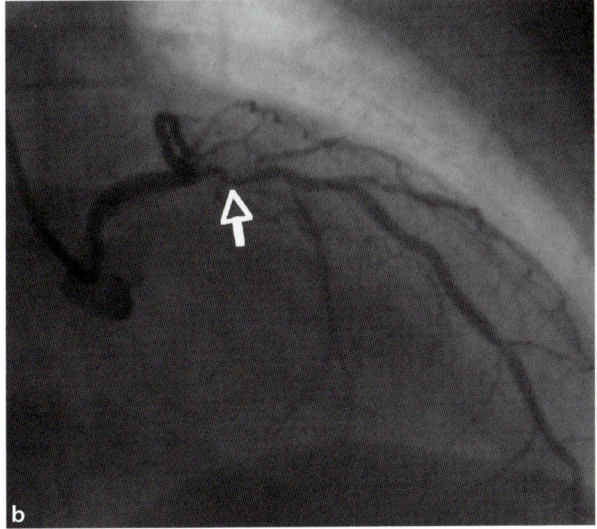
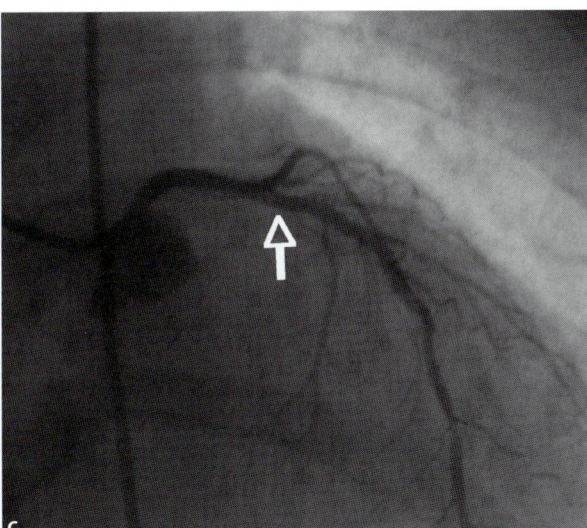

Fig. 15.5a,b,c CT coronary angiogram in a 57-year-old hypertensive female, with family history of CAD. The calcium score was 82 A. CT coronary angiogram demonstrates predominantly a non-calcified plaque, responsible for significant stenosis of proximal LAD (*arrow*), and confirmed by cardiac catheterization (**b**). The obstruction was relieved by percutaneous intervention, with a stent implantation (**c**). CT coronary angiography is helpful in screening intermediate risk, asymptomatic patients for early detection of disease

perfusion SPECT imaging has always been favoured for this purpose due to the additional benefit of risk stratification. However, it cannot diagnose non-cardiac origins of chest pain. Conversely, MDCT has the ability to discriminate non-coronary sources of chest pain, such as pericarditis, pericardial effusion, aortic dissection, pneumonias and pulmonary embolism [40–42]. Therefore, the incorporation of MDCT imaging into the diagnostic approaches to acute chest pain would help in the recognition of non-cardiac pathologies and would also identify patients who would benefit from priority intervention, with a positive impact on patient management (Fig. 15.8a–15.8c).

ECG gated cardiac CT can also assess ventricular function and regional wall motion abnormalities secondary to myocardial stunning in an acute setting as well as myocardial perfusion [43]. However, further clinical experience and validity of the technique is required before accepting it into clinical routine, particularly when echocardiography can accomplish such an evaluation at the patient's bedside, without any radiation.

15.2.3
Revascularization

The fundamental strategy of CAD treatment involves risk factor modification, with either pharmacotherapy or coronary revascularization or both. Percutaneous interventional procedures and coronary artery bypass graft (CABG) surgery remain the methods of choice for coronary revascularizations, with relatively sharp

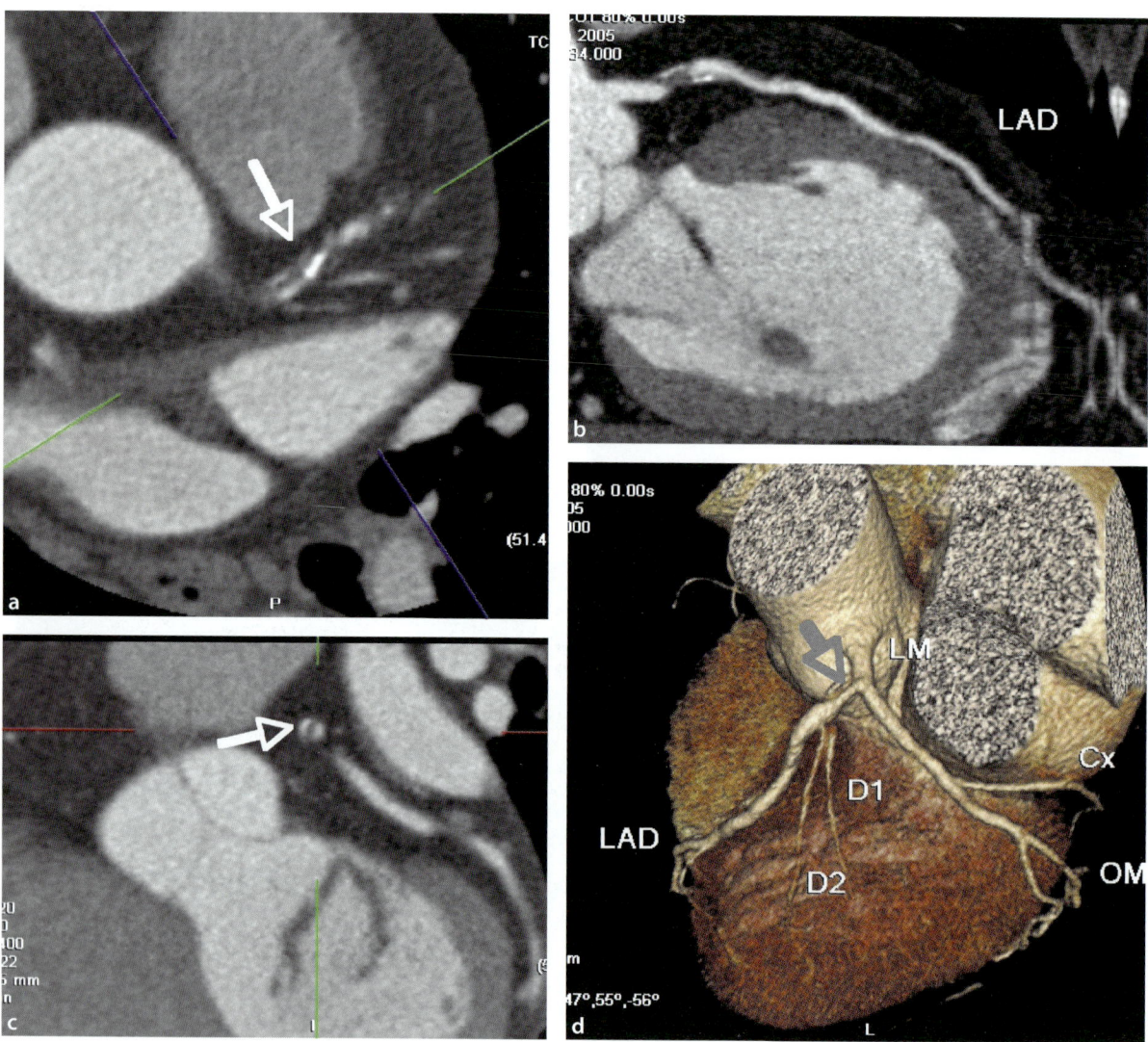

Fig. 15.6 Coronary CT angiogram in a middle-aged male with risk factors of DM and smoking. Calcium score was only 23 A. However, at least 50% stenosis of proximal LAD, just after its origin, is evident on the axial (**a**), orthogonal (**b**), cross sectional (**c**) and 3D-VR images (**d**). CT coronary angiography could also be helpful in screening asymptomatic diabetic patients

increase in percutaneous interventions [44]. Post-interventional re-stenosis of the targeted arterial lumen and of the implanted stent remains a clinical problem. The introduction of new drug-eluting stents to impede cellular proliferation and adjunctive pharmacological therapies with drugs such as clopidogrel and glycoprotein IIb/IIIa inhibitors are responsible for the increased number of percutaneous coronary interventional procedure [45–47]. However, recent data demonstrates that re-stenosis still remains a challenging task [48].

MDCT coronary angiography has the potential for non-invasive imaging of arterial lumen, stent lumen and stent-patency, permitting early and definitive detection of re-stenosis [49, 50]. The absence of contrast in the lumen of the stent suggests significant in-stent re-stenosis. Non-visualization of contrast in the arterial lumen distal to the stent is another sign of stent occlusion. In the past, relatively poor resolution and metal artefacts from the stent-struts made coronary stent evaluation difficult with MDCT angiography. However, the recent introduction of 64-slice MDCT scanners can often detect in-stent re-stenosis as well as neointimal hyperplasia [5] (Fig. 15.9). Therefore, MDCT coronary angiography is likely to become the methodology of choice for post-stent placement follow-up (Fig. 15.10a, 15.10b and 15.10c).

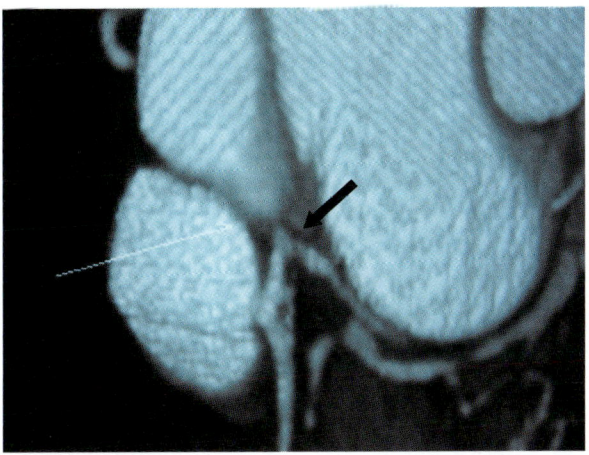

Fig. 15.7 CT coronary angiogram of a female patient, who presented with repeated episode of chest pain. Initial cardiac catheterization did not reveal evidence of disease. Two months later, CT angiography during an episode of chest pain revealed evidence of left main spasm (*arrow*)

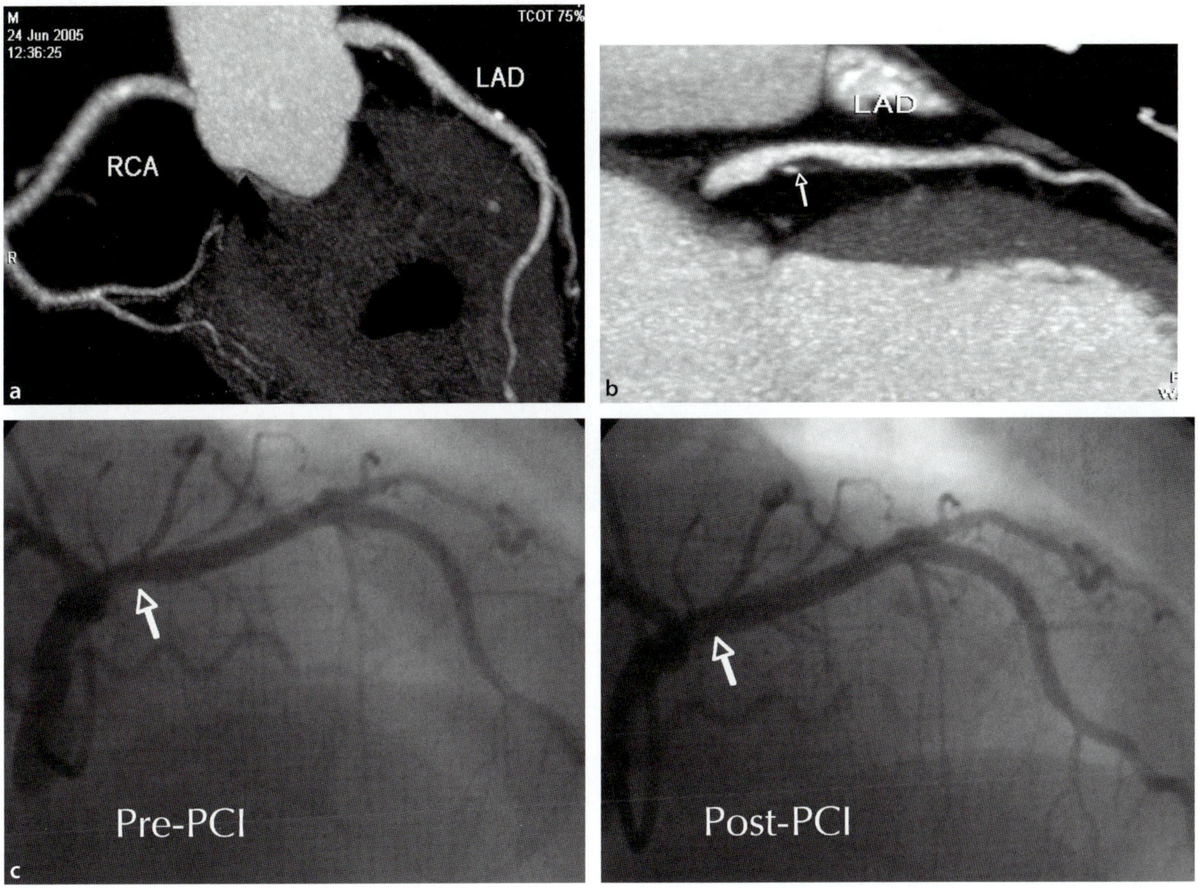

Fig. 15.8 55-year-male had an episode of acute chest pain while playing golf. ECG was normal. Coronary CT angiogram demonstrates a small bright spot in a soft plaque, indicative of an area of haemorrhage signifying acute plaque rupture (**a, b**). Emergency cardiac catheterization confirmed the findings, and per-cutaneous intervention with a stent placement was performed, stabilizing patient condition (**c**). Plaque rupture is most frequent cause of acute coronary syndrome but is a diagnostic challenge. A localized extraluminal accumulation of contrast or penetrating into the artery wall, surrounded by soft plaque would be indicative of plaque rupture on CT. CT coronary angiography has the potential for non-invasive diagnosis and assessment of acute coronary syndromes

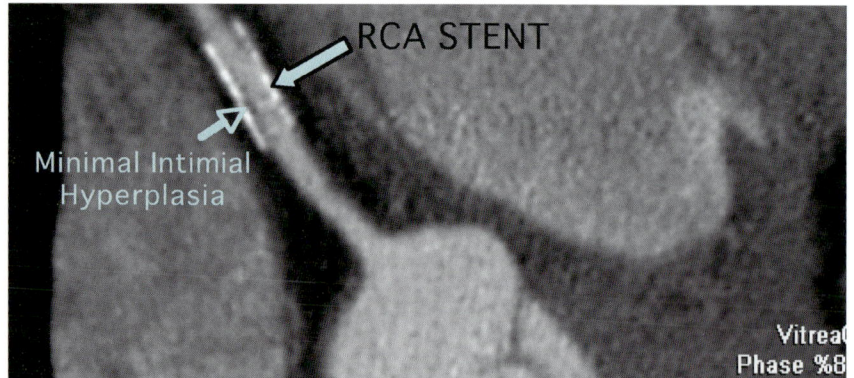

Fig. 15.9 High resolution CT coronary angiography demonstrating a patent stent, with minimal hyperplasia

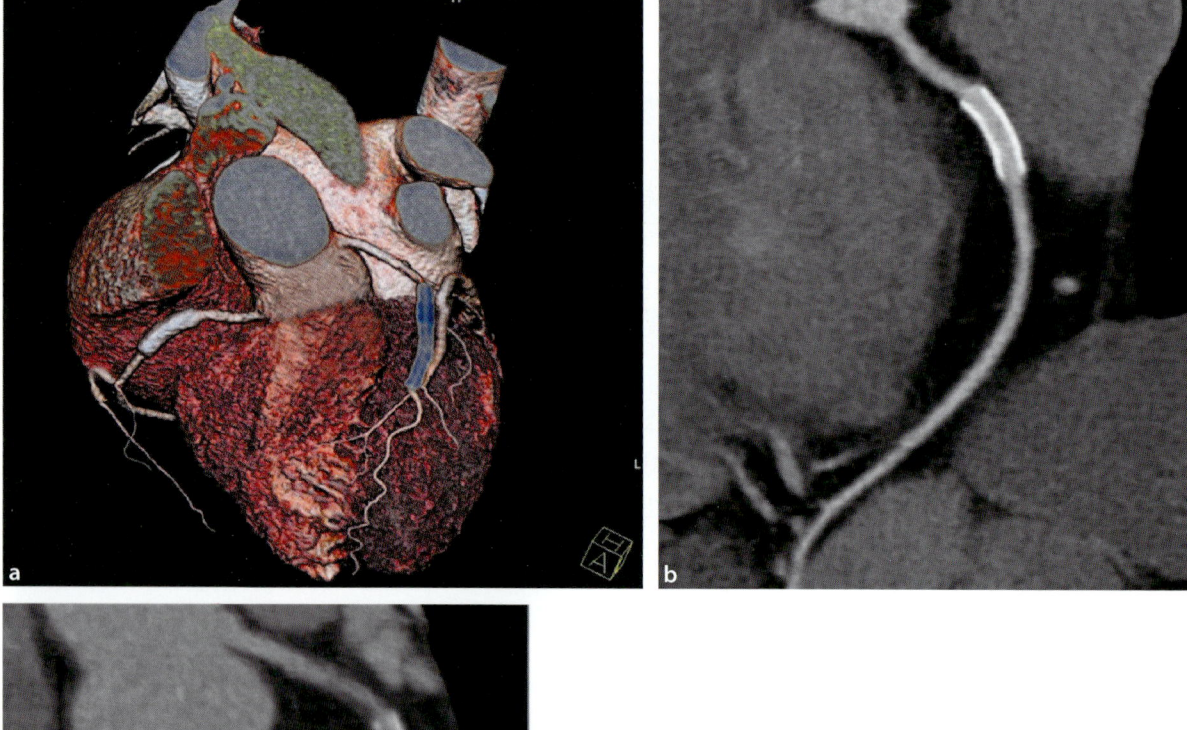

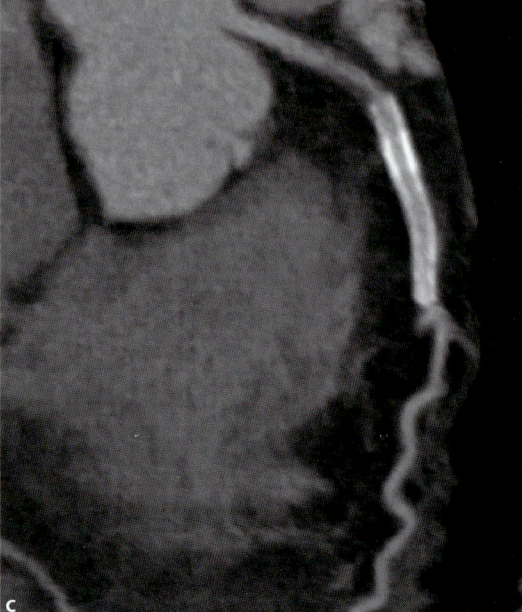

Fig. 15.10 (a) Volume rendered CT image showing stents in the proximal-to-mid LAD and mid-RCA. The images were acquired at a heart rate of 76 bpm, without any beta-blockers, using a dual-source MSCT scanner, SOMATOM definition. (b,c) Curved multiplanar CT images demonstrating excellent visualization of the in-stent lumen of RCA and LAD (Courtesy; Siemens Medical Solutions. Erasmus Medical Center, Rotterdam, the Netherlands)

The possible causes of worsening of symptoms after surgical revascularization include either progression of native coronary disease or occlusion of bypass grafts [52]. During the last decade, there have been many improvements in the surgical approaches to coronary revascularization. Arterial conduits using the internal mammary artery offer a better patency than venous grafts [53]. Moreover, less invasive procedures such as "off-pump" CABG surgery are being used more commonly [54].

CT coronary angiography was found to be helpful for the evaluation of patency of bypass grafts in the very initial stages of the technology, with a sensitivity of more than 90%, both for EBCT and single slice spiral CT [55–57]. A sensitivity of 97% and specificity of 98% was achieved with 4-slice CT scanners, making bypass graft evaluation the first clinical indication of CT angiography [58].

With the current generation of MDCT, not only accurate depiction of bypass graft conduits, but also simultaneous high resolution imaging of the native coronary tree has become feasible (Fig. 15.11) [59–61]. This helps to differentiate between conduit occlusion and the progression of disease in the native coronary arteries.

In early days post-CABG patients, chest pain could occur due to surgical wound, pleural effusion, sternal infection or problems with anastomosis. MDCT can identify the exact underlying cause in such cases.

Surgeons in certain countries have already started using MDCT coronary angiography for preoperative evaluation and surgical planning [61, 62]. However, wider use and switching from conventional cardiac angiography for pre-operative planning to CT angiography for such purposes will take a longer time.

15.2.4
Prognosis and Plaque Imaging

Coronary calcifications represent the process of coronary atherosclerosis and have been associated with a higher risk for coronary events [19, 20, 63]. However, studies have shown that the vulnerable soft plaques are responsible for acute coronary events and are composed of a thin fibrous cap with a large lipid pool and are mostly non-calcified. These "soft plaques" are unstable and likely to rupture, occluding the coronary artery lumen with consequent myocardial infarction (Fig. 15.8a–15.8c). Therefore, the identification of soft unstable plaques is more crucial than identification of stabilized calcified plaques, for prognosis, risk stratification and management decisions. These soft plaques cannot be visualized by routine catheter angiography, except intravascular ultrasound, which is an invasive and

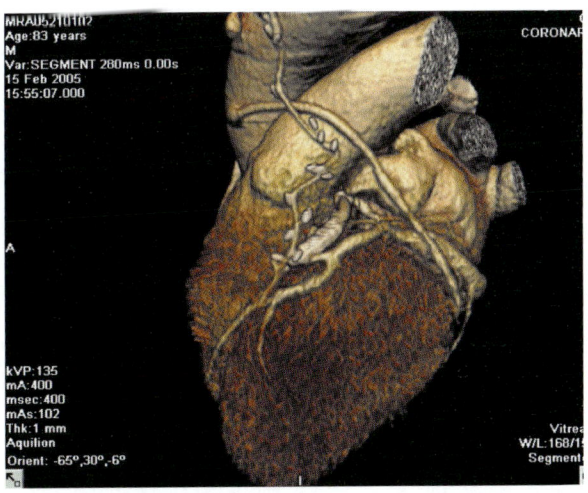

Fig. 15.11 One patent LIMA to LAD graft with a stent in proximal LAD and another saphenous graft to OM. Anatomical information is crucial at times in post-revascularization procedures, particularly if the myocardial perfusion SPECT is highly abnormal

costly procedure. Different plaque components have different CT attenuation values (lipids <50 HU; fibrous tissue 50–130 HU; calcifications >130 HU). Therefore, high resolution MDCT imaging permits cross-sectional evaluation of arterial lumen, helping in the identification and characterization of atherosclerotic plaque (Fig. 15.12a and 15.12b) [64–67]. Pharmacologioal therapy with drugs such as statins could help to stabilize such plaques, reducing the possibility of rupture.

MDCT coronary angiograhy provides both anatomical and morphological information about coronary atherosclerosis. Current generation 64 MDCTs have demonstrated good correlation with IVUS for plaque detection and characterization, identifying lipid-rich, fibrous and calcified plaques [67]. Accurate quantification of the plaque burden is objective of future MDCT enhancement [68]. Development and testing of various software techniques is in progress for clinical use. Absolute and reproducible quantitation could help to study the natural course of coronary plaques and their response to various therapies, helping better risk-stratification.

15.3
Role in Congenital Heart Diseases

There is a steady rise in the number of persons with congenital heart diseases surviving into adult life, with or without treatment [69]. Many of these adults, particularly from the underdeveloped countries, have no pre-

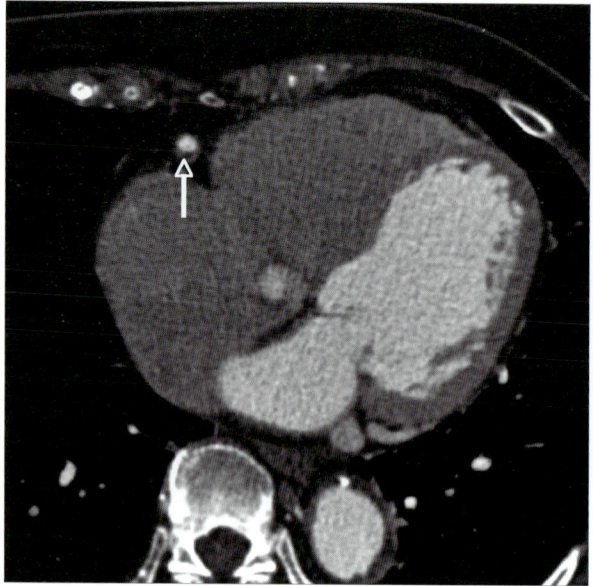 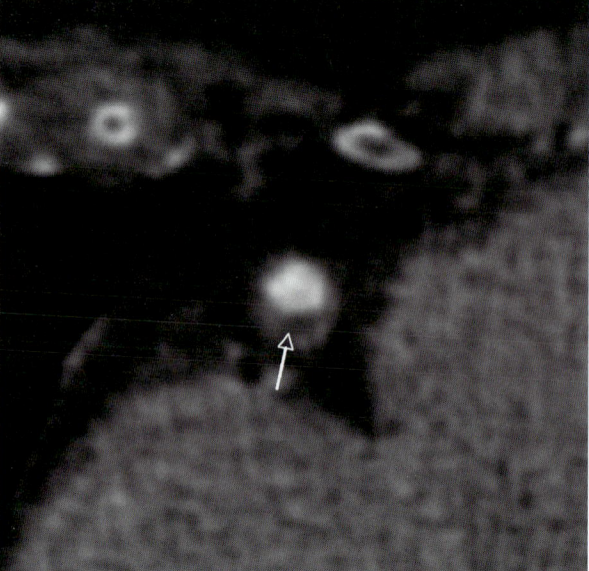

Fig. 15.12 CT coronary angiogram demonstrating a soft vulnerable plaque in proximal RCA, and well-visualized in cross-sectional images (**b**). A soft plaque is considered vulnerable if it has more than 40% lipid component, a fibrous cap <150 mm and the presence of inflammation. Vulnerable plaques are the major cause of major coronary events, even in non-significant obstructive lesions (<50%)

vious surgical correction procedure performed. Aortic valve disease, coarctation, pulmonary stenosis, atrial septal defect, and patent ductus arteriosus are the most common lesions in this group of patients.

Transthoracic echocardiography is the first-line diagnostic imaging technique for congenital defects, except anomalous coronary arteries. Coronary anamolies occur in approximately 1% of the general population [70, 71]. Coronary anomalies are usually discovered incidentally, during coronary angiography. However, X-ray angiography has limited ability to provide information regarding the spatial orientation of the anomalous artery with regard to the surrounding cardiovascular structures. MDCT permits high resolution non-invasive detection of anomalous coronary arteries (Fig. 15.13). MDCT is also helpful in the evaluation of congenital heart diseases of complicated anatomy. Furthermore, the larger field of view of CT helps to cover a bigger body, which is helpful to diagnose any extra cardiac abnormalities.

15.4 Hybrid Imaging

Functional information such as myocardial perfusion has a well-established role in risk-stratification. Com-

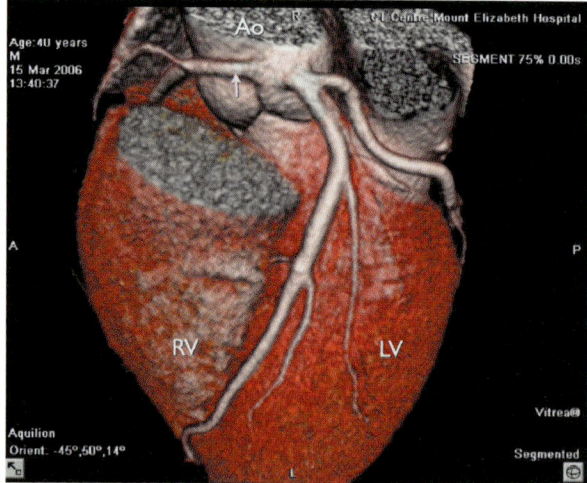

Fig. 15.13 MDCT in a 40-year-old male with complaint of occasional typical chest pain. The image demonstrates anamolous origin of RCA from the left coronary sinus (*arrow*), with an acute bend to course between the aorta and pulmonary trunk. Such an anomalous origin of RCA, is associated with angina, myocardial infarction and sudden death even in the absence of atherosclerosis (LV = left ventricle, RV = Right ventricle, Ao = Aorta)

bining anatomical data from MDCT with functional information is likely to improve patient management [72]. With 16-slice hybrid PET CT devices it is possible to perform coronary CT angiography and stress-rest myocardial perfusion assessment. The negative predictive value and accuracy of combined PET and 16-slice coronary CT angiography has been reported as 99% and 97%, respectively [73]. With improvement in technology and the launch of 64-slice PET-CT, the clinical role will be expanded. Such an approach may gain wider acceptance with easier availability of Rubidium generators, which do not require an on-site cyclotron.

A combination of SPECT with multislice CT is likely to be an economical alternative to PET-CT. Initially SPECT-CT devices were launched as 2-, 6- and 10-slice CT scanners. With these systems it is possible to quantify and localize coronary calcifications and correlate them precisely with perfusion abnormalities. However, for coronary angiography, at least 16-slice SPECT CT devices are mandatory, leading to recent launch of 16 and 64 slice SPECT-CT. It is too early to comment on the clinical feasibility of such systems. MDCT scanners acquire data much faster during part of the cardiac cycle, whereas myocardial perfusion SPECT images are averaged over time and this could generate fusion artefacts.

There will be an increased use of proteomics and genomics for early diagnosis and preventative therapies in high-risk patients. Hybrid imaging devices could be of potential help providing anatomical and functional/metabolic information in future for such management strategies.

15.5
Conclusion

MDCT angiography is likely to have a role in screening intermediate risk patients for early detection and follow-up of coronary artery disease. Its current main role in view of its higher negative predicative value is in the assessment of patients with atypical chest pain and symptoms, and in those with equivocal or borderline treadmill stress tests. MDCT is also useful for the evaluation of acute chest pain, triaging patients to appropriate treatment strategies. Non-invasive assessment of non-calcified plaque burden by MDCT is an exciting future application, likely to re-define high-risk patients with potential clinical implications. MDCT should not be used indiscriminately.

Improvements in spatial and temporal resolutions have been ongoing areas of technical research. With the introduction of flat-panel detectors, it is possible to image fifth-degree coronary artery branches [74, 75]. However, increased noise and higher radiation dose factors have limited the commercial launch of thease equipments. Alternatively, Phillips has very recently launched a 256-slice CT, providing 8 cm coverage, covering the entire heart in two scans (Fig. 15.14) and including a rotation speed of 0.27 s, which is currently the fastest in the world. It has been claimed to reduce the radiation dose by 80%, compared with 64-slice CT. Toshiba has launched a 320-slice CT, with coverage area of 16 cm. This permits coverage of the entire heart in a single rotation, with a resolution of 0.5 mm. Data can be acquired and reconstructed into full cardiac volume over a single heartbeat, thereby eliminating step artefacts often seen with 64-slice scanners. Another unique feature is the gantry design, which turns the kinetic energy of the scan into electricity to put back into the system. It is predicted that MDCT scanners will continue to be in clinical use, with more installations in cardiac and emergency departments as part of coronary artery disease management, moving away from "probability" to "definitive" diagnosis of CAD. However, the economic efficiency and impact on clinical management of the latest generation of expensive 256- and 320-slice CT canners has yet to be established.

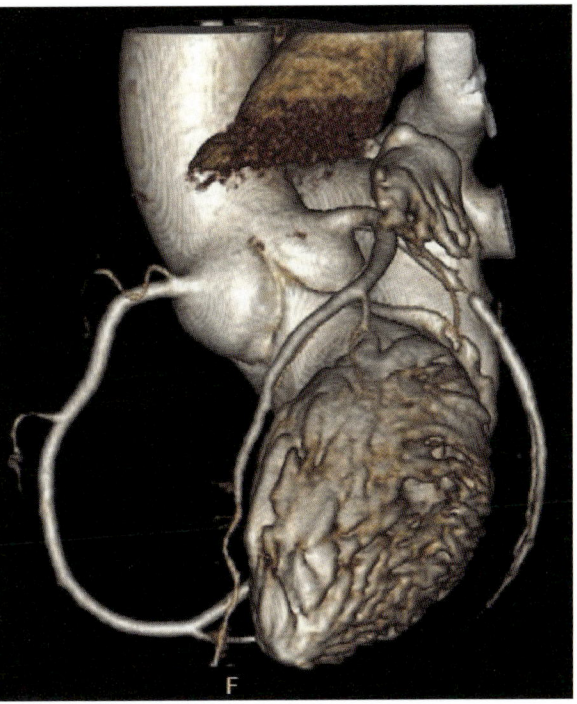

Fig. 15.14 CT coronary angiography using recent generation 256-slice CT (Courtesy: Philips Medical)

References

1. Prasad SK, Assomull RG, Pennell DJ (2004) Recent developments in non-invasive cardiology. BMJ 329:1386–1389.
2. Kohl G (2005) The evolution and state-of-the-art principles of multislice computed tomography. Proc Am Thoracic Soc 2:470–476.
3. Schoenhagen P, Halliburton SS, Stillman AE et al. (2004) Noninvasive imaging of coronary arteries: current and future role of multi–detector row CT. Radiology 232:7–17.
4. Hounsfield GN (1973) Computerized transverse axial scanning (tomography). Description of system. Br J Radiol 46:1016–1022.
5. Bushberg JT, Seibert JA, Leidholdt EM Jr et al. (2002) The Essential Physics of Medical Imaging, 2nd edn. Lippincott Williams & Wilkins, Philadelphia, PA, pp. 331–339.
6. Kalender WA, Seissler W, Klotz E et al. (1990) Spiral volumetric CT with single-breath-hold technique, continuous transport, and continuous scanner rotation. Radiology 176:181–183.
7. Woodhouse CE, Janowitz WR, Viamonte M Jr (1997) Coronary arteries: retrospective cardiac gating technique to reduce cardiac motion artifact at spiral CT. Radiology 204:566–569.
8. Budoff MJ, Raggi P (2001) Coronary artery disease progression assessed by electron-beam computed tomography. Am J Cardiol 88:46E–50E.
9. Bielak LF, Peyser PA, Sheedy PF (2003) Electronbeam computed tomography screening for asymptomatic coronary artery disease. Semin Roentgenol 38:39–53.
10. Achenbach S, Moshage W, Bachmann K (1998) Noninvasive coronary angiography by contrast-enhanced electron beam computed tomography. Clin Cardiol 21:323–330.
11. Kalender W (2000) Computed Tomography: Fundamentals, System Technology, Image Quality, Applications. MCD Verlag, Munich, Germany, pp. 35–81.
12. Flohr T, McCullough C, Bruder H et al. (2006) First performance evaluation of a dual source CT (DSCT). Eur Radiology 16:256–268.
13. Hausleiter J, Meyer T, Hadamitzky M et al. (2006) Radiation dose estimates from cardiac Multislice Computed Tomography in daily practice: Impact of different scanning protocols on effective dose estimates. Circulation 113:1305–1310.
14. Ropers U, Ropers D, Pflederer T et al. (2007) Influence of heart rate on the diagnostic accuracy of dual-source computed tomography coronary angiography. J Am Coll Cardiol 50:2393–2398.
15. Husmann L, Valenta I, Gaemperli O et al. (2008) Feasibility of low-dose coronary CT angiography: first experience with prospective ECG=gating. Eur Heart J 29:191–197.
16. Gianrossi R et al. (1989) Exercise induced ST depression in the diagnosis of coronary artery disease - a meta-analysis. Circulation 80:87–98.
17. Beller GA, Zaret BL (2000) Contributions of nuclear cardiology to diagnosis and prognosis of patients with CAD. Circulation 101:1465–1478.
18. Rich S, McLaughlin VV (2002) Detection of subclinical cardiovascular disease: the emerging role of electron beam computed tomography. Prevent Med 34:1–10.
19. Rumberger JA, Simons DB, Fitzpatrick LA et al. (1995) Coronary artery calcium area by electron-beam computed tomography and coronary atherosclerotic plaque area. A histopathologic correlative study. Circulation 92:2157–2162.
20. Greenland P, La Bree L, Azen T et al. (2004) Coronary artery calcium score combined with Framingham Score for risk prediction in asymptomatic individuals. J Am Med Assoc 291:210–215.
21. Nieman K, Oudkerk M, Rensing B J et al. (2001) Coronary angiography with multi-slice computed tomography. Lancet 357:599–603.
22. Achenbach S, Giesler T, Ropers D et al. (2001) Detection of coronary artery stenoses by contrast-enhanced, retrospectively electrocardiographically-gated, multislice spiral computed tomography. Circulation 103:2535–2538.
23. Schmermund A, Erbel R (2005) Non-invasive computed tomographic coronary angiography: the end of the beginning. Eur Heart J 26(15):1451–1453.
24. Bhatt (2005) To cath or not to cath: that is no longer the question. J Am Med Assoc 293:2935–2937.
25. Gracia MJ (2005) Noninvasive coronary angiography. Hype or new paradigm? J Am Med Assoc 293:2531–2533.
26. Kuettner A, Beck T, Drosch T et al. (2005) Image quality and diagnostic accuracy of non-invasive coronary imaging with 16 detector slice spiral computed tomowith 188 ms temporal resolution. Heart 91:938–941.
27. Hoffmann M HK, Shi H, Schmitz BL et al. (2005) Non-invasive coronary angiography with multislice computed tomography. J Am Med Assoc 293:2471–2478.
28. Leschka S, Alkadhi H, Plass A et al. (2005) Accuracy of MSCT coronary angiography with 64-slice technology: first experience. Eur Heart J 26:1482–1487.
29. Mollet N R, Cademartiri F, van Mieghem C AG et al. (2005) High-resolution spiral computed tomography coronary angiography in patients referred for diagnostic conventional coronary angiography. Circulation 112(15):2318–2323.
30. Margolis JR, Kannel WS, Feinleib M et al. (1973) Clinical features of unrecognized myocardial infarction-silent and symptomatic: eighteen-year follow-up: the Framingham Study. Am J Cardiol 32:1–7.
31. Weiner DA, Ryan TJ, Parsons L et al. (1991) Significance of silent myocardial ischemia during exercise testing in patients with diabetes mellitus: a report from the Coronary Artery Surgery Study (CASS) registry. Am J Cardiol 68:729–734.
32. Raggi P, Bellasi A, Ratti C (2005) Ischemia Imaging and plaque imaging in diabetes: complementary tools to im-

prove cardiovascular risk management. Diabetes Care 28:2787–2794.
33. Haffner SM, Lehto S, Rönnemaa T, Pyörälä K, Laakso M (1998) Mortality from coronary heart disease in subjects with type 2 diabetes and in non-diabetic subjects with and without prior myocardial infarction. N Engl J Med 339:229–234.
34. Anand DV, Lim E, Lahiri A et al. (2006) The role of non-invasive imaging in the risk stratification of asymptomatic diabetic subjects. Eur Heart J 27(8):905–912.
35. Bugiardinii R, Bairey Merz CN (2005) Angina with "normal" coronary arteries: a changing philosophy. J Am Med Assoc 293:477–484.
36. Reyes et al. (2005) Angina with "normal" coronary arteries. J Am Med Assoc 293:2468–2469.
37. Sicari et al. (2005) Long-term survival of patients with chest pain syndrome and angiographically normal or near-normal coronary arteries: the additional prognostic value of dipyridamole echocardiography test (DET). Eur Heart J 26:2136–2141.
38. Gasper T, Halon D, Rabinstein R, Peled N.(2005) Clinical application and future trends in cardiac CTA. Eur Radiology 15(Supplement 4) D10–D14.
39. Pope JH, Aufderheide TP, Ruthazer R et al. (2000) Missed diagnoses of acute cardiac ischemia in the emergency department. N Engl J Med 342(16):1163–1170.
40. White CS, Kuo D, Kelemen M et al. (2005) Chest pain evaluation in the emergency department: can MDCT provide a comprehensive evaluation? Am J Radiol 185:533–540.
41. Lawler LP, Fishman EK (2003) Multidetector row computed tomography of the aorta and peripheral arteries. Cardiol Clin 21:607–629.
42. Schoepf UJ, Costello P (2003) Multidetector-row CT imaging of pulmonary embolism. Semin Roentgenol 38:106–114.
43. Larlo A, Cardeiro M, Silva C et al. (2006) Constrast enhanced multidetector computed tomography viability after Myocardial Infarction. Circulation 113:394–404.
44. Faris P, Grant C, Galbraith D et al. (2004) Diagnostic cardiac catheterization and revascularization rates for coronary heart disease. Can J Cardiol 20(4): 391–397.
45. Schluter M, Schofer J, Gershlick AH et al. (2005) Direct stenting of native de novo coronary artery lesions with the sirolimus-eluting stent: a post hoc subanalysis of the pooled E- and C-SIRIUS trials. Overview J Am Coll Cardiol 45(1):10–13.
46. Werner GS, Krack A, Schwarz G et al. (2004) Prevention of lesion recurrence in chronic total coronary occlusions by paclitaxel-eluting stents. J Am Coll Cardiol 44(12):2301–2306.
47. The EPISTENT Investigators (1998) Randomised placebo-controlled and balloon-angioplasty-controlled trial to assess safety of coronary stenting with use of platelet glycoprotein-IIb/IIIa blockade. Evaluation of Platelet IIb/IIIa Inhibitor for Stenting. Lancet 352:87–92.
48. Price MJ, Cristea E, Sawhney N et al. (2006) Serial angiographic follow-up of sirolimus-eluting stents for unprotected left main coronary artery revascularization. J Am Coll Cardiol 47(4):871–877.
49. Nieman K, Cademartiri F, Raaijmakers R et al. (2003) Noninvasive angiographic evaluation of coronary stents with multi-slice spiral computed tomography. Herz 28:136–142.
50. Funabashi N, Komiyama N, Komuro I (2003) Patency of coronary artery lumen surrounded by metallic stent evaluated by three dimensional volume rendering images using ECG gated multislice computed tomography. Heart 89:388.
51. Cademartiri F, Mollet N, Lemos P et al. (2005) Usefulness of multislice computed tomographic coronary angiography to assess in-stent re-stenosis. Am J Cardiol 96:799–802.
52. Alderman EL, Kip KE, Whitlow PL et al. (2004) Native coronary disease progression exceeds failed revascularization as cause of angina after five years in the Bypass Angioplasty Revascularization Investigation (BARI). J Am Coll Cardiol 44:766–774.
53. Goldman S, Zadina K, Moritz T et al. (2004) Long-term patency of saphenous vein and left internal mammary artery grafts after coronary artery bypass surgery: results from a Department of Veterans Affairs Cooperative Study. J Am Coll Cardiol 44:2149–2156.
54. Khan NE, De Souza A, Mister R et al. (2004) A randomized comparison of off-pump and on-pump multivessel coronary-artery bypass surgery. N Engl J Med 350:21–28.
55. Lu B, Dai R P, Jing B L et al. (2000) Evaluation of coronary artery bypass graft patency using three-dimensional reconstruction and flow study on electron beam tomography. J Comput Assist Tomogr 24: 663–670.
56. Ha J, Cho S, Shim W et al. (1999) Noninvasive evaluation of coronary artery bypass graft patency using three-dimensional angiography obtained with contrast-enhanced electron beam CT. Am J Radiol 172: 1055–1059.
57. Godwin J, Califf R, Korobkin M et al. (1983) Clinical value of coronary bypass graft evaluation with CT. Am J Radiol 140:649–655.
58. Engelmann M, von Smekal A, Knez A et al. (1997) Accuracy of spiral computed tomography for identifying arterial and venous coronary graft patency. Am J Cardiol 80:569–574.
59. Schlosser T, Konorza T, Hunold et al. (2004) Noninvasive visualization of coronary artery bypass grafts using 16-detector row computed tomography. J Am Coll Cardiol 44(6):1224–1229.
60. Marano R, Storto M L, Merlino B et al. (2005) A pictorial review of coronary artery bypass grafts at multidetector row CT. Chest 127:1371–1377
61. Robert CG, Markowitz A, Peter S (2005) Society of Thoracic Radiology: Consensus Statement. Evaluation of the

Cardiac Surgery Patient With MSCT. J Thoracic Imaging 20(4):265–272.
62. Letter to the Editor (2005) Recent advances in non-invasive cardiology: Coronary angiography using computed tomography has been underplayed. BMJ 330:731–732.
63. Kondos GT, Hoff JA, Sevrukov A (2003) Electron-beam tomography coronary artery calcium and cardiac events: a 37-month follow-up of 5635 initially asymptomatic low- to intermediate-risk adults. Circulation 107:2571–2576.
64. Schroeder S, Kopp AF, Baumbach A et al. (2001) Non-invasive characterisation of coronary lesion morphology by multi- slice computed tomography: a promising new technology for risk stratification of patients with coronary artery disease. Heart 85:576–578.
65. Kopp AF, Schroeder S, Baumbach A et al. (2001) Non-invasive characterisation of coronary lesion morphology and composition by multislice CT: first results in comparison with intracoronary ultrasound. Eur Radiol 11:1607–1611.
66. Leber A, Knez A, White C et al. (2002) Composition of coronary atherosclerotic plaques in patients with acute myocardial infarction and stable angina pectoris determined by contrast-enhanced multislice computed tomography. Am J Cardiol 91:714–718.
67. Becker C, Nikolaou K, Muders M et al. (2003) Ex vivo coronary atherosclerotic plaque characterization with multi-detector-row CT. Eur Radiol 13:2094–2098.
68. Leber A, Becker A, Knez A et al. (2006) Accuracy of 64-slice computed tomography to classify and quantify plaque volumes in the proximal coronary system. J Am Coll Cardiol 47:672–677.
69. Brickner M, Hillis L, Lange R (2000) Congenital heart disease in adults. N Engl J Med 324:256.
70. Angelini P, Velasco JA, Flamm S (2002) Coronary anomalies: incidence, pathophysiology, and clinical relevance. Circulation 105:2449–2454.
71. Taylor AJ, Rogan KM, Virmani R (1992) Sudden cardiac death associated with isolated congenital coronary artery anomalies. J Am Coll Cardiol 20:640–647.
72. Hacker M, Jakobs T, Matthiesen F et al. (2005) Comparison of spiral multidetector ct angiography and myocardial perfusion imaging in the noninvasive detection of functionally relevant coronary artery lesions: first clinical experiences. J Nucl Med 46(8):1294–1300.
73. Namdar M, Hany T, Koepfli P et al. (2005) Integrated PET/CT for the assessment of coronary artery disease: a feasibility study. J Nucl Med 46(6): 930–935.
74. Knollmann F, Pfoh A (2003) Image in cardiovascular medicine: coronary artery imaging with flat-panel computed tomography. Circulation 107:1209.
75. Knollmann FD, Edic PM, Cesmeli E et al. (2002) Coronary artery imaging with flat-panel computed tomography. Radiology 225(P):538–539 (Abstract).

Chapter 16

Current Status of Cardiovascular MR Imaging

Shahid Mahmood and Robert Kwok

Contents

16.1	Introduction	177
16.1.1	Principal Concepts of MR Imaging	178
16.1.2	Cardiovascular MRI Techniques	178
16.2	Clinical Application	180
16.2.1	Coronary Artery Disease	180
16.2.2	Cardiomyopathies	183
16.2.3	Arrhythmogenic Right Ventricular Dysplasia	184
16.2.4	Myocarditis	185
16.3	Conclusions	185
	References	185

16.1 Introduction

The technique of cardiac magnetic resonance imaging (MRI) has been used for a long time for the evaluation of pericardial disease, cardiac masses and complex congenital heart diseases [1–4]. MRI has the ability to quantify pulmonary and systemic flow, valvular regurgitation, and pulmonary-to-systemic ratios across shunts. During recent years there have been impressive advances in technology, particularly in resolution and imaging speed, enabling MRI to enter into the mainstream of diagnostic imaging for coronary artery disease. However, despite its overwhelming advantages in imaging, it still has certain limitations (Table 16.1).

Table 16.1 Advantages and disadvantages of cardiac MR imaging

Advantages	Limitations
• 3-dimensional tomographic images	• Contraindicated in certain implants like pacemakers
• High resolution	• Lengthy acquisition time
• Intrinsic high contrast	• ECG distortion by magnetic field
• No radiation	
• Anatomical and functional information in a single study	• Difficulty in breath holding for very sick and old patients
	• Some patients could be claustrophobic
	• Lack of clinical prognostic data

16.1.1
Principal Concepts of MR Imaging

The property of nuclear magnetic resonance of atoms, first described in 1946 [5, 6] is the basic principle of magnetic resonance imaging [7, 8]. During MR imaging, protons in the body align themselves to an external magnetic field. A radio frequency wave is then applied through the body. The protons absorb this energy and change their direction and alignment. This leads to the induction of current in a receiver coil (similar to an aerial). When the radio frequency wave is turned off, the protons return to their original position, and during this process they release the absorbed energy. This energy decreases the signals in the receiver coil. Computers acquire the changes in signals digitally and form an image. Gradient fields help to localize these signals correctly in the X, Y and Z directions in the spatial frequency (k-space), through fast multi-dimensional Fourier transformations, usually preceded by interpolation and re-sampling techniques.

Although the magnetic field of each proton is very small, the combined effect of a large number of these protons enables an image to be formed. Fortunately, our body is made of a large number of hydrogen protons (1H), which makes magnetic resonance imaging possible. The subtle differences in the concentration of hydrogen protons in fat, muscle, blood and water gives rise to differences in the signal intensities received from these tissues. The contrast resolution of the images can be improved further by use of additional extrinsic protons, in the form of contrast agents.

Two terms are basic and an integral part of all MR images, i.e., T1 and T2 properties. Different tissues appear differently in the two images. White matter light grey in T1 and dark grey in T2. Grey matter appears grey in both images. The cerebrospinal fluid appears black in T1 and white in T2. The background to the image (air) appears black in both (T1 and T2) images.

Switching off the radio frequency causes the protons to return to their original state. The time taken for a proton to return to its original value of longitudinal magnetization is known as the T1 value, and differs from tissue to tissue, e.g., fat has a shorter T1 value than water. At the same time, the protons will also return to their haphazard original states in terms of phase. This time is known as T2 and is a measure of its transverse relaxation. In general this can be compared to the example of a classroom of students: when the teacher enters the class (similar to the RF signal) the students stand and face the teacher. When the teacher leaves the classroom, the students sit (return to their original position – T1) and also face their classmates (T2).

There are several ways to emphasize T1 or T2 values by applying different pulses, e.g., to emphasize T1, a 180° pulse is first applied. This is similar to asking the class to turn to face the back of the class before the teacher enters the room.

The time from one 90° pulse to the next is known as the repetition time (TR). The time from the 90° pulse to when the echo is received is known as the echo time (TE). Depending on the value of these times, the T1 or T2 characteristic is emphasized and different images can be obtained; e.g., for TR and TE short, a T1 image is obtained; for TR and TE long, a T2 image is obtained; for TR long and TE short, the image represents the amount of protons – thus a proton density image is obtained.

Initially, MR imaging started with conventional spin echo, using a 90° pulse followed by a 180° pulse, generating T1 and T2 images. During subsequent years, with the advances in technology, more advanced pulses and sequences were introduced into clinical use (e.g., fast spin echo, inversion recovery, short T1 inversion recovery, coherent gradient echo, incoherent gradient echo with RF spoiled or gradient spoiled, steady state free precession, ultra fast imaging), helping to generate different types of MR images for different clinical applications in orthopaedics, neurology and cardiovascular imaging.

16.1.2
Cardiovascular MRI Techniques

For cardiac applications, the commonly used techniques include:

16.1.2.1 Black Blood Imaging

The blood appears black, due to decreased signal from blood with reference to the myocardium, making it easier to perform cardiac chamber segmentation (Fig. 16.1). This enables:
a) visualization of cardiac anatomic structure
b) assessment of valvular structure
c) assessment of masses.

Fast spin echo (FSE), with a pre-saturation pulse, can produce such images. Commercially, all manufacturers term this differently, e.g., double/triple IR FSE, TSE, HASTE.

As the name implies, the fast spin echo (FSE) is a spin echo pulse sequence but its scan time is much shorter than the conventional spin echo. FSE uses a turbofactor (number of 180° rephasing pulses) to reduce its

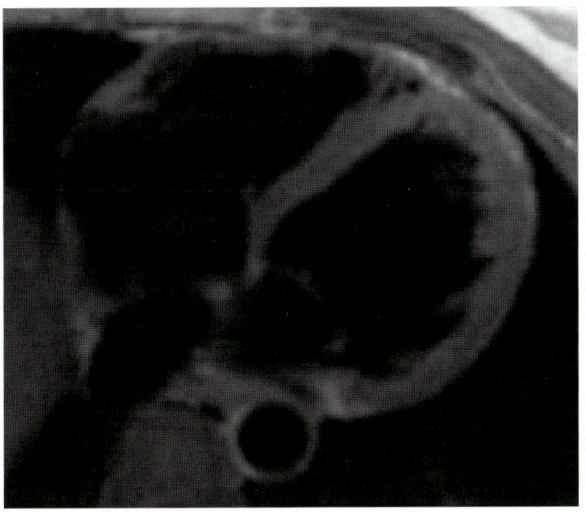

Fig. 16.1 An example of black blood imaging, in which blood appears black

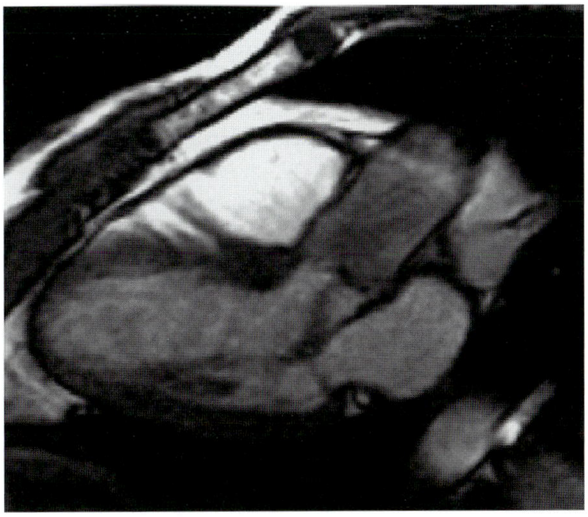

Fig. 16.2 Bright blood imaging (SSFP). LVOT view demonstrating moderate aortic valve regurgitation

scan time. Instead of the conventional 90°–180° pulse sequence, in FSE a 90° pulse is followed by a series of 180° rephrasing pulses giving the corresponding number of phase encoding steps. This enables more K space to be filled, reducing scan time. The addition of a pre-saturation pulse enables the moving protons to give no signal, resulting in the dark blood appearance.

Currently, it is common to apply a non-selective 180° pulse followed by a selective 180° de-inversion pulse. This sequence is often done in orthogonal planes–axial, coronal and sagittal for best visualization of anatomy.

ECG gated spin echo sequences with pre-saturation pulses for magnetization preparation reveal strong intravascular signal loss due to flow effects when appropriate imaging conditions, including spatial pre-saturation are used.

16.1.2.2 Bright Blood Imaging

In this technique, the pulses and sequences used are such that blood appears bright, instead of black, for visualization of:
a) cardiac anatomic structure
b) intra-cardiac thrombus.

In cardiac applications these types of images are usually displayed in cine mode, in short axis, long axis, 4-chamber, 2-chamber and LVOT (Fig. 16.2). The bright blood appearance may be obtained through various techniques – gradient echo/gradient moment rephrasing, and the latest sequence of steady state free precession (SSFP). Currently, SSFP is the method of choice for acquisition in cine mode. It is called different names by different vendors – True FISP cine, FIESTA and T2 FFE.

SSFP is a gradient echo sequence used to acquire images that show true T2 characteristics. It uses a 180° pulse to rephrase and a rewinder to move the spin echo before the pulse, such that the echo can be received. Spatial and temporal resolution are substantially improved with this technique, however, contrast on the basis of the ratio of T2 to T1 is not sufficiently high in soft tissues.

16.1.2.3 Myocardial Tagging

The technique of myocardial tagging has been used for evaluation of wall motion abnormalities. In myocardial tagging, a thin plane of myocardial tissue is saturated with a sequence of radiofrequency pulses. A saturated myocardium does not give any MR signal during myocardial contraction. Thus, myocardial tags move with the underlying myocardium during systole and diastole and relax with the T1 of the heart, and are regenerated at the onset of each contraction. It is possible to estimate accurately the displacement of the tag to within 0.1 mm, and to compute full 3D myocardial strain maps [9, 10].

Tagging has made it possible to understand some important aspects of cardiovascular dynamics and physiology. Besides simple short- and long-axis motions, tagging also demonstrates the twisting component of the ventricular contraction, whereby the base moves clockwise and the apex, counterclockwise. This torsion reverses during isovolumic relaxation, just prior to the opening of the mitral valve, generating ventricular suction, and is responsible for early diastolic filling.

16.1.2.4 Phase Contrast Angiography

Phase contrast sequencing provides a velocity map of blood flow. It is therefore excellent to demonstrate valvular function and provides information on regurgitation, shunt quantification and other related functional information.

16.1.2.5 Perfusion and Viability Imaging

Table 16.2 Use of Cardiac MR imaging in myocardial infarction

Acute MI	Old (Chronic) MI
Size/Prognosis	Hibernating myocardium detection
Wall motion	Wall motion abnormalities
Wall thickness normal	Wall thinning (+/−)
LV function	LV function
(Acute dysfunction)	(Chronic dysfunction)
Delayed enhancement	Delayed enhancement
(Dead myocytes)	(Fibrous scar)

In order to demonstrate cardiac perfusion and viability, a multi-phase multi-slice cine sequence is performed. The pulse sequence is a fast gradient echo sequence with an echo-planar readout. This sequence is done with contrast administration of 0.2 mmol/kg in order to demonstrate any filling defects due to ishaemic changes in the myocardium. Temporal resolution of about 150 ms per frame ensures good images. Additionally, a breath–hold inversion recovery prepared gated fast gradient echo technique is also used for demonstration of myocardial delayed enhancement. In this sequence, after a nonselective inversion pulse, the TI time for the myocardial nulling signal is collected. This TI value may range from 130–275 ms depending upon the quantity of residual contrast and speed of washout of contrast from the myocardium.

An important factor for diagnostic high quality cardiac MR imaging is an appropriate ECG gating. However, at times within the MR gantry the ECG signal is degraded by the superimposed electrical potential of flowing blood in the magnetic field. Currently, new systems gate using vectrocardiography, thereby limiting the problem of signal degradation and reducing such artefacts. Many techniques even without gating are also being evaluated, particularly with T-3 MR systems. Breath holding is another factor affecting cardiac MR images. With new coils and high gradients, image acquisition without breath holding has almost become a reality.

16.2 Clinical Application

16.2.1 Coronary Artery Disease

Cardiovascular MR imaging has the unique potential of assessment of a wide variety of anatomical and physiological parameters associated with coronary artery disease, ranging from coronary anatomy to myocardial viability (Table 16.2).

16.2.1.1 Coronary MR Angiography

Coronary arteriography has remained the gold standard for coronary artery disease evaluation. However, with recent advancements it is likely that coronary CT angiography with multi-detector CT (MDCT) will become a non-invasive alternative in many clinical scenarios.

In contrast to coronary CT angiography, good quality fast coronary MR angiography has been a challenge, due to smaller diameters, tortuousity, and cardiac and respiratory motion. The recent provisions of non-breath hold and non-ECG gated imaging on the new 3-T systems, probably provides one justification for the use of such nonradiation technique. However, due to the limited number of installations, these have not been clinically validated very well and therefore experience remains limited.

On the "black-blood" MR images, the walls of coronary arteries appear white and blood as black, making it easier to differentiate between normal and atherosclerotic vessels. Coronary MR angiography is still behind coronary CT angiography in clinical practice on a routine basis. However, in patients with extensive coronary calcifications, coronary MR angiography results in better quality images than CT. It is also possible to gain additional information regarding the status of myocardial perfusion.

In the past, the most commonly accepted applications of coronary MR angiography have been the evaluation of anomalous coronary arteries and the assessment of bypass-graft patency. Accuracies ranging from 93% to 100% have been reported for identification and definition of anomalous coronary arteries [11–13]. Coronary

MR angiography has also been used in children with Kawasaki disease, as coronary artery ectasia and aneurysm occur in more than 15% of cases of Kawasaki disease [14]. Coronary artery bypass grafts have a larger lumen, less tortuousity and motion, making MR angiography a feasible alternative to evaluate the patency of bypass conduits. Various techniques and imaging sequences have been used, with sensitivities and specificities ranging from 86% to 100% and 56% to 90%, respectively [15, 16]. 3D contrast-enhanced MR angiography further enhances its accuracy and image quality.

16.2.1.2 Plaque Imaging

MRI has the potential to differentiate between "stable" and "vulnerable" atherosclerotic plaques. Vulnerable plaques are prone to rupture, and are a major cause of sudden cardiac death and myocardial infarction. Detection of vulnerable (unstable) plaques would be of help in making treatment decisions and also to prioritize such patients. However, recent advances in multi-detector CT technology have also shown some initial impressive capabilities in this regard.

16.2.1.3 LV Function and Wall Motion Abnormalities

Echocardiography and cardiac MRI are the two standard methods accepted to assess global and regional myocardial function and wall motion abnormalities. In a deformed left ventricle due to myocardial infarction and remodelling, accurate assessment of function is tedious by echocardiography. Similarly, echocardiography is of limited use in accurate calculations of atrial volumes and function. Recent further enhancements in Doppler echocardiography have enabled some improvement in the assessment of such cases. On the other hand, cardiac MRI has no limitations for direct and accurate assessment of all chambers (Fig. 16.3) [17–20]. Ejection fraction and volumes calculated from cardiac MRI are considered to be the most accurate, compared with other modalities.

Regional wall motion abnormalities are indicators of myocardial ischaemia and may precede ECG abnormalities and chest pain. Cardiac MR imaging, with or without myocardial tagging provides a precise quantitative estimate of motion as well as myocardial wall shortening and thickening [21]. In clinical routine, however due to rapidity and ease of use only two-dimensional evaluation in the circumferential and radial directions are commonly preferred, rather than 3-D tagging.

Regional wall motion abnormalities, thickening and LV function can be assessed by MRI both under resting conditions as well as in response to various stress agents like dobutamine.

16.2.1.4 Assessment of Perfusion

MR myocardial perfusion at rest and during post-stress testing can be considered as an analogue to gated

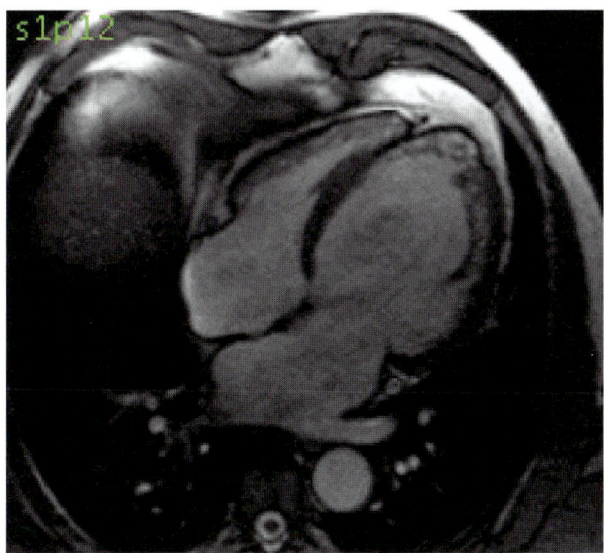
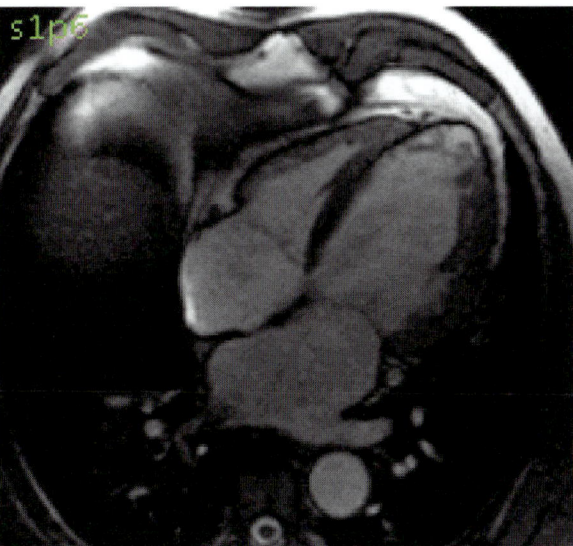

Fig. 16.3 Assessment of LV function: post-MI LV remodeling on SSFP images. Four chambers ED and ES frames, demonstrating dilated LV, with thinning of apex and anterior wall (remodeling) due to old MI. Moreover, the apex appears to be dyskinetic. LV remodeling after MI reduces effectiveness of contraction

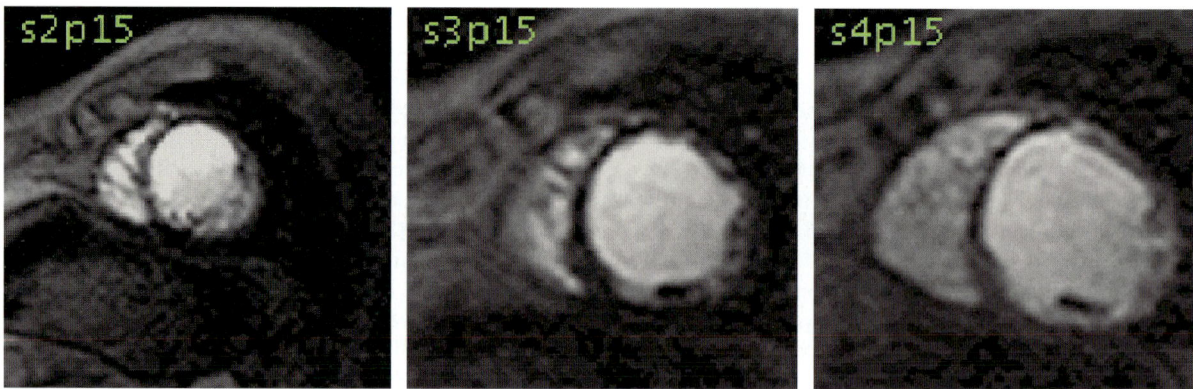

Fig. 16.4 Assessment of perfusion: first pass post-contrast images in short axis demonstrating an area of absent flow in the antero-septal region and one small area in the inferior wall. This does not improve on subsequent images and would be consistent with an infarction

myocardial perfusion SPECT imaging. However, MRI is likely to demonstrate more infarcts than PET and SPECT, correlating with histopathological findings [22, 23]. Multiple first pass contrast-enhanced images from apex to the base of LV are acquired, post-coronary vasodilatation, using adenosine or dipyridamole infusion. A flow-limiting stenosis demonstrates a region of hypoperfusion in the related vascular territory under stress, while an infarcted region demonstrates almost absent flow, with no subsequent improvement (Fig. 16.4). A flow reserve index can be calculated, proportional to the degree of coronary narrowing. However, more clinical validation is required to define its role in the evaluation of coronary artery disease.

16.2.1.5 Myocardial Viability

The detailed pathophysiology and clinical implications of hibernating myocardium have been discussed elsewhere in the book. The hibernating myocardium can be identified by the presence of myocardial metabolism, assessed using positron-emission tomography (PET); by cell membrane integrity or preserved cellular metabolism as in myocardial perfusion SPECT imaging using thallium-201 or Tc-99m MIBI; or by demonstrating preserved contractile reserve, assessed using dobutamine stress echocardiography or MRI [24–26]. Cardiac MRI using conventional gadolinium contrast agents is probably the latest and simplest approach for assessment of myocardial viability with the most superior spatial resolution (Fig. 16.5a and 16.5b)(Table 16.3) [27].

The superior spatial resolution of cardiac MRI compared with other imaging techniques like PET, SPECT, and echocardiography, makes it possible not only to delineate between transmural and non-transmural infarction, but also to identify small focal infarctions [28]. Comparative studies have demonstrated not only good agreement between PET and MR, but also its ability to identify additional non-viable areas, not seen by PET [22]. It has also been shown that patients with equivocal myocardial perfusion SPECT results could benefit from contrast-enhanced cardiac MR, particularly in the setting of non-transmural infarction [29, 30]. An area of myocardial infarctions involving less than 50% of the wall thickness on cardiac MRI is most likely to benefit from coronary revascularization, and to improve function. Delayed myocardial contrast enhancement sequences used for myocardial viability also assess intra-cardiac thrombi accurately, commonly present in patients with CAD, post-MI.

There is a wide range of time-consuming options available for cardiac MR imaging. It is therefore important to define precisely for any given clinical situation (Table 16.4). For example, it has been shown that a simple protocol consisting of baseline contractility and delayed enhancement cardiac MR study is adequate to differentiate dysfunctional, but viable from nonviable myocardium.

Table 16.3 Causes of delayed contrast enhancement

Fibrosis (MI, LV hypertrophy, Chagas disease)
Tumours
Myocarditis
Sarcoidosis

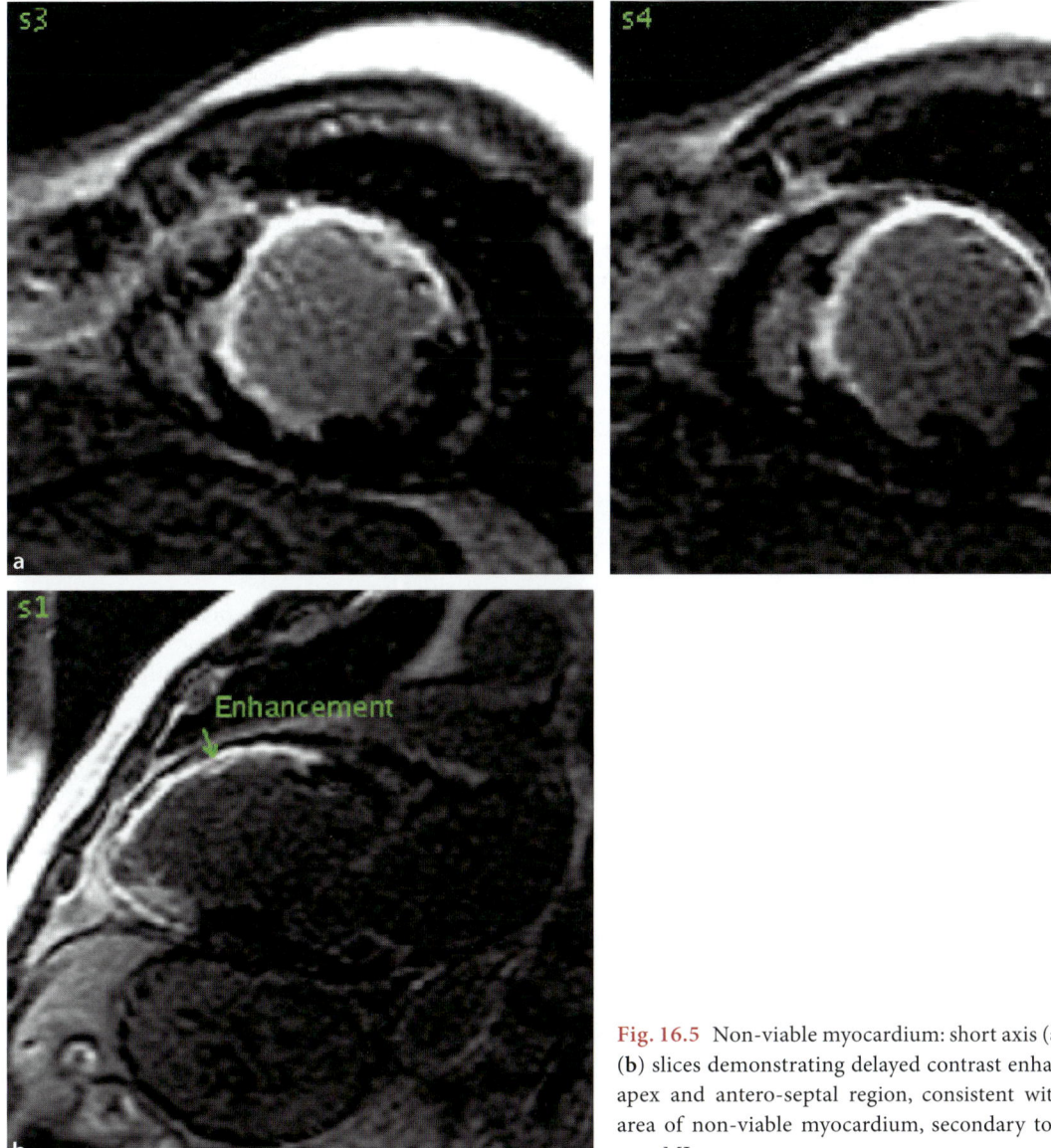

Fig. 16.5 Non-viable myocardium: short axis (**a**) and long axis (**b**) slices demonstrating delayed contrast enhancement of the apex and antero-septal region, consistent with an extensive area of non-viable myocardium, secondary to old full thickness MI

Table 16.4 Typical fast MRI protocol for myocardial viability

Long axis cine (SSFP)	: 5 minutes
First-pass contrast	
Short axis perfusion (Gad. First dose)	: 5 minutes
(Second Dose of Gad)	
Short axis cine SSFP	: 10 minutes
Delayed enhancement images	: 5 minutes

The addition of Dobutamine stress for wall motion abnormalities and perfusion cardiac MR studies appear to offer little or no additional information [22].

16.2.2
Cardiomyopathies

Cardiac MR is an excellent non-invasive imaging technique for hypertrophic cardiomyopathy [31, 32]. It is helpful to identify the degree of sub-aortic obstruction being caused by systolic anterior motion of the mitral leaflet, calculating LV mass, assessing diastolic function and demonstrating speckled delayed enhancement in septum and apex associated with hypertrophic cardiomyopathy (Fig. 16.6a–c). The sub-aortic obstruction can be relieved by percutaneous transluminal septal ablation using ethanol. Delayed enhancement imaging and cine sequences are helpful to document success of the ablation therapy [33, 34].

Cardiac MR imaging also has the ability to differentiate restrictive cardiomyopathy from constrictive pericarditis. Constrictive pericarditis has usually pericardial thickening of more than 4 mm, with the presence of pericardial calcifications at times, not present in the case of restrictive cardiomyopathy [35, 36].

16.2.3
Arrhythmogenic Right Ventricular Dysplasia

Arrhythmogenic right ventricular dysplasia (ARVD) is an autosomal dominant type of cardiomyopathy and normally affects young adults between the ages of 20 and 40 years. Partial or total thinning with fibro-fatty infiltration of the right ventricular free wall are typical characteristics of the disease. The symptoms mostly occur during exercise, causing sudden death [37, 38]. Due to excellent soft-tissue contrast and the ability to depict morphology and function, cardiac MRI may identify some of the major/minor criteria in many patients, successfully establishing diagnosis of ARVD.

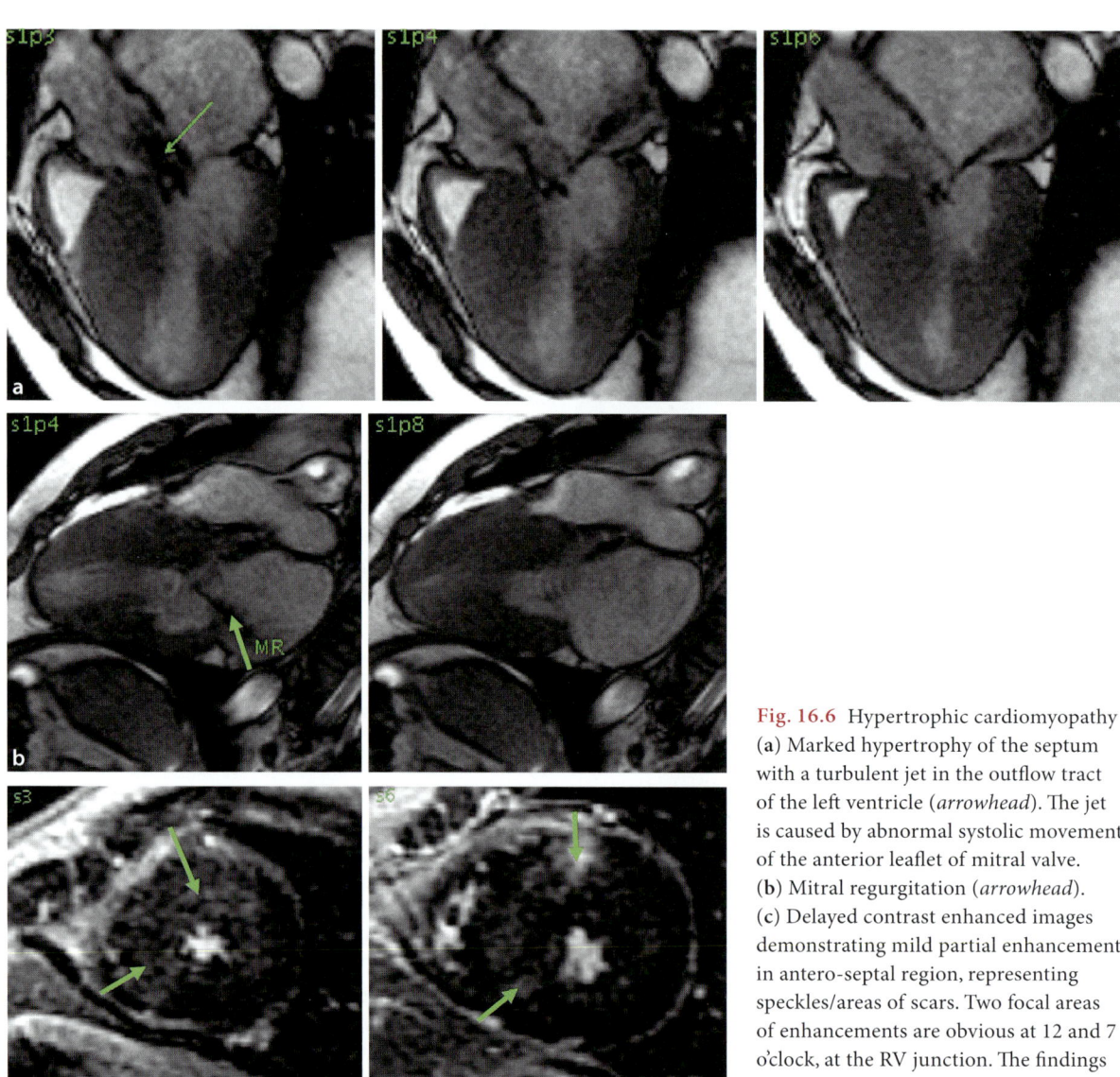

Fig. 16.6 Hypertrophic cardiomyopathy (a) Marked hypertrophy of the septum with a turbulent jet in the outflow tract of the left ventricle (*arrowhead*). The jet is caused by abnormal systolic movement of the anterior leaflet of mitral valve. (b) Mitral regurgitation (*arrowhead*). (c) Delayed contrast enhanced images demonstrating mild partial enhancement in antero-septal region, representing speckles/areas of scars. Two focal areas of enhancements are obvious at 12 and 7 o'clock, at the RV junction. The findings are consistent with idiopathic hypertrophic obstructive cardiomyopathy

In order to evaluate right-ventricle morphology, black-blood, double inversion recovery, fast spin echo sequences are used. Steady-state free precession cine images are used for the evaluation of function. It is important to give particular attention to the RV free wall, RV apex, inflow, and outflow tracts. In normal subjects, there is always a clear line of demarcation between the epicardial fat and the right ventricular myocardium. Disruption of this line would be suggestive of fatty infiltration. Thinning of the right ventricular wall is difficult to detect due to artefacts and the intrinsic limitations of spatial resolution [39, 40]. Other characteristic morphological features easy to identify on MRI are RV and RA dilatations, scalloping of the RV free wall, and prominent trabeculations, dyskinesia, RV free-wall systolic bulging and aneurysms. Dyskinesia limiting to the right ventricular outflow tract only is suggestive of RVOT tachycardia, and not of ARVD [41].

16.2.4
Myocarditis

Contrast cardiac MR is a valuable tool for the evaluation and monitoring of inflammatory heart disease [42]. In a given clinical setting, contrast enhancement is a frequent finding of suspected myocarditis and is associated with active inflammation defined by histopathology (Fig. 16.7) [43]. Myocarditis occurs predominantly in the lateral free wall. T2 images, although not of excellent quality, may demonstrate oedema in the myocardium [39]. Therefore, serial cardiac MR imaging appears to be an excellent non-invasive test to define the course of disease and to assess the effect of therapy in acute myocarditis [44, 45].

16.3
Conclusions

Magnetic resonance (MR) imaging, with its already established role in complex congenital heart disease, is also gradually emerging as one of the noninvasive tests of choice for many cardiovascular disorders in adults. It has good capability for assessing perfusion, LV remodelling, and myocardial viability. However, more clinical studies are required to establish its role in prognosis and risk stratification in patients with coronary artery disease. Despite the advantage of lack of non-ionizing radiation, Coronary MR angiography has yet to achieve a reasonable level of acceptance in clinical, compared to Coronary CT angiography. With advancement of MR technology, newer therapeutic applications, including MR compatible catheters for electrophysiological and interventional procedures are likely to become available in the near future.

MR has entered an era of molecular imaging, with anticipated capabilities of imaging at molecular levels for the detection of vulnerable plaque, apoptosis, angiogenesis and stem cell transplantation, thereby refining management of cardiovascular diseases in the years ahead.

References

1. Boxt LM (1996) MR imaging of congenital heart disease. Magn Reson Imaging Clin N Am 4:327–359.
2. Ho VB, Kinney JB, Sahn DJ (1996) Contribution of newer MR imaging strategies for congenital heart disease. Radiographics 16:43–60.
3. Brickner ME, Hillis LD, Lange RA (2000) Congenital heart disease in adults. N Engl J Med 342:256-63.
4. Fogel MA, Hubbard A, Weinberg PM (2001) Simplified approach for assessment of intracardiac baffles and extracardiac conduits in congenital heart survey with two- and three-dimensional magnetic resonance imaging. Am Heart J 142:1028–36.
5. Bloch F (1946) Nuclear induction. Phys Rev 70:460-473.
6. Purcell E, Torrey H, Pound R (1946) Resonance absorption by nuclear magnetic moments in a solid. Phys Rev 69:37–38.
7. Garroway A, Grannell P, Mansfield P (1974) Image formation in NMR by a selective irradiative pulse. J Phys C: Solid State Phys 7:L457–L462.
8. Lauterbur L (1973) Image formation by induced local interactions: examples employing nuclear magnetic resonance. Nature 242:190–191.

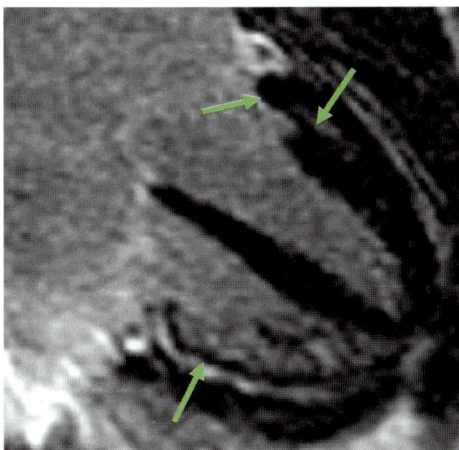

Fig. 16.7 Myocarditis: linear area of delayed contrast enhancement in a 27-year-old young male, compatible with myocarditis

9. Moore CC, O'Dell WG, Mcweight ER et al. (1992) Calculation of three-dimensional left ventricular strains from biplanar tagged images. J Magn Reson Imaging 2:165–75.
10. O'Dell WG, Moore CC, Hunter WC et al. (1995) Three-dimensional myocardial deformations: calculation with displacement field fitting to tagged MR images. Radiology 195:829–35.
11. Engel HJ, Torres C, Page HJL (1975) Major variations in anatomical origin of the coronary arteries: angiographic observations in 4250 patients without associated congenital heart disease. Catheterization Cardiovas Diagn 1:157–69.
12. McConnell MV, Ganz P, Sewyn AP et al. (1995) Identification of the anomalous coronary arteries and their anatomic course by magnetic resonance angiography. Circulation 92:3158–62.
13. Post JC, Van Rossum AC, Bronzwaer JG et al. (1995) Magnetic resonance angiography of anomalous coronary arteries. A new gold standard for delineating the proximal course? Circulation 92:3163–3171.
14. Greil GF, Stuber M, Botnar RM et al. (2002) Coronary magnetic resonance angiography in adolescents and young adults with Kawasaki disease. Circulation 105:908–911.
15. Vrachliotis TG, Bis KG, Aliabadi D et al. (1997) Contrast enhanced breath hold MR angiography for evaluating patency of coronary artery bypass grafts. Am J Roentgenol 168:1073–1080.
16. Wintersperger BJ, Engelmann MG, Von Smekal A et al. (1998) Patency of coronary bypass grafts: assessment with breath hold contrast enhanced MR angiography—value of a non-electrocardiographically triggered technique. Radiology 208:345–351.
17. Dulce MC, Mostbeck GH, Friese KK et al. (1993) Quantifications of left ventricular volumes and function with cine MR imaging: comparison of geometrical models with three-dimentional data. Radiology 188:371–376.
18. Chuang ML, Hibberd MG, Salton CJ et al. (2000) Importance of imaging method over imaging modality in noninvasive determination of left ventricular volumes and ejection fraction: assessment by two and three dimensional echocardiography and magnetic resonance imaging. J Am Coll Cardiol 35:477–484.
19. Matheijssen NA, Baur LH, Reiber JH et al. (1996) Assessment of the left ventricular volume and mass by cine magnetic resonance imaging in patient with anterior myocardial infarction: intraobserver and interobserver variability on contour detection. Int J Card Imaging 12:11–19.
20. Niwa K, Uchishiba M, Aotsuka H et al. (1996) Measurements of ventricular volumes by cine magnetic resonance imaging in complex congenital heart disease with morphologically abnormal ventricles. Am Heart J 131:567–575.
21. Zerhouni EA, Parish DM, Rogers WJ et al. (1988) Human heart: tagging with MR imaging – a method for noninvasive assessment of myocardial motion. Radiology 169:59–63.
22. Klein C, Nekolla SG, Bengel FM et al. (2002) Assessment of myocardial viability with contrast enhanced magnetic resonance imaging: comparison with positron emission tomography. Circulation 105:162–167.
23. Kim RJ, Fieno DS, Parrish TB et al. (1999) Relationship of MRI delayed contrast enhancement to irreversible injury, infarct age, and contractile function. Circulation 100(19):1992–2002.
24. Schelberd HR (2002) F-18 deoxyglucose and the assessment of myocardial viability. Semin Nucl Med 32:60-69.
25. Stillman AE, Wilke N, Jerosch-Herold M (1999) Myocardial viability. Radiol Clin North Am 37:361–378.
26. Lauerma K, Niemi P, Hanninen H et al. (2000) Multimodality MR imaging assessment of the myocardial viability: combination first pass and late contrast enhancement to wall motions dynamics and comparison with FDG-PET: initial experience. Radiology 217:729–736.
27. Simonetti OP, Kim RJ, Fieno DS et al. (2001) An improved MR imaging tecnique for the visualization of the myocardial infarction. Radiology 218:215–233.
28. Earls JP, Ho VB, Foo TK et al. (2002) Cardiac MRI: recent progress and continued challenges. J Magn Reson Imaging 16:111–127.
29. Lee VS, Resnick D, Tiu SS et al. (2004) MR imaging evaluation of myocardial viability in the setting of equivocal SPECT results with Tc-99m sestamibi. Radiology 30:191–197.
30. VanHoe L, Vanderheyden M (2004) Ischemic cardiomyopathy: value of different MRI techniques for prediction of functional recovery after revascularization. Am J Roentgenol 182:95–100.
31. Devlin AM, Moore MR, Ostman-Smith I et al. (1999) A comparison of the MRI and echocardiography in hypertrophic cardiomyopathy. Br J Radiol 72:258–264.
32. Pons-Llodo G, Carreras F, Borras X et al. (1997) Comparison of morphologic assessment of hypertrophic cardiomyopathy by magnetic resonance versus echocardiographic imaging. Am J Cardiol 79:1651–1656.
33. Schulz-Menger J, Strohm O, Waigand J et al. (2000) The value of magnetic resonance imaging of the left ventricular outflow tract in patient with hypertrophic obstructive cardiomyopathy after septal artery embolizations. Circulation 101:1764–1766.
34. Van Dockum WG, ten Cate FJ, ten Berg JM et al. (2004) Myocardial infarction after percutaneous transluminal septal myocardial ablation in hypertrophic obstructive cardiomyopathy: evaluation by contrast-enhanced magnetic resonance imaging. J Am Coll Cardiol 43:27–34.
35. Masui T, Finck S, Higgins CB (1992) Constructive pericarditis and restrictive cardiomyopathy: evaluation with MR imaging. Radiology 182:369–373.

36. Sechtem U, Higgins CB, Sommerhoff BA et al. (1987) Magnetic resonance imaging of restrictive cardiomyopathy. Am J Cardiol 59:480–482.
37. Thiene G, Nava A, Corrado D et al. (1988) Right ventricular cardiomyopathy and sudden death in young people. N Engl J Med 318:129–133.
38. Fontain G, Fontaliran F, Hebert JL et al. (1999) Arrhythmogenic right ventricular dysplasia. Annu Rev Med 50:17–35.
39. Blake L, Scheinman B, Higgins C (1994) MR features of arrhythmogenic right ventricular dysplasia. AJR Am J Roentgenol 162:809–812.
40. Burke AP, Fabr A, Tashko G et al. (1998) Arrhythmogenic right ventricular cardiomyopathy and fatty replacement of the right ventricular myocardium: are they different diseases? Circulation 97:1571–1580.
41. Carlson M, White R, Throhman R et al. (1994) Right ventricular outflow tract ventricular tachycardia: detection of previously unrecognized anatomic abnormalities using cine magnetic resonance imaging. J Am Coll Cardiol 24:720–727.
42. Laissy JP, Hyafil F, Feldman JL et al. (2005) Differentiating acute myocardial infarction from myocarditis: diagnostic value of early- and delayed-perfusion cardiac MR imaging. Radiology 237:75–82.
43. Mahrholdt H, Goedecke C, Wagner A et al. (2004) Cardiovascular magnetic resonance assessment of human myocarditis. A comparison to histology and molecular pathology. Circulation 109:1250–1258.
44. Friedrich M, Strohm O, Schulz-Menger J et al. (1998) Contrast media-enhanced magnetic resonance imaging visualizes myocardial changes in the course of viral myocarditis. Circulation 97:1802–1809.
45. Martin NT, Groenning AB, Dargie JH (2006) Diagnosing acute myocarditis using cardiac MRI. Eur Heart J 27(4):468.

Part III Nuclear Cardiology

Principles of Myocardial SPECT Imaging

Kathryn Adamson

Contents

17.1	Introduction	191
17.2	The Ideal Perfusion Tracer	191
17.3	Imaging Protocol	192
17.3.1	Stress and Rest Tests	192
17.3.2	Planar or SPECT MPI?	193
17.4	Imaging Systems	193
17.4.1	The Gamma Camera	193
17.4.2	Collimators	194
17.5	Image Quality	196
17.6	Data Acquisition	197
17.6.1	Matrix and Pixel Size	198
17.6.2	Orbit	198
17.6.3	Number of Projections	199
17.6.4	Acquisition Time	199
17.7	SPECT Reconstruction, Image Reorientation and Interpretation	199
17.7.1	Filtered Back Projection	199
17.7.2	Iterative Reconstruction	201
17.7.3	Image Reorientation	202
17.7.4	Interpretation	203
17.8	Other Factors Affecting MPI SPECT Images	203
17.8.1	Hepatobiliary Clearance and Gut Uptake	203
17.8.2	Photon Attenuation	203
17.8.3	Variable Resolution	205
17.8.4	Patient Motion	205
17.9	Quality Control	205
17.9.1	Uniformity of Response	205
17.9.2	Centre of Rotation	206
17.9.3	SPECT Performance	206
17.10	Recent Advances	206
17.10.1	Gated MPI SPECT	206
17.10.2	Non-Uniform Attenuation Correction (NUAC) in SPECT	207
17.11	Future Developments	209
17.12	Conclusions	209
	References	210

17.1 Introduction

The most widely used nuclear cardiology procedure is myocardial perfusion imaging (MPI) using single photon emission computed tomography (SPECT). It is a non-invasive imaging modality routinely used in the diagnosis of and for assessing the prognosis of coronary artery disease and heart muscle damage following an infarction. MPI SPECT images provide a visual three-dimensional image of the perfused myocardium for assessment. In addition, if the MPI SPECT studies are gated to the electrocardiogram (ECG) it is possible to make a functional assessment of the perfusion images.

The clinical success of MPI SPECT, and gated MPI SPECT, relies on an understanding of the physics and technical aspects of SPECT imaging, as well as the technical limitations and quality assurance requirements of the system.

The aim of this chapter is to bring together the most important points of myocardial perfusion imaging, with particular emphasis on the physics of SPECT applied to MPI, together with the relevant technical and practical limitations.

17.2 The Ideal Perfusion Tracer

To perform MPI a patient is intravenously given a radiopharmaceutical or tracer (a pharmaceutical labelled with a small amount of radioactivity, which emits gamma rays). The ideal tracer would have the following desirable properties: distribute in the myocardium in linear proportion to blood flow; efficient myocardial extraction from the blood on the first pass through the heart; stable retention within the myocardium during the scan but also rapid elimination allowing repeat studies under different conditions; be readily available; and have good imaging characteristics, e.g., emit gamma rays with energy of 100 to 200 keV [1]. Unfortunately, no tracer has all these properties, and compromises must be made.

The radiopharmaceuticals most commonly used for MPI are ^{201}Tl thallous chloride, ^{99m}Tc sestamibi or ^{99m}Tc tetrofosmin. The use of the former gold standard ^{201}Tl has decreased in favour of the ^{99m}Tc labelled radiopharmaceuticals. This is because the ^{99m}Tc radiopharmaceuticals produce higher quality images due to the higher energy photons produced and with a shorter half life than ^{201}Tl, which in turn allows larger amounts of radiopharmaceutical to be administered with a lower radiation dose to the patient (Table 17.1). Further advantages of ^{99m}Tc sestamibi or tetrofosmin are that imaging can be delayed for a short while after injection and scans can also be repeated without loss of sensitivity.

17.3 Imaging Protocol

17.3.1 Stress and Rest Tests

MPI scans are acquired under resting and stressing conditions, and comparison of the stress and rest images allows relative myocardial perfusion to be assessed. The stress condition can be induced either physically by performing an exercise task, or pharmacologically by intravenous injection of a vasoactive drug to the patient, e.g., adenosine, dipyridamole or dobutamine. This pharmacological stress makes it possible to test patients who are unable to achieve maximal cardiovascular stress using exercise. During periods of stress, areas of the myocardium supplied by normal healthy arteries will increase their blood supply, and therefore radiopharmaceutical delivery and uptake, more than areas of myocardium supplied by permanently or temporarily stenosed arteries.

^{201}Tl is administered at peak stress, and the patient is imaged as soon as possible after administration. To minimise the effects of redistribution the stress scan should be started within 5 minutes of the injection and should be completed within 30 minutes. Redistribution images are taken 3–4 hours after the stress images.

Unlike ^{201}Tl, ^{99m}Tc radiopharmaceuticals do not significantly redistribute, so the ^{99m}Tc tracer must be injected before both stress and rest imaging. Due to the 6 hour half life of ^{99m}Tc, if the stress and rest images are to be acquired on the same day, it is necessary to inject a larger amount (typically three to five times larger) of ^{99m}Tc sestamibi or ^{99m}Tc tetrofosmin in the second injection, in order to swamp activity from the first injection. In such a 1 day protocol, the rest study is normally performed before the stress.

Table 17.1 Characteristics of common perfusion agents [1]

Property	^{201}Tl	^{99m}Tc sestamibi	^{99m}Tc tetrofosmin
Photopeak energy (keV)	80, 167	140	140
Energy window (%)	20	20	20
Physical half life (hours)	73	6.02	6.02
Number of injections	1	2	2
Typical administered activity (MBq)	80	250 + 750 (1 day) 400 + 400 (2 day)	250 + 750 (1 day) 400 + 400 (2 day)
Effective dose (mSv)*	18	7.6 (1 day) 6.2 (2 day)	6.2 (1 day) 5.1 (2 day)
Initial myocardial uptake (%)	4	1.5	1.2
Extraction fraction (%)	85	65	54
Uptake relation to flow increase	Good	Adequate	Adequate
Redistribution	Yes	Minimal	No
Gated ventricular function	No	Yes	Yes
Excretion	Kidney	Gut	Gut and kidney

* Calculated using μSv/MBq factors outlined in the 2004 European Association of Nuclear Medicine (EANM) publication "Myocardial Perfusion Imaging, A Technologist Guide"

17.3.2
Planar or SPECT MPI?

Conventional planar imaging portrays a 3D distribution of radioactivity as a 2D image. Structures at any one depth in the patient are obscured by superimposition of overlying and underlying structures, which results in a loss of contrast (Fig. 17.1).

SPECT (tomography) imaging produces full 3D images and has several advantages over planar imaging (Table 17.2). In particular, tomography allows separation of target regions from overlying structures, and therefore gives improved diagnostic results over planar imaging. By performing MPI SPECT, it is possible to create a 3D volume representation of the perfused myocardium. By selecting appropriate planes through the myocardium, the cardiac shape can be assessed, together with regional and global perfusion patterns.

The sensitivity of CAD detection has been shown to be far superior with SPECT (93%) than with planar imaging (77%) [1]. Specificity is also improved in SPECT compared with planar imaging (88% and 82%, respectively). SPECT is, however, a much more complex technique, and there is scope for more image artefacts to appear during the image acquisition and subsequent image processing. However, by paying strict attention to detail throughout the whole imaging procedure (acquisition and processing) and by regularly performing quality control tests on the gamma camera, the chance of these image artefacts appearing is much reduced.

17.4
Imaging Systems

17.4.1
The Gamma Camera

MPI SPECT scans are acquired using a gamma camera. There are a number of different camera–detector configurations that are commercially available for MPI SPECT (Fig. 17.2), and the principal components of a gamma camera are shown in Fig. 17.3. The gamma camera consists of a large, relatively thin (9–25 mm) sodium iodide scintillation crystal that is doped with a small amount (~0.7%) of thallium to form NaI(Tl). NaI(Tl) has a density of 3.67 g/cm³ and a moderate response time of 230 nanoseconds. The crystal is optically coupled to an array of photomultipler tubes, which detect light, and are used to measure the position and energy of the incident photon.

A patient is injected with a radiopharmaceutical, which emits gamma rays in all directions, eventually escaping from the patient. Some of these gamma rays pass through the collimator and enter the gamma camera detector where they strike the NaI(Tl) scintillation crystal and are converted to flashes of light (burst of light

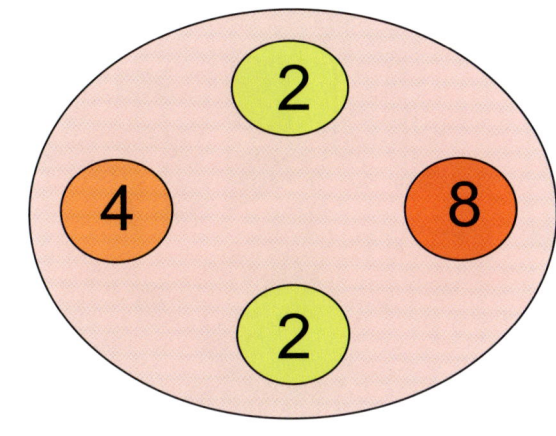
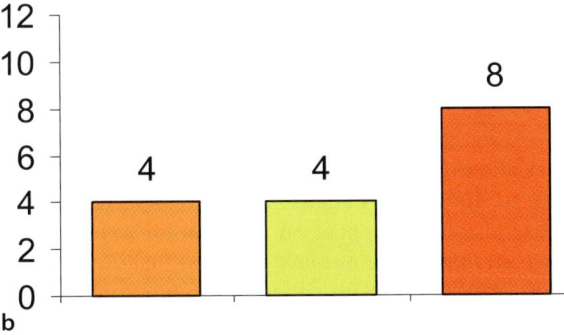

Fig. 17.1a,b In planar imaging the relative apparent contrast between areas with differing uptake of radioactivity is generally lower than the true value due to overlying and underlying tissues, which may also contain radioactivity. a Object containing localised areas of differing amounts of radioactivity. b Relative apparent contrast in 2D image

Table 17.2 Advantages of SPECT over planar MPI [1]

Property
Improved resolution
Ability to differentiate overlying and underlying tissues
Improved sensitivity and specificity of diagnosis
Ability to reconstruct images in same orientation irrespective of cardiac position
Ability to reconstruct images in a format comparable with other cardiological images

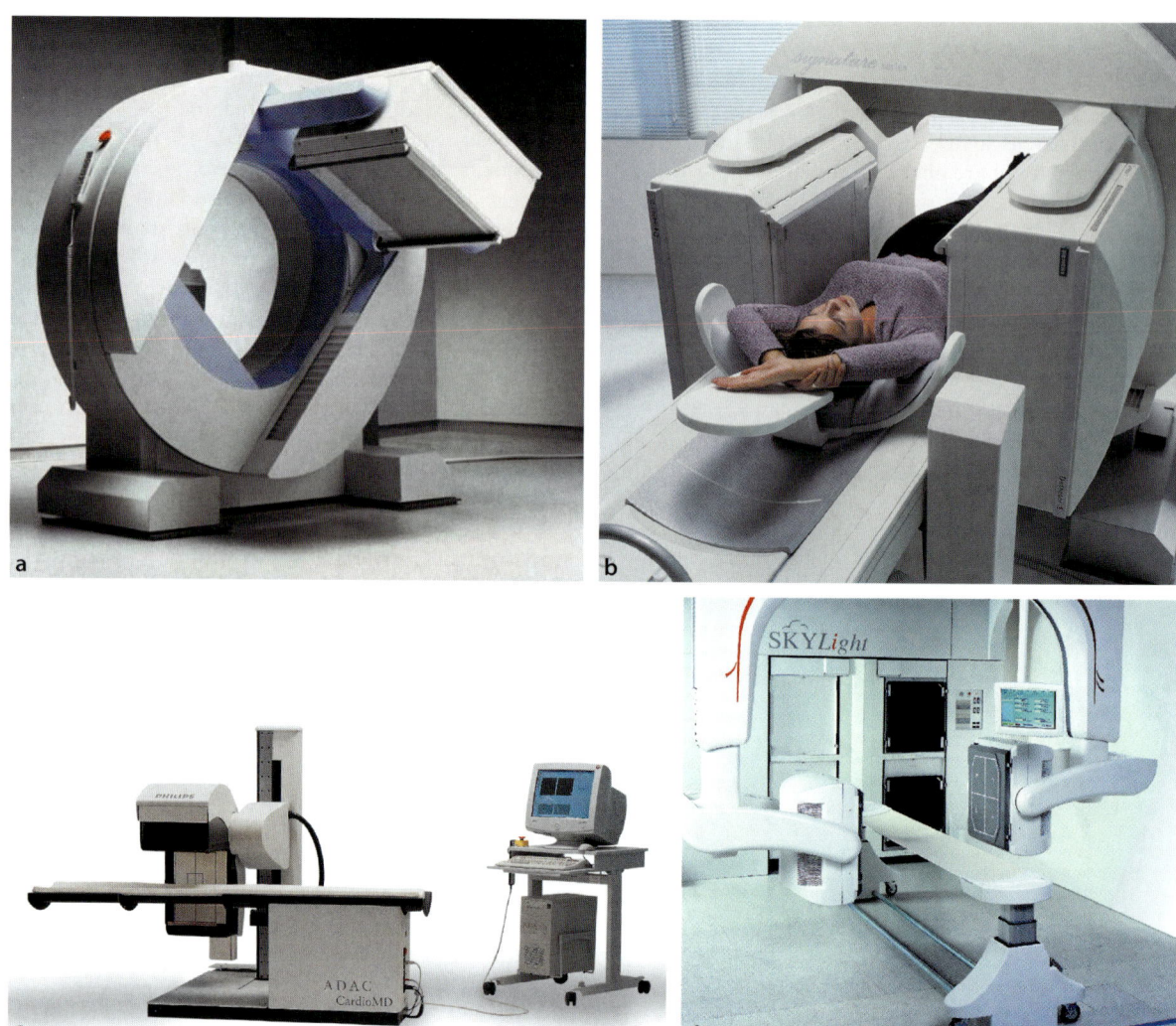

Fig. 17.2a–d Commercially available gamma cameras. a, b Photos courtesy of Siemens Medical Systems. c, d Photos courtesy of Philips Medical Systems

photons). The light photons are then viewed by all of the photomultiplier tubes (PMTs), some to a greater extent than others, depending on their proximity to the point of interaction between the gamma ray and scintillation crystal. By measuring the amount of light detected by each PMT the event can be localised to a relatively high degree of accuracy. The amount of light detected by the array of PMTs is transformed into three electronic signals (called X, Y and Z). The X and Y signals represent the spatial location of where the gamma ray hit the crystal. The Z signal represents the gamma ray energy deposited in the crystal, and is passed through a pulse height analyser to determine if it is within the range of values expected for the specific radiopharmaceutical used. If the Z signal is acceptable, then the X and Y signals are easily digitised for interfacing with a computer, and a dot is displayed at that given location on the monitor. Thousands of gamma rays are detected, and so thousands of dots appear on the monitor to eventually create an image. The number of individual dots at each co-ordinate (or pixel) is called the counts in that pixel. A high number of counts within a small pixel area is termed a high count density.

17.4.2
Collimators

The gamma rays from the radiopharmaceutical are emitted from the patient in all directions and cannot be fo-

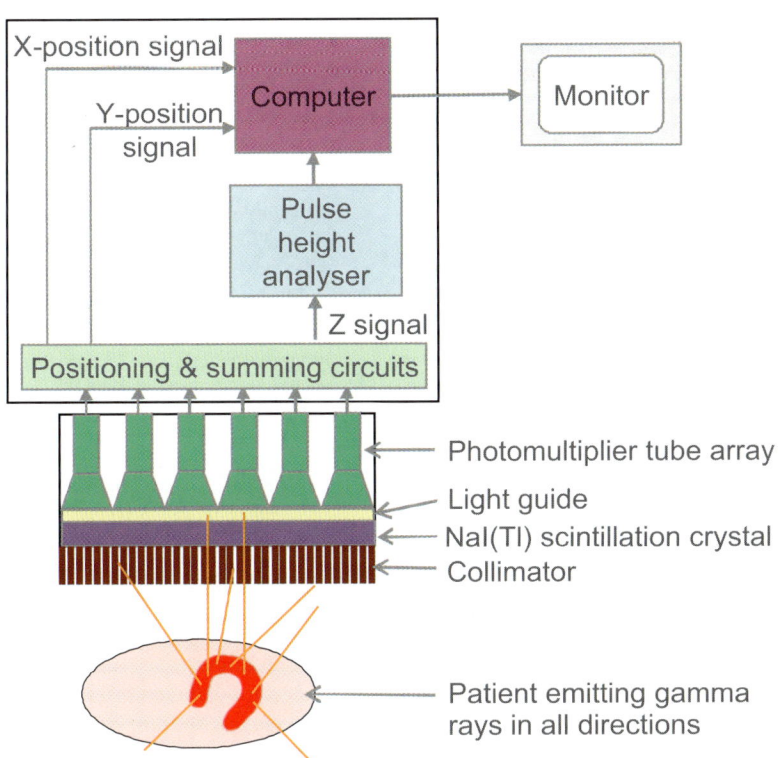

Fig. 17.3 Schematic diagram of a gamma camera

cused. A collimator is therefore used to selectively absorb or transmit gamma rays into the detector. The collimator consists of a lead plate with thousands (30 000 to 60 000) of tiny holes (0.8 to 1.5 mm diameter) through it. The lead walls between the holes are called septa. Each hole accepts gamma rays from only a limited angle, and those gamma rays not travelling in the preferred direction are absorbed by the lead septa and never reach the detector. This means that a large proportion of emitted gamma rays do not contribute to the imaging process.

Two principal parameters describing collimator performance are spatial resolution (the detail or sharpness of the image) and sensitivity (the proportion of gamma rays incident on the collimator that actually pass through to the detector). Unfortunately it is not possible to optimise both sensitivity and resolution simultaneously (Table 17.3) [2], and so collimators are designed to a particular specification, for a specific application, by varying the number of holes in the collimator, the direction of the holes, the diameter of the holes and the length of both holes and septa.

The most common type of collimators manufactured are parallel hole collimators (Fig. 17.4a), and most gamma cameras are supplied with a range of parallel hole collimators with different resolution and sensitivity properties. The septal thickness is determined by the energy of the gamma ray to be imaged, and is chosen to prevent gamma rays from crossing from one hole to the next. High resolution collimators with thin (short) septa and small holes are used for ^{99m}Tc high resolution cardiac imaging, whereas for ^{201}Tl scans, due to the low energy of the ^{201}Tl gamma rays, a low energy general purpose collimator is more appropriate. One very important characteristic of parallel hole collimators is that the field of view of the collimator is independent of the collimator to patient distance and so the detected image is always the same size as the object.

Although the parallel hole collimator is the most widely used collimator, other types of collimators have been designed for various specific applications. Converging collimators have a field of view that decreases

Table 17.3 Parallel hole collimator sensitivity versus resolution. It is not possible to optimise sensitivity and resolution simultaneously

Collimator parameter: Increase in…	Sensitivity	Resolution
Hole size	Increases	Deteriorates
Hole length	Decreases	Improves
Number of holes	Increases	No change
Septal thickness	Decreases	No change

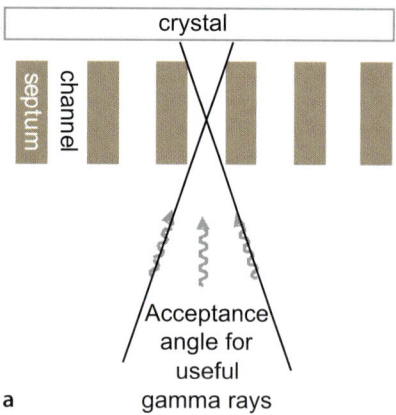
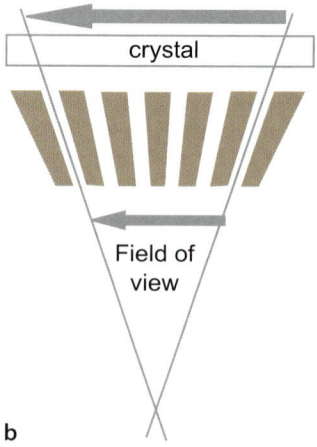

Fig. 17.4a,b Types of gamma camera collimators. **a** A parallel hole collimator is the most common collimator used. It has a field of view that is independent of the object distance from the collimator, and the image produced is always the same size as the object. **b** A converging collimator has a field of view that decreases with distance from the collimator. The image created is a magnification of the object within the field of view

with distance from the collimator (Fig. 17.4b). The image created is a magnification of the object within the field of view, but there is also some image distortion due to the fact that different planes of the object are at different distances from the collimator and are therefore magnified by different amounts. However, the collimator does provide improved spatial resolution and sensitivity with depth compared with the parallel hole collimator. Although converging collimators are rarely used now, a modification of it (the fan beam collimator) has been developed for cardiac SPECT imaging. The fan beam collimator [3] has holes in each row that converge, but the holes in each column are parallel. This means that the collimator focuses to a line rather than a point, but it still retains increased sensitivity and resolution compared with the parallel hole collimator.

17.5
Image Quality

Image quality refers to how well the acquired gamma camera image represents the object being imaged. In order for scans to be clinically useful it is necessary to have good quality scans. The quality of gamma camera images is limited by several factors relating to the properties of the radiopharmaceutical used for imaging as well as the performance of the camera. However, it is possible to characterise gamma camera image quality by summarising physical parameters that can be quantitatively measured, e.g., spatial resolution and contrast.

Spatial resolution is important when assessing spatial dimensions in the image, such as the extent of the myocardial defect, the cardiac shape or wall thickness. The spatial resolution of the image is comprised of intrinsic resolution (resolution of detector alone) and the collimator resolution. The intrinsic resolution is determined by the thickness of the scintillation crystal. Manufacturers build scintillation crystals of different thicknesses, since the optimum crystal thickness is a compromise between resolution and detection efficiency (sensitivity); as crystal thickness increases, the spatial resolution deteriorates but detection efficiency increases. The standard 3/8 inch (9.5 mm) is ideal for ^{99m}Tc imaging, whereas the slightly thicker 1/2 inch (12.7 mm) is better for higher energy isotope imaging. Thinner crystals are less sensitive, as gamma rays are more likely to penetrate the crystal without interacting. The resolution of the gamma camera is primarily limited by the geometric resolution of the collimator (Fig. 17.5), typically 6 to 9 mm at a distance of 10 cm from the collimator. The combination of intrinsic resolution and collimator resolution is often referred to as system resolution, and this is a function of a number of parameters, such as the distance from the emitting source to the collimator, the energy of the radionuclide, and the size and density of the object being imaged.

Spatial resolution is easily measured by measuring the profile across an image of a point source or thin line of radioactivity. It is measured in terms of the full width at half maximum (FWHM) counts and full width at tenth maximum (FWTM) counts (Fig. 17.6). The intrinsic resolution (FWHM) of a modern gamma camera is typically 3 to 4 mm. For clinical SPECT studies, the system spatial resolution (intrinsic plus collimator resolution) FWHM is typically 8 to 14 mm.

Image contrast refers to the differences in intensity of areas of the image representing different amounts of radioactivity. The true contrast will usually be masked by a contribution of scatter to the image. The energy resolution of the NaI(Tl) crystal is typically 10% FWHM in the energy range 0.1–1 MeV. This energy resolution pre-

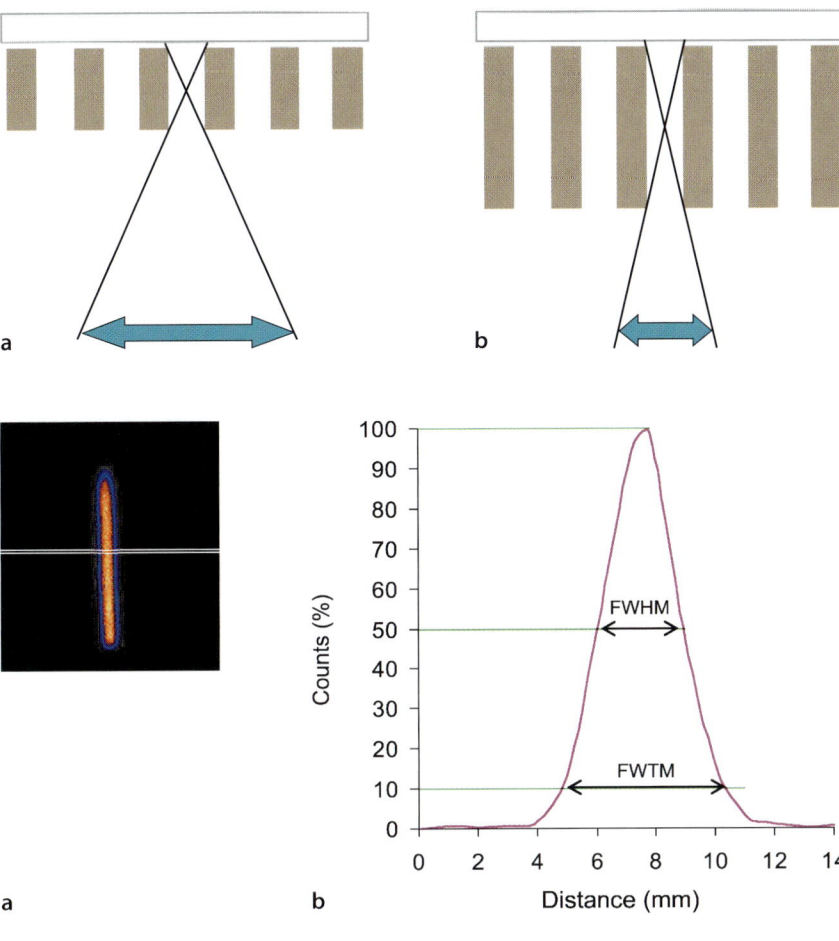

Fig. 17.5a,b Spatial resolution deteriorates with increasing distance from the collimator. It is not possible to optimise both the sensitivity and resolution of a parallel hole collimator. A general purpose collimator (**a**) has shorter bores than a high resolution collimator (**b**), leading to increased sensitivity, but a decrease in resolution

Fig. 17.6a,b An image of a line source of radioactivity (**a**) and the associated line spread function (**b**) at the position on the image shown by the white line. The line spread function (LSF) may be represented by the full width at half maximum (FWHM) and full width at tenth maximum (FWTM)

vents discriminating against photons that have undergone an interaction in the body, have been scattered and lost a small amount of energy. The resulting effect is that around 20 to 50% of all events detected by the gamma camera have been scattered within the body. This degrades the image quality by increasing the background level and therefore giving decreased contrast.

A major determining factor of image contrast is the radiopharmaceutical used, a desirable feature of which is to have a high uptake within the target organ, e.g., viable cardiac muscle, compared with the surrounding organs or tissue. MPI SPECT will increase the contrast resolution (how true contrast is represented in the image), which is advantageous in perfusion imaging since it gives improved detection of smaller or subtler perfusion defects.

Spatial resolution and contrast, as well as noise (statistical variations in counts due to random fluctuations in radioactive decay) are fundamental properties of an image, and their measurement contributes to the assessment of image quality. Unfortunately it is not possible to optimise all these physical parameters simultaneously while keeping the radiation dose to the patient at an acceptable level. An improvement in one is often made at the expense of one or more of the other parameters.

17.6
Data Acquisition

SPECT imaging requires the gamma camera to acquire 2D projection images around the patient at equally spaced angular intervals. However, in order to decrease scanning time and increase patient throughput, gamma cameras with multiple detectors are often used. Cameras with two or even three detectors allow two or three angular projections to be acquired simultaneously. This allows the image to be acquired in half or one-third of the time required for a single detector camera. Another important advance in the development of gamma cameras is the use of elliptical, rather than, circular orbits. This ensures that the detector passes as close as possible to the patient, which gives significant improvements in image spatial resolution. Factors that affect the quality of the SPECT images are the size of the acquisition matrix and pixel size, the detector orbit, the number of projections and the time spent at each projection angle [4].

17.6.1
Matrix and Pixel Size

The pixel size should be chosen to match the collimator resolution at the depth of the organ of interest, e.g., the heart. This pixel size should ideally be less than half the value of the measured FWHM of a line of radioactivity or point source. Larger pixels will result in a loss of spatial information but possibly a decrease in noise. If the pixel size is smaller than the optimum, there will be an increase in noise but no increase in spatial information. For cardiac imaging a 128 by 128 matrix is therefore typically used, giving a pixel size of approximately 2.5 mm for a 50 cm gamma camera detector.

17.6.2
Orbit

SPECT data may be acquired over 360° as a series of equally spaced angular steps around the patient. However, as the heart is positioned anteriorly in the body, the posterior views are seriously affected by gamma ray attenuation and scatter. To reduce the effects of this attenuation and scatter, the angular range used for MPI SPECT scans is generally 180°, ranging from 45° right anterior oblique to 45° left posterior oblique [5, 6]. An additional advantage of scanning over a 180° orbit is that it is possible to raise the scanning bed so that the heart is in the centre of the field of view of the camera. By doing this, the detector is closer to the body, improving the spatial resolution of the image. Furthermore, if an elliptical, rather than circular, orbit is chosen, the detector may move closer to the body, thus improving spatial resolution of the image even more (Fig. 17.7). An elliptical orbit may cause image artefacts when reconstructing the data [7], due to combining projection data with different resolution characteristics. To overcome this, a depth-dependent collimator response correction is required [8]. Elliptical orbits are required for attenuation correction methods to prevent body truncation. In order to compare both stress and rest MPI SPECT images, it is important that both the stress and rest studies are acquired with the same orbit.

Projection data can be acquired in two modes, "step and shoot" and "continuous" mode. In step and shoot mode the detector moves to a pre-selected angle and then acquires an image for a pre-selected period of time, before moving on to the next angle. This is repeated until all the projections are acquired. In continuous mode, the detector rotates at a constant speed and acquires data the

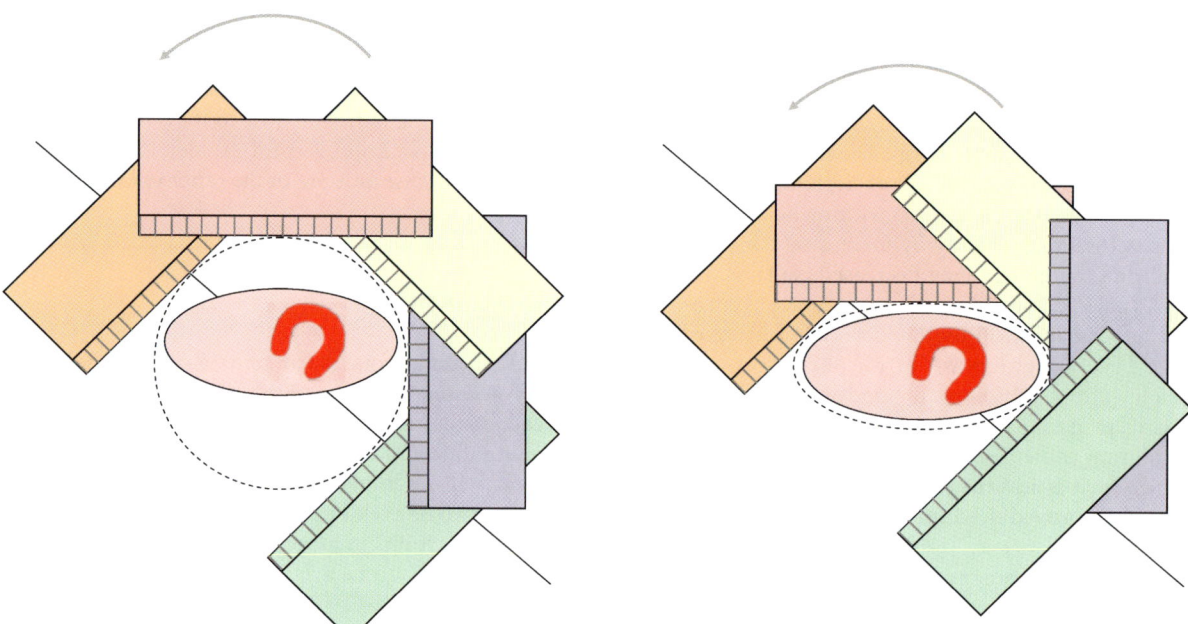

Fig. 17.7 180° circular and elliptical orbit. The elliptical orbit minimises the distance of the detector from the patient, improving the spatial resolution of the image

entire time. A continuous mode acquisition is faster than a step and shoot acquisition, but has the disadvantage of losing spatial resolution as the detector is moving during the acquisition. Although it takes longer to acquire a SPECT study in step and shoot mode, it is currently the most common method of image acquisition.

17.6.3
Number of Projections

The number of projections acquired during MPI SPECT (typically 32) affects the image quality. More projections will improve the image quality, but will also increase the acquisition time. The acquisition time is often constrained by patient comfort and so more projections can only be accommodated by reducing the time per projection. This will reduce the count density and increase the noise content per projection, reducing the overall image quality. Image noise can be reduced by more filtering during the image reconstruction process, but only at the expense of decreasing the spatial resolution.

17.6.4
Acquisition Time

The acquisition time for a study is determined by considering the need for having adequate counts in the image, and the ability of the patient to remain comfortable and still throughout the scan. The amount of ^{99m}Tc that can be administered to a patient with sestamibi or tetrofosmin is much greater than that allowed for ^{201}Tl thallous chloride [9]. This means that it is possible to have shorter acquisition times for the ^{99m}Tc perfusion studies and still produce high count densities in the images. The length of time it takes to acquire a ^{99m}Tc MPI SPECT scan will vary due to the type and age of the gamma camera, and the number of detectors. However, for a modern dual headed gamma camera, the scan should take approximately 15 to 20 minutes to perform. Acquisition times longer than 20 to 30 minutes can be counterproductive as the patient is likely to move during the scan.

17.7
SPECT Reconstruction, Image Reorientation and Interpretation

The projection data needs to be reconstructed to create a set of 2D images, which represent cross-sectional slices through the patient. This reconstruction process can be approached in two ways, either using filtered back projection (FBP) or an iterative algorithm [3, 10]. FBP is the most widely used method, however, iterative reconstruction is often used when implementing non-uniform attenuation correction methods.

17.7.1
Filtered Back Projection

FBP is a two-step process consisting of filtering of the data and backprojection. During the FBP process, the projection data are spread back along a line through the image space ("back-projected") at an angle corresponding to the angle of the acquired projection. The data from each back projection are added and interpolated on the image matrix, and a crude image of the object is formed (Fig. 17.8). After doing this from a large number of angles, the areas of the object with the highest count rate have the most counts, but unfortunately areas of the object without any activity will also be represented by some counts in the image.

Regions of high uptake of radiopharmaceutical show up well on the image, but the image is blurred with an obvious star-like artefact. This artefact can be reduced by increasing the number of projection angles and the number of data samples along the projection profile. However, even with an infinite number of projections the image will still be blurred. With no noise in the image, this blurring could be completely corrected, but it is never possible to create an image without noise and this will always limit the accuracy of reconstruction. These are problems that are fundamental to SPECT, but filtering the projections before performing back projection (filtered back projection) will reduce the noise and therefore improve the ability to correct the data without introducing further artefacts.

Images are filtered to suppress image noise while preserving, and possibly enhancing, useful image information. Improper filtering can lead to a poor quality image that could ultimately be incorrectly reported by the physician. The design and use of filters is best appreciated in terms of the mathematical "frequency space", as opposed to "real" space [2]. In frequency space it is possible to describe an image in terms of its spatial frequencies. Lower spatial frequencies are associated with larger structures and higher spatial frequencies represent smaller detail. A very blurred image contains only low spatial frequencies. Noise is constant at all frequencies, but generally predominates at the high spatial frequencies in the image.

FBP blurs images by increasingly suppressing higher and higher spatial frequencies. This can be corrected by amplification of frequencies in proportion to the value of each frequency. Such a correction looks like a ramp in frequency space and is therefore called a ramp filter. Clinical data contains noise as well as a true signal. Noise is usually constant at all frequencies, but at fre-

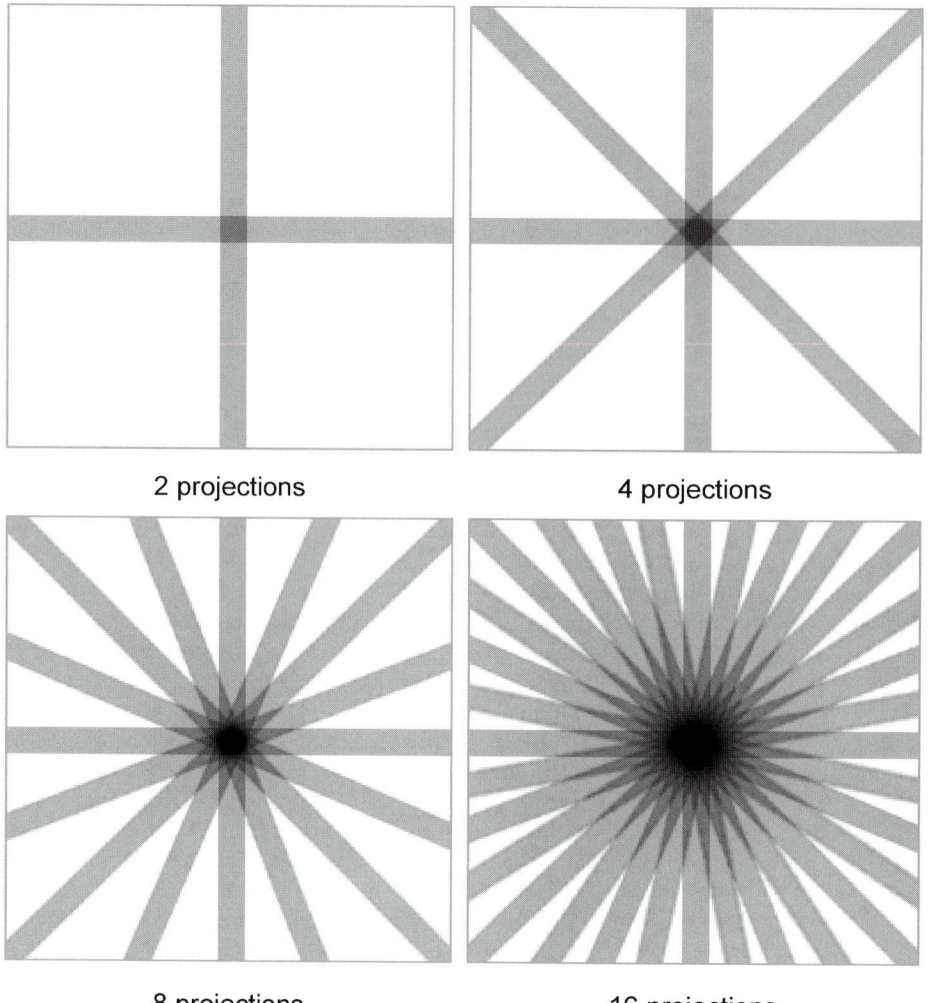

Fig. 17.8 Diagram showing filtered back projection of a point source. Data projections of the point source are spread back through the image space. The resulting image is blurred and has a star-like artefact. In practice back projection is not carried out over 360°. If projections have been acquired over 360°, it is usual to average opposite projections, and then back project only over 180°. If projection data has only been acquired over 180°, as is often the case for MPI SPECT, then back-projection is performed without averaging

quencies above the resolution of the system there is only noise and no true signal. A simple ramp filter on clinical data would therefore increasingly amplify noise at higher frequencies creating artefacts and a poor quality image. To avoid excessive amplification of this noise, the ramp filter function is "rolled off" to zero above a chosen frequency, the "cut-off frequency". The exact shape of this roll off can be altered, as represented by many filter functions (Hanning, Shepp-Logan, Butterworth, Hamming, etc.) and the point (and for some filters the rate) where "roll-off" occurs, are parameters that may be varied (Fig. 17.9a). The values chosen depend on the system resolution, the required image resolution and the count density in the reconstructed image. The same projection data can be used to produce vastly different tomographic images depending on the filter used (Fig. 17.9b). For MPI SPECT scans, a Butterworth filter is generally applied to the raw projection data and then a ramp filter is applied during the back projection reconstruction of the 2D cross-sectional slice data.

The optimum filter preserves spatial resolution with the least amount of noise in the image, and is determined by the count density in the area of interest, e.g. myocardium in MPI SPECT. As ^{201}Tl studies generally have fewer counts than ^{99m}Tc images, they require a smoother filter, with a lower cut-off frequency.

It is often difficult to determine the optimum filter, and it is usually established for each application on phantom and patient studies. For MPI SPECT, significant ischaemia or infarction is demonstrated by a few large defects in the images. Small defects are not usually seen since constant heart motion during the acquisition will blur them, rendering them unnoticeable. If multiple small irregularities are seen on the reconstructed image, then the filter is too sharp (i.e. has a high cut-off frequency) allowing too much noise in the image. Conversely, it is possible to over-smooth the image, which may be more difficult to detect. An adequately smoothed image should show just a slight irregularity at the edge of the myocardium, caused by the FBP star artefact. All studies of the same type should be reconstructed using the same filters and filter parameters to ensure that all the images have consistent levels of noise and resolution. This will then allow for consistent reporting of the images, and also give the reporting physician confidence in determining if any perceived defect is real.

The advantage of reconstructing SPECT data using FBP is that it is computationally efficient, and data can be reconstructed within seconds. The disadvantages are that due to statistical noise, attenuation, and scattering, the projection data are inconsistent with respect to each other, and if this is not corrected for prior to reconstruction it will cause artefacts in the reconstructed image. However, it is not possible to build into the reconstruction process any models of the data acquisition process which affect the final reconstruction. For these reasons FBP may be considered a simplistic approach to reconstructing an image from projection data.

17.7.2 Iterative Reconstruction

Iterative reconstruction techniques provide a more accurate representation of the radiopharmaceutical distribution in the patient than FBP. This is because iterative reconstruction more accurately compensates for physical sources of error, such as noise, scatter and collimator blurring.

The iterative reconstruction process works by creating the final image by successive approximations or estimates. An initial estimate of the image is often very simple, e.g., a blank or uniform image. The projection data for this estimate is then calculated using a tech-

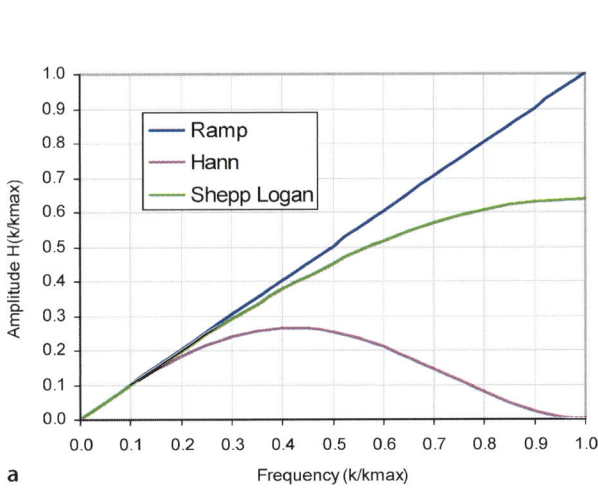
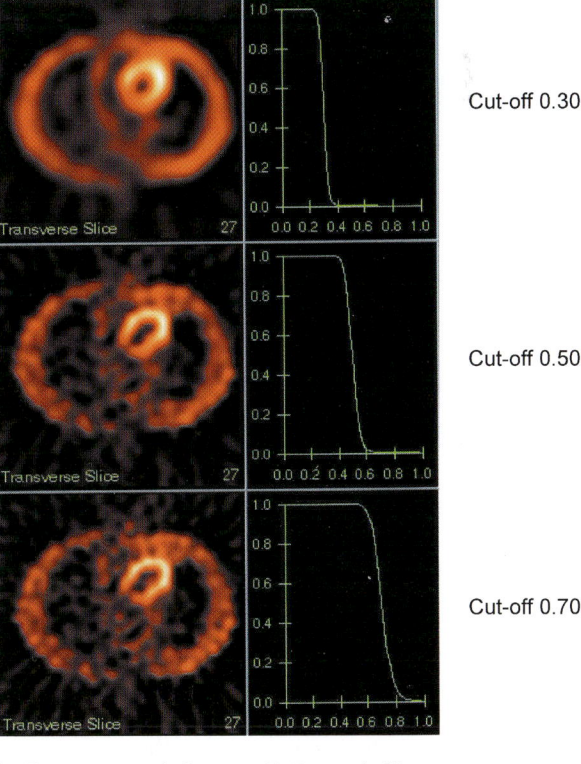

Fig. 17.9a,b a Ramp filter response, compared with two other reconstruction filters (Hann and Shepp Logan) that roll off gradually at higher frequencies minimising artefacts and noise amplification caused by the sharp cut-off of the ramp filter at maximum frequency $k$max. All filters have the same response at lower frequencies, and cut-off frequencies are set so that cut-off frequency $k$cut-off = $k$max. b 2D cross-sectional slice through the myocardium reconstructed with a Butterworth filter. Different cut-off values smooth the image by different amounts

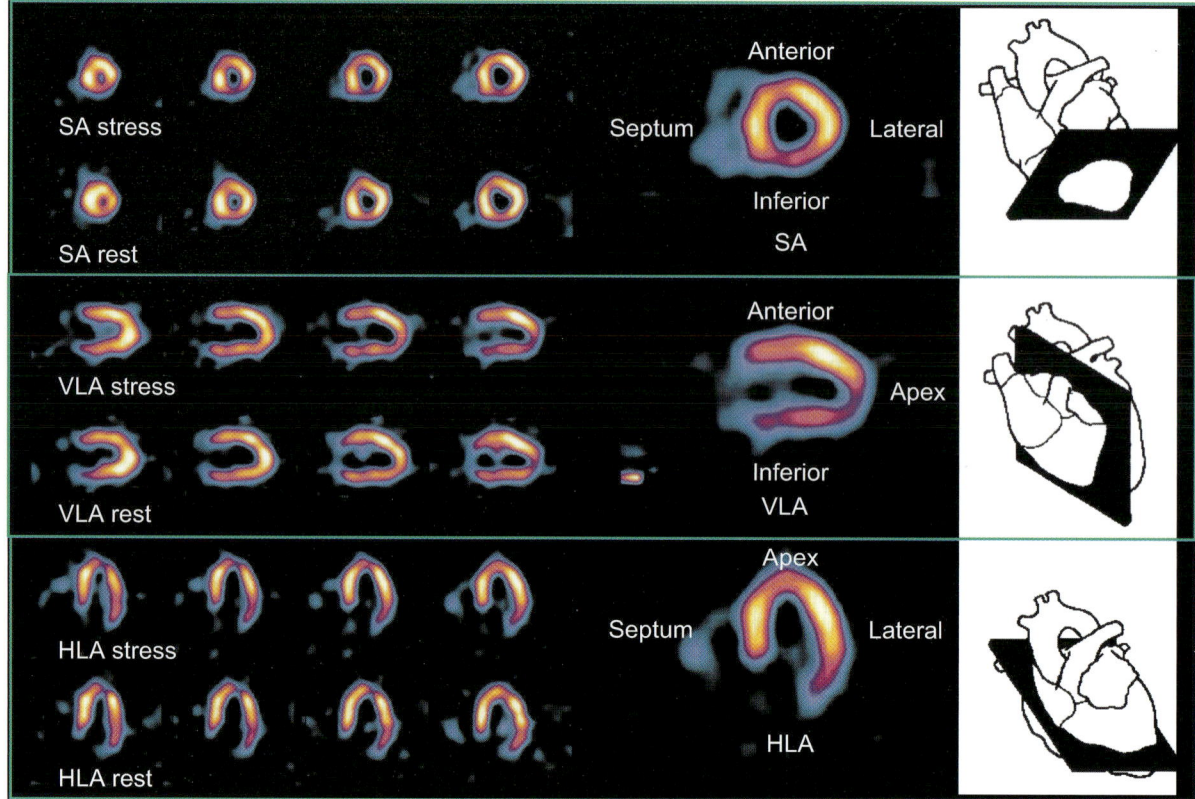

Fig. 17.10 Standard tomographic heart slices, orientated at 90° angles to each other. SA: short axis image is perpendicular to the long axis of the left ventricle (LV) of the heart. VLA: Vertical long axis image is parallel to the long axis of the LV and to the septum. HLA: Horizontal long axis image is parallel to the long axis of the LV and perpendicular to the septum

nique called "forward projection", which is the reverse of back projection. The forward projected data is then compared with the measured (actual) projection data. If these do not agree, the differences between the two sets of projection data are used to update the estimated image. This update and compare process is repeated until the current estimated image is as close as possible to the ideal image.

Iterative reconstruction is computationally more intensive than FBP because most iterative algorithms require several iterations to converge to an acceptable image, and each of these iterations is equivalent to one FBP procedure. New iterative algorithms are being developed to speed up the reconstruction process. However, as the iterative reconstruction techniques are harder to implement than FBP and take longer to reconstruct the data, they are not yet routinely used in the clinical environment.

17.7.3
Image Reorientation

Reconstruction of planar projections produces 2D transaxial images, which are images perpendicular to the long axis of the patient. It is common practice to reorient these transaxial images into short axis (SA) images, which are perpendicular to the long axis of the left ventricle (LV) of the heart. This reorientation is performed because the orientation of the heart relative to the patient's long axis varies from patient to patient. It also makes it easier to visually assess myocardial perfusion defects.

To produce a standardization of all forms of tomographic imaging of the heart, it is recommended that all tomographic imaging modalities define, orient and display the heart in the same manner [11], resulting in the formation of short axis (SA), vertical long axis (VLA) and horizontal long axis (HLA) slices, which are orientated at 90° angles to each other (Fig. 17.10). Reorientation of myocardial SPECT images has traditionally required manual selection of a mid-ventricular transaxial image and manual drawing of the long axis of the LV in that plane. The transaxial dataset is then resampled to generate a vertical long axis (VLA) image. By defining the long axis of the LV on the VLA image it is possible to generate a horizontal long axis (HLA) image [12]. The position of the LV long axis in these two reference images defines its location in 3D space. This means that it is possible to define the matrix necessary to reorient and display the data in a coordinate system perpendicular to the long axis of the LV. Due to the subjective nature of this procedure, particularly when perfusion defects are present, software has been developed to automate the reorientation process. This automation, allows the long axis of the LV to be extracted accurately and reproducibly directly from the three-dimensional transaxial image volume.

17.7.4
Interpretation

Reconstructed MPI SPECT scans are generally interpreted visually. Comparison of the stress and rest images allows relative myocardial perfusion to be assessed. A normal myocardium, with no clinically significant muscle damage or CAD, is demonstrated by images showing a uniform distribution of radiopharmaceutical throughout the myocardium (Fig. 17.11a). An area of reduced, or no, uptake of radiopharmaceutical on the images represents a defect in the myocardium. Defects appearing on both the stress and rest images indicate areas of loss of viable myocardium, such as myocardial infarction (Fig. 17.11b), whereas an area of reduced uptake at stress that improves at rest indicates an inducible perfusion abnormality corresponding to inducible ischaemia (Fig. 17.11c).

Problems in reporting MPI scans and diagnosing CAD occur when there are localised areas of soft tissue, such as breasts or diaphragm. These areas attenuate the gamma rays emitted from the radiopharmaceutical, which can result in areas of reduced uptake of radiopharmaceutical on the image. Attenuation artefacts may appear as defects in the myocardium, which can mimic true myocardial perfusion abnormalities. Although an experienced physician is familiar with these image artefacts, and can allow for them, recent advances in applying non-uniform attenuation correction methods and the use of MPI SPECT studies gated to the electrocardiogram signal from the heart, may help decrease problems in reporting scans.

17.8
Other Factors Affecting MPI SPECT Images

The quality of the final reorientated SPECT images depends on the original projection images. The quality of projection images is affected by gamma camera characteristics and choice of radiopharmaceutical, but will also be affected by hepatobiliary clearance and gut uptake of the ^{99m}Tc based radiopharmaceuticals, photon attenuation, variable resolution and patient motion.

17.8.1
Hepatobiliary Clearance and Gut Uptake

^{99m}Tc sestamibi or ^{99m}Tc tetrofosmin are excreted through the hepatobiliary system into the duodenum and bowel [13]. Exercise stress studies result in lower liver activity when compared with rest images [14], whereas pharmacological stress tests result in higher liver and gut uptake with slower clearance than exercise stress imaging. However, ^{99m}Tc sestamibi or ^{99m}Tc tetrofosmin are cleared from the liver at a faster rate than from the myocardium, so by increasing the delay between the injection and the scan it is possible to acquire an image with less liver uptake. As the heart is positioned near the left lobe of the liver and the bowel, scattered radiation from these organs may cause a significant, but artificial, increase or decrease in uptake in the inferior wall when using FBP or iterative reconstruction algorithms.

17.8.2
Photon Attenuation

All SPECT images are compromised by attenuation of the photons within the emitting volume. Photon attenuation refers to the combined effects of photoelectric absorption and Compton scattering [15]. However, in the energy range 0.1 to 1.0 MeV the predominant mode of interaction is by Compton scattering. Compton scatter occurs when photons interact in the patient and detector prior to detection; the photon loses energy to the electron it scatters off and changes direction. This causes incorrect assignment of the photon's line of response, and if these Compton scattered photons are included in the projection data, it will result in a loss of resolution and reduced contrast in the projection data, and consequently the reconstructed data.

Absorption of photons, via the photoelectric effect, result in photons that are emitted from the myocardium becoming totally absorbed in the body. If a gamma ray is absorbed it will not reach the gamma camera, and there-

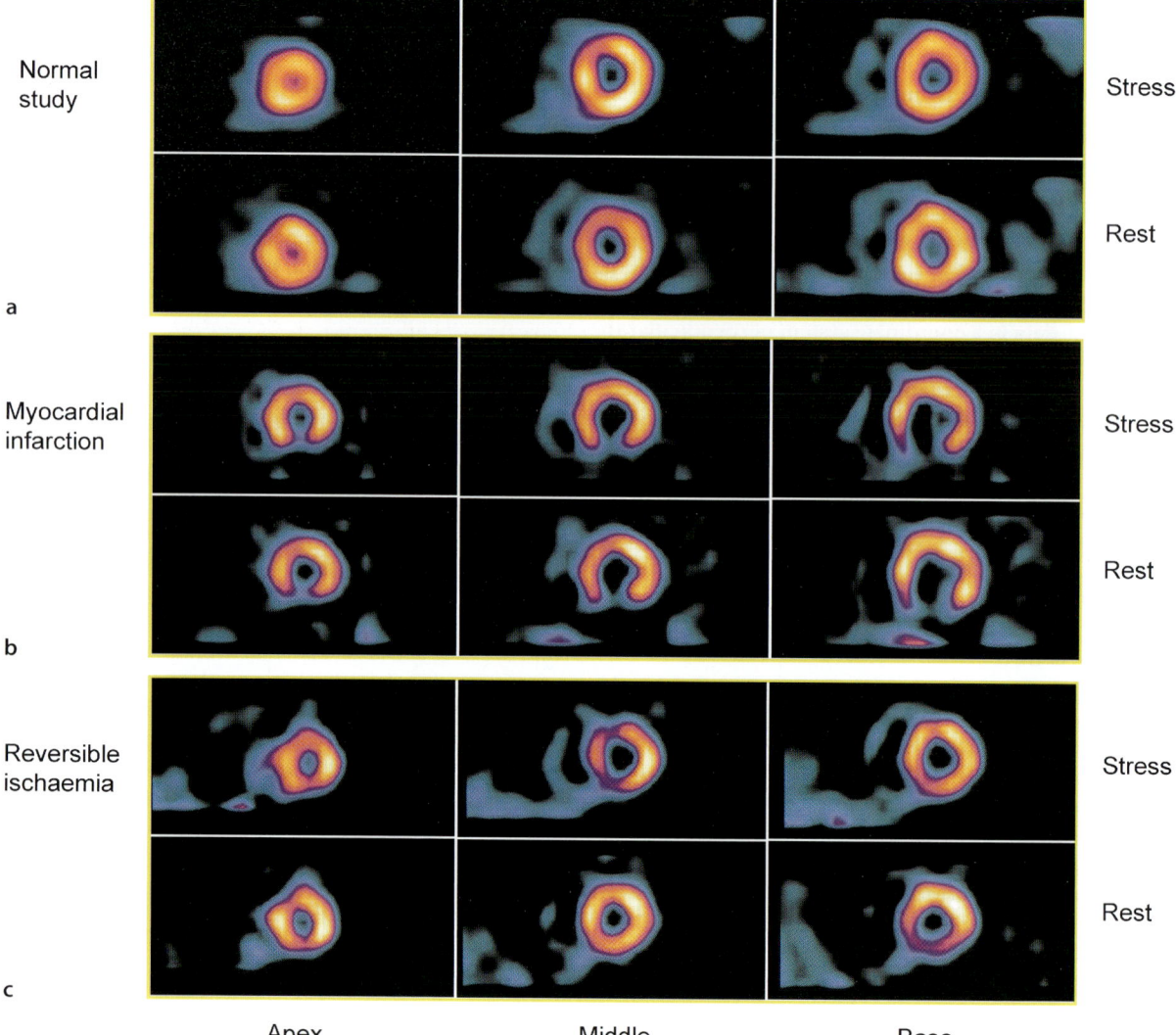

Fig. 17.11a,b MPI SPECT cross-sectional slices through the short axis of the myocardium (from the apex of the heart to the base) under both stress and rest conditions. a A normal study. There is a uniform distribution of radiopharmaceutical throughout the myocardium. b An example of a myocardial infarction. All slices have defects (no uptake in some areas of the myocardium) appearing on both stress and rest images. c An example of reversible ischaemia. Areas of reduced uptake at stress improve on the rest images

fore will not contribute to the resulting image. Absorption of photons via the photoelectric effect is dependent on the atomic number (Z) of the tissue and varies as $1/Z^3$. The probability of absorption occurring decreases as the photon energy increases; this is why ^{99m}Tc attenuation artefacts are less severe (but still significant) than the lower energy ^{201}Tl images.

Attenuation is described by Equation (1), where A_0 is the true activity (amount of tracer), and A_x is the activity measured after attenuation through a thickness of tissue x:

$$A_x = A_0 e^{-\mu x} \tag{1}$$

The exponential term $e^{-\mu x}$ represents the fraction of photons that are attenuated (absorbed and scattered) over a distance x; μ is referred to as the attenuation coefficient, and is a unique value depending on the tissue. When no scatter is present in the gamma camera photopeak energy window, the μ value is referred to as the narrow beam attenuation coefficient. When scattered photons are present, the μ value is referred to as broad beam.

The most frequent artefacts caused by photon attenuation are apparent perfusion defects in the anterior or lateral myocardial wall in large breasted women (breast attenuation) and defects in the inferior wall secondary to diaphragmatic attenuation.

17.8.3
Variable Resolution

As discussed in Sect. 17.6.2 non-circular orbits of the gamma camera around the patient, used to ensure the detectors are always close to the patient, lead to the collection of projection data at different resolutions. When reconstructing this data, artefacts can be introduced due to combining projection data with different resolution characteristics. Several approaches have been proposed to compensate for this effect [16].

17.8.4
Patient Motion

Patient or organ motion is believed to affect as many as 10% to 20% of all cardiac SPECT studies [12]. Motion can occur in any direction. The patient can move parallel to the camera axis (shift up or downwards) or rotate about the axis. There can also be a relative upward movement of the heart within the thorax ("cardiac creep") after stress ^{201}Tl.

It is common practice to check for patient movement prior to reconstruction by visually checking the rotating planar projection images. Movement parallel to the camera axis is usually easy to detect, but rotations are more difficult to see. When patient movement occurs, during FBP the back projected rays will not intersect correctly. If the motion is small (less than half a pixel in a 64 x 64 matrix) this will result in a small loss of spatial resolution and contrast resolution, which an experienced reporting physician can usually tolerate. However, if the motion is significant (more than half a pixel in a 64 x 64 matrix) and occurs in more than one projection, artefacts in the reconstructed image can occur that may manifest as areas of increased or decreased uptake.

There are motion correction software packages available which correct for motion parallel to the camera axis (a shift up or down the bed), by adjusting (moving) the projection data to the correct position prior to reconstruction. Although software packages make a reasonable attempt at correcting movement, it is best to ensure that patient motion is limited as much as possible throughout the scan. One way in which to do this is by using arm-holding devices, or by imaging the patient in the prone position, instead of the conventional supine position. Prone imaging is associated with less cardiac creep [17] than supine imaging, and may also be helpful in reducing left ventricle wall attenuation.

17.9
Quality Control

Routine gamma camera quality control (QC) is designed to assess the performance of the gamma camera and determine if there has been any deterioration in its imaging capabilities. It is important to ensure that the QC measurements are made as regularly, accurately and as reproducibly as possible if subtle changes are to be detected. The type and frequency of QC tests will be defined locally, and will be based on a series of measurements performed during the formal acceptance testing of the new gamma camera in the hospital [18]. However, the tests must be regularly reviewed and modified with time, as systems tend to become less stable with age.

There are many QC procedures that can be performed on gamma cameras, most of which are performed in the conventional 2D planar mode. However, there are additional QC tests that should be made when the gamma camera is used for SPECT imaging. These tests vary with complexity, but the most useful are those that are simple and easy to accurately reproduce, e.g. uniformity, centre of rotation and SPECT performance.

17.9.1
Uniformity of Response

When performing SPECT imaging it is necessary to obtain a consistent and uniform response from the detector, regardless of the angular position of the detector and the position of the incident gamma rays on the detector. For SPECT imaging, it is desirable to have a variation in intrinsic (no collimator) planar non-uniformity of less than 2%. If the detector has any significant area of non-uniform response, then each planar data projection will have an area of increased or decreased counts corresponding to the non-uniform area. During reconstruction the regions of non-uniformity will produce a circular ring artefact of decreased or increased intensity in the 2D cross-sectional slices. It is possible to reduce these non-uniformities by creating uniformity correction maps and applying them to the acquired projection data.

To check SPECT uniformity, a plain Perspex cylinder filled with a solution of ^{99m}Tc is imaged and reconstructed into 2D cross-sectional slices, correcting for gamma ray attenuation within the phantom. These slices are visibly inspected to ensure that there are no ring artefacts.

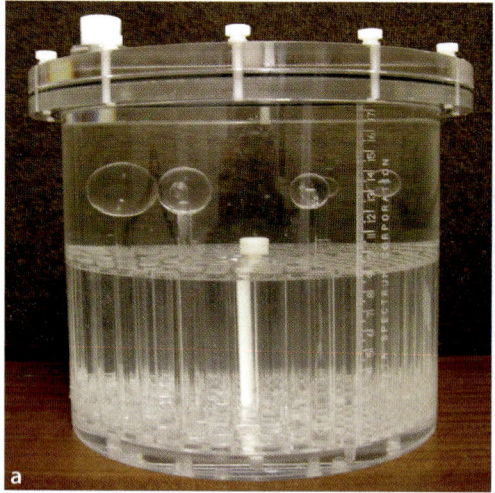 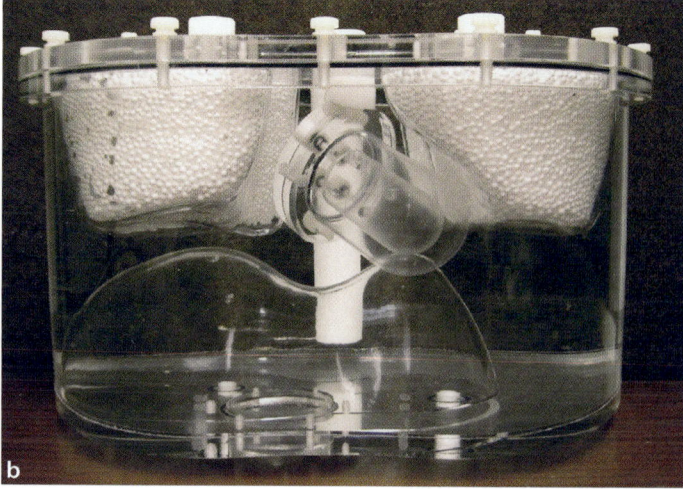

Fig. 17.12a,b Complex phantoms, such as the Data Spectrum Jaszczak Phantom™ (a) and the Data Spectrum cardiac phantom (b) have been developed to assess multiple aspects of SPECT performance

17.9.2
Centre of Rotation

It is critical that the mechanical centre of rotation (COR) of the rotating gamma camera gantry coincides with the mathematical centre of rotation as used in the SPECT reconstruction algorithms. If a detector sags as it rotates around the patient, blurring or ring artefacts may be seen on the image. Most manufacturers have software that corrects for any small deviations from the COR on a projection by projection basis. The validation of the mechanical and mathematical COR can easily be tested by performing a SPECT scan of a point source of ^{99m}Tc placed in air and along the axis of rotation. Software supplied with the gamma camera is then used to calculate various COR offset parameters and these are usually displayed together with acceptable limits.

17.9.3
SPECT Performance

Complex phantoms, such as a Jaszczak phantom™ (Fig. 17.12a), have been developed to assess multiple aspects of SPECT performance. These can be filled with a solution of ^{99m}Tc and scanned using clinical protocols to assess system performance. By varying individual acquisition and reconstruction parameters, an objective assessment of the effects can be made by inspecting the resulting images. This provides a useful indicator of the SPECT performance achievable with a given system under specific test conditions.

As well as general SPECT performance phantoms, it is possible to buy SPECT phantoms to assess specific image applications, for instance myocardial perfusion (Fig. 17.12b). By imaging the cardiac phantom, parameters such as minimum detectable lesion size and minimum detectable contrast ratio may be measured and investigated using different clinical protocols.

17.10
Recent Advances

17.10.1
Gated MPI SPECT

Gated MPI SPECT scans are created by acquiring several image sets corresponding to different phases or intervals of the cardiac cycle. Gated MPI SPECT scans have increased temporal resolution, and so it is possible to analyse individual phases of the cardiac cycle. In a gated acquisition, counts from each phase of the cardiac cycle are associated with a temporal frame within the computer (Fig. 17.13). Reconstruction of each interval of a gated MPI SPECT into a tomographic image set allows for visual or quantitative estimation of functional parameters, such as myocardial motion and thickening. The most common gating rate is eight frames per R–R interval per projection, although 16 frames are sometimes used. Some camera manufacturers provide an extra frame in which counts from all rejected beats are accumulated. Counts from this extra frame can be added to counts from the individual gating frames to produce

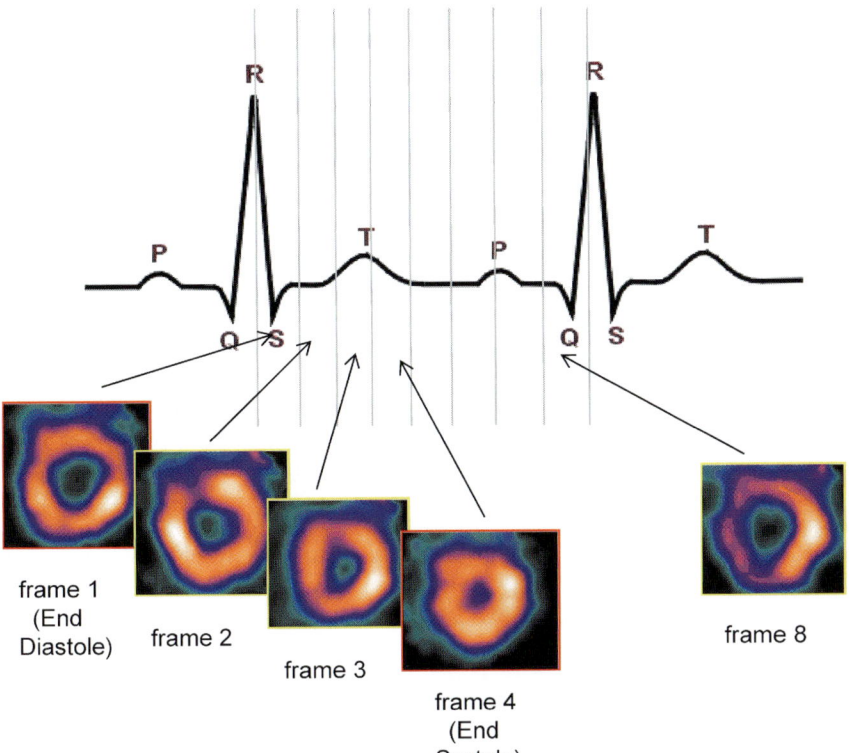

Fig. 17.13 ECG-gated MPI SPECT. SPECT data is acquired in step and shoot mode, and for each angular projection separate temporal frames are acquired at different phases of the cardiac cycle. Usually 8 frames are used, with frame 1 normally corresponding to the heart at end diastole and frame 4 to end systole. Counts from all the frames can be added together to produce an "un-gated" or summed SPECT perfusion projection data set

an "un-gated" or summed SPECT perfusion projection data set.

To optimise protocols for gated MPI SPECT it is necessary to consider both gated and ungated image quality. There must be high count statistics in each temporal frame at each projection angle, since each image of the cardiac cycle is individually reconstructed for calculation of LVEF. To achieve a high count density it may be necessary to increase the total acquisition time compared with conventional MPI SPECT. An acceptance window for bad-beat rejection must also be specified. A narrow window will reject most of the ectopic beats, and the count density will therefore decrease in proportion to the number of rejected beats. This makes the value of the LVEF (left ventricular ejection fraction) more reliable, but perfusion data will suffer. Conversely a wide window will preserve perfusion data, but functional gated information will deteriorate. A 20% window (±10%) is often used.

Gated MPI SPECT wall motion is often visualised using bulls eye plots or a 3D surface display or mesh method (Fig. 17.14), and allows the reporting physician to distinguish between fixed defects from artefacts. End-diastolic and end-systolic images or polar map displays also help assess apparent perfusion abnormality. Another advantage of gated MPI SPECT data is that it can be used to calculate the end-diastolic and end-systolic volumes, and as a result, calculate the left ventricular ejection fraction (LVEF) [19], which is a fundamental diagnostic and prognostic predictor of CAD.

Gated MPI SPECT may not be suitable for all patients, as changes in heart rate due to a variety of factors can result in temporal "blurring" or mixing of counts from adjacent planes. These factors may be patient related, e.g., patient anxiety, normal sinus rhythm or arrhythmia, or due to technical problems related to a poor ECG connection. However, gated MPI SPECT is a promising method for examining myocardial perfusion and wall motion and is rapidly gaining popularity in the UK.

17.10.2
Non-Uniform Attenuation Correction (NUAC) in SPECT

Many gamma rays emitted from the radiopharmaceutical are attenuated (absorbed or scattered) in areas of soft tissue, such as breast tissue, and never actually reach the gamma camera detector. Attenuation can result in reduced counts in areas of the myocardium, mimicking myocardial perfusion abnormalities (Fig. 17.15a),

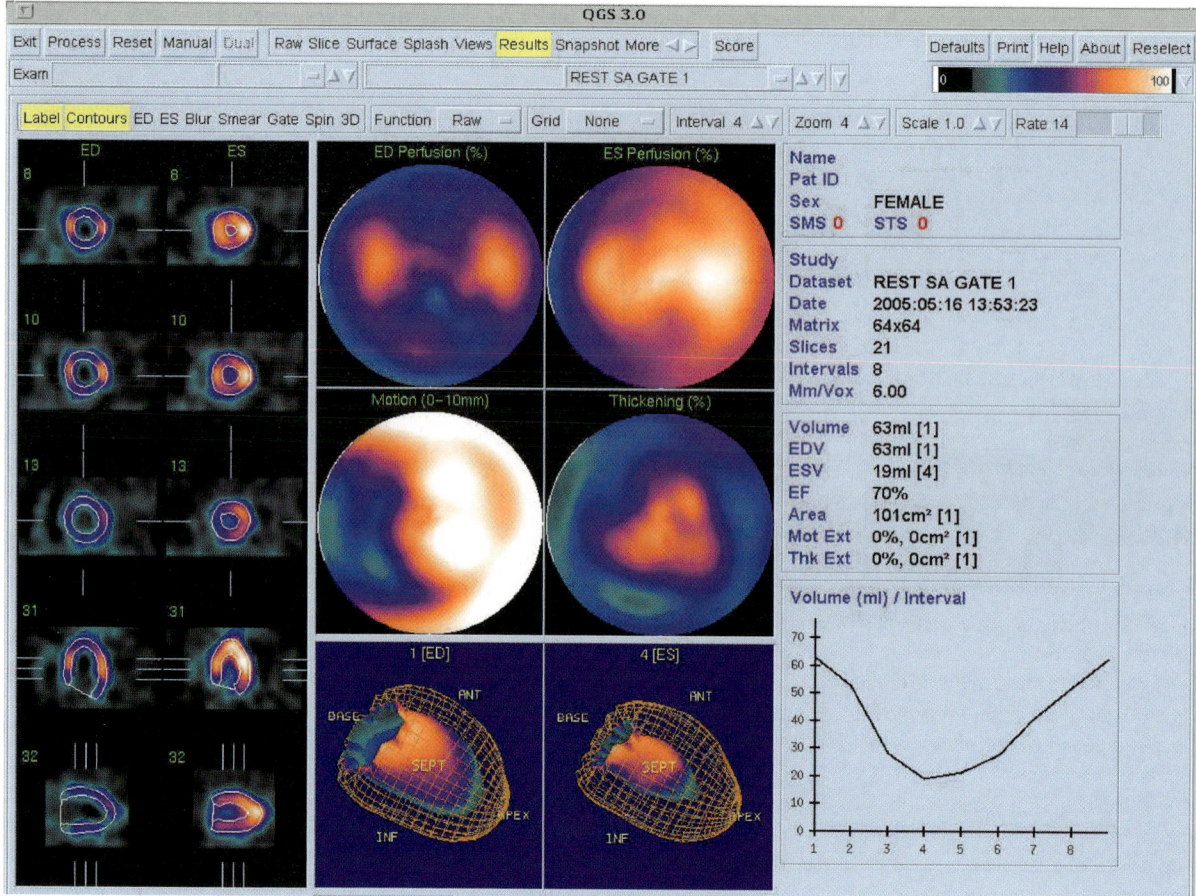

Fig. 17.14 A screen display of a commercially available quantitative gated MPI SPECT analysis program, QGS (Quantitative Gated SPECT). QGS is an interactive application for the automatic segmentation, quantification, analysis and display of gated myocardial perfusion SPECT studies. (The algorithms were developed at Cedars-Sinai Medical Center.)

reducing the specificity of MPI SPECT. Although an experienced physician is familiar with the characteristic appearance of these artefacts, it is better to remove them from the myocardium perfusion images, making these easier to interpret (Fig. 17.15b). Many research groups around the world have been developing ways to achieve this goal by acquiring and implementing a non-uniform attenuation map specific to each patient. This can be attained by using transmission scanning techniques, either by scanning the patient with an external radioactive source, such as ^{153}Gd [16], or by a basic CT scan [20]. The transmission scan gives the specific attenuation information required. It is hoped that by implementing a non-uniform attenuation correction (NUAC) the specificity and sensitivity for the detection of coronary stenosis and viability will be increased. However, not all UK centres using MPI SPECT with NUAC have achieved this, and the nuclear medicine community is still undecided on whether NUAC is ready to be used for routine clinical use [21–24]. It is recommended that NUAC images should only be used when reviewed alongside the uncorrected images [25].

If NUAC is performed, it is important that QC of the transmission scan is also performed. This may include checking such things as the uniformity, variability and temporal drift of the reference transmission scan, as well as ensuring there are adequate transmission scan counts in all images.

17.11
Future Developments

Nuclear cardiology developing rapidly, and the future is dependent on the technical advancement of gamma cameras, processing computers and associated software, as well as the development of biological advancements, such as targeted imaging.

The future for nuclear cardiology may lie in its ability to image physiological processes at a molecular level and explore many mechanisms involved in CAD. For example, Annexin-V is a protein that binds to cells undergoing apoptosis, and when labelled with ^{99m}Tc, gamma cameras images can be used to identify the site and extent of apoptotic cell death. Applications of this tracer in nuclear cardiology include visualisation of cell death in patients with acute myocardial infarction and in vivo detection of transplant rejection [26].

Another topical area of cardiology research is myocardial fatty acid metabolism. In patients with multi-vessel disease or with unstable angina it is not always possible to perform stress MPI SPECT, and rest only MPI SPECT scans have limited value for identifying ischaemic disease, particularly when chest pain has subsided and the image shows normal findings. However, research groups have discovered that the iodinated fatty acid analogue, 15-(p-[123I] iodophenyl)-3-(R,S) methylpentadecanoic acid (BMIPP) SPECT scans can identify ischaemic myocardium, without evidence of myocardial infarction, as a region of reduced tracer uptake [27]. It has been found that a resting BMIPP SPECT is more useful than a rest only ^{99m}Tc tetrofosmin MPI SPECT, for patients who are unable to undergo a stress test. However, the role of this agent in routine clinical practice is still to be defined.

Dual modality imaging of SPECT and diagnostic CT (in the form of SPECT/CT cameras) offers great potential as a cardiac imaging technique [28]. It is likely that CT based non-uniform attenuation correction with perfusion imaging will improve the detection of severe and extensive CAD. In addition, CT data may be used to help produce accurate measures of quantitative tracer uptake and retention. The ability to co-register SPECT and CT data also makes SPECT/CT cameras an ideal tool for molecular imaging, although the exact clinical value of these methods is not yet defined.

17.12
Conclusions

The National Institute for Clinical Excellence (NICE) have recently published guidelines for the management of chronic heart failure in adults [29]. These guidelines recognise the importance of MPI in the field of cardiology and recommend it as the initial diagnostic tool for

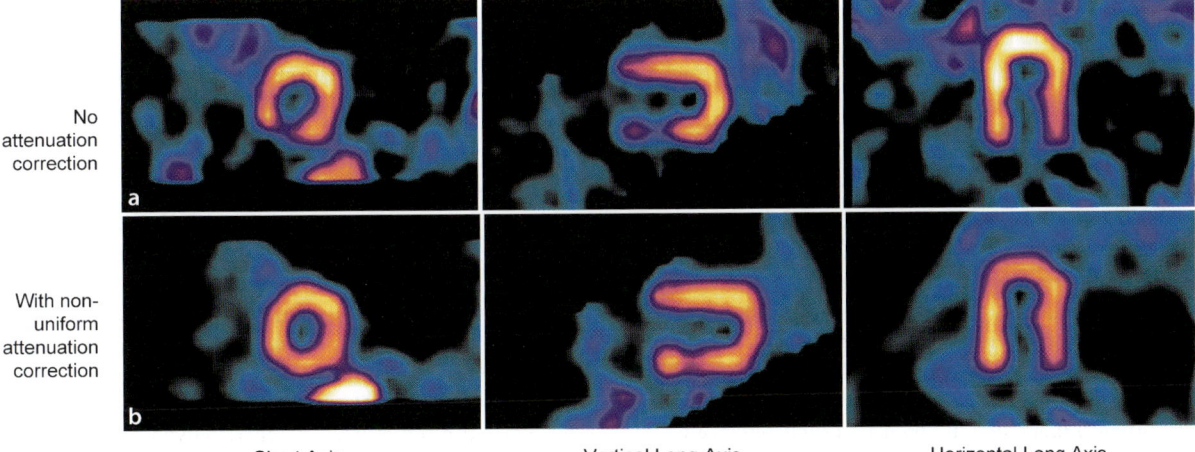

Fig. 17.15a,b A cardiac phantom, with no myocardial defects and simulated breast attenuation, was scanned and reconstructed without (**a**) and with (**b**) using a non-uniform attenuation correction (NUAC). The NUAC has improved the quality of the images as there is a much more uniform representation of the distribution of radiopharmaceutical throughout the heart

people with suspected CAD for whom stress ECG poses problems of poor sensitivity or difficulties in interpretation. NICE also recommend it as part of the investigational strategy in the management of established CAD patients who remain symptomatic following myocardial infarction or revascularisation.

In order to recognise the full potential of MPI SPECT, research groups are actively working in all areas of gamma camera hardware and software design. Reconstruction protocols and full quantitative processing software packages are getting ever more sophisticated, taking advantage of the increased computing power now available.

References

1. Pennel DJ, Prvulovich E (1995) Clinicians Guide to Nuclear Medicine: Nuclear Cardiology, 1st edn. London, BNMS.
2. Sharp PF, Gemmell HG, Smith FW (1998) Practical Nuclear Medicine, 2nd edn. New York, Oxford University Press.
3. Cherry SR, Sorenson JA, Phelps ME (2003) Physics in Nuclear Medicine, 3rd edn. Philadelphia, PA, WB Saunders.
4. Webb S (1988) The Physics of Medical Imaging. Bristol, Institute of Physics Publishing.
5. DePuey EG, Garcia EV, Berman DS (2001) Cardiac SPECT Imaging, 2nd edn. Philadelphia, PA, Lippincott, Williams and Wilkins.
6. O'Connor MK, Hruska CB (2005) Effect of tomographic orbit and type of rotation on apparent myocardial activity. Nucl Med Commun 26:25–30.
7. Maniawki PJ, Morgan HT, Whackers FJTh (1991) Orbit related variation in spatial resolution as a source of artificial defects in thallium-201 SPECT. J Nucl Med 32(5):871–875.
8. Fakhri GN, Buvat I, Pelegrini M et al. (1999) Respective roles of scatter, attenuation, depth-dependent collimator response and finite spatial resolution in cardiac single photon emission tomotgraphy quantitation: a Monte Carlo study. Eur J Nucl Med 26:437–446.
9. Administration of Radioactive Substances Advisory Committee (1988) Notes for guidance on the clinical administration of radiopharmaceuticals and use of sealed radioactive sources, December 1988.
10. Bruyant P (2002) Analytic and Iterative Reconstruction Algorithms in SPECT. J Nucl Med 43(10):1343–1358.
11. Association Writing Group on Myocardial Segmentation and Registration for Cardiac Imaging, Cerqueira MD, Weissman NJ, Dilsizian V et al. (2002) Standardized Myocardial Segmentation and Nomenclature for Tomographic Imaging of the heart A statement for healthcare professionals from the cardiac imaging committee of the council on clinical cardiology of the American Heart Association American Heart. Circulation 105:539–542.
12. Germano G (2001) Technical Aspects of Myocardial SPECT Imaging. J Nucl Med 42(10):1499–1507.
13. Peace RA, Lloyd JL (2005) The effect of imaging time, radiopharmaceutical, full fat milk and water on interfering extra-cardiac activity in myocardial perfusion single photon emission computed tomography. Nucl Med Commun 26:17–24.
14. Shih WJ, McFarland KA, Keifer V et al. (2005) Illustrations of abdominal abnormailities on ^{99m}Tc tetrofosmin gated cardiac SPECT. Nucl Med Commun 26:119–127.
15. Johns HE, Cunningham JR (1983) The Physics of Radiology, 4th edn. Illinois, Charles C Thomas.
16. Galt JR, Cullon J, Garcia EV (1999) Attenuation and scatter compensation in Myocardial Perfusion SPECT. Seminars Nucl Med XXIX(3):204–220.
17. Peterson P, Parker JA, Tepper MR et al. (2005) Prone SPECT myocardial perfusion imaging is associated with less cardiac drift during the acquisition duration than imaging in the supine position. Nucl Med Commun 26:115–117.
18. IPEM Report No. 86 (2003) Quality Control of Gamma Camera Systems. York, UK, York Publishing Services Ltd.
19. Lee DS, Cheon GJ, Ahn JY et al. (2000) Reproducibility of assessment of myocardial function using gated 99Tcm-MIBI SPECT and quantitative software. Nucl Med Commun 21:1127–1134.
20. Tonge CM, Manoharan M, Lawson RS et al. (2005) Attenuation correction of myocardial SPECT studies using low resolution computed tomography images. Nucl Med Commun 26:231–237.
21. Corbett JR, Ficaro EP (2000) Attenuation corrected cardiac perfusion SPECT. Curr Opin Cardiol 15:330–336.
22. Chouraqui P, Livschitz S, Baron J et al. (2004) The Assessment of infarct size in post myocardial infarction patients undergoing thallium-201 tomographic imaging is improved using attenuation correction. Clin Nucl Med 29:352–357.
23. Ficaro EP, Wackers FJT (2002) Should SPECT attenuation correction be more widely employed in routine clinical practice? Eur J Nucl Med 29;409–415.
24. Heller GV, Links J, Bateman TM et al. (2004) American Society of Nuclear Cardiology and Society of Nuclear Medicine joint position statement: Attenuation correction of myocardial perfusion SPECT scintigraphy. J Nucl Cardiol 11:229–230.
25. Procedure Guidelines for Radionuclide Myocardial Perfusion Imaging (2003) Adopted by the British Cardiac Society, the British Nuclear Cardiology Society, and the British Nuclear Medicine Society, Writing Group: Anagnostopoulos C, Harbinson M, Kelion A, K Kundley, Loong CY, Notghi A, Reyes E, Tindale W, Underwood SR.

26. Narula J, Acio F, Narula N et al. (2001) Annexin-V imaging for non-invasive detection of cardiac allograft rejection. Nature Med 7(12):1347–1352.
27. Kawai Y, Morita K, Nozaki Y et al. (2004) Diagnostic value of 123I-Betamethyl-p-Iodophenyl-Pentadecanoic Acid (BMIPP) Single Photon Emission Computed Tomography (SPECT) in patients with chest pain. Circ J 68:547–552.
28. American Society of Nuclear Cardiology (2005) Computed tomography imaging with nuclear cardiology. Information statement – approved November 2004. J Nucl Cardiol 12:131–142.
29. National Institute for Clinical Excellence (NICE) (2003) Technology Appraisal Guidance 73; Myocardial perfusion scintigraphy for the diagnosis and management of angina and myocardial infarction; November 2003; www.nice.org.uk/TA073guidance

Radionuclides in Nuclear Cardiology: Current Status and Limitations

Chapter 18

Richard Fernandez

Contents

18.1	Introduction	213
18.2	From Atoms to Solar Systems	213
18.3	Radiation	214
18.4	Isomers and Misnomers	215
18.5	Modes of Radioactive Decay	215
18.5.1	Alpha Decay	215
18.5.2	Beta Decay: Beta Emission	216
18.5.3	Beta Decay: Positron Emission	216
18.5.4	Electron Capture	216
18.5.5	Gamma Decay (Isomeric Transition)	216
18.6	Half-Life: To Decay or not Decay?	217
18.7	Ideal Properties of a Radionuclide	217
18.8	Decisions, Decisions …Radionuclides Used for Imaging in Nuclear Cardiology	217
18.9	Method of Production	217
18.9.1	The Molybdenum-99/Technetium-99m Generator	218
18.10	Current Diagnostic Applications	218
18.10.1	Technetium-99m	218
18.10.2	Thallium-201	219
18.10.3	Iodine-123	219
18.10.4	Indium-111	219
18.10.5	Gallium-67	219
18.11	Future Development of Radionuclides in Nuclear Cardiology	219
	References	220

18.1 Introduction

Nuclear cardiology has evolved significantly since its first reported use in the mid-1920s. Blumgart and Weiss described a method for collecting radon gas dissolved in saline and investigated its use in measuring central circulation transit times in humans [1, 2]. Although the concept of using radionuclides to study cardiology is by no means new, many of the developments in this field have occurred only in the past decade or so. Massive advances in camera technology and computational power have generated sophisticated functional imaging techniques, from 3-D imaging of myocardial perfusion and wall motion in SPECT to imaging of metabolism and viability in PET.

Fundamental to the evolution of nuclear cardiology, and indeed nuclear medicine as a whole, has been the advances made in radionuclide production and pharmaceutical preparation. Radiopharmaceuticals used in cardiovascular nuclear medicine will be dealt with subsequently (Chapters 19). The focus of this chapter will primarily be on non-positron emitting radionuclides used in nuclear cardiology for diagnosis and therapy. The reader is referred to Chapter 32 for discussion of positron emitting radionuclides used in nuclear cardiology.

18.2 From Atoms to Solar Systems

All matter consists of molecules. Molecules are in turn formed from a combination of elements. The smallest constituent of an element with the same chemical properties is the atom. The atom itself consists of three elementary particles; protons, neutrons and electrons. Classically the atom consists of a positively charged nucleus, comprised of positively charged protons and electrostatically inert neutrons, surrounded by negatively charged electrons. A neutral atom has no overall charge as the number of electrons is equal to the number of protons (also termed the *atomic number*, Z).

In the simplest model, first proposed by Bohr in 1913, electrons occupy discrete energy states or 'shells' around the nucleus, analogous to the planets orbiting the sun. When the atom is in its most stable, lowest energy state, also termed the 'ground' state, electrons occupy the lowest possible shells, closest to the nucleus. The attractive electrostatic force binds electrons to the nucleus. Energy is therefore required to excite electrons to higher, unoccupied energy levels (this energy may be supplied for example, by an incident particle striking the atom). Electrons, if given sufficient energy, can be removed completely from the atom. This process is termed *ionisation*.

The energy required to ionise electrons is referred to as the binding energy and is measured in electronvolts (eV). Electrons in different shells have different binding energies, with electrons closest to a particular nucleus having the greatest binding energy and electrons in higher shells, further from that nucleus having a lower binding energy. This is analogous to when two opposing poles of a magnet are placed close together. The closer they are brought to each other, the greater the amount of effort required to pull them apart.

Figure 18.1 illustrates a model of atomic structure (a) and the process of ionisation (b). The term *nuclide* is used to describe a aprtikular composition of neutrons and protons that constitute a nucleus.

The characteristics of a particular nuclide with chemical symbol X, can be described by the notation, $^A_Z X$. The atomic number, Z denotes the number of protons. The mass number, A denotes the total number of protons and neutrons (the number of neutrons can be calculated by A−Z). For example, $^{16}_{8}O$ contains eight protons and eight neutrons. Atomic and nuclear structure are dealt with more thoroughly elsewhere in the literature [3–5].

18.3 Radiation

There are two forms of radiation, particulate and electromagnetic radiation. Alpha and beta particles, discussed in more detail subsequently, are examples of particulate radiation. X-rays are an example of electromagnetic radiation.

Ionisation of an inner shell electron results in an outer shell electron filling the vacancy created. The dif-

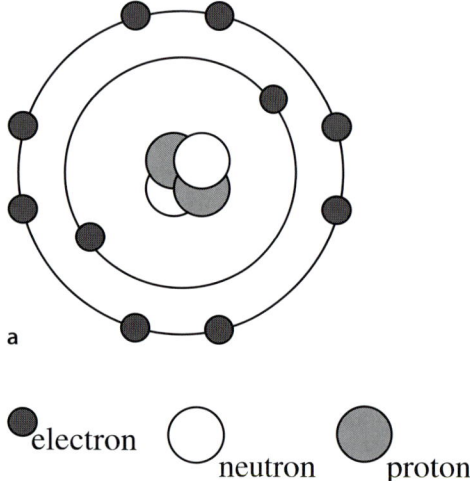
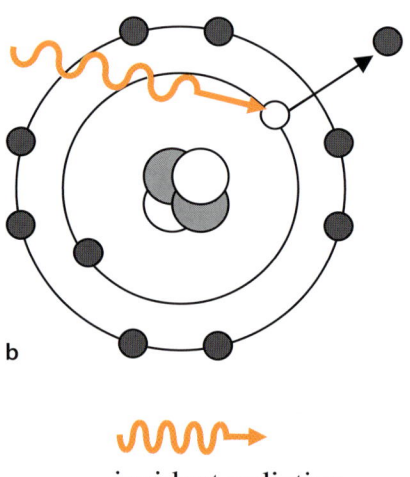

Fig. 18.1 a Simple model of atomic structure. Discrete electron shells surrounding the nucleus are designated by the letters, K, L M…, etc. with the K-shell closest to the nucleus. **b** The process of ionisation. Incident radiation ejects an electron from the K-shell

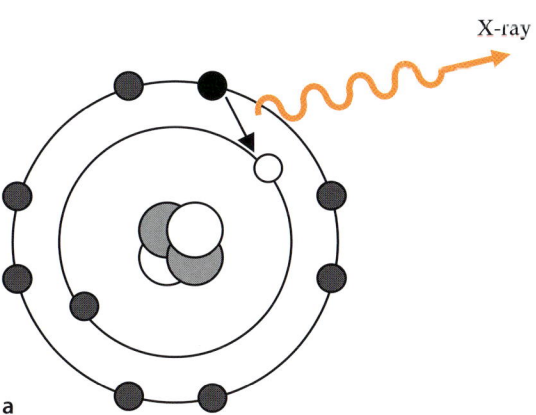 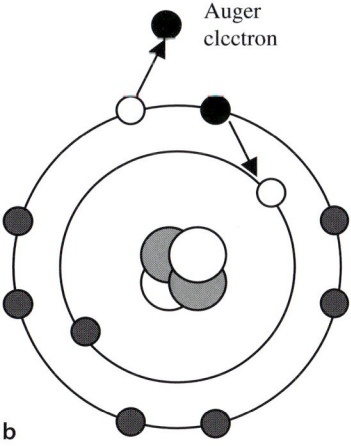

Fig. 18.2 a Characteristic X-ray emission. **b** Auger electron emission

ference in binding energy between the two shells results in energy released in the form of an X-ray. These X-rays are termed *characteristic* X-rays as they are specific to each element since different elements, with differing nuclei, have differing electron binding energies.

As an alternative to characteristic X-ray emission, the energy released when an outer shell electron fills a vacancy in a lower shell can be transferred to *another* outer electron. This ionised electron (or *Auger electron*) results in a second vacancy in the outer shell.

Figure 18.2 illustrates the process of characteristic X-ray (a) and Auger electron emission (b).

In the same way that electrons have different energy states, the nucleus can also exist in discrete energy states. When the nucleus converts from an unstable, more energetic, state into a more stable state radiation can be emitted. These energetically unstable nuclei are termed *radionuclides* and can occur naturally (e.g., $^{14}_{6}C$) or they can be produced artificially in a nuclear reactor or cyclotron. The stability of a nucleus is determined by the ratio of neutrons to protons in the nucleus. For stable, low atomic number nuclei the neutron/proton ratio is approximately 1. For higher atomic number nuclei the neutron/proton ratio necessary for stability increases to approximately 1.5, i.e., more neutrons are required to ensure nuclear stability.

The term *radioisotope* refers to a radioactive isotope of a specific element. For example ^{131}I, ^{125}I and ^{123}I are all radioisotopes of iodine. Sometimes in nuclear medicine the term 'radioisotope' is used erroneously in place of 'radionuclide'. Technically, the term radioisotope refers to a radioactive isotope of a specific element.

Isomers is a term used to describe nuclides with identical numbers of protons and neutrons but with differing nuclear energy states, e.g., $^{A}_{Z}X*$ is an excited state of $^{A}_{Z}X$.

18.5 Modes of Radioactive Decay

Unstable nuclides undergo transformation to a more stable state by the process of releasing energy through radioactive decay. The unstable or radioactive nuclide is referred to as the *parent*, and the more stable product nucleus is referred to as the *daughter* nucleus. In some cases the parent nuclide decays via a *series* of daughter nuclides and emissions to eventually reach a stable ground state.

There are a number of modes of radioactive decay; alpha decay, beta decay, electron capture and gamma decay. In all of theses modes there can also be characteristic X-ray emission as well as Auger electron emission.

18.4 Isomers and Misnomers

Isotopes are nuclides with the same atomic number, and therefore have the same chemical properties, but which have different numbers of neutrons (e.g., $^{238}_{92}U$, $^{235}_{92}U$)

Isotones refers to nuclides with the same number of neutrons. Isobars are nuclides which have different atomic numbers but which have the same mass number.

18.5.1 Alpha Decay

Emission of an alpha particle can occur in unstable nuclei with a high atomic number (Z > 83). This process may be written as

$$^{A}_{Z}X \rightarrow\, ^{A-4}_{Z-2}Y + ^{4}_{2}\alpha$$

Note that the total mass number and total atomic number on both sides of the equation are identical, satisfying the requirement for conservation of both mass and charge.

Alpha particles are essentially helium nuclei (A = 4, Z = 2) and because they are massive and doubly charged they cause large amounts of ionisation. Consequently the range of alpha particles is very small (typically a few microns in tissue) and deposition of energy occurs in a small volume. The high dose resulting from emission of alpha particles therefore excludes their use in diagnostic nuclear cardiology.

18.5.2
Beta Decay: Beta Emission

This mode of decay occurs when an unstable nucleus has an excess of neutrons, relative to more stable neighbouring nuclei. A more stable state is achieved by a neutron in the nucleus converting to a proton. This results in emission of a beta particle, β, a high energy electron necessary for the conservation of charge, together with the emission of an antineutrino, v. The neutrino (and antineutrino) have neither mass nor charge and are not discussed further as they have no relevance to nuclear medicine. The process of beta emission may be written as

$$^{A}_{Z}X \rightarrow ^{A}_{Z+1}Y + ^{0}_{-1}\beta + v$$

The excess energy resulting from the nuclear transition is characteristic to the nucleus, and is shared between the beta particle and the antineutrino. Beta particles are therefore emitted with a spectrum of energies from zero up to this finite maximum.

Due to their short range in tissue (typically a few millimetres) beta particles are used in therapeutic applications, such as vascular brachytherapy [6], rather than for in-vivo diagnostic imaging.

18.5.3
Beta Decay: Positron Emission

The converse of beta decay occurs in positron emission. An unstable nucleus with a higher proton to neutron ratio than more stable neighbouring nuclei, converts to a more stable energy state through the conversion of a proton to a neutron with the emission of a positron and neutrino. The process of positron emission may be written as

$$^{A}_{Z}X \rightarrow ^{A}_{Z-1}Y + ^{0}_{+1}\beta + v$$

A positron is the anti-particle of an electron, having identical mass but opposite charge to the electron. As with beta particles, positrons are emitted with a range of energies up to a finite maximum. The positron loses its kinetic energy through interactions and subsequently annihilates with a free electron, yielding two gamma ray photons. These two photons are emitted at 180° to each other, each with initial energy 511 keV (equivalent to the rest mass of an electron). The coincident detection of these two gamma rays is the objective of PET imaging.

18.5.4
Electron Capture

When a nucleus does not have sufficient energy for positron emission, the excess of protons may be reduced by the process of 'capture' of an orbital electron. A proton in the nucleus combines with an orbital electron and converts to a neutron with the emission of a neutrino. Since the neutrino is charge-less and mass-less it is virtually undetectable and consequently the process of electron capture would be externally undetectable. However the vacancy left by the orbital electron usually results in additional characteristic X-ray emission from the daughter nucleus.

18.5.5
Gamma Decay (Isomeric Transition)

In this process a daughter radionuclide in an excited state (isomer) decays to a more stable state through the emission of a gamma ray. The transition is not necessarily instantaneous and the nucleus can exist in the excited state for a measurable length of time. This prolonged state is referred to as an isomeric state, or more commonly, a metastable state and is usually denoted by the letter m following the mass number (A) in the notation, ^{Am}X, e.g., ^{99m}Tc.

Gamma rays are similar to X-rays in that they are also part of the electromagnetic spectrum. However they differ in their mode of production; X-rays are produced by transitions of orbital electrons whereas gamma rays are produced from *nuclear* transitions.

An alternative to the emission of a gamma ray by the isomer is the process of internal conversion in which the excited nucleus transfers its excess energy directly to an orbital electron. The vacancy, created by ejection of an electron in internal conversion, is filled by an electron from a higher orbital shell. This results in subsequent characteristic X-ray or Auger electron emission.

Gamma rays are essential for diagnostic imaging in nuclear cardiology and nuclear medicine as a whole. However internal conversion, an alternate process to gamma ray emission, is undesirable as the electron emission adds to the effective dose of the patient without imparting any diagnostic information. For this reason a low internal conversion to gamma emission ratio is desirable in diagnostic imaging.

18.6
Half-Life: To Decay or not Decay?

The rate at which radionuclides decay is specific to each nuclide. Radioactive decay is a random process and for each type of nuclide is characterised by a decay constant. The decay constant can be related to a more physically meaningful quantity called the *half-life*. The half-life of a particular radionuclide is the time taken for half of the nuclei to decay. Some radionuclides such as $^{14}_{6}C$ have a half-life of the order of years, whereas other radionuclides have a half-life of the order of microseconds. The decay constant λ, is related to the half-life $T_{1/2}$ by the equation

$$\lambda = \frac{\ln(2)}{T_{1/2}}$$

When radionuclides are labelled with pharmaceuticals and administered in-vivo, as well as the physical half-life of the radionuclide, the biological half-life of the radiopharmaceutical needs also to be considered. The combination of physical and biological half-life gives rise to the *effective half-life* of the radiopharmaceutical.

The effective half-life, $T_{EFFECTIVE}$, is obtained by summation of the physical and biological decay constants, and is given by the following equation [7]:

$$\frac{1}{T_{EFFECTIVE}} = \frac{1}{T_{PHYSICAL}} + \frac{1}{T_{BIOLOGICAL}}$$

18.7
Ideal Properties of a Radionuclide

The ideal properties required of a radionuclide depend on the application it is intended for. Radionuclides used for diagnostic imaging necessarily have very different properties to those intended for therapeutic use. A significant proportion of nuclear cardiology involves diagnostic imaging and so primary focus will be on radionuclides used in this application. Table 18.1 lists the properties required of the ideal radioisotope for diagnostic imaging [8].

Radionuclides intended for diagnostic applications should emit gamma radiation with no particulate emissions. This is because alpha and beta radiation contribute to the patient dose without providing diagnostic information. The gamma ray energy should be sufficient

Table 18.1 Ideal properties of a radionuclide used for diagnostic imaging

Gamma emission only, no particulate (alpha/beta) emissions
Gamma ray energy 100–200 keV
Physical half-life comparable with length of investigation (typically few hours)
Short physical half-life to minimise waste disposal/storage issues
Non-toxic
Chemically suitable for incorporation into biologically relevant pharmaceuticals without altering their behaviour
Readily available at the hospital site
Inexpensive

to allow the radiation to penetrate tissue and be detected efficiently by a gamma camera.

The physical half-life of the radionuclide should be comparable to the length of the investigation, again to minimise radiation burden to the patient. As discussed previously, the effective half-life of the radiopharmaceutical administered in-vivo depends on *both* the biological half-life and the physical half-life. However it is not sufficient to rely solely on biological half-life as this may be altered in pathological states; a short *physical* half-life is therefore essential for the ideal diagnostic imaging radionuclide.

In therapeutic applications, such as vascular brachytherapy, the converse of the above applies. Particulate emission and a sufficiently long half-life are usually required for effective therapy.

18.8
Decisions, Decisions …Radionuclides Used for Imaging in Nuclear Cardiology

Table 18.2 lists radionuclides routinely used for imaging in nuclear cardiology. The use of the plural form indicates that unfortunately there is no singular radionuclide that satisfies all the requirements specified in Table 18.1.

18.9
Method of Production

Radionuclides manufactured in a cyclotron, in which a target nucleus is bombarded by positively charged par-

Table 18.2 Radionuclides routinely used for imaging in nuclear cardiology

Radionuclide	Half-life	Principle photon emissions (keV)	Type of decay*	Mode of production
^{67}Ga	78.2 h	92, 182, 300, 390	EC	Cyclotron
^{99m}Tc	6.0 h	140	IT	Generator
^{123}I	13.2 h	159	EC	Cyclotron
^{111}In	67 h	173, 247	EC	Cyclotron
^{201}Tl	73 h	68–80$^\$$	EC	Cyclotron

*EC = electron conversion, IT = isomeric transition
$^\$$Characteristic X-rays

ticles, typically have an excess of protons. This excess is reduced by subsequent decay, typically by either positron emission or electron capture.

Radionuclides produced in a nuclear reactor typically have an excess of neutrons due to the process of neutron capture in the reactor. Molybdenum-99 (^{99}Mo), the parent radionuclide of technetium-99m (^{99m}Tc), is produced in a nuclear reactor. Instability caused by an excess of neutrons results in ^{99}Mo decaying by beta emission to form Tc-99m.

All radionuclide generators operate on the principle that a relatively long-lived parent radionuclide decays to a produce a daughter radionuclide. The chemical properties of the daughter radionuclide differ from that of the parent to facilitate effective separation.

18.9.1
The Molybdenum-99/Technetium-99m Generator

The ^{99}Mo-^{99m}Tc generator is the most commonly used radionuclide generator system in nuclear medicine. The generator consists of ^{99}Mo absorbed onto an alumina column. ^{99}Mo decays by beta emission to ^{99m}Tc with a half-life of 67 hours. To minimise radiation exposure from the emitted beta particles and gamma radiation, the alumina column is shielded, typically by depleted uranium. The ^{99m}Tc can be removed from the column, as sodium pertechnetate (Na^{99m}TcO$_4$) by drawing a solution of sodium chloride through the column. This process is known as elution or 'milking' of the generator.

^{99m}Tc decays by isomeric transition to ^{99}Tc with the emission of a 140 keV gamma ray. Technetium-99 has an extremely long half-life of 2.1×10^5 years and eventually decays to a stable nuclide, ruthenium-99, with the emission of a beta particle.

The full nuclear transformation process of the ^{99}Mo-^{99m}Tc generator may be written as

$$^{99}_{42}\text{Mo} \rightarrow {}^{99m}_{43}\text{Tc} + \beta + \gamma \rightarrow {}^{99}_{43}\text{Tc} + \gamma_{140} \rightarrow {}^{99}_{44}\text{Ru} + \beta$$

18.10
Current Diagnostic Applications

Below are examples of diagnostic applications of radionuclides listed in Table.18.2 relevant to nuclear cardiology.

18.10.1
Technetium-99m

^{99m}Tc is the closest to achieving the requirements of the ideal tracer. This is due to its relatively short half-life, comparable with the duration of the majority of nuclear medicine tests. ^{99m}Tc only emits gamma radiation, the energy of which is optimal for detection by a gamma camera. ^{99m}Tc radiopharmaceuticals are produced by combining the radionuclide, as sodium pertechnetate, with the required pharmaceutical. This is usually achieved by a process as simple as addition of pertechnetate to the vial containing the pharmaceutical and shaking to dissolve the contents. Production of ^{99m}Tc by a generator ensures it is available on-site and is therefore cost-effective.

^{99m}Tc is used extensively throughout nuclear medicine and has a number of applications in diagnostic nuclear cardiology. Red blood cells labelled in-vivo with ^{99m}Tc are used to investigate equilibrium ventriculography through multiple gated acquisition. Due to its ease of preparation and rapid blood clearance, ^{99m}Tc DTPA is used in first-pass ventriculography. Nowadays, ^{99m}Tc is the radionuclide of choice for myocardial perfusion imaging. ^{99m}Tc labelled Sestamibi and Tetrofosmin are used extensively to investigate myocardial ischaemia and infarction. The physical properties of ^{99m}Tc, such as its high photon flux and gamma ray energy, enable it to be used for gated SPECT imaging. This enables information on regional wall motion and thickening to be obtained concurrently with the perfusion study.

18.10.2
Thallium-201

Thallium-201 (^{201}Tl) is produced in a cyclotron and decays by electron capture to the stable nuclide, mercury-201 with a half-life of 73 hours. This decay is accompanied by a low abundance of gamma ray emissions together with characteristic mercury-201 X-ray emissions of energy between 68 and 80 keV. The decay process for ^{201}Tl has the form

$$^{201}_{81}Tl + e \rightarrow ^{201}_{80}Hg + \gamma$$

^{201}Tl thallous chloride, an analogue of potassium, was the most commonly used radionuclide for investigation of myocardial viability and perfusion. Increasingly ^{99m}Tc labelled pharmaceuticals have been used as an alternative to ^{201}Tl for myocardial perfusion [9, 10]. This is due to the higher radiation burden associated with ^{201}Tl due to the longer physical half-life and characteristic X-ray emission. Additionally image quality is inherently poorer due to the increased scatter and attenuation of the lower energy ^{201}Tl photons compared to ^{99m}Tc.

18.10.3
Iodine-123

Iodine-123 (^{123}I) also decays by electron capture with the emission of a 159 keV gamma ray to 'stable' tellurium-123 (half-life 1.2×10^{13} years). The energy of the emitted gamma is suitable for diagnostic imaging. The decay process for ^{123}I is given by

$$^{123}_{53}I + e \rightarrow ^{123}_{52}Te + \gamma$$

^{123}I labelled with MIBG can be used to investigate the sympathetic nervous system, in particular cardiac innervation [11]. MIBG has a structure analogous to noradrenaline and its retention reflects neuronal uptake. Cardiac neurotransmission imaging enables the assessment of innervation and neuronal status in dilated cardiomyopathy and coronary artery disease.

18.10.4
Indium-111

Indium-111 (^{111}In) has a half-life of 67 hours and decays by electron capture to stable cadmium-111 with gamma ray emissions of energy 173 keV and 247 keV. The decay process for ^{111}In is of the form

$$^{111}_{49}In + e \rightarrow ^{111}_{48}Cd + \gamma$$

Myocardial infarction can be investigated through ^{111}In labelled monoclonal antibodies such as anti-myosin [11, 12]. Since this antibody binds exclusively to intra-cellular myosin, which is only exposed upon death of the cell, areas of myocardial infarction can be localised.

18.10.5
Gallium-67

Gallium-67 (^{67}Ga) is produced in a cyclotron and decays by electron capture to stable Zinc-67 with a number of gamma emissions and a half-life of 78.2 hours. ^{67}Ga citrate can be used in the detection of inflammatory disease and sarcoidosis.

18.11
Future Development of Radionuclides in Nuclear Cardiology

There are many new advances on the horizon for the field of nuclear cardiology. Some of the development will be driven by advances in imaging technology. Image fusion is now realisable and in the ascendancy. Although the benefits of image fusion are clearly evident in the field of oncology, it is unclear whether the surge of PET/CT and SPECT/CT systems will benefit nuclear cardiology. The myocardium is in constant motion making registration between modalities inherently more difficult. While advances in hybrid camera technology are unsubtle, with different modalities almost simply 'welded' together, conversely, advances in radiopharmaceuticals are directed towards the infinitesimal. Radiopharmaceutical development is striving towards molecular diagnostics with the aim of targeting specific molecules or components of the cell.

Advances in radiopharmaceuticals will primarily be driven by the development of pharmaceuticals providing the targeting, rather than the development of new radionuclides. A comprehensive discussion of emerging radiopharmaceuticals in nuclear cardiology is given by Narula et al. [13].

Many new pharmaceuticals currently under development will be labelled with ^{99m}Tc as this radionuclide has optimal labelling and imaging characteristics as well as availability.

^{99m}Tc labelled tracers such as sestamibi and tetrofosmin are the principal radiopharmaceuticals used for investigation of myocardial perfusion, although it is unclear whether they will completely replace ^{201}Tl. Although ^{99m}Tc labelled tracers benefit from the physical characteristics of the radionuclide, higher photon energy and photon flux enabling better image quality and lower patient dose, ^{201}Tl has a higher myocardial extraction and can be used to assess myocardial viability. ^{99m}Tc N-NOET is a tracer currently under development for assessment of myocardial perfusion. It has a higher extraction efficiency than either ^{201}Tl or ^{99m}Tc labelled sestamibi or tetrofosmin but further investigation is required to determine if it provides comparable diagnostic accuracy. It is important to realise that ^{99m}Tc N-NOET has its own unique properties. It is not simply a ^{99m}Tc labelled version of ^{201}Tl, and being neutral will behave differently to the cationic ^{99m}Tc sestamibi and tetrofosmin. Therefore effort should be directed at finding the particular use for ^{99m}Tc N-NOET in myocardial perfusion rather than competing for applications that already exist.

^{99m}Tc labelled glucarate is currently under investigation as an alternative to ^{111}In antimyosin for the detection of myocardial necrosis. Imaging of myocardial necrosis is valuable in the assessment of myocardial infarction as well as in the detection of heart transplant rejection.

^{99m}Tc FMISO is a tracer under development for the localisation of myocardial hypoxia – useful in assessment of ischaemia. Although ^{99m}Tc has greater availability and is more cost-effective, some research indicates that later imaging times are more beneficial and so I-123, with its longer physical half-life, may be used instead.

A more detailed discussion of emerging radiopharmaceuticals in nuclear cardiology is given in a subsequent chapter.

References

1. Blumgart H, Weiss S (1927) Studies on the velocity of blood flow VI. The method of collecting the active deposit of radium and its preparation for intravenous injection. J Clin Invest 4:389–398.
2. Blumgart H, Weiss S (1927) Studies on the velocity of blood flow VII. The pulmonary circulation time in normal resting individuals. J Clin Invest 4:399.
3. Sorenson J, Phelps M (1987) Physics in Nuclear Medicine, 2nd edn. Philadelphia, PA, W B Saunders Company.
4. Chandra R (2004) Nuclear Medicine Physics, 6th edn. Philadelphia, PA, Lippincott Williams & Wilkins.
5. Short M (1994) Basic principles of radionuclide physics. In Sampson C (ed). Textbook of Radiopharmacy: Theory and Practice, 2nd edn. Yverdon, Switzerland, Gordon & Breach Science Publishers.
6. Waksman R, King S, Crocker I, Mould R (1996) Vascular Brachytherapy. AX Veenendaal, Holland: Nucletron B.V.
7. Sharp P (1998) Nuclear medicine imaging. In Sharp P, Gemmel H, Smith F (eds). Practical Nuclear Medicine, 2nd edn. Oxford, Oxford University Press.
8. Ire-Celltarg (1989) Fundamentals of Radiopharmacy. Huntingdon, UK, Transart Pharmaceutical Ltd.
9. Larock M-P, Braat S, Sochor H, Maisey M, Rigo P (1993) New Developments in Myocardial Imaging: Technetium ^{99m}Tc Sestamibi. London, Martin Dunitz Ltd.
10. Ellestad M (2003) Stress Testing: Principles and Practice, 5th edn. Oxford, Oxford University Press.
11. Rigo P, Braat S (1994) Radiopharmaceuticals for the study of the heart. In: Murray I, Ell P (eds). Nuclear medicine in Clinical Diagnosis & Tereatment, 2nd edn. London, Chapman & Hall.
12. Lazarus C (1994) Radiopharmaceuticals. In Maisey M, Britton K, Gilday D (eds). Clinical Nuclear Medicine, New York, Churchill Livingstone.
13. Narula J, Flotats A, Nunn A, Carrio I (2003) Development of newer radiotracers for evaluation of myocardial and vascular disorders. In Iskandrian A, Verdani M (eds). Nuclear Cardiac Imaging, 3rd edn. Oxford, Oxford University Press.

Planar and SPECT Radiopharmaceuticals in Nuclear Cardiology: Current Status and Limitations

Chapter 19

Gopinath Gnanasegaran, Akhtar Ahmed, Jilly Croasdale and John R. Buscombe

Contents

19.1	Introduction	221
19.2	Common Radiopharamaceuticals Used in Nuclear Cardiology	222
19.2.1	201Thallium: Physical Characteristics, Biodistribution and Dosimetry	222
19.2.2	^{99m}Tc-Sestamibi [^{99m}Tc-Methoxyisobutyl Isoinitrile]: Physical Characteristics, Biodistribution and Dosimetry	224
19.2.3	^{99m}Tc-Tetrofosmin [^{99m}Tc-1, 2-bis [bis (2-Ethoxyethyl) Phosphino] Ethane]: Physical Characteristics, Biodistribution and Dosimetry	224
19.3	Miscellaneous Radiopharmaceuticals in Nuclear Cardiology	225
19.3.1	^{99m}Tc-Teboroxime(Cardiotec): Physical Characteristics, Biodistribution and Dosimetry	225
19.3.2	^{99m}Tc-Furifosmin: Physical Characteristics, Biodistribution and Dosimetry	225
19.3.3	^{99m}TcN-NOEt (N-Ethoxy-N-Ethyl-Dithiocarbamate) Nitrido: Physical Characteristics, Biodistribution and Dosimetry	227
19.3.4	Iodophenylpentadecanoic Acid (I-123 IPPA, and I-123-BMIPP)	227
19.3.5	Metaiodobenzylguanide (MIBG)	227
19.4	Conclusion	227
	References	227

19.1 Introduction

The branch of nuclear cardiology is ever expanding with newer indications for imaging the heart. Technical advancement in the instrumentation together with better radiopharmaceuticals has revolutionized the field of nuclear cardiology. Assessment of myocardial perfusion, function and metabolism using radiopharmaceuticals is a well-established method. There is a volume of literature supporting the role of radionuclide imaging in the assessment of a patient with suspected or diagnosed heart disease. Many different classes of radionuclide myocardial imaging agents are available. However, all these compounds have some advantages and disadvantages [1–6], and the final responsibility for choosing the right agent and protocols depends on the physician in charge. In general the team involved in providing a nuclear cardiology service should be made aware of the procedural guidelines for the use of radiopharmaceuticals [7] (Table 19.1).

The agents used to image perfusion and function of the myocardium should possess some ideal or near ideal properties [1,8–10] (Table 19.2). The radiopharmaceutical or radiotracer should be taken up by the myocardium in proportion to the regional myocardial blood flow. The myocardial uptake should be high and long enough in the myocardium to detect the difference over different regions of the myocardium [1, 8–10]. Most importantly the initial distribution should remain stable until the imaging is completed. The final product should have physical characteristics providing adequate photon flux and counting statistics for gamma camera imaging [1, 8–10]. Myocardial uptake of the tracer is affected by various factors; the commonest are variations in myocardial blood flow and myocardial extraction. An ideal radiopharmaceutical should not only possess these characteristics, but more importantly it should be cost-effective and easy to label or handle. In spite of all the wonderful advances, the quest to find an ideal radiopharmaceutical continues.

Table 19.1 Summary of Society of Nuclear Medicine (SNM) procedure guidelines for the use of radiopharmaceuticals. (Reprinted by permission of the Society of Nuclear Medicine from: Ronald J. Callahan, Henry M. Chilton, David A. Goodwin, Donald J. Hnatowich, James A. Ponto, Dennis P. Swanson, and Henry J. Royal. Procedure Guideline for Imaging with Radiopharmaceuticals: 1.0. J Nucl Med. 1996 37(12): 2092-2094.)

- The prescribing physician is responsible for: safety, quality, and correctness of all radiopharmaceuticals prepared and dispensed for administration under his/her direction.
- A comprehensive radiopharmaceutical quality control programme should be in place and implemented.
- The nuclear pharmacist is responsible for: safety, quality and correctness of radiopharmaceuticals prepared and dispensed under his/her supervision.
- The preparation, quality control, dispensing and patient administration of radiopharmaceuticals and adjunctive drugs may be delegated to qualified personnel, in accordance with local laws.
- Prior to administration, the identity of the radiopharmaceutical, patient and route of administration should be verified.
- Female patients who are post-menarche and pre-menopause should be asked about pregnancy, lactation and breast-feeding prior to administration.
- The quantity of radioactivity dispensed should be within 10% of the prescribed dose or dosage range and the actual quantity administered must be recorded in the patient's medical record.
- Radiopharmaceuticals should not be used beyond the manufacturer's recommended expiration date/time.
- Radiopharmaceuticals should be prepared according to manufacturer's instructions (aseptic procedures must be followed).
- Records of receipt, usage, administration and disposal of all radiopharmaceuticals shall be kept
- For all radiopharmaceuticals, the identity of the radiopharmaceutical, the amount of radioactivity administered, patient identity, identity of individual performing the administration, route of administration, and date and time of use must be recorded.
- Records of radionuclide dose calibrator testing (constancy, accuracy, linearity and geometric variation) should be maintained.
- Disposal of all radioactive material must be accomplished in accordance with institutional, state regulations.
- Adverse reactions associated with administration of radiopharmaceuticals should be investigated and documented.
- Misadministration of radiopharmaceutical should be reported and documented.
- Policies and procedures should be developed which assure that the correct patient receives the correct drug (at the correct time, correct dose and by the correct route).

Table 19.2 Basic characteristics of a myocardial perfusion tracer [1]

- Myocardial uptake of the tracer should be proportional to the regional myocardial blood flow (over wide range of blood flow)
- Myocardial uptake should be high to allow accurate discrimination between normal and abnormal areas
- Myocardial distribution should be stable from the time of injection until the time/completion of acquisition
- The tracer should be labelled to a ideal radionuclide having adequate physical characteristics (high photon flux and optimal counting statistics)

19.2
Common Radiopharmaceuticals Used in Nuclear Cardiology

19.2.1
201Thallium: Physical Characteristics, Biodistribution and Dosimetry

201-Thallium (201Tl) is a metallic element in-group IIIA of the periodic table. Thallium is a monovalent cation produced in the cyclotron [11] (Table 19.3). It decays by electron capture to Mercury 201 with a half-life of 73.1 hours [1]. It emits gamma photons with energies of 135 keV and 167 keV, and 201-Mercury emits mainly

Table 19.3 Summary and salient features of ^{201}Thallium [1, 11–14]

- ^{201}Thallium is a metallic element in group IIIA of the periodic table
- Biological similarities to potassium
- Monovalent cation
- Cyclotron produced
- Decays by electron capture (EC) to mercury (^{201}Hg)
- Physical half-life is 73.1 hours
- Biological half life is 10 days
- Emits predominantly mercury X-rays at 67–82 keV
- Principle photo peaks at 135 and 167 keV (12%)
- Requires no in-house preparation
- Single injection for stress and rest imaging
- First pass extraction is 60–70% (stress injection), 80-90% (rest injection)
- Maximum myocardial uptake is approximately 3.7–4% of injected dose
- Extraction decreases at higher flow rates
- Accumulation and retention depends on coronary blood flow and cellular viability
- Redistributes
- Critical organs: ovaries (0.73 mSv/MBq), kidneys (0.48 mSv/MBq), large intestine (0.32 mSv/MBq)
- Myocardial uptake has two components: early component (80% with half life of 4 hours) and delayed component (20% with half life of 40 hours)
- Disappearance from the blood compartment rapid and has two components: 92% disappears with a half life of 5 minutes and 8% with a half life of 40 hours
- Requires stringent imaging protocol (stress imaging should be completed by 30 minutes post- injection)
- Whole body effective dose is 0.22 mSv/MBq (rem/mCi) [80 MBq study =18 mSv]
- Excretion: faeces (80%), urine (20%)
- Limitations: Relatively long physical half life [high radiation burden], relatively low injected activity [low-signal to noise ratio, sub optimal images (obese), low counts levels [impairs high quality ECG-gating SPECT], relatively low energy emission [low resolution images and attenuation by soft tissues]

X-rays between 67 and 82 keV. At the time of calibration, contaminants such as ^{200}Tl, ^{202}Tl and ^{202}Pb can be present [1], however, they represent only about 2% of the total activity. 201Tl is a potassium analogue and uptake is mainly dependent upon a functioning sodium/potassium ATPase pump. There is also uptake via a non-energy-dependent facilitated diffusion (or co-transport system). Thallium is rapidly cleared from the blood with a myocardial first pass extraction efficiency of approximately 85% under normal basal flow/resting conditions [13]. Extraction of 201Tl decreases at higher flow rates; however, extraction is still superior to sestamibi and tetrofosmin [1, 13]. Approximately 3.7– 4% of the injected dose is taken up by the myocardium and peak myocardial activity usually occurs around 5–15 minutes post-injection [1]. The highest concentration is found in the kidneys, heart and liver. Myocardial uptake of thallium is by two components, with nearly 80% of the uptake by an early component and 20% by a delayed component [1]. Disappearance from the blood compartment is also by two components. About 92% of the activity disappears with a half-life of 5 minutes, the remaining activity clears with a half-life of 40 hours and kidneys are the target organs [1, 8, 9, 14]. According to European Commission guidelines, interruption of breast-feeding is not essential if the admintred activity is less than 80 MBq. If the injected activity is going to be more than 80 MBq, it is recommended that breast milk be expressed days beforehand and stored for use. Once 201Tl is injected, the first breast milk should be expressed and discarded [13, 16].

19.2.2
^{99m}Tc-Sestamibi [^{99m}Tc-Methoxyisobutyl Isoinitrile]: Physical Characteristics, Biodistribution and Dosimetry

Sestamibi is a lipophilic monovalent cation (an isonitrile compound) with a trade name of cardiolite. The myocardial uptake of ^{99m}Tc-sestamibi is dependent on multiple factors like mitochondrial-derived membrane electrochemical gradient, intact energy production pathways and cellular PH [1, 2, 8, 9, 15] (Table 19.4). Sestamibi will not be extracted by non-viable myocardium and in plasma, less than 1% is protein bound. A hyperpolarized state of plasma membrane and mitochondrial potentials increases the uptake and retention of ^{99m}Tc-sestamibi. The first pass extraction fraction for ^{99m}Tc-sestamibi is approximately 65%, which is lower than that for thallium [9, 17]. Only about 1–2% of the injected dose localizes to the myocardium at rest. However, this lower extraction fraction is overcome by injecting a larger dose, which in turn results in a higher count rate. The uptake in myocardium is proportional to blood flow in the physiologic flow range. However, at higher flow rates there is a plateau in extraction [9, 18]. The extraction plateau at high flow rates is reported to underestimate the blood flow. Myocardial clearance of ^{99m}Tc-sestamibi is slow and the agent does not redistribute like 201Tl. The main route of excretion is hepatobiliary (approximately 33%) with a half-life of approximately 30 minutes. The organs at risk are the gallbladder and kidneys. Although the breast takes up ^{99m}Tc-sestamibi, there is only minimal transfer to breast milk and cessation of breast-feeding is not essential [13, 16, 19].

19.2.3
^{99m}Tc-Tetrofosmin [^{99m}Tc-1, 2-bis [bis (2-Ethoxyethyl) Phosphino] Ethane]: Physical Characteristics, Biodistribution and Dosimetry

Tetrofosmin is a lipophilic, cationic compound, which is rapidly cleared from the blood following intravenous administration (Table 19.5) [9, 20, 21–26]. Approximately 1 to 1.5% of the injected dose is taken up by the myocardium. The uptake mechanism is membrane-potential driven diffusion independent of cation chan-

Table 19.4 Salient features of ^{99m}Tc-sestamibi [1, 10–14]

- Lipophilic monovalent cation
- Generator produced
- Emits gamma rays at 140 keV (89%)
- Decays by isomeric transition (IT)
- Physical half-life is 6 hours
- The biological half-life is approximately 11 hours
- Favourable myocardium to background radiation for myocardial imaging
- High energy photons decreases the problems of photon attenuation
- Myocardial uptake depends on normal mitochondria
- Distribution depends on plasma membrane and mitochondrial membrane potentials
- Once accumulated, it is bound in a relatively stable fashion
- Redistribution is negligible or partial [10–15%] (does not redistribute to a degree that can be imaged clinically)
- First pass extraction fraction is approximately 60% (rest injection), 40% (stress injection)
- 1–2% of the injected dose localizes to the myocardium at rest
- Higher dose compensates for lower extraction
- Flexible imaging protocols
- Separate injections for stress and rest imaging
- At higher flow rates there is a plateau in extraction
- Blood clearance is rapid and bi-exponential
- Whole body effective dose is 0.009 mSv/MBq at rest, 0.008 mSv/MBq at stress
- In a 1000 MBq study the effective dose will be 8.7 mSv
- The primary route of excretion is hepatobiliary (33%)
- Critical organs: gallbladder, kidneys and colon
- Preparation takes longer (includes a boiling step in water bath)
- Reconstituted shelf life is about 10 hours

Table 19.5 Salient features of ^{99m}Tc-tetrofosmin [1, 10–14]

- Lipophilic, cationic compound
- Generator produced
- Emits gamma rays at 140 keV
- Physical half-life is 6 hours
- Biological half-life is approximately 5 hours
- Approximately 1 to 1.5% of the injected dose is taken up by the myocardium
- Enters myocytes/myocardial cells by a passive transport mechanism driven by the intact cell with a negative membrane potential
- The agent accumulates within mitochondria similar to Tc-sestamibi. However, it is localized mostly in the cytosol and only a fraction passes into the mitochondria
- Rapid blood clearance
- Does not redistribute
- Flexible imaging protocols
- Separate injections for stress and rest imaging
- Hepatic uptake is lower than with Tc-Sestamibi and it also clears more quickly
- First pass extraction fraction is about 54%
- The myocardial extraction plateaus at higher flow rate
- Overestimates flow at low flow rates (0.2 mL/min/g)
- Higher dose compensates for lower extraction
- Whole body effective dose is 0.008 mSv/MBq at rest, 0.007 mSv/MBq at stress
- In a 1000 MBq study the effective dose will be 7.5 mSv
- Critical organs: gallbladder, bladder and colon
- Preparation requires no boiling in water bath
- Reconstituted shelf life is about 10 hours

nel transport [6]. The agent accumulates within mitochondria similar to ^{99m}Tc-sestamibi [9]. This agent, like ^{99m}Tc-sestamibi, does not redistribute to any significant degree. However, higher lipophilicity of the compound may explain its higher initial uptake and faster washout [6, 23–26]. The biological half-life for tetrofosmin in normal myocardium is around 5 hours, which is shorter than sestamibi (11 hours) [6]. Hepatic uptake is lower than with Tc-sestamibi and it also clears more quickly [1, 6, 22]. The mean first pass extraction fraction is about 54% [9]. ^{99m}Tc-tetrofosmin also has decreased tracer extraction compared with 201Tl at high flow rates. The myocardial extraction of ^{99m}Tc-tetrofosmin plateaus at a higher flow rate. Both at stress and rest the gallbladder is the target organ followed by the colon, bladder wall and small intestine [1, 6, 10, 20].

19.3
Miscellaneous Radiopharmaceuticals in Nuclear Cardiology

19.3.1
^{99m}Tc-Teboroxime(Cardiotec): Physical Characteristics, Biodistribution and Dosimetry

^{99m}Tc-teboroxime is a cationic compound (Table 19.6). It is a highly liphophilic and neutral compound. The molecular size of teboroxime is smaller that ^{99m}Tc-sestamibi and larger than 201Tl [1, 2, 10, 27]. ^{99m}Tc-teboroxime is reported to be one of the best compounds for both planar and SPECT imaging. The extraction fraction of ^{99m}Tc-teboroxime is higher than that of ^{99m}Tc-sestamibi and 201Tl [1, 2]. Myocardial uptake of ^{99m}Tc-teboroxime is independent of the metabolic status of the cells [1, 2, 10]. The myocardial uptake and clearance of ^{99m}Tc-teboroxime is rapid, myocardium is visualized in 1–2 minutes post-injection [1, 2, 27]. Clearance from the myocardium is bi-exponential, with 68% of the injected activity cleared with a half-life of 2 minutes, and the remainder in 78 minutes [1, 2, 27]. The large intestine and gallbladder are reported to be the target organs. Currently, this compound is not used clinically because of its technical limitations, such as rapid myocardial washout, early hepatic uptake, early imaging (to obtain high quality images, the imaging should begin within 2 minutes post-injection, and should be completed in less than 5–10 minutes post-injection) [1, 2, 27]. Further, due to rapid washout, the possibility of performing good quality gated SPECT studies may be limited [1]. To satisfy all these factors, we also require an ultrafast acquisition system [1, 27].

19.3.2
^{99m}Tc-Furifosmin: Physical Characteristics, Biodistribution and Dosimetry

^{99m}Tc-furifosmin is a cationic compound that is structurally different from ^{99m}Tc-tetrofosmin (Table 19.6) [1]. Unlike other ^{99m}Tc-MPS agents, the preparation kit does not contain stannous ion. The uptake and retention mechanism of ^{99m}Tc-furifosmin is similar to ^{99m}Tc-sestamibi and ^{99m}Tc-tetrofosmin [1]. The plasma clearance

Table 19.6 Salient features of miscellaneous MPS radiopharmaceuticals [1, 11, 13, 27–31]

Tc-Teboroxime (Cardiotec)	^{99m}Tc-furifosmin
• Neutral lipophilic boronic acid adduct of technetium dioxime (BATO) complex	• Belongs to the class of schiff base phosphine
• Myocardial extraction fraction is about 90% higher than thallium)	• Cation
• The extraction falls off less rapidly at high flow rates (than sestamibi or thallium)	• 2–2.2% of the injected activity is taken up by the myocardial uptake
• Rapid myocardial washout- the myocardial T1/2 is 10 to 11 minutes (>70% washout)	• Requires labelling (boiling/heating)
• Because of rapid washout, high speed imaging devices are required	• Does not redistribute
• 3–4% of the injected activity is taken up by the myocardial uptake	• Gallbladder is the target organ
• Requires labelling (boiling/heating)	**I-123 IPPA**
• Redistributes	• Synthetic long chain fatty acid with kinetics similar to palmitate
• Proximal/upper large intestine are the target organs	• First pass extraction of I-123 IPPA is less than that for thallium
• Timing of imaging is crucial to obtain high quality images.	• 4 to 5% of the injected localizes to the myocardium
• Acquisition should begin within 2 minutes of tracer injection and should be completed in less than 5 to 10 minutes after injection	• Lugol's solution should be given prior to the study (protect the thyroid)
^{99m}TcN-NOEt	• Myocardial ischemia inhibits fatty acid beta oxidation and will result in reduced uptake of the agent
• Belongs to the class of nitrodo compounds	• Metabolites rapidly excreted by the kidneys
• Neutral charge	**I-123-BMIPP**
• 3–3.5% of the injected activity is taken up by the myocardial uptake	• Iodine-123-BMIPP is a beta-methyl fatty acid analogue
• Requires labelling (boiling/heating)	• Prolonged myocardial residence time
• Redistributes	• Injected under fasting conditions
• Kidneys are the target organs	• Imaging is performed 20–30 minutes after administration
• High pulmonary activity	• Areas with reduced uptake represent ischemic, but viable myocardium

is bio-exponential with fast and slow clearance components. The myocardial uptake is 2.2% and 2.5% of the injected activity at 1 hour following rest and stress injections, respectively [1]. The principle target organs are the gallbladder, large and small intestine, kidneys and urinary bladder [1].

19.3.3
^{99m}TcN-NOEt (N-Ethoxy-N-Ethyl-Dithiocarbamate) Nitrido: Physical Characteristics, Biodistribution and Dosimetry

^{99m}TcN-NOEt belongs to the class of neutral MPS agents named ^{99m}Tc-nitrido dithiocarbamates (Table 19.6) [1]. ^{99m}TcN-NOEt is a highly lipophilic compound and is reported to overestimate coronary blood flow in the low flow range and underestimate it in the high flow range. The first extraction in an animal model was 75%+4% (basal conditions) and 85%+2% (hyperaemic conditions) [1]. Structural membrane integrity is important for retention of ^{99m}TcN-NOEt in the myocardium. The cell membranes are reported to be the most probable site of subcellular localization of ^{99m}TcN-NOEt [1]. The principal target organ is the kidney [1]. Although, its characteristics are reported to be similar to thallium, the high lung uptake may compromise the image quality [11].

19.3.4
Iodophenylpentadecanoic Acid (I-123 IPPA, and I-123-BMIPP)

19.3.4.1 I-123 IPPA

I-123 IPPA is a single photon-labelled synthetic long chain fatty acid with kinetics similar to palmitate [28, 29]. In general the free fatty acids circulate in the plasma bound to albumin and cross the cell membrane by passive diffusion. Once inside the cell, fatty acids can either back diffuse or become activated by acyl-CoA synthetase [28, 29]. Once the latter step occurs, fatty acids become polar and are trapped inside the cell where they can either undergo beta-oxidation (within the mitochondria) or be incorporated into the intracellular lipid pool [28, 29]. Myocardial ischaemia inhibits fatty acid beta-oxidation and will result in reduced uptake (due to diminished perfusion) and delayed clearance of tracer activity from these regions [28, 29]. Infarcted myocardium demonstrates markedly reduced initial uptake of the agent, and no significant metabolism over time [28–31].

19.3.4.2 123Iodine Labelled 15-(p-Iodophenyl)3-R, S-Methylpentadecanoic Acid (BMIPP)

BMIPP is a beta-methyl fatty acid analogue in which methyl branching is introduced to inhibit beta oxidation [28, 29]. BMIPP undergoes slower oxidation and clearance by incorporation into the endogenous lipid pool, which results in prolonged residence time. Because the agent is retained in the myocardium for some time, it is more useful for SPECT imaging with a conventional gamma camera. BMIPP is usually injected under fasting conditions and imaging is performed 20–30 minutes after administration [28, 29]. BMIPP is a very sensitive indicator of metabolic alterations in ischaemic myocardium. The areas with reduced uptake of BMIPP are felt to represent ischaemic, but viable myocardium, and these areas have been shown to demonstrate a metabolic-perfusion mismatch on PET studies [28–31].

19.3.5
Metaiodobenzylguanide (MIBG)

Metaiodobenzyl guanidine is an analogue of guanethidine and behaves in a manner that is qualitatively similar to norepinephrine, a transmitter of the adrenergic system in the heart [32–34]. MIBG is labelled with 123 Iodine and the half-life and energy is 13.3 hours and 159 keV (83%), respectively [11]. 123I-MIBG is the most commonly used tracer for cardiac innervation imaging. After MIBG injection, the tracer is internalized by presynaptic nerve endings of postganglionic neuronal cells through the energy-dependent uptake-1 system. In addition, MIBG enters the presynaptic nerve endings through the uptake-2 system, the activity of which is low in the human heart [35]. After neuronal depolarization, MIBG is released in the synapse cleft but is not metabolized by enzymes as norepinephrine [32–35].

19.4
Conclusion

Different radiopharmaceuticals are available for imaging the myocardium. They all play an important role in the diagnosis and management of ischaemic heart disease. The choice of radiopharmaceuticals should be based on the clinical questions to be answered. The choice of compound used depends on a weighing up of the advantages and disadvantages of each tracer and making a clinical decision on which will give the best information.

References

1. Taillefer R (2001) Radiopharmaceuticals, in Cardiac SPECT Imaging, 2nd edn, DePuey EG, Garcia EV, Berman DS (eds). Lippincot Williams and Wilkins, Philadelphia, PA, pp. 117–154.
2. Leppo JA, DePuey EG, Johnson LL (1991) A review of cardiac imaging with sestamibi and teboroxime. J Nucl Med 32:2012–2122.

3. Jain D, Wackers FJTh, Mattera J, McMahon M, Sinusas AJ, Zaret BL (1993) Biokinetics of technetium-99m-tetrofosmin: myocardial perfusion imaging agent: implications for a one day imaging protocol. J Nucl Med 34:1254–1259.
4. Kelley JD, Forster AM, Higley B, Archer CM et al. (1993) Technetium-99m-tetrofosmin a new radiopharmaceutical for myocardial perfusion imaging. J Nucl Med 34:222–227.
5. Brown KA, Altland E, Rowen M (1994) Prognostic value of normal technetium-99m-sestamibi cardiac imaging. J Nucl Med 35:554–557.
6. Munch G, Neverve J, Matsunari I, Schroter G, Schwaiger M (1997) Myocardial technetium-99m-tetrofosmin and technetium-99m-sestamibi kinetics in normal subjects and patients with coronary artery disease. J Nucl Med 38:428–432.
7. Callahan RJ, Chilton HM, Goodwin DA, Hnatowich DJ, Ponto JA, Swanson DP, Royal HJ (1996) Procedure guideline for imaging with radiopharmaceuticals: 1.0. Society of Nuclear Medicine. J Nucl Med 37(12):2092–2094.
8. Beller GA, Watson DD (1991) Physiological basis of myocardial perfusion imaging with the technetium 99m agents. Semin Nucl Med 2:173–181.
9. Beller GA, Bergmann SR (2004) Myocardial perfusion imaging agents: SPECT and PET. J Nucl Cardiol 11:71–86.
10. Jain D (1999) Technetium labeled myocardial perfusion imaging agents. Semin Nucl Med 29:221–236.
11. Prvulovich L (2004) Radiopharmaceutical for the study of the heart. In Nuclear Medicine In Clinical Diagnosis and Treatment, 3rd edn, Ell PJ, Gambhir SS (eds). Churchill Livingstone, pp. 1015–1022.
12. Atkins HL, Budinger TF, Lebowitz E, Ansari AN, Greene MW, Fairchild RG, Ellis KJ. (1977) Thallium-201 for medical use. Part 3: Human distribution and physical imaging properties. J Nucl Med 18(2):133–140.
13. Hesse B, Tagil K, Cuocolo A et al. (2005) EANM/ESC procedural guidelines for myocardial perfusion imaging in nuclear cardiology. Eur J Nucl Med Mol Imaging 32(7):855–897.
14. International Commission on Radiological Protection (1998) IRCP publication 80. Radiation dose to patients from radiopharmaceuticals. Elsevier Science, Oxford.
15. Mandalapu BP, Amato M, Stratmann HG (1999) Technetium Tc 99m Sestamibi myocardial perfusion imaging. Current role for evaluation of prognosis. Chest 115:1684–1694.
16. EC (1998) Radiation Protection 100. Guidance for protection of unborn children and infants irradiated due to parental medical exposures. European Commission on line publication catalogue 1998.
17. Wackers FJTh, Berman DS, Maddahi J et al. (1989) Technetium-99m hexakis 2-methoxyisobutyl isonitrile: human biodistribution, dosimetry, safety and preliminary-comparison to thallium-201 for myocardial perfusion imaging. J Nucl Med 30:301–311.
18. Taki J, Fujino S, Nakajima K, Matsunari I, Okazaki H, Saga T, Bunko H, Tonami N (2001) ^{99m}Tc-sestamibi retention characteristics during pharmacologic hyperemia in human myocardium: comparison with coronary flow reserve measured by doppler flowire. J Nucl Med 42:1457–1463.
19. Klopper RS et al. (1994) The excretion of radiopharmaceuticals in human breast milk: Additional data and dosimetry. Eur J Nucl Med 21:144–153.
20. Jain D, Zaret BL (1998) Technetium 99m tetrofosmin. In New Developments in Cardiac Nuclear Imaging, 1st edn. Iskandrian AE, Verani MS (eds). Futura Publishing, Armonk, NY, pp. 29–58.
21. Higley B, Smith FW, Smith T et al. (1993) Technetium-99m-1,2 bis[bis(2-ethoxyethyl)phosphino]ethane: human biodistribution, dosimetry and safety of a new
22. myocardial perfusion imaging agent. J Nucl Med 34:30–38.
23. Cuocolo A, Soricelli A, Nicolai E, Squame F et al. (1995) Technetium-99m-tetrofosmin regional myocardial uptake at rest: relation to severity of coronary artery stenosis in previous myocardial infarction. J Nucl Med 36:907–913.
24. Sinusas AJ, Shi Q, Saltzberg MT, Vitols P, Jain D, Wackers FJ, Zaret BL (1994) Technetium-99m-tetrofosmin to assess myocardial blood flow: experimental validation in an intact canine model of ischemia. J Nucl Med 35(4):664–671.
25. Arbab AS, Koizumi K, Toyama K, Arai T, Araki T (1998) Technetium-99m-tetrofosmin, technetium-99m-MIBI and thallium-201 uptake in rat myocardial cells. J Nucl Med 39(2):266–271.
26. Platts EA, North TL, Pickett RD, Kelly JD (1995) Mechanism of uptake of technetium-tetrofosmin. I: Uptake into isolated adult rat ventricular myocytes and subcellular localization. J Nucl Cardiol 2(4):317–326.
27. Younès A, Songadele JA, Maublant J, Platts E, Pickett R, Veyre A (1995) Mechanism of uptake of technetium-tetrofosmin. II: Uptake into isolated adult rat heart mitochondria. J Nucl Cardiol 2(4):327–333.
28. Hendel RC, McSherry B, Karimeddini M, Leppo JA (1990) Diagnostic value of a new myocardial perfusion agent, teboroxime (SQ 30,217), utilizing a rapid planar imaging protocol: preliminary results. J Am Coll Cardiol 16:855–861.
29. Hansen CL, Heo J, Oliner C, Van Decker W, Iskandrian AS (1995) Prediction of improvement in left ventricular function with iodine-123-IPPA after coronary revascularization. J Nucl Med 36:1987–1993.
30. Tamaki N, Tadamura E, Kawamoto M et al. (1995) Decreased uptake of iodinated branched fatty acid analog indicates metabolic alterations in ischemic myocardium. J Nucl Med 36:1974–1980.

31. Tamaki N, Morita K, Kuge Y, Tsukamoto E (2000) The role of fatty acids in cardiac imaging. J Nucl Med 41:1525–1534.
32. Shi CQ, Young LH, Daher E et al. (2002) Correlation of myocardial p-123-iodophenylpentadecanoic acid retention with 18F-FDG accumulation during experimental low-flow ischemia. J Nucl Med 43:421–431.
33. Kline RC, Swanson DP, Wieland DM, Thrall JH, Gross MD, Pitt B et al. (1981) Myocardial imaging in man with I-123 meta-iodobenzylguanidine. J Nucl Med 22:129–32.
34. Wieland DM, Brown LE, Rogers WL, Worthington KC, Wu JL, Clinthorne NH et al. (1981) Myocardial imaging with a radioiodinated norepinephrine storage analog. J Nucl Med 22:22–31.
35. Sisson JC, Wieland DM, Sherman P, Mangner TJ, Tobes MC, Jacques S Jr (1987) Metaiodobenzylguanidine as an index of the adrenergic nervous system integrity and function. J Nucl Med 28:1620–1624.
36. Dae MW, De Marco T, Botvinick EH, O'Connell JW, Hattner RS, Huberty JP et al. (1992) Scintigraphic assessment of MIBG uptake in globally denervated human and canine hearts--implications for clinical studies. J Nucl Med 33:1444–1450.

Further Reading

1. DePuey EG, Garcia EV, Berman DS (2001) Cardiac SPECT Imaging, 2nd edn. Lippincot Williams and Wilkins, Philadelphia, PA.
2. Heo J, Iskandrian AS (1994) Technetium-labelled myocardial perfusion agents. Cardiol Clinics 12(2):187–198.
3. Maddahi J, Rodrigues E, Berman DS, Kiat H (1994) State of the art myocardial perfusion imaging. Cardiol Clinics 12:199–222.
4. Hesse B, Tagil K, Cuocolo A et al. (2005) EANM/ESC procedural guidelines for myocardial perfusion imaging in nuclear cardiology. Eur J Nucl Med Mol Imaging 32(7):855–897.

Myocardial Perfusion Imaging for Risk Stratification in Suspected or Known Coronary Artery Disease: Current Status and Limitations

Firas A. Ghanem and Assad Movahed

Contents

20.1	Introduction	231
20.2	Chronic Stable Angina	231
20.3	Acute Coronary Syndrome (ACS)	232
20.4	Asymptomatic Patients	234
20.5	MPI in Women	234
20.6	Limitations	234
20.7	Conclusion	234
	References	235

20.1 Introduction

Coronary artery disease (CAD) remains the leading cause of morbidity and mortality in the western world. Early detection and risk stratification of underlying (CHD) is a major step in clinical decision-making. As discussed in the other chapters, myocardial perfusion imaging (MPI) using thallium-201(Tl-201) or technetium-99m (Tc-99m) sestamibi or tetrofosmin, is used in various clinical settings to provide invaluable information on myocardial perfusion, left ventricular volumes and left ventricular function, and prognosis. MPI has the ability to localize hemodynamically important coronary stenosis; thus yielding positive results by increasing demand myocardial ischemia during exercise or inducing inhomogeneous distribution of radiotracers during pharmacological stress testing with dipyridamole or adenosine [1].

20.2 Chronic Stable Angina

Significant CAD is defined angiographically as CAD with greater than or equal to 70% diameter stenosis of at least one major epicardial artery segment or greater than or equal to 50% diameter stenosis of the left main coronary artery. Although lesions of less stenosis can cause angina, they have much less prognostic significance [2]. For patients with chronic chest pain syndromes, testing is directed towards establishing the presence or absence of CAD to guide therapy and determine prognosis. Special consideration needs to be given to establishing the pre-test probability of CAD based on the patient's history, physical examination and risk factor assessment [3]. Those with an intermediate to high pre-test probability of CAD are considered the best candidates for single-photon emission computed tomography myocardial perfusion imaging (SPECT MPI) whereas it is deemed inappropriate for patients with low pre-test probability [4]. The referral bias can influence the sensitivity and specificity of MPI. While most patients with an abnormal scan undergo coronary angiography, few patients with a normal MPI are referred for invasive procedures. Referral bias may result in an overestimation of test sensitivity and an underestimation of test specificity. Reported sensitivities (the percentage of abnormal images in patients with significant CAD) of exercise and vasodilator stress SPECT MPI are 87% and 89% respectively; while specificities (the percentage of normal images in patients without significant CAD) are 73% and 75% [1]. In patients with stable symptoms, a normal stress Tc-99m sestamibi SPECT MPI was associated with a very low risk of death or nonfatal myocardial infarction (0.6% annually) in contrast to a 12-fold higher event rate (7.4% annually) in patients with abnormal images (fixed or reversible defects) [5]. Similar results were reported using Tl-201 [6]. Moreover, a normal stress MPI study carries similar satisfactory outcomes in stable angina patients with significant angiographic disease. The annual rate of cardiac death or nonfatal myocardial infarction in these patients, remains less than 1% per year, comparable with the overall event rate in patients with a normal scan who had documented CAD [7].

MPI in high risk or low risk patients may not be appropriate for prognostic purposes, because they are already risk stratified sufficiently for clinical decision making [1]. A clear paradox exists in that most acute coronary syndromes occur in lesions causing less than <50% stenosis as a result of a rupture of high-risk and vulnerable plaque [8]. A potential explanation is coronary endothelial dysfunction that may lead to differential response of minimally obstructive CAD lesions to stress, leading to temporal myocardial perfusion defects [9]. Supporting this theory is the improvement in MPI with the use of statins. Schwartz et al. showed that serial SPECT MPI demonstrated improved stress myocardial perfusion in 48% of patients treated for six months with pravastatin, despite poor correlation with improvements in lipids [10]. Another potential explanation is that patients with severe CAD, and hence extensively abnormal MPI, may have other small lesions susceptible to rupture [8]. Therefore, stress perfusion imaging identifies the patient at risk for acute coronary events regardless of the anatomic significance of the lesion. Given the likelihood of CAD progression with time, the prediction of low-risk outcome following a normal MPI extends to probably no more than two years after testing [11].

Patients with remote myocardial infarction may also benefit from stress MPI for prediction of subsequent cardiac events. Zellweger et al. found that patients with mildly, moderately, or severely abnormal scans based on the summed stress score had annual hard event rates of 2.4%, 3.7%, and 5.9%, respectively [12].

In general, stress imaging procedures are preferable to exercise electrocardiography (ECG) when resting ECG abnormalities (left ventricular hypertrophy, digoxin, more than one millimeter ST depression) preclude adequate interpretation of the exercise ECG. Also, if the resting ECG shows an electronically paced ventricular rhythm or left bundle-branch block, dipyridamole or adenosine myocardial perfusion imaging is preferred [2]. Dobutamine stress does not provoke as great an increase in coronary flow as do coronary vasodilators (dipyridamole or adenosine) and is less ideal for stress MPI and should generally be restricted to patients with contraindications to direct coronary vasodilators [1]. Integration of the severity of ischemia, left ventricular functional status, lung-to-heart ratio and the presence of transient ischemic dilatation of the left ventricle (LV) improves post-test stratification of patients into low, intermediate, and high risk of cardiac death, and help guide clinical decision-making and referral for coronary angiography and revascularization [13–15].

20.3
Acute Coronary Syndrome (ACS)

In the emergency department (ED), the differentiation between cardiac and noncardiac chest pain is often difficult despite meticulous initial evaluation. Acute coronary syndrome refers to any constellation of clinical symptoms that are compatible with acute myocardial ischemia. It includes ST-segment elevation myocardial infarction (STEMI), non-ST-segment elevation myocardial infarction (NSTEMI), as well as unstable angina (UA). Using a careful history, physical examination, 12-lead ECG, and initial cardiac marker tests, chest pain can be divided according to risk level into a noncardiac diagnosis, chronic stable angina, possible ACS, and definite ACS. It also identifies those who need immediate reperfusion therapy [16]. In the absence of markers of ischemia or obvious abnormalities on initial ECG (possible ACS), rest Tc-99m sestamibi perfusion imaging is appropriate and can reduce unnecessary hospitalizations among patients without acute ischemia [17]. Tc-99m-sestamibi or tetrofosmin are suitable for acute imaging at the ED as they remain trapped in the myocardium and do not redistribute, enabling later imaging. Tl-201, on the other hand, is not a practical tracer for the imaging of acute chest pain patients in the ED as it redistributes in the myocardium over time and needs immediate imaging after injection [1]. While rest MPI is useful for diagnosis of an acute myocardial infarction by identifying perfusion defects, such defects do not distinguish between acute ischemia, acute infarction, or previous infarction. The sensitivity of rest MPI in patients with acute chest pain is similar to serial creatine kinase–MB and troponin analysis but is maximal at the onset of acute infarction and immediately reflects the status of regional myocardial blood flow at the time of tracer injection [1]. The negative predictive value (NPV) of SPECT MPI to exclude myocardial infarction in these patients ranges from 99% to 100% and the NPV for excluding future cardiac events during medium-term follow-up is approximately 97% [18]. Current practice favors using coronary angiography for delineation of coronary anatomy as the basis for decision management in acute coronary syndrome.

The American College of Cardiology and the American Heart Association (ACC/AHA) recommends an early invasive strategy in UA/NSTEMI for any of the following high-risk patients: (a) recurrent angina/ischemia at rest or with low level activities despite intensive anti-ischemic therapy; (b) elevated ischemic markers; (c) new or presumably new ST-segment depression; (d) hemodynamic instability, heart failure signs or symptoms, or depressed LV systolic function (e.g., left ventricular ejection fraction < 0.40 on noninvasive study; (e) high-risk findings on noninvasive stress testing; (f) sustained ventricular tachycardia; (g) percutaneous coronary intervention within 6 months or prior coronary artery bypass graft surgery [16]. In the absence of these findings, the guidelines suggest that either an early conservative or invasive approach is reasonable. Dakik et al. evaluated the prognostic value of pre-discharge quantitative stress nuclear MPI in an unstable angina cohort without high-risk indicators of elevated biomarkers or ischemic electrocardiographic changes on presentation. Over a mean 31-month follow-up, they found that the best multivariate predictors of death or MI were total perfusion defect size, the presence of reversible perfusion defects, and the presence of multiple perfusion defects. Notably, cardiac events were much more likely to develop in patients with defects involving 15% or more of the left ventricle [19] In medically stabilized US/NSTEMI patients, stress gated. SPECT MPI is appropriate for (1) detection of inducible ischemia in the distribution of the "culprit lesion" or in remote areas in patients at intermediate or low risk for major adverse cardiac events; (2) recognition of the severity/extent of inducible ischemia; (3) identification of hemodynamic significance of coronary stenosis after coronary arteriography; and (4) measurement of baseline LV function [1]. In patients with STEMI, MPI remains an accurate method for risk-stratifying patients after acute reperfusion therapy. The importance of MPI in this setting emerges from the common recurrence of cardiac events, and the prevalence of scintigraphic ischemia vs. ischemic ST-segment depression during exercise (38% vs. 15%) in patients who underwent thrombolytic therapy [20]. Exercise and pharmacologic stress MPI can predict the outcome in patients following thrombolytic therapy. Travin et al. reported that the presence of either ischemia as seen on SPECT or defects in multiple vascular territories identified 92% of patients who subsequently experienced an event after hospital discharge [21]. Brown et al. reported that dipyridamole ^{99m}Tc-sestamibi MPI performed 2–4 days after admission for STEMI was superior to predischarge (day 6 to 12) submaximal exercise MPI. Dipyridamole MPI showed that the extent and severity of defect reversibility had significant prognostic value for predicting early and late cardiac events [22]. Similarly, by using adenosine Tl-201MPI, Mahmarian et al. showed that the predictors of all cardiac events were perfusion defect size, absolute extent of left ventricular ischemia and ejection fraction. Death was best predicted by total perfusion defect size [23]. As post-thrombolysis patients who lack ischemia by noninvasive testing have an excellent prognosis, it seems unlikely that routine late coronary revascularization in this population would further improve outcomes [24]. The adenosine sestamibi post-infarction evaluation (INSPIRE) trial is currently underway using adenosine SPECT for risk assessment of post-infarction patients. A high-risk subgroup of this cohort with inducible ischemia was then randomized to maximal medical therapy or maximal medical therapy plus revascularization. Preliminary results demonstrated that the greater the SPECT perfusion defect size, the greater the subsequent cardiac event rate. Interestingly, in the high-risk randomized population, intensive medical therapy or intensive medical therapy plus revascularization yielded a comparable change in total defect size and ischemic defect size [25]. Current guidelines recommend exercise or pharmacological MPI before or early after discharge in patients with STEMI who are not undergoing cardiac catheterization to look for inducible ischemia. MPI is also reasonable in hemodynamically and electrically stable patients 4 to 10 days after STEMI to assess myocardial viability when required to define the potential efficacy of revascularization. A small fixed perfusion defect indicates an excellent prognosis, and probably low benefit from revascularization. On the other hand, patients with markers of increased risk (number and severity of myocardial perfusion defects, transient LV dilation, and increased tracer lung uptake) could be referred for coronary angiography and revascularization [1].

20.4
Asymptomatic Patients

Using the Bayesian principles in establishing pretest probability, the relatively low prevalence of CAD in the general asymptomatic population will translate into low positive predictive value even in the presence of abnormal MPI [1]. The American College of Cardiology Foundation (ACCF) and the American Society of Nuclear Cardiology (ASNC) recommend against routine stress imaging studies in asymptomatic patients without chest pain syndrome with the exception of patients with moderate to high CHD risk and the presence of new-onset or diagnosed heart failure, new-onset atrial fibrillation, ventricular tachycardia, those with high-risk occupation (e.g., airline pilot) or evaluation of ventricular function with the use of potentially cardiotoxic therapy (e.g., Doxorubicin) [4]. SPECT MPI is of particular importance in the evaluation of silent myocardial ischemia in moderate risk patients undergoing major vascular surgery, type II diabetics, chronic hemodialysis patients and transplant recipients [26–28].

20.5
MPI in Women

Cardiovascular disease is one of the principal causes of death in women. Women have been generally underrepresented in the major trials of coronary artery diagnosis, contributing to the paucity of gender-specific data on the performance of MPI. It is well perceived that exercise electrocardiography (ECG) has lower diagnostic accuracy in women, in particular because of the occurrence of ≥1 mm of ST segment depression. In women, exercise ECG has an average sensitivity and specificity of 61% and 70% [29]. Critical factors that have been reported to affect test accuracy in women include age at presentation, inability to attain maximal exercise, resting ST-T-wave changes in hypertensive women, lower electrocardiographic voltage, and hormonal factors [30]. These limitations have led to increased interest in the potential additive benefit of stress MPI in women, particularly those with an intermediate–high pretest likelihood of CAD. A retrospective analysis of more than 4000 men and women, who underwent rest Tl-201/exercise Tc-99m-sestamibi SPECT imaging reported incremental prognostic value of MPI compared with clinical and exercise variables in women as well as men. This modality identified relatively high risk women more accurately than relatively high risk men [31]. Factors associated with suboptimal accuracy are small heart size, breast artefact, and the prevalence of single-vessel disease. The use of ^{99m}Tc-sestamibi, or tetrofosmin improves SPECT accuracy [30]. Women incapable of performing a minimum of 5 METS of exercise should be considered candidates for myocardial perfusion imaging with pharmacologic stress. Using adenosine technetium-99m sestamibi MPI, Amanullah et al. reported 91% sensitivity and 86% specificity for detecting coronary disease in 130 women without prior MI, and documented a normalcy rate of 93% in 71 women with a low likelihood of coronary disease [32]. In women undergoing exercise myocardial perfusion imaging, the number of abnormal territories remained the strongest correlate of mortality after adjustment for exercise variables [33].

20.6
Limitations

As discussed earlier, the use of MPI has inherent major limitations to its accuracy mainly tissue attenuation artefacts, photon scatter, motion artefacts, and limited spatial resolution. Medications such as beta-blockers, calcium channel blocking agents and long-acting nitrates may limit the development of ischemia during the exercise test or decrease the extent of perfusion defects [1]. The level of exercise may also affect the sensitivity of SPECT MPI in the localization and evaluation of the extent of coronary artery disease and the detection of ischemia [34]. In the setting of ACS, the availability of alternative methods and the logistics and time demands of performing MPI in the setting of AMI have limited its widespread clinical application [1]. STEMI patients treated with thrombolysis have a low overall mortality and as a result the ability of a positive early scan to predict poor outcomes may be inadequate [35]. In extensive CAD, SPECT MPI may not show the typical pattern of multi-vessel disease and may not necessarily reflect involvement of more than one vessel [36]. Some scintigraphic features such as transient ischemic dilatation and increased lung uptake of tracer (201Tl) represent useful predictors of extensive CAD [37, 38].

20.7
Conclusion

Stress SPECT MPI provides incremental diagnostic and prognostic value in patients at an intermediate or high pretest likelihood of CAD or patients with known CAD. Patients who exhibit normal myocardial perfusion and function or have a small defect with normal left ventricular function have an excellent prognosis. Patients with a high-risk scan may benefit from an invasive strategy and possible revascularization. In women SPECT MPI is superior to stress ECG for detection of CAD when patients are unable to exercise or with the presence of resting ECG abnormalities.

References

1. Klocke FJ, Baird MG, Lorell BH et al. (2003) ACC/AHA/ASNC guidelines for the clinical use of cardiac radionuclide imaging. A report of the American College of Cardiology/American Heart Association Task Force on Practice Guidelines (ACC/AHA/ASNC Committee to Revise the 1995 Guidelines for the Clinical Use of Cardiac Radionuclide Imaging). American College of Cardiology Web Site. Available at: http://www.acc.org/clinical/guidelines/radio/index.pdf. Accessed June 04, 2006.
2. Gibbons RJ, Chatterjee K, Daley J et al. (2002) ACC/AHA 2002 guideline update for the management of patients with chronic stable angina: a report of the American College of Cardiology/American Heart Association Task Force on Practice Guidelines (Committee to Update the 1999 Chronic Stable Angina Guidelines). American College of Cardiology Web Site. Available at:http://www.acc.org/clinical/guidelines/stable/stable_clean.pdf. Accessed June 4, 2006.
3. Koller D (2002) Assessing diagnostic performance in nuclear cardiology. J Nucl Cardiol 9(1):114–123.
4. Brindis RG, Douglas PS, Hendel RC, Peterson ED et al. (2005) ACCF/ASNC appropriateness criteria for single-photon emission computed tomography myocardial perfusion imaging (SPECT MPI): a report of the American College of Cardiology Foundation Quality Strategic Directions Committee Appropriateness Criteria Working Group and the American Society of Nuclear Cardiology endorsed by the American Heart Association. J Am Coll Cardiol 46(8):1587–1605.
5. Iskander S, Iskandrian AE (1998) Risk assessment using singlephoton emission computed tomographic technetium-99m sestamibi imaging. J Am Coll Cardiol 32:57–62.
6. Brown KA (1991) Prognostic value of thallium-201 myocardial perfusion imaging: a diagnostic tool comes of age. Circulation 83:363–381.
7. Brown K (1996) Prognostic value of myocardial perfusion imaging: state of the art and new developments. J Nucl Cardiol 3:516.
8. Little WC, Constantinescu M, Applegate RJ (1988) Can coronary angiography predict the site of a subsequent myocardial infarction in patients with mild-to-moderate coronary artery disease? Circulation 78(5Pt 1):1157–1166.
9. Hasdai D, Gibbons RJ, Holmes DR Jr, Higano ST, Lerman A (1997) Coronary endothelial dysfunction in humans is associated with myocardial perfusion defects. Circulation 96(10):3390–3395.
10. Schwartz RG, Pearson TA, Kalaria VG et al. (2003) Prospective serial evaluation of myocardial perfusion and lipids during the first six months of pravastatin therapy: coronary artery disease regression single photon emission computed tomography monitoring trial. J Am Coll Cardiol 42:600–610.
11. Hachamovitch R, Hayes S, Friedman JD et al. (2003) Determinants of risk and its temporal variation in patients with normal stress myocardial perfusion scans. What is the warranty period of a normal scan? J Am Coll Cardiol 41:1329.
12. Zellweger MJ, Dubois EA, Lai S, et al. (2002) Risk stratification in patients with remote prior myocardial infarction using rest-stress myocardial perfusion SPECT: prognostic value and impact on referral to early catheterization. J Nucl Cardiol 9:23–32.
13. Sharir T, Germano G, Kang X et al. (2001) Prediction of myocardial infarction versus cardiac death by gated myocardial perfusion SPECT: risk stratification by the amount of stress-induced ischemia and the poststress ejection fraction. J Nucl Med 42: 831–837.
14. Leslie WD, Tully SA, Yogendran MS et al. (2005) Prognostic value of lung sestamibi uptake in myocardial perfusion imaging of patients with known or suspected coronary artery disease. J Am Coll Cardiol 45(10):1676–1682.
15. Abidov A, Bax JJ, Hayes SW et al. (2003) Transient ischemic dilation ratio of the left ventricle is a significant predictor of future cardiac events in patients with otherwise normal myocardial perfusion SPECT J Am Coll Cardiol 42(10):1818-1825.
16. Braunwald E, Antman E, Beasley J, et al. ACC/AHA 2002 guideline update for the management of patients with unstable angina and non-ST-segment elevation myocardial infarction: a report of the American College of Cardiology/American Heart Association Task Force on Practice Guidelines A Report of the American College of Cardiology/American Heart Association Task Force on Practice Guidelines (Committee on the Management of Patients With Unstable Angina); Available at: http://www.acc.org/clinical/guidelines/unstable/unstable.pdf. Accessed June 04, 2006.
17. Udelson JE, Beshansky JR, Ballin DS, et al. (2002) Myocardial perfusion imaging for evaluation and triage of patients with suspected acute cardiac ischemia: a randomized controlled trial. J Am Med Assoc 288:2693–2700.
18. Wackers FJTh, Brown KA, Heller GV et al. (2002) American Society of Nuclear Cardiology position statement on radionuclide imaging in patients with suspected acute ischemic syndromes in the emergency department or chest pain center. Am J Nucl Cardiol 9:246–250.
19. 19 Dakik HA, Hwang WS, Jafar A, Kimball K, Verani MS, Mahmarian JJ (2005) Prognostic value of quantitative stress myocardial perfusion imaging in unstable angina patients with negative cardiac enzymes and no new ischemic ECG changes. J Nucl Cardiol 12:32–36.
20. Dakik HA, Mahmarian JJ, Kimball KT et al. (1996) Prognostic value of exercise thallium-201 tomography in patients treated with thrombolytic therapy during acute myocardial infarction. Circulation 94:2735–2742.

21. Travin MI, Dessouki A, Cameron T, Heller GV (1995) Use of exercise technetium-99m sestamibi SPECT imaging to detect residual ischemia and for risk stratification after acute myocardial infarction. Am J Cardiol 75:665–669.
22. Brown KA, Heller GV, Landin RS et al. (1999) Early dipyridamole ^{99m}Tc-sestamibi single photon emission computed tomographic imaging 2 to 4 days after acute myocardial infarction predicts in-hospital and postdischarge cardiac events: comparison with submaximal exercise imaging. Circulation 100:2060–2066.
23. Mahmarian JJ, Mahmarian AC, Marks GF, Pratt CM, Verani MS (1995) Role of adenosine thallium-201 tomography for defining long-term risk in patients after acute myocardial infarction. J Am Coll Cardiol 25:1333–1340.
24. Ellis SG, Mooney MR, George BS et al. (1992) Randomized trial of late elective angioplasty versus conservative management for patients with residual stenoses after thrombolytic treatment of myocardial infarction. Treatment of Post Thrombolytic Stenoses (TOPS) Study Group. Circulation 86:1400–1406.
25. Beller GA (2004) Nuclear cardiology in randomized multicenter clinical trials. J Nucl Cardiol 11(3):235–236.
26. Eagle KA, Coley CM, Newell JB et al. (1989) Combining clinical and thallium data optimizes preoperative assessment of cardiac risk before major vascular surgery. Ann Internal Med 110(11):859–866.
27. Wackers FJ, Young LH, Inzucchi SE et al. Detection of silent myocardial ischemia in asymptomatic diabetic subjects: the DIAD study. Diabetes Care 27(8):1954–1961.
28. Derfler K, Kletter K, Balcke P, Heinz G, Dudczak R (1991) Predictive value of thallium-201-dipyridamole myocardial stress scintigraphy in chronic hemodialysis patients and transplant recipients. Clin Nephrol 36(4):192–202.
29. Kwok YS, Kim C, Grady D et al. (1999) Meta-analysis of exercise testing to detect coronary artery disease in women. Am J Cardiol 83:660–666.
30. Mieres JH, Shaw LJ, Hendel RC et al. (2003) A report of the American Society of Nuclear Cardiology Task Force on Women and Heart Disease (Writing Group on Perfusion Imaging in Women). J Nucl Cardiol 10:95–101.
31. Hachamovitch R, Berman DS, Kiat H et al. (1996) Effective risk stratification using exercise myocardial perfusion SPECT in women: gender-related differences in prognostic nuclear testing. J Am Coll Cardiol 28:34–44.
32. Amanullah AM, Kiat H, Friedman JD et al. (1996) Adenosine technetium-99m sestamibi myocardial perfusion SPECT in women: diagnostic efficacy in detection of coronary artery disease. J Am Coll Cardiol 27:803–809.
33. Marwick TH, Shaw LJ, Lauer MS et al. (1999) The noninvasive prediction of cardiac mortality in men and women with known or suspected coronary artery disease. Economics of Noninvasive Diagnosis (END) Study Group. Am J Med 106:172–178.
34. Iskandrian AS, Heo J, Kong B, Lyons E (1989) Effect of exercise level on the ability of thallium-201 tomographic imaging in detecting coronary artery disease: analysis of 461 patients. J Am Coll Cardiol 14:1477–1486.
35. Miller TD, Gersh BJ, Christian TF et al. (1995) Limited prognostic value of thallium-201 exercise treadmill testing early after myocardial infarction in patients treated with thrombolysis. Am Heart J 130(2):259–266.
36. Benoit Th, Vivegnis D, Lahiri A et al. (1996) Tomographic myocardial imaging with technetium-99m tetrofosmin. Eur Heart J 17:635–642.
37. Daou D, Delahaye N, Lebtahi R et al. (2000) Diagnosis of extensive coronary artery disease: intrinsic value of increased lung Tl-201 uptake with exercise SPECT. J Nucl Med 41:567–574.
38. Ho K-T, Miller TD, Christian TF et al. (2001) Prediction of severe coronary artery disease and long-term outcome in patients undergoing vasodilator SPECT. J Nucl Cardiol 8:438–444.

Imaging Protocols in Myocardial Perfusion Scintigraphy

Shobhan Vinjamuri

Contents

21.1 Introduction 237
21.2 Stress Mechanism 237
21.2.1 Exercise Stress 237
21.2.2 Pharmacological Stress 238
21.3 Important Factors in MPS SPECT Protocols [4–13] 238
21.3.1 Choice of Radiotracer 238
21.3.2 Image Acquisition 239
21.4 Protocols 239
21.4.1 Tc-99m-based Protocols 239
21.4.2 Tl-201-based Protocols 242
21.4.3 Dual Isotope Protocols 242
21.5 Future Trends and Conclusion 243
References 243

21.1 Introduction

Imaging protocols for stress myocardial perfusion imaging (MPI) are subject to huge variation in clinical practice primarily due to a tendency to "customise" protocols. The components of imaging protocols for MPI include the "stress" procedure; choice of radiopharmaceuticals; mechanism of data acquisition; and "data analysis" for reporting. Finally, the logistics of patient attendance, such as inability to attend on two separate days, and the logistics of the department, whereby slots for MPI need to fit in with the overall nuclear medicine service, also need to be taken into account. However, protocol parameters other than those listed may be preferred at other institutions and research into corrections for attenuation, scatter and newer cameras may result in forming new protocols in the future. Although each of these components is distinct and has a clear identifiable role, the choice of a particular component frequently influences the other components, and a multidisciplinary team in each nuclear medicine department should ideally review the completely customised protocol (Table 21.1).

21.2 Stress Mechanism

21.2.1 Exercise Stress

This is usually performed with a treadmill or bicycle ergometer with continuous patient monitoring and it is the preferred stress modality in patients who can exercise to an adequate workload. Exercise testing has a limited value in patients who cannot achieve an adequate heart rate and blood pressure response due to non-cardiac physical limitations such as pulmonary, peripheral vascular, musculoskeletal abnormalities or due to a lack of motivation. A treadmill is the most widely used exercise modality, with Bruce and modified Bruce being the most widely used exercise protocols. Departments may decide not to offer exercise stress MPI routinely if

Table 21.1 Factors related to choosing a protocol

Type of patients referred: diagnosis, prognosis, viability, screening, low risk, intermediate or high risk patients
Type of dept: dedicated nuclear cardiology, nuclear medicine, radiology dept
Type of stressing: treadmill, pharmacological
Type of MPS: planar, stress only (if stress is normal), stress and rest, ± gating, ±attenuation correction (AC)
Stress scheduling
Staffing
Urgent/regular request
Inpatient or outpatient
Choice of radionuclide/radiopharmaceutical
Information/clinical question requested
Costing
Camera type; single head, multihead detector

the patient population within the catchment area of the department is likely to include a high proportion of patients with non-cardiac physical limitation.

21.2.2
Pharmacological Stress

The pharmacological stress test has proven to be an excellent alternative to the physical exercise test and can be performed using vasodilator agents (such as Dipyridamole or Adenosine) or Dobutamine. Adenosine is a direct coronary vasodilator and leads to a 3.5 to 4-fold increase in myocardial blood flow and is routinely given as a continuous infusion at a rate of 140 μg/kg/min over 6 minutes [1, 2]. Patients who cannot perform exercise stress for various reasons and those who are on concomitant treatment with medications which blunt the heart rate response (such as beta-blockers and calcium channel blockers) are better suited to Adenosine stress. Dipyridamole is an indirect coronary artery vasodilator that increases the tissue levels of Adenosine by preventing the intracellular reuptake and deamination of Adenosine [1, 2]; it induces hyperemia, which lasts for more than 15 minutes. Although the incidence of side effects is less than with Adenosine, they last for a longer period and additional intervention such as IV Aminophylline may be required to reverse side effects. This warrants a

relatively higher degree of surveillance in the immediate "post-stress" period than with Adenosine [3].

Dobutamine is usually a secondary pharmacological stressor and is used in patients who cannot undergo exercise stress and have contraindications to using vasodilator stress. It increases regional myocardial blood flow and results in direct β1 (beta) and β2 receptor stimulation, with a dose-related increase in heart rate, blood pressure and myocardial contractility [1–3].

21.3
Important Factors in MPS SPECT Protocols [4–13]

21.3.1
Choice of Radiotracer

The choice of radiotracer depends on the clinical scenario and availability. The dose injected also depends on patient type, radiotracer and the local licensing authorities. The commonly used radiotracers currently are Thallium-201 (Tl-201) and ^{99m}Tc-labelled compounds such as ^{99m}Tc- Sestamibi and ^{99m}Tc-Tetrofosmin.

21.3.1.1 Thallium-201

This is used in a dose of 2 to 3 mCi (74 to 111 MBq). A single dose of Tl-201 is used for stress and redistribution imaging performed 2.5 to 4 hours apart. An additional reinjection of Tl-201 can be considered in patients with fixed perfusion defects on stress and redistribution images [4–7]. Tl-201 is injected at the peak of the exercise and the imaging is performed 10–15 minutes later [4–15].

21.3.1.2 ^{99m}Tc-Sestamibi

This is used in a dose of 15 to 30 mCi (555 to 1110 MBq). Two separate injections are required for stress and rest imaging. In order to allow adequate hepatobiliary clearance of the radiotracer, a minimum delay of 15 to 20 minutes for exercise, 45 to 60 minutes for rest and 60 minutes for pharmacological stress is advised [4–15].

21.3.1.3 ^{99m}Tc-Tetrofosmin

This is used in a dose of 15 to 30 mCi (555 to 1110 MBq). Two separate injections are again required for stress and rest imaging. In order to allow adequate hepatobiliary clearance of the radiotracer, a minimum delay of 10 to

Table 21.2 Important factors in MPS SPECT protocols [5–13]

1. Acquisition protocols

Dose: average, heavier patients, gating

Position: supine versus prone

Delay time: ^{99m}Tc-sestamibi and ^{99m}Tc-tetrofosmin

Energy windows

Collimators: low-energy all purpose (LEAP) for thallium, low-energy high-resolution (LEHR) for Technetium labeled compounds

Orbit: 180° versus 360°

Orbit type: circular versus noncircular (elliptical)

Pixel size.

Acquisition type: step-and-shoot, continuous, continuous step-and-shoot,

Number of projections.

Matrix.

Time/projection and total time

Gated SPECT.

Multidetector systems

2. Quality control

Uniformity, sensitivity, center of rotation (COR), multiple detector head alignment, detector head tilt

3. Processing protocols

Filtering

4. Reconstruction

Analytic, iterative

5. Reorientation

6. Display

7. Perfusion quantitation

Data sampling.

Normalization.

Analysis

Variables

Display

15 minutes for exercise, 30 to 45 minutes for rest and 45 minutes for pharmacological stress is advised [4–15].

21.3.2
Image Acquisition

21.3.2.1 Image

Planar imaging, although not considered "state-of-the-art", may be the only possible means of data acquisition in acutely ill patients and very obese patients who are too heavy for the imaging table of a SPECT camera [5, 6]. Reproduction of the same patient position between stress and rest images requires skill. Even minor differences in angulations of the camera, positioning of the breasts, or pressure of the camera on the chest wall can produce artefacts and inaccuracies in the comparison of stress and rest images. Single photon emission computed tomography (SPECT) is the default and routinely used data acquisition technique and some important factors in image acquisition are summarised in Table 21.2 [4–24].

21.3.2.2 Collimator Choice

In general, parallel hole collimators are routinely used for cardiac SPECT acquisitions. low energy all purpose (LEAP) collimators are routinely used along with Tl-201 and low energy high resolution (LEHR) collimators are used along with ^{99m}Tc radiotracers [5, 6]. LEHR collimators have longer bores, thinner septa, and smaller holes, and provide better resolution at the expense of reduced sensitivity, therefore these are better suited for use with imaging agents providing high count rates, such as ^{99m}Tc [4–13].

21.3.2.3 180° versus 360° Data Acquisition

Generally, 180° data acquisition (from 45° RAO to 45° LPO) is preferred to 360° data acquisition in both single and multiple head gamma camera systems. The avoidance of posterior projections lessens noise contamination due to significant attenuation and decreased image resolution owing to the greater distance between the heart and the detector [4–13].

21.4
Protocols

21.4.1
Tc-99m-based Protocols

The ^{99m}Tc-labelled compounds such as Sestamibi and Tetrofosmin have good properties for imaging. The

Table 21.3 Common indications for choosing a one day or two day protocol

1 day protocol:

Elderly/ill patients

Coming from too far (transportation, accompanying relative, etc.)

Patients with high likelihood of CAD

Inpatients

Patients who need a very urgent report

Renal patients on dialysis (scheduling problems due to dialysis)

2 day protocol:

Busy dept/few cameras/scheduling problems

Patients with low likelihood of CAD

Obese patients

property of no or minimal redistribution is helpful in making the protocols or imaging time flexible. Currently existing protocols are one day (rest/stress or stress/rest), two-day stress/rest. Some common indications (clinical scenarios), advantages and limitations of these protocols are summarised in Tables 21.3 and 21.4 [4–13].

21.4.1.1 One-Day Imaging Protocol

Ideally, stress and rest imaging with ^{99m}Tc-labelled agents should be performed on two separate days. However, for logistical reasons, both stress and rest studies can be performed on the same day (Table 21.3). This requires the use of unequal radiotracer doses whereby a smaller dose of 7 to 10 mCi (250 to 370 MBq) is followed by a larger dose of 20 to 30 mCi (740 to 1110 MBq) 2 to 3 hours later on the same day [4–13].

21.4.1.2 Two-Day Imaging Protocol

This is the protocol of choice in patients who are overweight and in whom a relatively lower dose of radiopharmaceutical will result in sub optimal images. This requires use of radiotracer doses of 15–30 mCi for rest and 15–30 mCi for stress [4–13].

21.4.1.3 Single Isotope Protocol

Departments may choose (for logistical reasons or due to non-availability of some isotopes) to use only one isotope for a particular test. The additional value of using a single isotope for stress and rest images is a perceived improvement in reproducibility between the two sets of images, whereas two identical slices of the myocardium may appear different when imaged with two different isotopes [4–13].

21.4.1.4 Dual Isotope Protocol

The advantage of a "dual isotope protocol" relies on the differences in the time between injection of the isotope and imaging, and the relative differences in the gamma ray energy photo peak between the two isotopes. The usefulness of these protocols is described below.

Table 21.4 Advantages and limitations of various protocols [5-13]

Same day rest–stress protocol:

Advantages:

- If the problem is to detect viable myocardium and reversibility in previous infarction
- Better image contrast
- Convenient for patients
- Provides diagnostic information quickly
- True rest study may improve ability to detect defect reversibility

Limitations:

- It provides less than ideal stress defect contrast due to resting background activity
- Tc-Sestamibi and Tc-tetrofosmin rest imaging have also been shown to underestimate the extent of viable tissue
- 2 tracer injections is necessary, even if the stress study is normal

Table 21.4 *(continued)* Advantages and limitations of various protocols

Same day stress-rest protocol:

Advantages

- Scheduling similar to thallium
- Convenient to patients
- Provides diagnostic information quickly
- Good choice of patients with low likelihood of CAD
- Rest study is not needed in stress MPS is normal

Limitations:

- Reversibility may be underestimated due to presence interference residual/remaining activity from the
- stress study
- Stress/rest sequence may result in an increased number of ischemic segments incorrectly being identified as fixed defects
- Rest portion of the exam may not be considered to be a "true" rest study as it follows a period of exercise

Two day stress–rest protocol:

Advantages

- Good quality images/optimal defect contrast with minimal background
- Images acquired using the same dosage
- Facilitates easy comparison
- No cross-talk or cross-contamination
- Radiation burden to patient and staff lower
- Ideal based of physical half-life of ^{99m}Tc
- Best for novice use of ^{99m}Tc-MIBI, Tetrofosmin
- Increased scheduling flexibility
- Ability to image obese patients
- Good choice of patients with low likelihood of CAD/better patient flow
- Rest study is not needed in stress MPS is normal

Limitations:

- Patient must come on two different days for imaging if the stress is abnormal or equivocal
- Relative delay in diagnosis

201Th Stress – 4 hours redistribution protocol:

Advantages:

- Single injection
- No labeling is required

Limitations:

- Scanning should begin 5–10 minutes post-injection/post-stress
- Scanning should completed by 30 minutes post-injection/post-stress
- Attenuation artefacts
- Evaluation of LVEF and wall motion is inferior to ^{99m}Tc-labeled compounds
- Radiation to patient is higher than with ^{99m}Tc-labeled compounds

21.4.1.5 Same Day Stress Rest ^{99m}Tc Acquisition Protocol

Same day protocols are attractive to patients and to medical teams as any perceived discomfort associated with hospital visits is not replicated on two or more occasions. This protocol is useful in patients with low likelihood of CAD. In general patients who are very ill or those who have to travel large distances should preferably be investigated by same day protocols [5–11], however, if these same patients are likely to be overweight, a two-day protocol is more useful. This protocol involves the administration of Tc99m-labelled radiopharmaceuticals (Sestamibi or Tetrofosmin) for both stress and rest components. Typically, the initial administered activity for the stress phase is of the order of 250 to 370 MBq (7 to 10 mCi). The administered activity for the rest phase of the study typically needs to be of the order of three to four times the initial activity. The relative advantage of this protocol is that if a preliminary analysis of the "stress" images reveals normal perfusion to all myocardial walls; this negates the need for further resting images (Table 21.4). The usefulness of this approach is lower in populations with a high incidence of cardiac disease, as more scans are likely to be abnormal (either fixed or reversible perfusion defects) in this population.

21.4.1.6 Same Day Rest Stress ^{99m}Tc Acquisition Protocol

This protocol involves switching the stress and rest components in the one-day protocol, whereby the rest study is done first and the stress component next [16]. By relying on the higher count rates from the heart during the stress study in comparison with the rest study, theoretically there is a higher accuracy of identifying abnormal areas of perfusion [5, 6]. On a practical and clinical note, this theoretical advantage has not been proven. The other relative advantage of this approach is that the stress process can start earlier in the day, thereby improving flexibility of planning the daily departmental workload.

Anxious patients may also prefer this protocol whereby they are gradually introduced to the stress component of the study, and they are therefore better-prepared and less likely to move during data acquisition.

21.4.1.7 Two Day Stress Rest ^{99m}Tc Protocol

This protocol allows the scheduling of overweight patients. As the administered activity is higher, the image quality especially in overweight patients is better. There is a possibility that some patients will not attend for the second component of the two day protocol [8–10].

21.4.2 Tl-201-based Protocols

A number of modifications in Tl-201 imaging protocol such as Tl-201 stress-delayed, Tl-201 rest-redistribution and Tl-201 reinjection imaging protocols have been suggested to overcome Tl-201 imaging shortcomings. The use of Tl-201 in a one or a two day protocol for both stress and rest components is limited by the photon flux and the maximum amount of Tl-201 that can be used for optimum imaging [4–14].

21.4.2.1 Stress–Rest Thallium 201 Protocol

Images should be acquired post-stress, 5–10 minutes pos-injection, with redistribution images 2.5–4 hours apart.

21.4.2.2 Reinjection Protocol

Tl-201 in a dosage of 1.5 to 2.0 mCi (up to 74 MBq) is useful for imaging the myocardium up to 24 hours after the initial Tl-201 injection (where the previous scans are abnormal) [4–13].

21.4.3 Dual Isotope Protocols

21.4.3.1 Rest Thallium and Stress Tc99m Dual Isotope Acquisition Protocol

This protocol involves using Tl-201 for the rest component, and this is followed by a Tc99m radiotracer along with the stress component. Other combinations (such as Tl-201 for the stress first, followed by Tc99m tracers for the rest, and ^{99m}Tc for stress first followed by Tl-201 for rest images later) are not feasible for technical reasons. The biggest advantage of this protocol is that all components of the study can be finished in 2 hours, which helps to increase throughput. The minor disadvantage is that using two different isotopes for two different phases (stress and rest) may identify some problems during comparison of the two datasets [5–9]. Experienced observers (with both Tl-201 and 99m Tc tracers) can usually account for this difference while reporting [12, 15]. The advantages and limitations of dual isotope separate and simultaneous acquisition protocols are summarised in Table 21.5 [4–13].

Table 21.5 Advantages and limitations of dual isotope protocols [5–13]

Dual-isotope separate-acquisition protocol

Advantages

- Short duration of the entire study (<2 hours)
- Contribution of counts from 201Tl to the ^{99m}Tc window is insignificant
- No need for cross-talk correction
- Optimal defect contrast
- Minimization of the problem of cross-contamination
- Comparable rest and stress images
- True rest study (which allows a better evaluation of reversible defects)
- Viability assessment
- Favorable dosimetry
- Patient convenience

Limitations

- Comparison of stress–rest images
- Differences in image resolution
- Variability in attenuation factors
- Greater Compton scatter of 201Tl than of ^{99m}Tc
- The myocardial wall thickness is greater with 201Tl than with ^{99m}Tc because of increased scatter
- Evaluation transient ischemic dilatation is suboptimal because of left ventricular cavity being larger with ^{99m}Tc
- Evaluating minimal reversible defects is difficult
- Not ideal for obese patients (low photon energy of 201Tl)

Dual-isotope simultaneous-acquisition protocol

Advantages

- No need for two separate imaging sessions
- The camera acquisition time is reduced
- The study duration is shorter
- Less or fewer motion artefacts than with separate rest and stress acquisitions
- The registration between images obtained with 201Tl and images obtained with ^{99m}Tc is exact and optimal

Limitations

- Cross-talk and downscatter
- There is contribution of scattered and primary photons from the first radionuclide into the photopeak window of the second radionuclide (significant degradation of image quality, image resolution, and quantitation)

21.5 Future Trends and Conclusion

MPS-SPECT imaging results in added value and enhanced patient care. With the increasing use of gated SPECT, there is a tendency towards more use of Tc99m-labelled isotopes and quantification of both stress and rest perfusion scores. The development of cardiac computed tomography (CT), especially with hybrid systems including SPECT-CT and PET-CT modalities, may have the potential for adding value to the practice of nuclear cardiology, especially in attenuation correction. However, careful and critical evaluation of these new modalities is important.

References

1. Iskandrian AS, Verani MS, Heo J (1994) Pharmacologic stress testing: mechanism of action, hemodynamic responses, and results in detection of coronary artery disease. J Nucl Cardiol 1:94–111.
2. Travain MI, Wexler JP (1999) Pharmacological stress testing. Semin Nucl Med 29:298–318.
3. Elhendy A, Bax JJ, Poldermans D (2002) Dobutamine stress myocardial perfusion imaging in coronary artery disease. J Nucl Med 43:1634–1646.
4. Anagnostopoulos C, Harbinson M, Kelion A et al. (2004) Procedure guidelines for radionuclide myocardial perfusion imaging. Heart 90(1):i1–i10.
5. American Society of Nuclear Cardiology (1996) Imaging guidelines for nuclear cardiology procedures, part1. Myocardial perfusion stress protocols. J Nucl Cardiol 3(3):G11–G15.
6. American Society of Nuclear Cardiology (1999) Imaging guidelines for nuclear cardiology procedures, part 2. Myocardial perfusion stress protocols. J Nucl Cardiol 6(2):G47–G84.
7. Hansen CL, Goldstein RA, Akinboboye OO, Berman DS, Botvinick EH, Churchwell KB (2007) American Society

of Nuclear Cardiology. Myocardial perfusion and function: single photon emission computed tomography. J Nucl Cardiol 14(6):e39–e60.
8. Hesse B, Tagil K, Cuocolo A et al. (2005) EANM/ESC procedural guidelines for myocardial perfusion imaging in nuclear cardiology. Eur J Nucl Med Mol Imaging 32(7):855–897.
9. Husain SS (2007) Myocardial perfusion imaging protocols: is there an ideal protocol? J Nucl Med Technol 35(1):3–9.
10. Henzlova MJ, Cerqueira MD, Mahmarian JJ, Yao SS (2006) Quality Assurance Committee of the American Society of Nuclear Cardiology. Stress protocols and tracers. J Nucl Cardiol 13(6):e80–e90.
11. Ritchie J, Bateman TM, Bonow RO et al. (1995) Guidelines for clinical use of cardiac radionuclide imaging. A report of the AHA/ACC Task Force on Assessment of Diagnostic and Therapeutic Cardiovascular Procedures, Committee on Radionuclide Imaging, developed in collaboration with the American Society of Nuclear Cardiology. Circulation 91:1278–1303.
12. Strauss HWD. Miller D, Wittry MD et al. (2002) Society of Nuclear Medicine Procedure Guideline for Myocardial Perfusion Imaging.
13. Port SC (1999) Imaging Guidelines for Nuclear Cardiology Procedures. J Nucl Cardiol 6:2.
14. Taillefer R (2001) Radiopharmaceuticals, in Cardiac SPECT Imaging. Anatomy and Techniques, 2nd edn, DePuey EG, Garcia EV, Berman DS (eds). Lippincot Williams and Wilkins, Philadelphia, PA, pp. 117–154.
15. DePuey GE, Garcia EV et al. (2001) Updated imaging guidelines for nuclear cardiology procedures, part 1. J Nucl Cardiol 8(1):G5–G58.
16. Siebelink HM, Natale D, Sinusas AJ, Wackers FJ (1996) Quantitative comparison of single-isotope and dual-isotope stress-rest single-photon emission computed tomographic imaging for reversibility of defects. J Nucl Cardiol 3(6 Pt 1):483–493.
17. DePuey EG, Parmett S, Ghesani M et al. (1999) Comparison of Tc-99m sestamibi and thallium-201 gated perfusion SPECT. J Nucl Cardiol 6:278–285.
18. Galt JR, Germano G (1994) Advances in instrumentation for cardiac SPECT. In Cardiac SPECT Imaging, DePuey EG, Berman DS, Garcia EV (eds). Raven Press, New York, pp. 91–102.
19. Segall GM, Davis MJ (1989) Prone versus supine thallium myocardial SPECT. A method to decrease artifactual inferior wall defects. J Nucl Med 30:548–555.
20. Maniawski PJ, Morgan HT, Wackers FJ et al. (1991) Orbit-related variation in spatial resolution as a source of artifactual defects in thallium-201 SPECT. J Nucl Med 32:871–875.
21. Cooper JA, Neuman PH, McCandless BK et al. (1992) Effect of patient motion on tomographic myocardial perfusion imaging. J Nucl Med 13:1566–1571.
22. Garcia EV, Cooke CD, Van Train KF et al. (1990) Technical aspects of myocardial SPECT imaging with Tc-99m sestamibi. Am J Cardiol 66:23E–31E.
23. Van Train K, Garcia EV, Maddahi J et al. (1994) Multicenter trial validation for quantitative analysis of same-day rest-stress technetium-99m-sestamibi myocardial tomograms. J Nucl Med 35:609–618.
24. Bateman TM, Berman DS, Heller GV et al. (1999) ASNC position statement on ECG-gating of myocardial perfusion SPECT scintigrams. J Nucl Cardiol 6:470–471.

Pharmacological Stress Myocardial Perfusion Imaging: Current Status and Limitations

Chapter 22

Gopinath Gnanasegaran,
Francis Sundram,
Margaret Hall and John R Buscombe

Contents

22.1	Introduction	245
22.2	Catecholamines	247
22.2.1	Dobutamine	247
22.2.2	Low-Dose Dobutamine SPECT for Identification of Viable Myocardium	248
22.2.3	Arbutamine	249
22.3	Vasodilators	253
22.3.1	Adenosine	253
22.3.2	Dipyridamole	254
22.4	Miscellaneous Agents	255
22.4.1	Atropine	255
22.4.2	Nitroglycerine/Nitroglycerin	256
22.4.3	Added Physical Stress	256
22.5	Newer Pharmacological Stress Agents	257
22.6	Conclusion	257
	References	257

22.1 Introduction

Stress myocardial perfusion imaging is based on the principle that flow heterogeneity in coronary vascular beds can be detected as a perfusion defect [1]. The addition of myocardial perfusion scintigraphy (MPS) to physical exercise improves the diagnostic accuracy [2, 3]. Stress MPS has become a central guide (gate keeper) in clinical decision making with regard to patients with coronary artery disease (CAD) and ischaemic heart disease (IHD). However, specific patient groups with conditions such as peripheral vascular, neurological, respiratory, renal or joint diseases always have difficulties performing adequate exercise. In these groups of patients exercise tests are often inconclusive with no objective evidence of myocardial ischaemia [4]. Further, reports have concluded that 50% of patients over 75 years of age and 33% of patients less than 75 years of age have difficulty in reaching the target heart rate (THR) specified in the physical exercise test protocols [5]. In such patients, pharmacological stress combined with MPS is a logical alternative [4]. In general, a pharmacological stress test has proven to be an excellent alternative to a physical exercise test. Pharmacological stress agents fall into two categories: (a) coronary vasodilating agents such as dipyridamole and adenosine, which act directly on the coronary vessels to increase blood flow [2, 4, 6, 7], and (b) cardiac positive ionotropic agents such as dobutamine and arbutamine (catecholamines), which act indirectly by increasing myocardial workload, leading to enhanced coronary blood flow [1, 6] (Fig. 22.1). Dobutamine is also reported to have a minor direct vasodilatory effect on coronary vessels [8]. The vasodilators have two types of effects; (a) a proischaemic effect and (b) a hyperaemic effect. The hyperaemic effect is useful in radionuclide myocardial perfusion studies [9]. In general, both groups of agents produce perfusion abnormalities resulting from heterogeneity of coronary blood flow re-

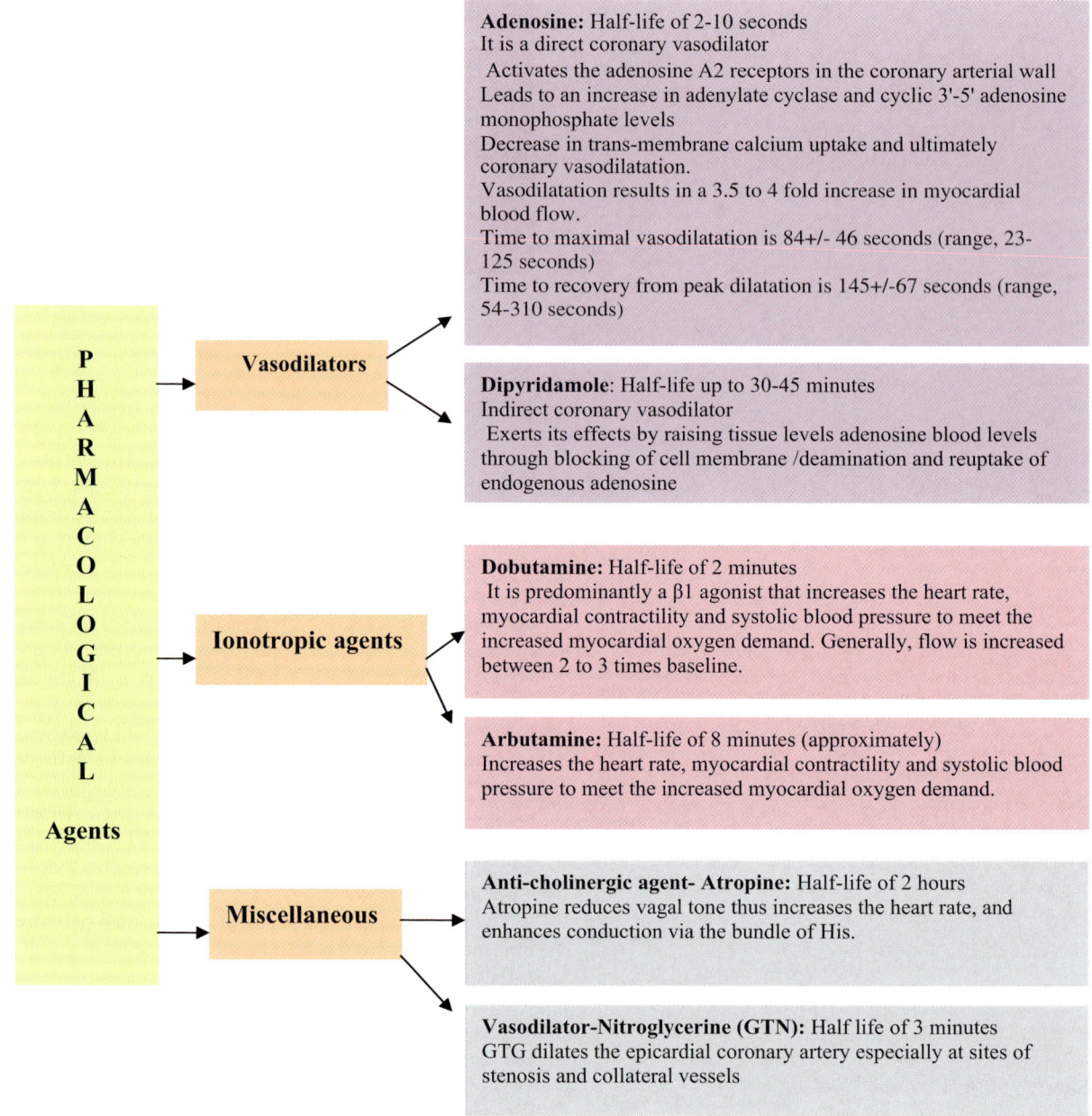

Fig. 22.1 Pharmacological stress agents and their mechanisms of action [6–9, 14, 15, 18, 21]

serve in the presence of coronary artery disease (CAD) [1]. Before carrying out MPS, as a routine, it is important to check patient details such as name, date of birth, address, etc. Taking a brief clinical history during the stress procedure and also while reporting the scans is very important (Table 22.1) [1–16].

Table 22.1 Important checklist before and during pharmacological stressing in MPS [15, 18]

Before the test:
Justification and authorisation for performing the test should be confirmed before starting.
In general, before the test, withdrawal of drugs that may interfere with physiological exercise responses should be considered unless medically contraindicated.
Patients should also avoid caffeine containing foods, beverages, and drugs as per the local guideline or protocol.
Patients should be instructed to dress appropriately for exercise.
Exercise testing must be undertaken by an appropriately trained healthcare professional.
The healthcare professional supervising the stress test should be up to date in immediate life support.
Emergency medical kit with emergency medicine should be in the stressing room.
Easy/rapid access to personnel trained in advanced life support (ALS) and appropriate assistance and emergency support should be available.
Initial evaluation should include a medical history (including symptoms, coronary risk factors, drug treatment, and previous diagnostic and therapeutic procedures) and a review of referral letters and other medical records if available.
Regardless of the exercise protocol used, an intravenous line should be secured.
The IV line should be flushed with 5–10 ml of 0.9% sodium chloride injection to ensure patency before starting the test.
Pregnancy form should be signed.
During the stress test
Heart rate and blood pressure and ECG should be monitored at rest and throughout the test and recorded at each stage.
Monitoring with a 12 lead ECG is required for the detection of ST segment/T wave changes/arrhythmias.
Exercise duration, symptoms/side effects, reason for stopping, and ECG changes should be noted.
After the stress test
Intravenous line should be secured until the imaging is completed and should be removed before the patient leaves the department.

22.2 Catecholamines

22.2.1 Dobutamine

Dobutamine is a positive inotropic agent reserved for patients who are unable to exercise adequately and have a contraindication to dipyridamole or adenosine infusion (Table 22.2) [17–19]. Dobutamine is used or applied to produce true ischaemic response and it increases regional coronary flow. However, this method is dependent on adequate augmentation of myocardial oxygen demands [19]. Mason et al. reported the use of dobutamine for stress testing in combination with 201Tl imaging [20].

Dobutamine is a synthetic catecholamine with a significant ionotropic and less chronotropic effect. Dobutamine increases the heart rate, systolic blood pressure, cardiac output and stroke volume [19, 21]. There is a two-three-fold increase in coronary flow, comparable with that occurring during physical exercise, but the peak heart rate is usually lower than that achieved with exercise [20].

Dobutamine has predominantly beta 1 (β1) activity with weak beta 2 (β2) and alpha 1 (α1) activity. Through its β2 activity it increases the heart rate and contractility with a resultant increase in cardiac output [9, 22,

Table 22.2 Inotropic stress indications and contraindications [1, 3, 6–9, 14, 15, 18, 21]

Indications
Dobutamine infusion is commonly used when dynamic exercise is not feasible and there are contraindications to vasodilator stress such as severe COPD/Asthma, high grade A-V block, arterial hypotension, or xanthine medication.
Contraindications to dobutamine administration
Unstable angina (USA) or recent (<1 week) MI
Critical or severe aortic stenosis
Haemodynamically significant left ventricular out flow tract obstruction
Prior history of ventricular tachycardia
Recent history of life threatening arrhythmias/supraventricular tachyarrhythmia (SVT)
Patients with aortic dissections
Patients with large aortic aneurysms
Hypertrophic obstructive cardiomyopathy (HOCM)
Recent pulmonary embolism or infarction
Thrombophlebitis or active deep vein thrombosis
Active endocarditis, myocarditis, or pericarditis
Known hypokalaemia
Uncontrolled hypertension/Severe systemic hypertension (systolic blood pressure >200 mm Hg and/or diastolic blood pressure >110 mm Hg)
LBBB, bifascicular block, and paced rhythm (relative contraindication)
Patients on beta-blockers
Contraindications to atropine administration
Patients with narrow-angle glaucoma, myasthenia gravis
Obstructive uropathy
Obstructive gastrointestinal disorders
Atrial fibrillation with uncontrolled heart rate
Prior adverse reaction to atropine

23]. The agent has more inotropic than chronotropic activity at low doses (4–8 µg/kg/min), which increases the rate and force of contraction. At high doses used for pharmacologic stress (greater than 10–20 µg/kg/min), it increases both inotropic and chronotropic action of the heart (additionally increasing heart rate and systolic blood pressure) [4]. The increase in heart rate and myocardial contractility as a result of dobutamine infusion results in an increase in myocardial oxygen demand, with subsequent hyperaemia. This causes secondary dilatation of coronary arteries, resulting in increased blood flow through normal coronary arteries [24]. After intravenous administration, dobutamine is metabolised by catechol-o-methyl transferase to inactive compounds that are excreted by the hepatobiliary system. Dobutamine is infused incrementally starting at a dose of 5 to 10 µg/kg/min, which is increased at 3 minute intervals to 20, 30, and 40 µg/kg/min (Fig. 22.2) [25]. Carefully monitored titration is required throughout the test and is often time consuming. Some use atropine in patients where the heart rate fails to reach 85% of age predicted heart rate or THR, even with the maximum dose of dobutamine [25] (Table 22.3). However, Secknus et al. in their dobutamine echocardiography studies have reported that only 73% of patients reached 85% of the THR in spite of atropine [26]. Although relatively safe, complications do occur and the common side effects of dobutamine include chest pain, dyspnoea, headache, palpitations and hypotension (Table 22.4) [27–29]. Beta-blockers are the antidotes used to counteract the side effects/complications of dobutamine.

22.2.2
Low-Dose Dobutamine SPECT for Identification of Viable Myocardium

In patients with myocardial infarction and impaired left ventricular function, differentiation of dysfunctional but viable myocardium from irreversibly damaged scar tissue is important and has important clinical implications [30, 31]. In a setting of severe narrowing, even low-dose dobutamine can bring about regional dysfunction [32]. Low-dose dobutamine echocardiography is widely used to assess the inotropic reserve of severely dysfunctional myocardium [33]. Initial results from Everaert et al. reported that low-dose dobutamine gated SPECT findings correlated well with dobutamine stress echocardiography (DSE) in identifying inotropic reserve in infarcted areas [34]. Further, Yoshinaga et al. also reported that low-dose dobutamine SPECT correlated well with DSE in detecting viable myocardium. In addition, the use of gated SPECT helps in evaluating regional wall motion and provides information that is often missed by routine perfusion scans (non-gated) [35].

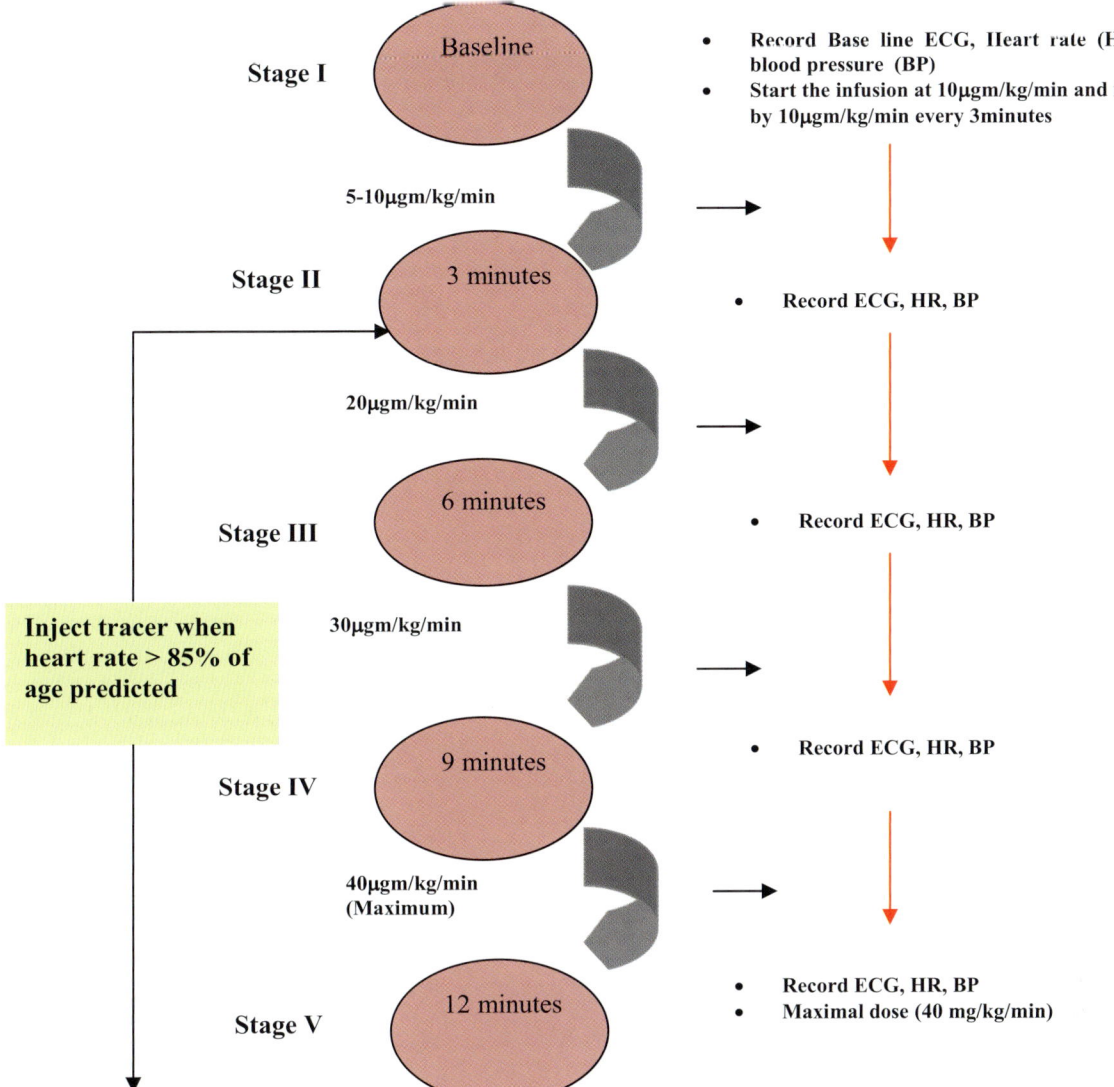

Fig. 22.2 Schematic representation of the standard Dobutamine stress protocol. 1. During the infusion inject the radiopharmaceutical if the patient achieves the target heart rate (THR) and continue the infusion for 2 minutes, stop the infusion and wait until the heart returns to the baseline. 2. Atropine may be given in the presence of submaximal heart rate response

22.2.3
Arbutamine

Arbutamine is a synthetic sympathomimetic agent developed for use as a pharmacological stress agent. It is a mixed β-1 and β-2 agonist with a mild affinity for α-1 receptors [36–38]. It has an inotropic and chronotropic activity similar to that of dobutamine, but it has less peripheral vasodilating activity. Arbutamine simulates exercise more closely than does dobutamine [36–38], and the onset of action is within 1–2 minutes, with a plasma half-life of about 8 minutes [39]. Arbutamine appears to elicit a more balanced inotropic and chronotropic response than dobutamine [40]. The infusion is by a delivery system (device) and the device calculates the dosing regimen according to the heart rate and adjusts the infusion to achieve the required target heart rate. The arbutamine delivery system includes a prefilled

Table 22.3 100% and 85% target heart rate (THR) for male and female

Male (220 – age)			Female (210 – age)		
Age	100%THR	85% THR	Age	100%THR	85% THR
30	190	162	30	180	153
31	189	161	31	179	152
32	188	160	32	178	151
33	187	159	33	177	150
34	186	158	34	176	149
35	185	157	35	175	148
36	184	156	36	174	148
37	183	155	37	173	147
38	182	154	38	172	146
39	181	154	39	171	145
40	180	153	40	170	144
41	179	152	41	169	143
42	178	151	42	168	143
43	177	150	43	167	142
44	176	149	44	166	141
45	175	148	45	165	140
46	174	148	46	164	139
47	173	147	47	163	138
48	172	146	48	162	138
49	171	145	49	161	137
50	170	144	50	160	136
51	169	143	51	159	135
52	168	143	52	158	134
53	167	142	53	157	133
54	166	141	54	156	132
55	165	140	55	155	131
56	164	139	56	154	131
57	163	138	57	153	130
58	162	138	58	152	129
59	161	137	59	151	128
60	160	136	60	150	127
61	159	135	61	149	126
62	158	134	62	148	126
63	157	133	63	147	125

Table 22.3 (continued) 100% and 85% target heart rate (THR) for male and female

Male (220 − age)			Female (210 − age)		
Age	100%THR	85% THR	Age	100%THR	85% THR
64	156	132	64	146	124
65	155	131	65	145	123
66	154	131	66	144	122
67	153	130	67	143	121
68	152	129	68	142	120
69	151	128	69	141	120
70	150	127	70	140	119
71	149	126	71	139	118
72	148	126	71	138	117
73	147	125	73	137	116
74	146	124	74	136	115
75	145	123	75	135	114
76	144	122	76	134	114
77	143	121	77	133	113
78	142	120	78	132	112
79	141	120	79	131	111
80	140	119	80	130	110
81	139	118	81	129	109
82	138	117	82	128	109
83	137	116	83	127	108
84	136	115	84	126	107
85	135	114	85	125	106
86	134	114	86	124	105
87	133	113	87	123	104
88	132	112	88	122	103
89	131	111	89	121	103
90	130	110	90	120	102

syringe of the agent, automatic dosing based on the patient's heart rate response, continuous monitoring of heart rate and blood pressure, a printout of test results, and safety features (visual and audible warnings and automatic discontinuation of drug after an alarm) [37, 41]. The infusion rate is from 0.8 µg/kg/min and can go up to a maximum of 10 µg/kg/min [9, 40]. Shehata et al. reported that although there were no differences in symptoms in patients stressed with dobutamine and arbutamine, a larger number of patients required treatment for symptoms with arbutamine than with dobutamine (Table 22.4). Even though a shorter infusion time has been observed with arbutamine, the overall test duration is longer due to a longer recovery time [40]. Results from larger studies are awaited and arbutamine has remained less popular than other stress agents.

Table 22.4 Patient instructions, and side effects of pharmacological agents [1, 3, 6–9, 14, 15, 18, 21]

Vasodilators

Patient instructions before stress:

A 24-hours abstention from coffee, tea, soft drinks and 36–48 hours abstention from slow release theophylline. Patients on dipyridamole should discontinue the drug at least for 24 hours prior to adenosine stress.

Early termination of infusion.

(a) Severe hypotension (systolic blood pressure < 80 mm of Hg), (b) development of symptomatic, persistent second degree or complete heart block, (c) wheezing, (d) severe chest pain associated with 2 mm ST depression, (e) signs of poor perfusion such as cold skin, pallor or cyanosis, (f) patient's request to stop, and (g) monitoring equipment failure

End protocol:

Adenosine: Approximately 8–10 minutes after stopping infusion or when stable (BP & HR returns to baseline)
Dipyridamole: approximately 15 minutes post- injection of radiopharmaceutical or when stable (BP & HR returns to baseline)

Common side effects:

Adenosine – Chest pain 35%, Dyspnoea 20–35%, Flushing 37%, Headache 14%, SVT/ventricular arrhythmias 3%, Bronchospasm 0.1%, Palpitations 1%, Dizziness 9%, Hypotension 2–5%, High degree AV block 5%

Dipyridimole – Chest pain 20 %, Dyspnoea 3%, Flushing 3 %, Hypotension 5%, High degree AV block 2 %, SVT/ventricular arrhythmias 5%, Bronchospasm 0.15%, Headache 12%, Palpitations 3% Dizziness 12%

Reversal of side effects:

Adenosine – Side effects are spontaneous and disappear after stopping the infusion
The side effects can be reversed by the administration of theophylline, an adenosine receptor antagonist [administer only as needed]

Dipyridamole – The side effects can be reversed by the administration of theophylline, an adenosine receptor antagonist [125–250 mg (1–2 mg/kg) slow IV]

Sensitivity and specificity

Adenosine MPS - 90% and 86%

Dipyridamole MPS - 89% and 71%

Iontropic agents

Patient instructions before stress:

Patients should stop beta-blockers for five half-lives or at least 24 hours before the test unless contraindicated.

Early termination

Similar to those for exercise stress [Chapt. 8]

End protocol:

Approximately 15–20 minutes post-stress (after stopping infusion) or if patient is stable (BP and HR returns to baseline)

Common side effects:

Dobutamine – Chest pain 31%, Dyspnoea 14%, Flushing 14%, Headache 14%, Palpitations 29%, Hypotension 15%, SVT/ventricular arrhythmias 8–10%. ST segment depression occurs in approximately one-third of patients
Arbutamine – Tremor (22%); Dizziness (11%); Headache (11%); Paraesthesia (7%); Arrhythmias (6%); Hypotension (4%)

Reversal of side effects:

Side effects of dobutamine can be reverted by metoprolol (1–5 mg) or esmolol, 0.5 mg/kg over one minute intravenously (also reverses the effects of atropine)

Atropine intoxication (is a central anticholinergic syndrome causing confusion or sedation) can be treated by physotigmine I.V 0.5–2.0 mg

Patients should be informed of possible difficulties while driving (in the 2 hours following atropine administration due to reduced ocular accommodation)

Sensitivity and specificity

Dobutamine MPS – 82% and 73–75%

22.3
Vasodilators

22.3.1
Adenosine

Adenosine is a coronary vasodilator and its infusion results in a modest increase in heart rate and a modest decrease in both systolic and diastolic blood pressures. Adenosine is an endogenous purine nucleotide, which slows atrioventricular conduction and dilates coronary and peripheral vessels [42]. Adenosine triphosphate (ATP) and the S-adenosyl homocysteine are the two pathways in which adenosine is produced intracellularly [8]. During ischaemia the ATP is broken down and adenosine is produced intracellularly and this crosses the cell membrane and enters the extra cellular space where it acts on the adenosine receptors found on the cell wall [7, 9, 43–45]. The exact mechanism of how adenosine causes vasodilatation is not known. At least four subtypes of adenosine receptors have been reported (A1, A2A, A2B and A3) [7, 9, 43]. These have been cloned from animal or human sources [9, 43]. Adenosine receptors are members of the G-protein coupled receptor (GPCR) family, and they are typically thought to mediate stimulation or inhibition of adenylate cyclase activity, and hence cyclic AMP levels [7, 9]. A1 receptor activation causes slowing of the heart rate and conduction through the atrioventricular node (Table 22.5). A2 receptor activation causes vasodilatation in most vascular beds except renal afferent arterioles and hepatic veins where it causes vasoconstriction [9]. The coronary vasodilatation is induced by the stimulation of adenosine A2A receptors, and the non-specific stimulation of the other receptors is thought to be the cause of the side effects. The plasma half-life of adenosine is approximately 2–10 seconds and hence needs a constant intravenous infusion during pharmacological stress test to maintain high plasma levels. Adenosine administered for pharmacological stress is rapidly removed from the circulation by the erythrocytes and vascular endothelial cells [1].

It is reported that during pharmacological stress, adenosine (140 μg/kg/min dose) increases heart rate by 11 ± 9 beats/minute, and mean arterial blood pressure decreases by – 16 ± 5 mmHg [7, 46].

The commonly used adenosine dosage protocol for pharmacological stress testing is 140 μg/kg/min for 6 minutes [7, 9]. This may be coupled with submaximal dynamic exercise when tolerated to reduce the frequency and severity of adverse effects encountered during infusion [47, 48]. This attenuates the adenosine-induced drop in blood pressure and also improves image quality by decreasing the artefacts due to increased splanchnic activity (which is common with pharmacological stress perfusion imaging) [25]. However, in general, exercise is not recommended for patients with left bundle branch block or ventricular paced rhythm. There are also reports of using a 3 minute protocol instead of the conventional 6 minute protocol to reduce side effects [11, 43]. However, further crossover study is required.

Adenosine is administered as an intravenous infusion using an infusion or syringe pump (an intravenous line is required and a three-way connector or a Y-connector should be used to allow tracer injection without interruption of adenosine infusion) (Fig. 22.1). To avoid a sudden bolus of adenosine, the tracer injection should be given over 10–20 seconds. This can be done via the other arm of the "Y" cannula or via a separate intravenous access. The infusion should be continued for 1–2 minutes after injection of the tracer. In patients with recent ischaemic event, borderline hypotension or possible or unproven asthma, the infusion can be started at a lower dose (50 μg/kg/min) [17, 18, 28]. If the patient tolerates this dose for 1 minute, then the rate can be increased to 75, 100 and 140 μg/kg/min at one-minute intervals [17,18]. The tracer in this situation should be

Table 22.5 Adenosine and its receptors [7, 9, 43, 44]

A1 receptor activation:
• Slowing of the heart rate and conduction through the atrioventricular node
• Believed to cause most of the side effects

A2 receptors activation:
• Stimulation of the cAMP production
• Decrease uptake of calcium by the sarcoplasmic reticulum
• Smooth muscle relaxation and vasodilatation

A2A receptors activation:
• Produces maximal or near-maximal coronary vasodilatation within 55 seconds to 2 minutes of intravenous infusion

A2B receptors activation:
• Appear to mediate the peripheral vasodilator effect
• Causes systemic hypotension

A3 receptors activation (mainly found in the lungs and liver):
• Responsible for causing bronchospasm

injection one minute after starting the 140 µg/kg/min dose and infusion is then continued for 3 minutes before stopping [18].

The safety and efficacy of adenosine pharmacological stress is good and it is commonly used in patients having difficulty in undergoing a treadmill test (TMT) (Tables 22.4 and 22.6). However, there are numerous side effects and contraindications for using this agent. Fortunately, these side effects are often short-lived and rarely require active intervention [49–53].

22.3.2
Dipyridamole

The vasodilator effect of dipyridamole is mediated through adenosine. Dipyridamole causes vasodilatation indirectly by inhibition of reuptake of adenosine by the vascular endothelial cells [54, 55]. The onset and duration of action of dipyridamole are usually prolonged. The peak pharmacological effects occur about 6 to 8 minutes following initiation of the infusion [56–58]. Effects persist for 15 to 30 minutes, but may last as long as 60 minutes [1]. The half-life of dipyridamole is approximately 12 hours [7, 8]. Prolonged pharmacological activity could occur in the setting of hepatic insufficiency [27].

The heterogeneity in blood flow in dipyridamole-induced ischaemia is probably due to the steal phenomenon, where the normal coronary arteries dilate and augment blood flow leaving a reduced pressure for flow of blood across the compromised arteries [59, 60]. It is reported that during pharmacological stress, dipyridamole (0.56 mg/kg dose) increases heart rate by 11 ± 7 beats/minute and the mean arterial blood pressure decreases by -10 ± 3 mmHg [46].

The dose of dipyridamole is 140 µg/kg/min, infused over 4 minutes. The radiopharmaceutical is then injected 3–5 minutes following completion of dipyridamole infusion [17, 18] (Fig. 22.3b). The indications and side effect profile of dipyridamole is similar to that of adenosine, but these are prolonged (Table 22.4). The side effects can be reversed by the administration of theophylline, an adenosine receptor antagonist. Aminophylline competitively blocks endothelial adenosine receptors [27]. However it does not reduce circulating adenosine levels,

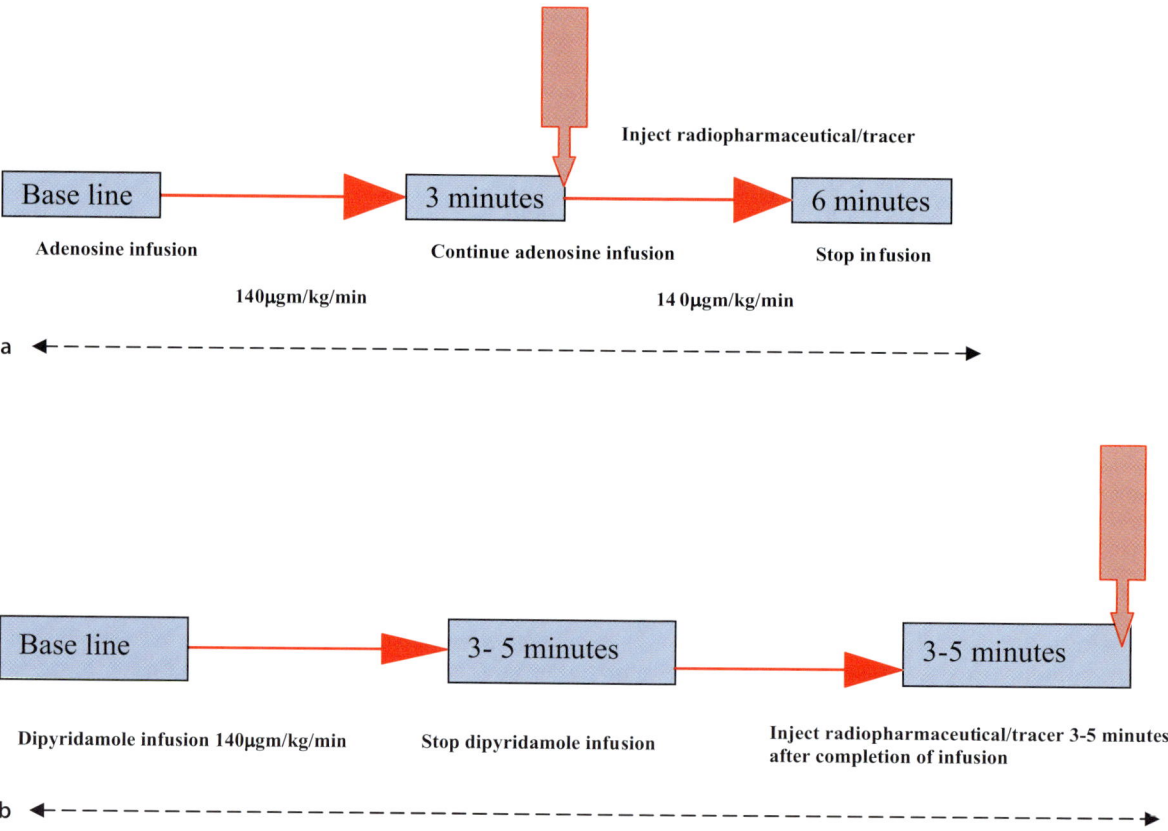

Fig. 22.3a,b Schematic representation of (a) the standard 6 minute adenosine stress protocol; (b) the dipyridamole stress protocol

Table 22.6 Vasodilator stress indications and contraindications [1, 3, 6–9, 14, 15, 18, 21]

Indications:	Contraindications:
Peripheral vascular disease	Suspected or known severe bronchospasm (patients with well controlled asthma can undergo adenosine stress after pre treatment with one or two puffs of albuterol or a comparable inhaler)
Neurological disease	
ESRD (end stage renal disease) on dialysis	
Musculoskeletal and joint diseases-poliomyelitis, arthritis	Hypotension (systolic < 90 mmHg)
Congestive heart failure	Recent acute coronary syndrome
Orthopaedic limitation - lower limb amputation or patients with artificial limbs	Second and third degree atrioventricular block in the absence of a functioning pacemaker
Poor patient motivation to exercise	Sick sinus syndrome.
LBBB-left bundle branch block	Recent cerebral ischaemia or infarction
Very soon after acute myocardial infarction in clinically stable patients (< 2 days)[Once stabilized, stress with vasodilators can be considered 24 to 72 hours after chest pain, depending upon clinically assessed risk] and soon after angioplasty/stent (<2 weeks)	Ingestion of cafeinated food in the last 12–24 hours
	Relative contraindications:
	Dipyridamole or adenosine hypersensitivity
Ventricular pre-excitation (Wolff–Parkinson–White syndrome) and electronically paced ventricular rhythm	Sinus bradycardia (less than 40 beats/min)
	Aminophylline intake or dipyridamole use in the last 24 hours
Medications that blunt the heart response (beta-blockers and calcium channel blockers)	Severe atherosclerotic lesion of extracranial artery
Chronic systemic illness and general debility	Unstable acute MI or acute coronary syndrome

which remain elevated as long as dipyridamole is present in the circulation. Further, half-life of dipyridamole is longer than that of aminophylline and side effects may recur after aminophylline has been metabolised. Therefore, patients should be monitored for a longer period of time [1, 6, 9, 19, 27].

22.4
Miscellaneous Agents

In addition to the commonly used vasodilators and catecholamine, there are a few other pharmacological agents used in myocardial perfusion scintigraphy.

22.4.1
Atropine

Atropine is an alkaloid from the plant atropa belladonna and has a half-life of 2 hours [42]. It reduces the vagal tone thus increasing the heart rate and enhances the bundle of His. Atropine is partly destroyed in the liver and some is excreted unchanged by the kidney [42]. Dobutamine has a sub-optimal chronotropic effect and therefore the target heart rate might not be reached in all patients. The addition of atropine has been shown to increase the heart rate and hence the sensitivity for detection of ischaemic heart disease without increasing the side effects [61–63]. Dobutamine–atropine myocardial perfusion scintigraphy is a feasible method for the evaluation of coronary artery disease with a safety profile and feasibility comparable to those reported for dobutamine stress echocardiography [8]. During dobutamine stress MPS; atropine is administered as 0.5–0.6 mg bolus injections intravenously at 1 minute intervals, up to a maximum dose of 2 mg [4, 64]. Timing of atropine administration with stress testing can be either before the test or during the test, as in dobutamine stress echocardiography [64]. The use of atropine is contraindicated in patients with narrow-angle glaucoma, myasthenia gravis, obstructive uropathy and obstructive gastrointestinal diseases.

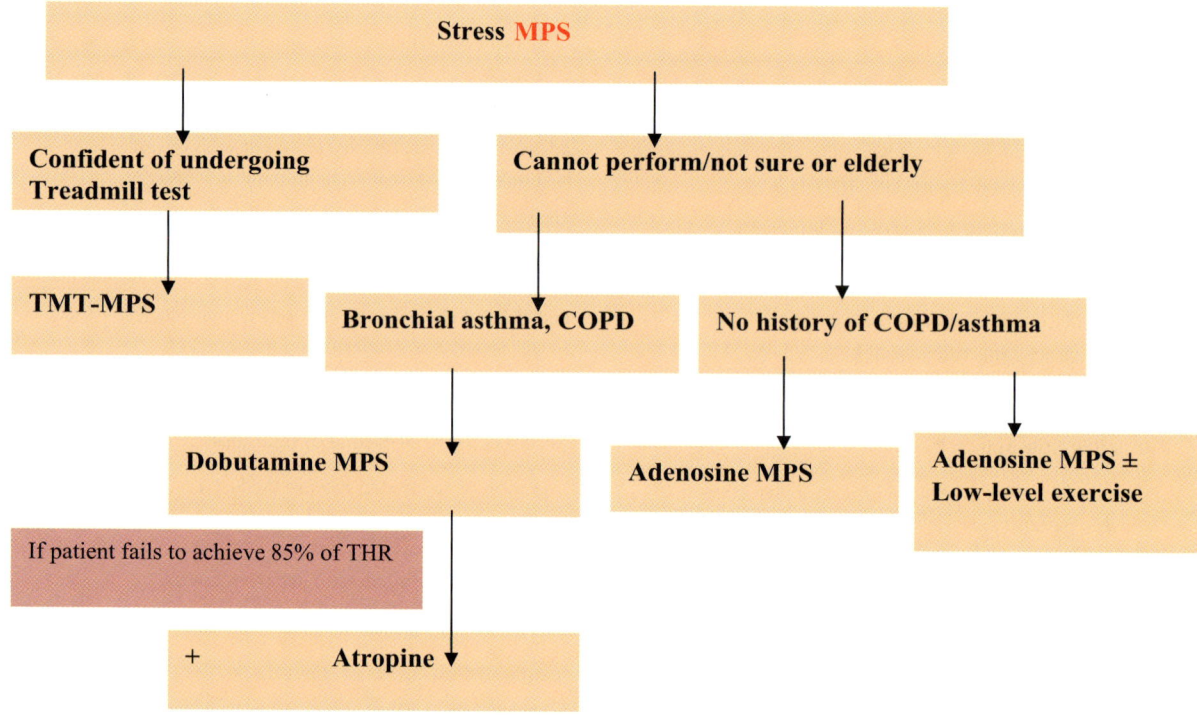

Fig. 22.4 Proposed algorithm for stress MPS

22.4.2
Nitroglycerine/Nitroglycerin

Nitroglycerine, a vasodilator, has been widely used in the treatment of acute and chronic heart failure to improve left ventricular function [65]. It has been observed that nitroglycerine dilates the epicardial coronary artery [66, 67], especially at sites of stenosis, and collateral vessels on coronary angiography [64, 66–68]. Assessment of myocardial viability is very important to identify those patients who would benefit from revascularisation procedure. Nitroglycerine is considered effective in identifying viable myocardium. Rest-redistribution Tl-201 imaging has been considered a method of choice for viability assessment [69–72]. Viability detection in nitroglycerine enhanced ^{99m}Tc-MIBI imaging offers significant prognostic value in patients with CAD after myocardial infarction [11]. During the assessment of viability, nitroglycerine is administered orally, sublingually or by intravenous infusion. One of the most common side effects of this agent is headache, which is probably due to stretching of pain-sensitive tissues around the meningeal arteries resulting from increased pulsation that accompanies local vasodilatation. However, this can be treated by paracetamol or ibuprofen [42].

Nitroglycerine has a biological half-life of 3 minutes in plasma [42].

22.4.3
Added Physical Stress

The impact of exercise combined with adenosine on sensitivity and defect severity remains inconclusive [48, 73–75]. Mahmood et al. [74] reported less non-cardiac side effects with combined exercise/adenosine 201Thallium-SPECT imaging but no differences in sensitivity and specificity. Pennell et al. [48] compared 201Thallium-SPECT imaging after adenosine alone, adenosine combined with submaximal bicycle exercise, or a continuous adenosine infusion combined with maximal bicycle exercise. Although there were no differences in sensitivity or specificity, the reversibility scores were greater with the continuous adenosine-maximal exercise protocol. However, Jamil et al. [76] results were different and they found that limited treadmill exercise combined with adenosine infusion does not increase myocardial perfusion defect severity compared with adenosine alone [76]. The general majority of reports suggest simultaneous low-level treadmill exercise with adenosine ^{99m}Tc-sestamibi imaging is safe and feasible, significantly reduces unfavorable side effects, and enhances image quality [75, 77, 78].

22.5
Newer Pharmacological Stress Agents

Selective adenosine A_{2A} receptor agonists (regadenoson) is currently under investigation as a pharmacological stress agent. The adenosine-regadenoson SPECT image agreement was reported to be good (86%) and was comparable with that reported for sequential dipyridamole and adenosine SPECT scans [79, 80]. These were compared in the same patients [77, 78]. These results were comparable with the previous study with A_{2A} agonist (binodenoson), which was administered as either a 3 minute 1.5 µg/kg IV infusion or as a range of 30 second IV boluses [81, 82]. However, further reports are awaited regarding the use of regadenoson.

22.6
Conclusion

Different agents are available for MPS using pharmacological stress. However, the choice of the agents should be based on the clinical questions to be answered and the patient's medical history. The diagnostic accuracy of these compounds not only depends on technical factors and indications, but also the patient population investigated. Pre-test assessment plays an important role in the evaluation of the correct stress or agent for the right patient (Fig. 22.4).

References

1. Iskandrian AS, Verani MS, Heo J (1994) Pharmacologic stress testing: mechanism of action, hemodynamic responses, and results in detection of coronary artery disease. J Nucl Cardiol 1:94–111.
2. Berman DS, Germano G, Shaw LJ (1999) The role of nuclear cardiology in clinical decision-making. Semin Nucl Med 29:280–297.
3. DePuey EG et al. (2002) Updated imaging guidelines for nuclear cardiology procedures, Part 1. J Nucl Cardiol 8:G5–G58.
4. Elhendy A, Bax JJ, Poldermans D (2002) Dobutamine stress myocardial perfusion imaging in coronary artery disease. J Nucl Med 43:1634–1646.
5. Hashimoto A, Palmer EL, Scott JA et al. (1999) Complications of exercise and pharmacological stress tests: differences in younger and elderly patients. J Nucl Cardiol 6:612–619.
6. Travain MI, Wexler JP (1999) Pharmacological stress testing. Semin Nucl Med 29:298–318.
7. Bokhari S, Ficaro EP, McCallister BD Jr (2007) Adenosine stress protocols for myocardial perfusion imaging. J Nucl Cardiol 14(3):415–416.
8. Elhendy A, Valkema R, van Domburg RT et al. (1998) Safety of dobutamine-atropine stress myocardial perfusion scintigraphy. J Nucl Med 39:1662–1666.
9. Ali Raza J, Reeves WC, Movahed A (2001) Pharmacological stress agents for evaluation of ischemic heart disease. Int J Cardiol 81:157–167.
10. American Society of Nuclear Cardiology (2001) Updated imaging guidelines for nuclear cardiology procedures. Part I. stress myocardial perfusion stress protocols. J Nucl Cardiol 8:G5–G58
11. Kostkiewicz M, Olszowska M, Przewlocki T, Podolec P, Tracz W (2003) Prognostic value of nitrate enhanced Tc99m MIBI SPECT study in detecting viable myocardium in patients with coronary artery disease. Int J Cardiovasc Imaging 19:129–135.
12. Kotler JA, Stewart J, Mand Kurzon JD (1992) Pharmacologic myocardial perfusion stress tests. J Florida Med Assoc 79:31–36.
13. Cheitlin MD, Alpert JS, Armstrong WF et al. (1997) ACC/AHA Guidelines for the Clinical Application of Echocardiography. A report of the American College of Cardiology/American Heart Association Task Force on Practice Guidelines (Committee on Clinical Application of Echocardiography). Circulation 95:1686–1744.
14. Bovinick EH, Verani MS, Leppo J, Alexander S (1998) Pharmacological Stress And Associated Topics-Nuclear Medicine, Self Study III. Nuclear Medicine Cardioliology. SNM Publications.
15. Anagnostopoulos C, Harbinson M, Kelion A et al. (2003) Procedure guidelines for radionuclide myocardial perfusion imaging. Nucl Med Commun 24:1105–1119.
16. Ranhosky A, Kempthorne-Rawson J (1990) The safety of intravenous dipyridamole thallium myocardial perfusion imaging. Circulation 81:1205–1209.
17. Strauss HW, Miller DD, Wittry MD, Cerqueira MD, Garcia EV, Iskandrian AS, Schelbert HR, Wackers FJ (1998) Procedure guideline for myocardial perfusion imaging. Society of Nuclear Medicine. J Nucl Med 39(5):918–923.
18. Hesse B, Tagil K, Cuocolo A et al. (2005) EANM/ESC procedural guidelines for myocardial perfusion imaging in nuclear cardiology. Eur J Nucl Med Mol Imaging 32(7):855–897.
19. Mamarian JJ, Verani MS (1994) Myocardial perfusion imaging during pharmacogical stress testing, Cardiol Clinic 12.223–245.
20. Mason JR, Palac RT, Freeman MC et al. (1984) Thallium scintigraphy during Dobutamine infusion: nonexercise-

dependent screening test for coronary disease. Am Heart J 107(3):481–485.
21. Gopinath G, Buscombe JR (2004) Pharmacological stress agents in nuclear cardiology. World J Nucl Med 4(1):64–72.
22. Ruffolo RR (1997) The pharmacology of dobutamine. Am J Med 294:244–248.
23. Meyer SL, Curry GC, Donsey MS, Twieg DB, Parkey RW, Willerson JT (1976) Influence of dobutamine on hemodynamics and coronary blood flow in patients with and without coronary artery disease. Am J Cardiol 38:103–108.
24. Fung AY, Gallagher KP, Buda AJ (1987) The physiologic basis of dobutamine as compared with dipyridamole stress interventions in the assessment of critical coronary stenosis. Circulation 76:943–951.
25. Pennel DJ, Ell PJ (1994) Whole body imaging of thallium-201 after six different stress regimens. J Nucl Med 35:425–433.
26. Secknus MA, Marwick TH (1997) Evolution of dobutamine echocardiography protocols and indications: safety and side effects in 3,011 studies over 5 years. J Am Coll Cardiol 29:1234–1240.
27. Botvinik EH et al. (1998) Nuclear Medicine: Cardiology – Topic 2. Pharmacological Stress, Self study program III.A publication of the society of Nuclear Medicin, pp. 1–59.
28. Leppo JA (1989) Dipyridamole-thallium imaging: the lazy man's stress test. J Nucl Med 30(3):281–287.
29. Heys JT, Mahmarian JJ, Cochran AJ et al. (1993) Dobutamine thallium201-tomography for evlauating patients with suspected coronary artery disease unable to undergo execrcise or pharmocological stress testing. J Am Coll Cardiol 21:1583–1590.
30. Gould KL (1991) Myocardial viability: what does it mean and how to measure it? Circulation 83:333–335.
31. 31.Wijns W, Vatner SF, Camici P (1998) Hibernating myocardium. N Engl J Med 339:173–181.
32. Birnbaum Y, Kloner RA (1996) Myocardial viability. West J Med 165:364–371.
33. Smart SC, Sawada S, Ryan T et al. (1993) Low dose dobutamine echocardiography detects reversible dysfunction after thrombolytic therapy of acute myocardial infarction. Circulation 88:405–415.
34. Everaert H, Vanhove C, Franken P (2000) Low-dose dobutamine gated single-photon emission tomography: comparison with stress echocardiography. Eur J Nucl Med 27:413–418.
35. Yoshinaga K, Morita K, Yamada S et al. (2001) Low-dose dobutamine electrocardiograph-gated myocardial SPECT for identifying viable myocardium: comparison with dobutamine stress echocardiography and PET. J Nucl Med 42:838–844.
36. Saremi F, Jadvar H, Siegel ME (2002) Pharmacologic interventions in nuclear radiology: indications, imaging protocols, and clinical results. Radiographics 22:477–490.
37. Marwick TH (1995) Arbutamine stress testing with closed loop drug delivery: toward the ideal or just another pharmacologic stress technique? J Am Coll Cardiol 26:1176–1179.
38. Lovell SL, Maguire SM, Turtle F, McDowell G, Campbell NP, Riley MS, Nicholls DP (2000) Comparative physiological study of arbutamine with exercise in humans. Clin Sci (London) 98:489–494.
39. Dennis CA, Pool PE, Perrins EJ et al. (1995) Stress testing with closed-loop arbutamine as an alternative to exercise. The International Arbutamine Study Group. J Am Coll Cardiol 26:1151–1158.
40. Shehata AR, Ahlberg AW, Gillam LD et al. (1997) Direct comparison of arbutamine and dobutamine stress testing with myocardial perfusion imaging and echocardiography in patients with coronary artery disease Am J Cardiol 80:716–720
41. Crouse (1998) Advances in pharmacological cardiac stress testing: arbutamine closed-loop feedback system. Echocardiography 15:393–400.
42. Laurence DR, Bennet PN, Brown MJ (1997) Text Book of Clinical Pharmacology, 8th edn. Churchill Livingstone, London.
43. Treuth MG, Reyes GA, He ZX et al. (2001) Tolerence and diagnostic accuracy of an abbreviated adenosine infusion for myocardial scintigraphy: A randomised, prospective study. J Nucl Cardiol 8:548–554.
44. Shryock JC, Snowdy S, Baraldi PG, Cacciari B, Spalluto G, Monopoli A et al. (1998) A2A-adenosine receptor reserve for coronary vasodilation. Circulation 98:711–718.
45. Salvatore CA, Jacobson MA, Taylor HE, Linden J, Johnson RG (1993) Molecular cloning and characterization of the human A3 adenosine receptor. Proc Natl Acad Sci USA 90:10365–10369.
46. Rossen JD, Quillen JE, Lopez AG, Stenberg RG, Talman CL, Winniford MD (1991) Comparison of coronary vasodilation with intravenous dipyridamole and adenosine. J Am Coll Cardiol 18,485–491.
47. Stein L, Burt R, Oppenheim B (1997) Syptom-limited arm exercise increases detection of ischaemia during dipyridamole tomographic thallium stress testing in patients with coronary artery disease. Am J Cardiol 29:531–536.
48. Pennell DJ, Mavrogeni SI, Forbat SM, Karwatowski SP, Underwood SR (1995) Adenosine combined with dynamic exercise for myocardial perfusion imaging. J Am Coll Cardiol 25:1300–1309.
49. Ardekani JM, Clowes P, Menash-Bonsu V and Nunan TO (2000) Time for abstention from caffeine before an adenosine myocardial perfusion scan. Nucl Med Commun 21:361–364.

50. Ogilby JD, Iskandrian AS, Untereker WJ, Heo J, Nguyen TN, Mercuro J (1992) Effect of intravenous adenosine infusion on myocardial perfusion and function. Hemodynamic/angiographic and scintigraphic study. Circulation 86:887–895.
51. Cerqueira MD, Verani MS, Schwaiger M, Heo J, Iskandrian AS (1994) Safety profile of adenosine stress perfusion imaging: results from the Adenoscan Multicenter Trial Registry. J Am Coll Cardiol 23:384–389.
52. Rochmis P, Blackburn H (1971) Exercise tests. A survey of procedures, safety, and litigation experience in approximately 170,000 tests. J Am Med Assoc 217:1061–1066.
53. Gibbons RJ, Heller GV, Wackers FJ, Johnson JR, Udelson JE (2003) SPECT image concordance between the new selective adenosine A2A receptor agonist, binodenoson and adenosine, A multi-centre randomized dose-selection trial. J Nucl Cardiol 10:ASNC abstracts.
54. Beller GA, Holzgrefe HH, Watson DD (1983) Effects of dipyridamole-induced vasodilation on myocardial uptake and clearance kinetics of thallium-201. Circulation 68:1328–1338
55. Knabb RM, Gidday JM, Ely SW (1984) Effects of dipyridamole on myocardial adenosine on active hyperaemia. Am J Physiol 247:804–810.
56. Ranhosky A, Kempthorne-Rawson J (1990) The safety of intravenous dipyridamole thallium myocardial perfusion imaging. Circulation 81:1205–1209.
57. Marchant E, Pichard A, Rodriguez JA, Casanegra P (1989) Acute effect of systemic versus intracoronary dipyridamole on coronary circulation. Am J Cardiol 57:1401–1404.
58. Moser GH, Schrader J, Deussen A (1989) Turnover of adenosine in plasma of human and dog blood. Am J Physiol 256:C799–C806.
59. Picano E, Sicari R, Varga A (1999) Dipyridamole stress echocardiography. Cardiol Clin 17:481–499.
60. Picano E (1989) Dipyridamole-echocardiography test: historical background and physiologic basis. Eur Heart J 10:365–376.
61. Poldermans D, Fioretti PM, Boersma E et al. (1994) Safety of dobutamine-atropine stress echocardiography in patients with suspected or proven coronary artery disease. Am J Cardiol 73:456–459.
62. Caner B, Karanfil A, Uysal U (1997) Effect of an additional atropine injection during dobutamine infusion for myocardial SPECT. Nucl Med Commun 18:567–573.
63. Variola A, Albiero R, Dander B, Buonanno C (1997) The exercise test with atropine. G Ital Cardiol 27:255–262.
64. Munagala VK, Guduguntla V, Kasravi B, Cummings G, Gardin JM (2003) Use of atropine in patients with chronotropic incompetence and poor exercise capacity during treadmill stress testing. Am Heart J 145:1046–1050.
65. Lahiri A, Crawley JC, Sonecha TN, Raftery EB (1984) Acute and chronic effects of sustained action buccal nitroglycerin in severe congestive heart failure. Int J Cardiol 5:39–48.
66. Feldman RL, Pepine CJ, Curry RC Jr et al. (1979) Coronary arterial responses to graded doses of nitroglycerin. Am J Cardiol 43:91–97.
67. Brown BG, Bolson E, Petersen RB, Pierce CD, Dodge HT (1981) The mechanisms of nitroglycerin action: stenosis vasodilatation as a major component of the drug response. Circulation 64:1089–1097.
68. Fujita M, Yamanishi K, Inoko M et al. (1994) Preferential dilation of recipient coronary arteries of the collateral circulation by intracoronary administration of nitroglycerin. J Am Coll Cardiol 24:631–635.
69. Dilsizian V, Perrone-Filardi P, Arrighi JA et al. (1993) Concordance and discordance between stress-redistribution-reinjection and rest-redistribution thallium imaging for assessing viable myocardium: comparison with metabolic activity by positron emission tomography. Circulation 88:941–952.
70. Ragosta M, Beller GA, Watson DD, Kaul S, Gimple LW (1993) Quantitative planar rest-redistribution 201Tl imaging in detection of myocardial viability and prediction of improvement in left ventricular function after coronary bypass surgery in patients with severely depressed left ventricular function. Circulation 87:1630–1641.
71. Udelson JE, Coleman PS, Metherall J et al. (1994) Predicting recovery of severe regional ventricular dysfunction:comparison of resting scintigraphy with 201Tl and ^{99m}Tc-sestamibi. Circulation 89:2552–2561.
72. Perrone-Filardi P, Pace L, Prastaro M et al. (1996) Assessment of myocardial viability in patients with chronic coronary artery disease: rest-4-hour-24-hour 201Tl tomography versus dobutamine echocardiography. Circulation 94:2712–2719.
73. Holly TA, Satran A, Bromet DS, Mieres JH, Frey MJ, Elliott MD, Heller GV, Hendel RC (2003) The impact of adjunctive adenosine infusion during exercise myocardial perfusion imaging: results of the Both Exercise and Adenosine Stress Test (BEAST) trial. J Nucl Cardiol 10:291–296.
74. Mahmood S, Gupta NK, Gunning M, Bomanji J B, Jarritt PH, Ell PJ (1994) 201 Tl myocardial perfusion SPECT: adenosine alone or combined with dynamic exercise. Nucl Med Commun 15:86–592.
75. Samady H, Wackers FJ, Joska TM, Zaret BL, Jain D (2002) Pharmacologic stress perfusion imaging with adenosine: role of simultaneous low-level treadmill exercise. J Nucl Cardiol 9:188–196.
76. Jamil G, Ahlberg AW, Elliott MD et al. (1999) Impact of limited treadmill exercise on adenosine Tc-99m sestamibi single-photon emission computed tomographic myocardial perfusion imaging in coronary artery disease. Am J Cardiol 84:400–403.

77. Thomas GS, Prill NV, Majmundar H, Fabrizi RR, Thomas JJ, Hayashida C, Kothapalli S, Payne JL, Payne MM, Miyamoto MI (2000) Treadmill exercise during adenosine infusion is safe, results in fewer adverse reactions, and improves myocardial perfusion image quality. J Nucl Cardiol 7:439–446.
78. Vitola JV, Brambatti JC, Caligaris F, Lesse CR, Nogueira PR, Joaquim AI, Loyo M, Salis FV, Paiva EV, Chalela WA, Meneghetti JC (2001) Exercise supplementation to dipyridamole prevents hypotension, improves electrocardiogram sensitivity, and increases heart-to-liver activity ratio on Tc-99m sestamibi imaging. J Nucl Cardiol 8(6):652–659.
79. Taillefe R, Amyot R and Turpin S et al. (1996) Comparison between dipyridamole and adenosine as pharmacologic coronary vasodilators in detection of coronary artery disease with thallium 201 imaging. J Nucl Cardiol 3,281–283.
80. Levine MG, Ahlberg AW, Mann A et al. (1999) Comparison of exercise, dipyridamole, adenosine, and dobutamine stress with the use of Tc-99m tetrofosmin tomographic imaging. J Nucl Cardiol 6:389–396.
81. Udelson E, Heller G, Wackers FJ et al. (2004) Randomized, controlled dose-ranging study of the selective adenosine A2a receptor agonist binodenoson for pharmacological stress as an adjunct to myocardial perfusion imaging. Circulation 109:457–464.
82. Barrett RJ, Lamson MJ, Johnson J et al. (2005) Pharmacokinetics and safety of binodenoson after intravenous dose escalation in healthy volunteers, J Nucl Cardiol 12:166–171.

Further Reading

1. Botvinick EH et al. (1998) Nuclear Medicine Cardiology Self Study Programme III, Pharmacological Stress and Associated Topics. SNM Publication, pp. 1–59.
2. American Society of Nuclear Cardiology (ASNC) (2001) Updated imaging guidelines for nuclear cardiology procedures. Part I. Stress myocardial perfusion stress protocols. J Nucl Cardiol 8:G5–G58.
3. Mamarian JJ, Verani MS (1994) Myocardial perfusion imaging during pharmacogical stress testing. Cardiology Clinics 12(2):223–245.
4. Anagnostopoulos C, Harbinson M, Kelion A et al. (2004) Procedure guidelines for radionuclide myocardialperfusion imaging. Heart 90:1–10.
5. Hesse B, Tagil K, Cuocolo A et al. (2005) EANM/ESC procedural guidelines for myocardial perfusion imaging in nuclear cardiology. Eur J Nucl Med Mol Imaging 32(7): 855–897.

Gated Single Photon Emission Computed Tomography (SPECT) Imaging: Current Status and Limitations

Sagir Ahmed and Assad Movahed

Contents

23.1 History 261
23.2 Evolution of ECG Gated SPECT and Current Status 261
23.3 Gated SPECT Acquisition 262
23.4 Cardiac Beat Length Acceptance Window . 262
23.5 Imaging Protocols 263
23.6 Quantification and Software 264
23.7 Diagnostic and Prognostic Value of Gated SPECT 265
23.8 Prognosis and Risk Stratification 266
23.9 Limitations 268
23.10 Conclusion 268
References 272

23.1 History

In 1925 Herrmann Blumgart performed the first test of cardiac function using radioactive indicators on human beings. Blumgart used himself as the first test subject. The concept of producing radioactive materials, rather than using those occurring naturally, came from the 1931 Nobel Prize-winning development of the cyclotron by Ernest Lawrence, at Berkeley, California in 1928. Lawrence's physician brother, John Lawrence, is called the "father of nuclear medicine" for his contribution in this field (Fig. 23.1) [1].

23.2 Evolution of ECG Gated SPECT and Current Status

Strauss et al. introduced the concept of using ECG to trigger image frame acquisition in 1971 [3]. Combined perfusion/function studies became commonplace in the late 1980s with the advent of Tc-99m labeled myocardial perfusion agents and has rapidly evolved into a standard for myocardial perfusion imaging in the USA. In its position paper in March 1999, The American Society of Nuclear Cardiology recommended the routine incorporation of ECG gating during SPECT cardiac perfusion scintigraphy [4]. Gated SPECT allows simultaneous assessment of *both* perfusion and function in a single-injection, single-acquisition sequence. Over 90% of all myocardial perfusion SPECT studies in the USA are now gated. The exponential growth of gated SPECT was fueled by the development of new radioisotopes, improvements in computer technology imaging hardware and by the development of automated algorithms to quantitatively measure left ventricular (LV) volume and ejection fraction (EF), regional myocardial wall motion (WM) and wall thickening (WT) from gated SPECT,

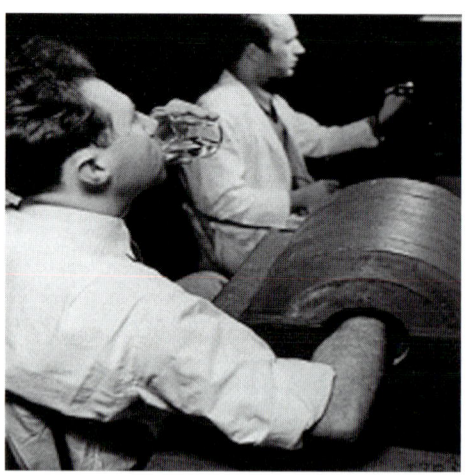

Fig. 23.1 One of John and Ernest Lawrence's colleagues, Joseph Hamilton, is shown drinking radiosodium in January 1939 with Robert Marshak to the right. Lawrence had made Na-24 efficiently by bombarding rock salt with deuterons. Distributing through the body like ordinary sodium, its half-life of 14.8 hours made it a potentially useful candidate for diagnosis and therapy. Most likely as a result of the high-energy emissions of Na-24, as well as repeated radiation exposure during his search for radioisotopes for medical uses, Hamilton subsequently died of leukemia in 1957 [1, 2]. Source: American Society of Nuclear Cardiology. J Nucl Cardiol 2005;12: 86–95 with permission

rapidly and accurately, and with minimal or no operator interaction [5–10].

The 99mTc-based perfusion tracers (sestamibi or tetrofosmin), because of their higher count rates and minimal redistribution, permit evaluation of regional myocardial wall motion and wall thickening throughout the cardiac cycle. It is also possible to have gated Tl-201 studies, but image quality is less optimal because of low counts [9].

23.3
Gated SPECT Acquisition

First the computer estimates the average R–R interval, based on five to ten beats. The interval is then broken into equal time segments. For an average R–R interval of 1000 ms, eight "gates" are opened, each gate of 125 ms. Eight tomograms are acquired that reflect eight equal parts of the heartbeat. Usually, the first tomogram is closest to end-diastole and the third or fourth is nearest to end systole. For non-gated SPECT, one image (instead of eight or 16 with gated SPECT) is acquired for every one-projection angle [11] (Fig. 23.2).

Count accumulation is triggered by the R wave and eight images are obtained, each representative of a specific phase of cardiac cycle. Traditionally 8-frame gating is used but a higher frame rate, such as 16, is possible. Gated SPECT acquisitions are performed in buffered frame mode, using classic filtered back projection (first described by Bracewell for astronomical application in 1967) or iterative reconstruction; all projection images of a specific time interval are reconstructed to form the SPECT image and are displayed in four-dimensional format (x, y, z and time). Image quality depends directly on count number of individual frames, no matter what radiopharmaceutical is used [5–9].

23.4
Cardiac Beat Length Acceptance Window

Most gated SPECT uses a "fixed temporal resolution framing" approach. In this approach all gating intervals

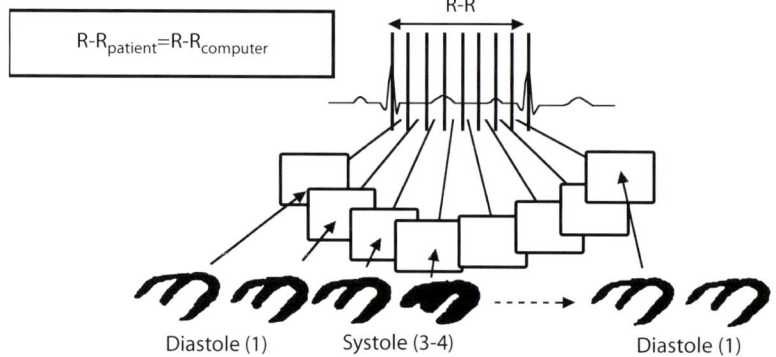

Fig. 23.2 Principle of ECG gated SPECT acquisition (8-frame model). For each angular projection, separate temporal frames are acquired corresponding to different phases of cardiac cycles. Perfusion projection images are obtained from summation of individual frames. (From Cullom SJ, Case JA, Bateman TM. Electrocardiographically gated myocardial perfusion SPECT. J Nucl Cardiol 1998;5(4): 418–425, with permission.)

will be set to the same temporal length. So in an 8-frame gating, each interval will span 125 ms, if the expected R–R interval is 1000 ms. However, in real life, the R–R interval varies during the acquisition, so tolerance needs to be built into the count collection process. Tolerance defines the acceptable deviation of each R–R interval from the expected value, and minimizes temporal blurring. The beat length acceptance window is defined as a percentage of the mean R–R interval and this eliminates those beats that are too long or too short. A 20% beat length acceptance window allows data accumulation from cardiac beats having R–R duration within ±10% of the expected duration. An acceptance window of 100% allows data accumulation from cardiac beats having duration within ±50% of the expected duration. This is *not* equivalent to accepting 100% of the beats. If you accept 100% of the beats (all beats), that is equivalent to a window of infinite width. For example, if the expected R–R duration is 1000 ms, then a 20% window will allow data from cardiac beats having durations 900–1100 ms. A window of 100% will allow data from cardiac beats having durations 500–1500 ms. Anything beyond these boundaries will be rejected [5–7] (Fig. 23.3).

Perfusion SPECT data is derived from summing the various intervals of the gated study. If too many counts are rejected due to gating problems or arrhythmias, not only will the gated data be invalid, it will also corrupt the perfusion data and make it unreliable. This issue can be resolved by collecting all rejected counts in an "extra" frame (9th frame in 8-frame gated study) and adding the extra frame back during the generation of the "summed" perfusion study. It is advisable to use a wide acceptance window when no extra frame is available to save the rejected counts, otherwise use a 20–30% window when the feature is available [7, 9].

Extra frame?	No	use 100% window
Extra frame?	Yes	use 20–30% window
Acquisition		
↓		
8–16 projection sets	> Reconstruction >	Gated short axis
Extra frame		
↓		
Σ	Summed ungated projection set >	Reconstruction > Short axis

23.5
Imaging Protocols

Several imaging protocols (Fig. 23.4) are used for gated SPECT imaging, with 99m Tc –sestamibi or tetrofosmin [12].

Generally, the stress study is performed first with the 2-day protocol. To improve target-to-nontarget ratios and eliminate artefacts due to "upward creep" of the heart, images are usually acquired 15–60 minutes after stress using 99m Tc sestamibi or tetrofosmin. The pharmacological stress test needs a longer delay to allow additional gut clearing. Circular orbits are used in either a *step-and-shoot* or *continuous* data acquisition mode. For single-detector gamma cameras and for cameras with two perpendicular detectors fixed at 90°, a total arc of 180° rather than a full 360° is used for cardiac acquisitions. The full range of motion of the 180° data acquisition arc is from 45° right anterior oblique to 45° left posterior oblique views. Although gating is usually performed at 8 frames/cardiac cycle, a greater number of frames can be acquired (for example, 16 frames/R–R interval). Because higher frame rates have fewer counts per frame, the ability to accurately identify endocardial borders and define regional functional abnormalities decreases. In addition, subtle wall motion (WM) and wall thickness (WT) abnormalities may not be appreciated. Use of 8 rather than 16 frames under-represents the dynamic aspect of the cardiac data. When too few cinematic frames are acquired, end-diastolic volumes

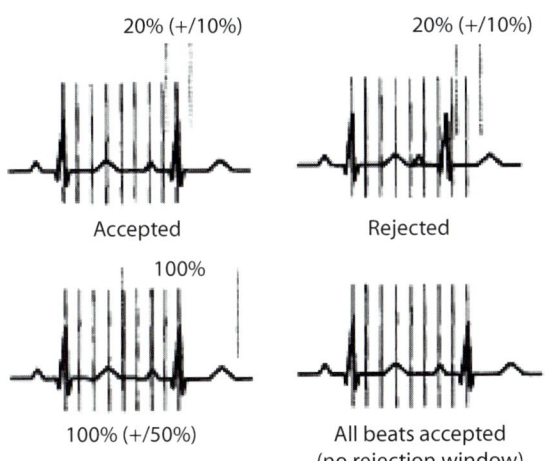

Fig. 23.3 Relation between cycle length and rejection criteria for some common setting. (Reprinted from Journal of Nuclear Cardiology, 5(4), Cullom SJ, Case JA, Bateman TM. Electrocardiographically gated myocardial perfusion SPECT. Technical principles and quality control considerations, 418–425 (1998), with permission from Elsevier.)

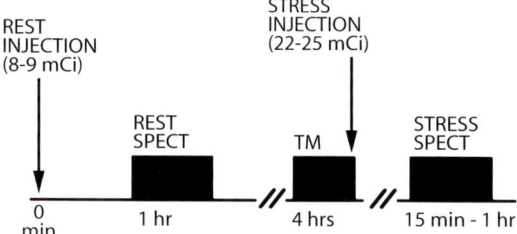
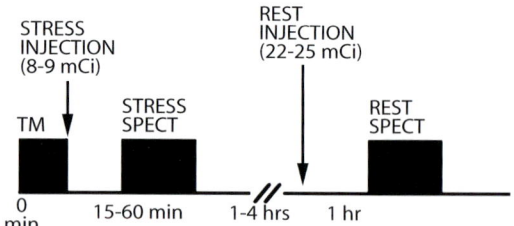
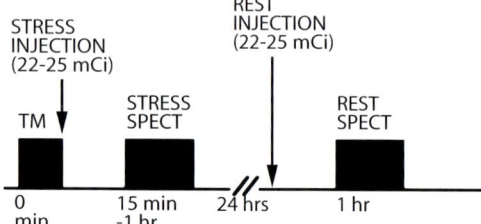
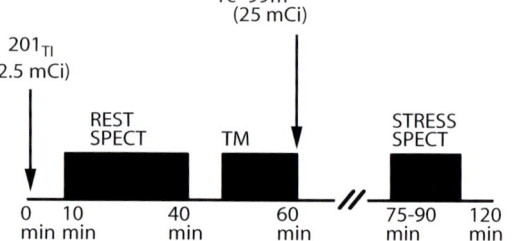

Fig. 23.4 Radionuclide myocardial perfusion imaging protocols. (From Journal of Nuclear Cardiology, 8(1), DePuey GE, Garcia VE. Updated imaging guidelines for nuclear cardiology procedures Part 1, G1–G58 with permission from Elsevier) (Note TM = Treadmill)

will be smaller and end-systolic volumes larger than they really are, resulting in low EF measurements. EF measurements calculated from 8-frame data are 3% to 4% lower, fairly constant, and predictable over a wide range of true EF measurements. Nevertheless, to speed data processing and to minimize requirements for data storage, most institutions use 8 frames for gated SPECT and acquire data in a buffered frame mode using a 100% rhythm acceptance window. For an R–R interval of 800 ms, the beat-acceptance windows are from 400 to 1200 ms.

23.6 Quantification and Software

Advances in nuclear cardiology software have been made: (1) automation of image processing has improved reproducibility, reduced operator time, and measurement of regional thickening and wall motion; (2) integration has helped to set up an optimal image display that includes most functions in one package; and (3) increased speed reduces technologist and physician time.

Gated SPECT can quantitatively measure regional, global and systolic parameters of cardiac function.

In addition, measured transient ischemic dilatation (TID), in its *ungated* form is a highly specific marker of severe and extensive CAD. Several algorithms have been developed for quantification of gated SPECT in recent years. They are based on different mathematical operations and principles, and reflect different degrees of validation and automation. EF measurement from gated SPECT has been extensively validated against other quantitative techniques such as MUGA or MRI. Gated SPECT for measuring LVEF is usually volume based rather than count based as in gated blood pool images. ECG gated SPECT provides robust and highly reproducible estimates of LVEF.

DePuey and Boonyaprapa described methods based on the automated or semi-automated detection of endocardial borders on the perfusion images [5]. Smith et al. used the partial volume effect to quantify regional thickening fractions and estimate LVEF, without the need for edge detection. However, Germano et al. at Cedars-Sinai Medical Center developed the first totally automated method (QGS; quantitative gated SPECT) of fitting geometric shapes to the endocardial borders to obtain systolic and diastolic volumes and EFs. The QGS methodology uses a Gaussian fit to determine endocardial and epicardial offsets, whereas ECT (Emory Cardiac Toolbox) is a count-based method. This technique rapidly became the industry standard. Other totally automated packages include packages from Emory University (Emory Cardiac Toolbox: ECT), University of Michigan (4D-MSPECT), and Yale University (Wackers-Liu CQ package). In a meta-analysis by Ioannidis et al. the values of end-diastolic volume and end-systolic volume generally correlated very well with volumes from magnetic resonance imaging.

23.7 Diagnostic and Prognostic Value of Gated SPECT

Gated SPECT helps to differentiate soft tissue attenuation artefact from scar. Artefact will show normal function and thickening, while scar will show as a fixed defect, with diminished or lack of wall thickening and motion. Gated SPECT thereby increases the specificity of perfusion SPECT (Fig. 23.5). DePuey and Rozanski demonstrated that false-positive perfusion studies could be reduced from 14% to 3% by incorporating regional wall motion data in the interpretation of perfusion imaging. In women, where the false-positive rate of stress ECGs is relatively high and breast soft-tissue attenuation artefact is common, ECG gating has been shown to further enhance the diagnostic specificity of 99mTc perfusion imaging from 84% to 94%. Smanio et al. demonstrated that the number of "borderline-normal" or "borderline-abnormal" interpretations was significantly reduced. In patients with a low likelihood of CAD, the normalcy rate increased from 74% to 93%. In patients with a high likelihood of CAD, the trend was also toward a higher number of unequivocally abnormal interpretations [13].

Perfusion SPECT images are normalized to the area of highest uptake within the myocardium. In the case of multivessel disease or left main disease, balanced global hypoperfusion comes into play. According to several reports, only 13–50% of patients with three-vessel CAD or left main disease actually have perfusion abnormalities in multiple territories. In the setting of diffuse ischemia, a perfusion defect may not be seen, because of image normalization. Transient ischemic dilatation (TID) in myocardial perfusion imaging (MPI) refers to a significant enlargement in left ventricular (LV) size on the stress images compared with the rest images. In the case of balanced ischemia, TID due to stunning results in an increase in ESV [15] and a decrease in EF. This is helpful to correctly identify significant CAD for predicting severe proximal left anterior descending artery or multivessel critical coronary lesion, even though there is no perfusion abnormality due to balanced ischemia [14]. The mechanism of TID is controversial. Myocardial thinning resulting from stress-induced diffuse subendocardial hypoperfusion produces a visually larger LV cavity. At rest, the subendocardium is better perfused and the LV cavity appears relatively smaller. So dilatation is apparent, not true dilatation. More recent thought is that TID is a combination of both apparent (visual) and true dilatation. Hung et al. provided evidence suggesting that TID in dipyridamole MPI was significantly correlated with stress-induced ischemic stunning by use of Tl-201 gated SPECT. Enlargement of ESV as a result of ischemic stunning was an important factor resulting in TID [15]. Several studies have clearly demonstrated the incremental value of using both functional and perfusion data in detecting multivessel disease or high-grade stenosis over perfusion data alone, and a clue may be diffuse post-stress stunning (decrease in post-stress EF when compared with baseline). Another important application is in severe cardiomyopathy. Gated SPECT can help in differentiating the etiology of severe cardiomyopathy (nonischemic vs ischemic).

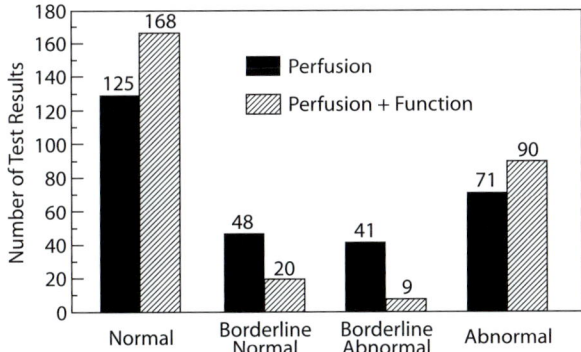

Fig. 23.5 Incremental value of gated SPECT relative to perfusion scan assessment alone is shown by the reduction of equivocal cases. (From Smanio PE, Watson DD, Segalla DL et al. Value of gating of technetium-99m sestamibi single photon emission computed tomography imaging. J Am Coll Cardiol 1997;30:1687, with permission)

23.8
Prognosis and Risk Stratification

Gated SPECT has superior sensitivity and specificity when compared with exercise ECG and provides information regarding the effect, severity and location of CAD. However its ability to stratify those patients who are at a high risk for subsequent cardiac events have helped to define nuclear cardiology as a tool beyond the establishment of clinical diagnosis. A normal exercise or pharmacological stress SPECT is associated with a 0.3–1.0% annual risk of MI or CAD, in comparison with an abnormal study where the risk is 5–10-fold increased. Further more, the risk for MI or CD is magnified when high risk scan findings are present, such as (1) transient ischemic dilatation of LV, (2) increase lung to heart radiotracer uptake, (3) extensive defect, (4) reversible defect, (5) perfusion abnormalities in multivessel or proximal LAD distribution, (6) reduced LV function, and (7) peri-infarction ischemia.

Gated SPECT imaging plays an important role in the risk assessment of patients with known or suspected CAD. Sharir et al. demonstrated in a large series of 1680 consecutive patients who underwent dual-isotope gated SPECT imaging, that those with EFs <45% were associated with reduced survival, irrespective of the perfusion defect size or severity. Additionally, those patients with normal end-systolic volumes <70 mL or an EF >45% had a very low cardiac mortality rate, despite severe perfusion abnormalities (Fig. 23.6) [16].

This group also examined the relative value of perfusion and function in risk stratification in 2686 patients into low-, intermediate-, and high-risk categories for cardiac death and MI [(17]. LVEF was most predictive of death and the amount of ischemia (summed difference score on perfusion imaging) was the best predictor of nonfatal MI (Fig. 23.7).

Functional information was found to be of incremental value in the prediction of cardiac death beyond the perfusion imaging parameters (Figs. 23.8–23.11).

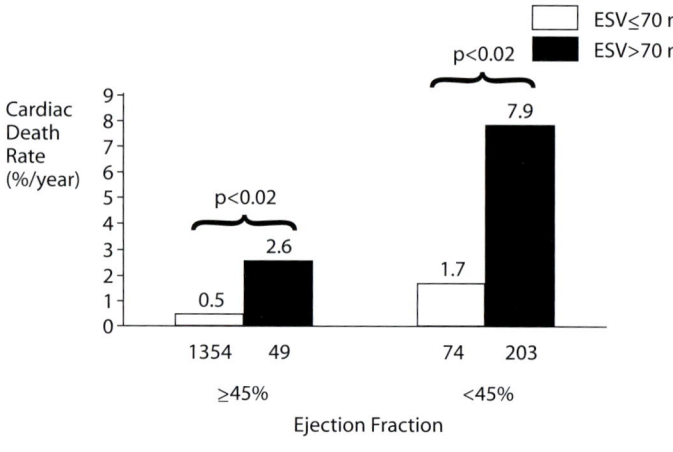

Fig. 23.6 Cardiac death rate (%/year) as a function of EF and ESV (Source: Sharir T, Germano G, Kabanaugh PB et al. Incremental prognostic value of post-stress left ventricular ejection fraction and volume by gated myocardial perfusion single photon emission computed tomography. Circulation 1999;100(10): 1035–1042, with permission)

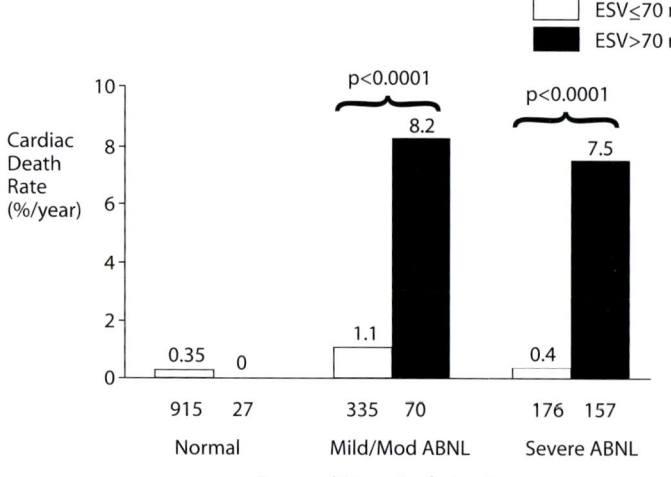

Fig. 23.7 Cardiac death rate (%/year) as a function of perfusion abnormality and ESV. The number of patients within each category is indicated below each column. The categories are summed stress score are normal (0–3), mild/moderate (4–13) and severe (>13). ABNL = abnormality, MOD = moderate. (From Sharir T, Germano G, Kabanaugh PB et al. Incremental prognostic value of post-stress left ventricular ejection fraction and volume by gated myocardial perfusion single photon emission computed tomography. Circulation 1999;100(10): 1035–1042, with permission)

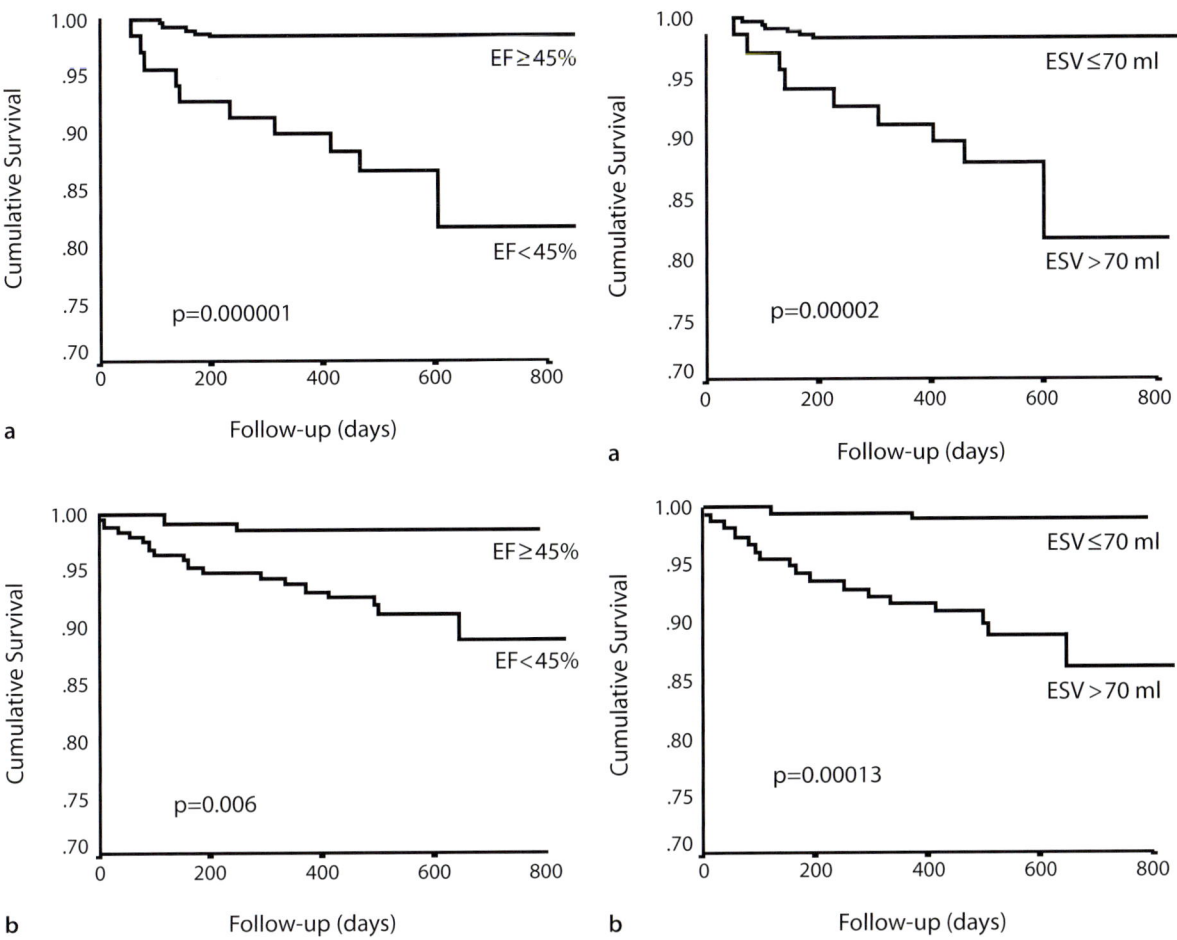

Fig. 23.8 Cumulative survival in (A) patients with mild/moderate perfusion abnormalities and (B) patients with severe perfusion abnormalities, stratified into EF>45% and EF<45%. (From Sharir T, Germano G, Kabanaugh PB et al. Incremental prognostic value of post-stress left ventricular ejection fraction and volume by gated myocardial perfusion single photon emission computed tomography. Circulation 1999;100(10): 1035–1042, with permission)

Fig. 23.9 Cumulative survival in (A) patients with mild/moderate perfusion abnormalities and (B) patients with severe perfusion abnormalities, stratified into ESV#70 mL and ESV.70 mL. (From Sharir T, Germano G, Kabanaugh PB et al. Incremental prognostic value of post-stress left ventricular ejection fraction and volume by gated myocardial perfusion single photon emission computed tomography. Circulation 1999;100(10): 1035–1042, with permission)

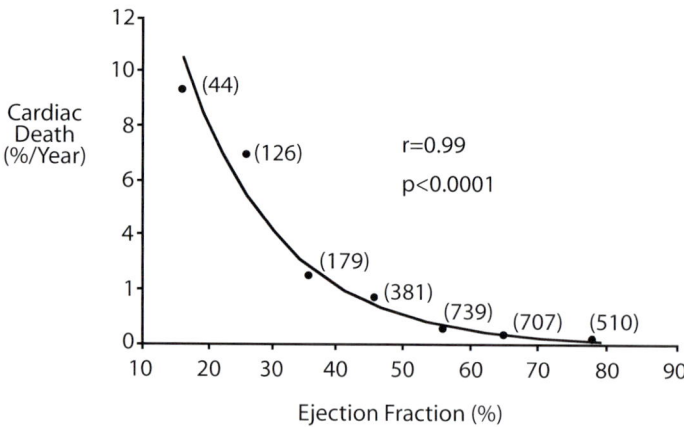

Fig. 23.10 Annual CD rate as a function of EF. Number of patients at each interval is indicated in parenthesis. (From Sharir T, Germano G, Kang X et al. Prediction of myocardial infarction versus cardiac death by gated myocardial perfusion SPECT: Stratification by the amount of stress-induced ischemia and the post stress ejection fraction. J Nucl Med 2001;42: 831–837, with permission from Elsevier)

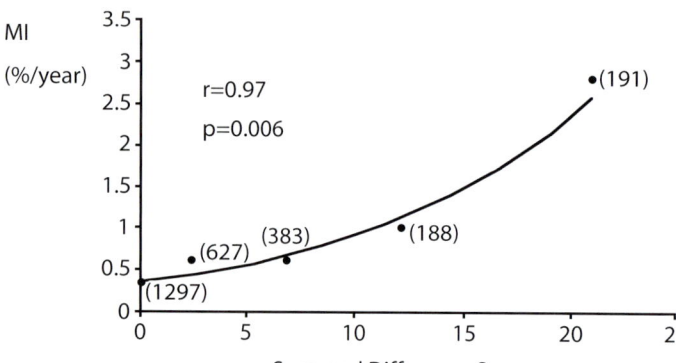

Fig. 23.11 Nonfatal MI rate as function of SDS (summed difference score) Number of patients at each 5-unit is indicated. (From Sharir T, Germano G, Kang X et al. Prediction of myocardial infarction versus cardiac death by gated myocardial perfusion SPECT: Stratification by the amount of stress-induced ischemia and the poststress ejection fraction, J Nucl Med 2001;42:831–837, with permission from Elsevier)

Interestingly, the presence of ischemia did not influence prognosis in patients with LVEFs of 30%, due to the already high mortality rate. After an acute MI, LV function has long been a key determinant for survival. A study done by Hashimoto et al. assessed the relationship between perioperative cardiac events and various predictors, including clinical factors, perfusion, and functional assessment using the QGS program to assess LV function and estimate regional wall motion. Multivariate analysis demonstrates functional analysis to be an independent predictor of perioperative cardiac events. Function and wall motion assessment proved especially useful in patients with normal perfusion scans [18].

The development of automated algorithms to quantitatively measure left ventricular (LV) volume and ejection fraction (EF), regional myocardial wall motion and thickening from gated SPECT, rapidly and accurately, and with minimal operator interaction, has also contributed to its widespread use. These innovations have made gated SPECT imaging a premier method of noninvasive evaluation of myocardial blood flow and cardiac function in a variety of clinical situations [3].

23.9
Limitations

Nuclear images have low spatial resolution. This could be a problem in a very small heart, specifically measuring the end systolic volume and overestimation of EF is a strong possibility. When perfusion to a given segment of myocardium is severely diminished or absent, detecting the cardiac surfaces is challenging and EF calculation may not be valid (Figs. 23.12 and 23.13). Automated selection of noncardiac structures in juxtaposition to the myocardium may also occur. Also in the case of severe arrhythmias, gating is not valid.

23.10
Conclusion

Quantitative analysis of myocardial perfusion and function from ECG gated SPECT must be performed at a high quality nuclear department. Using the proper software tool, quantitative analysis promotes the standardization of quality control, acquisition, processing,

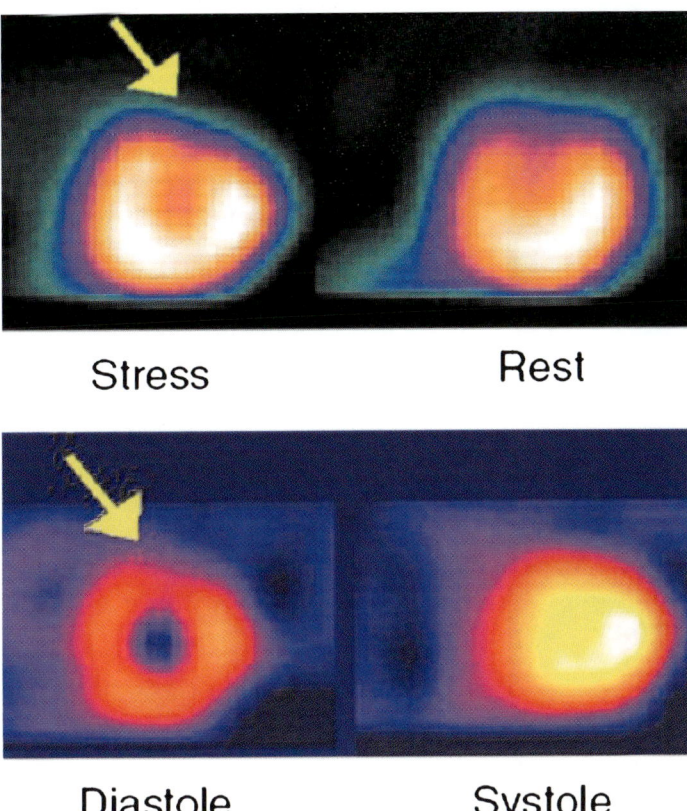

Fig. 23.12 Breast attenuation artefact. Top row: a mild fixed anterior defect related to a possible breast attenuation artefact. In the bottom row, diastolic and systolic frames from an electrocardiographic-gated single-photon emission computed tomography (SPECT) acquisition demonstrating preserved wall thickening in the territory of the mild anterior fixed defect. The preserved wall thickening supports the conclusion that the mild defect is an attenuation artefact. Source: Odelson JE, Dilsizian V, Bonow RO. Nuclear cardiology. In Zipes DP, Libby P, Bonow RO, Braunwald E (eds), Braunwald's Heart Disease – a Textbook of Cardiovascular Medicine, 7th edn. Philadelphia, PA, Elsevier Saunders, p. 294, Figure 13–10, with permission

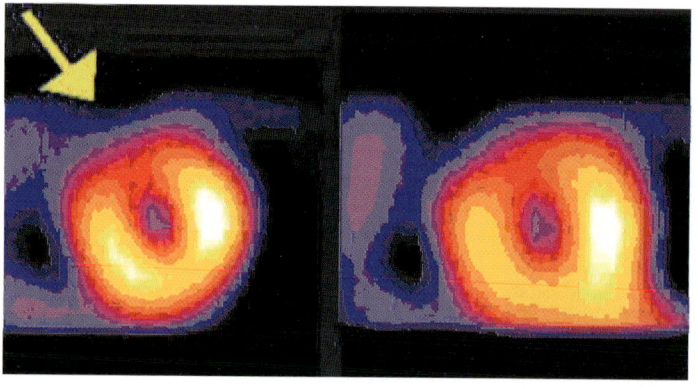

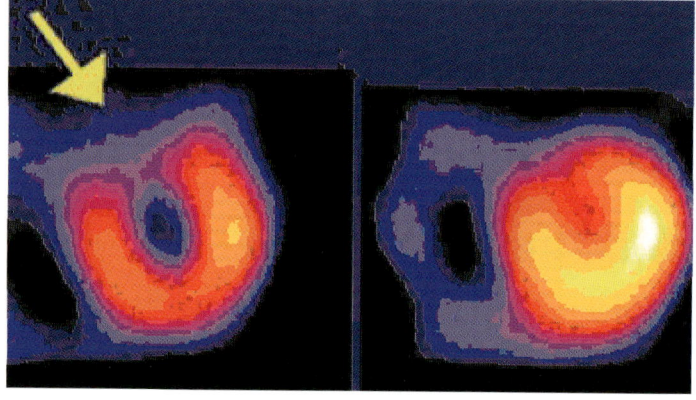

Fig. 23.13 A more severe anterior fixed defect is unlikely to represent an artefact on the basis of the severity and is more likely to represent myocardial infarction. In the bottom row, diastolic and systolic frames from the gated SPECT acquisition demonstrate abnormal thickening, supporting the interpretation of infarct rather than artefact. Source: Odelson JE, Dilsizian V, Bonow RO. Nuclear cardiology. In Zipes DP, Libby P, Bonow RO, Braunwald E (eds), Braunwald's Heart Disease – a Textbook of Cardiovascular Medicine, 7th edn. Philadelphia, PA, Elsevier Saunders, p. 294, Figure 13–10, with permission

interpretation, and reporting. There are many commercial packages available (Figs. 23.14 and 23.15). The most integrated and popular packages are (1) the QGS/QPS packages developed at Cedars–Sinai in Los Angeles; (2) the Emory cardiac Toolbox TM (ECTB TM) developed at Emory University; and (3) 4-D MSPECT developed at the university of Michigan. Quantitative analysis should always be used as a second objective interpretation of the status of the patient's perfusion and function.

Gated SPECT imaging has attained widespread acceptance. It increases the specificity of perfusion SPECT by its ability to improve artefact recognition; the use of functional information also improves the detection of severe and extensive coronary artery disease. TID provides independent and incremental prognostic information. There is better survival with EF > 45% and ESV < 70 mL, irrespective of perfusion abnormalities.

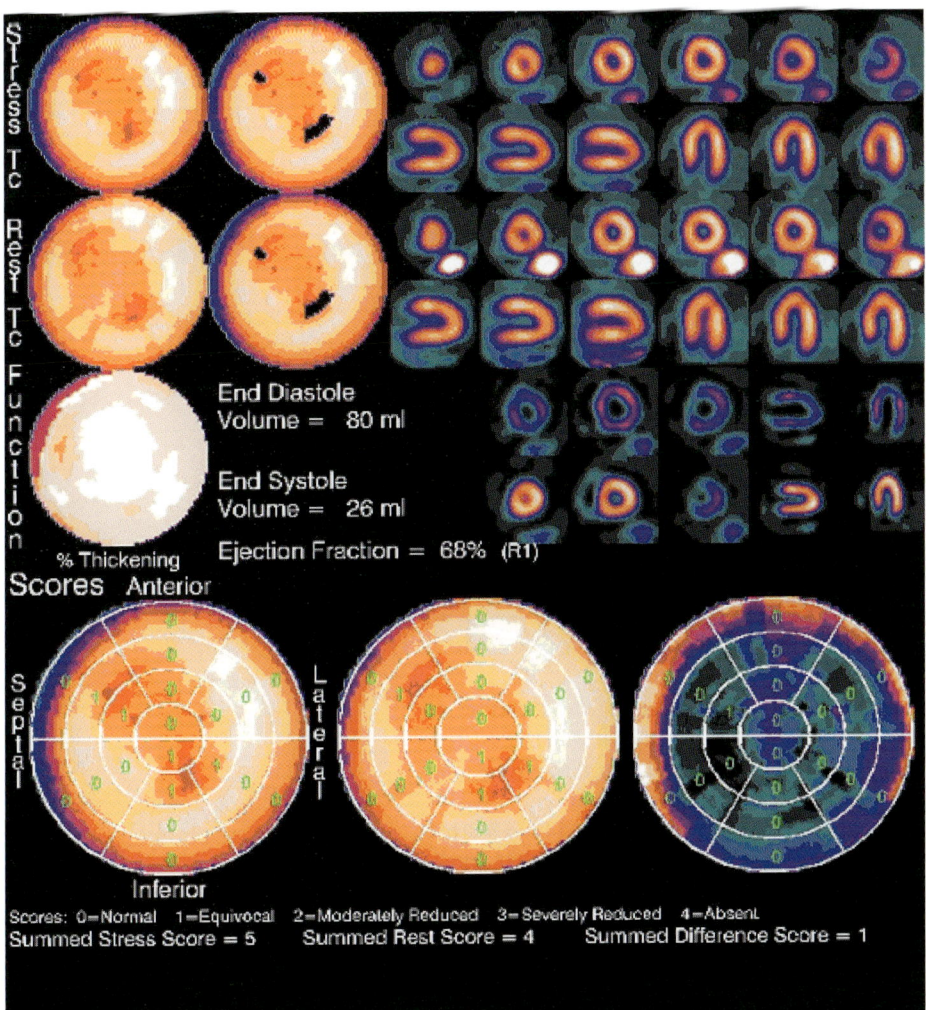

Fig. 23.14 *Top*: Emory Cardiac Toolbox™ integrated display which includes CEqual® quantitative output, the Emory Gated SPECT functional output, and selected tomograms demonstrating both perfusion (stress and rest) and function (end-diastolic and end systolic) showing no evidence of perfusion abnormalities. Functional parameter include percentage wall thickening, end-diastolic and end-systolic volumes, and ejection fraction. Global LVEF was 68%. *Bottom*: The visual scores for 20 myocardial perfusion segments of the CEqual® stress and rest polar maps are generated and displayed in this output. The visual scores are based on a five-point scoring system and key for this system is listed at the bottom of the display. The summed stress score (SSS) represents the sum of the visual score for the stress, the summed rest score (SRS) represents the sum of the visual scores for rest, and the summed difference score represents the difference between the SSS and SRS values. This display allows for the integration of visual scores and the quantitative analysis of myocardial perfusion. Source: Ahmed and Movahed. ECU Cardiology, Greenville, NC, USA

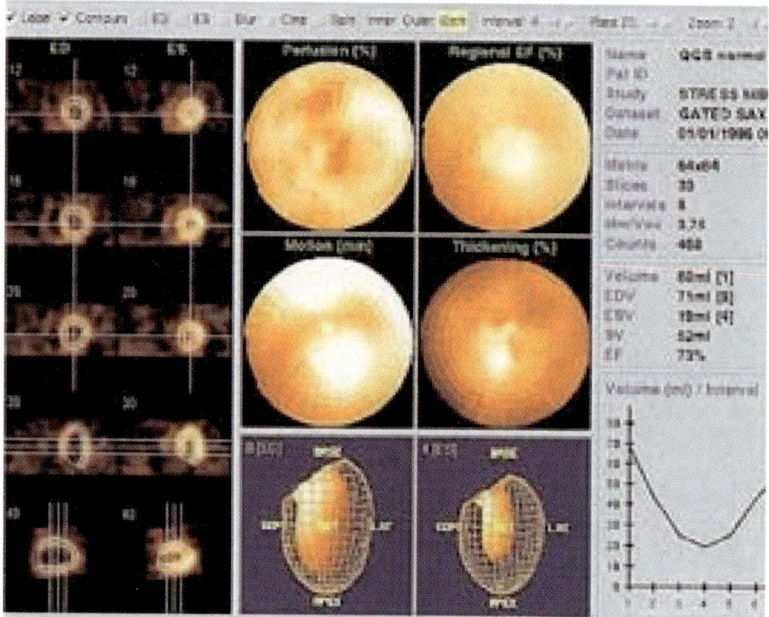

Fig. 23.15 Gated-SPECT myocardial perfusion using Gaussian edge detection fit. Another example of gated-SPECT myocardial perfusion is shown, with LVEF determination using a Gaussian edge detection fit on horizontal long axis, vertical long axis, and three levels of short axis images, with perfusion, regional EF, thickening and motion polar maps, and a ventricular volume curve. (Reprinted from Journal of the American College of Cardiology, 42(7), FJ Klocke, MG Baird, BH Lorell, TM. Bateman, JV Messer, DS Berman, PT O'Gara, BA Carabello, RO Russell, MD Cerqueira, MG St John Sutton, AN DeMaria et al. ACC/AHA/ASNC Guidelines for the Clinical Use of Cardiac Radionuclide Imaging – Executive Summary: A Report of the American College of Cardiology/American Heart Association Task Force on Practice Guidelines (ACC/AHA/ASNC Committee to Revise the 1995 Guidelines), 1318–1333, 2003, with permission from Elsevier.)

References

1. Williams KA (2005) Measurement of ventricular function with scintigraphic techniques: Part I-Imaging hardware, radiopharmaceuticals, and first-pass radionuclide angiography. J Nucl Cardiol 12:86–95.
2. Available from: URL:http://dynaweb.oac.cdlib.org: 8088/dynaweb/uchist/public/inmemoriam/inmemoriam 1959/503.
3. Strauss HW, Zaret BL, Hurley PJ, Natarajan TK, Pitt B (1971) A scintiphotographic method for measuring left ventricular ejection fraction in man without cardiac catheterization. Am J Cardiol 28:575–580.
4. Bateman TM, Berman DS, Heller GV et al. (1999) American Society of Nuclear Cardiology position statement on electrocardiographic gating of myocardial perfusion SPECT scintigrams. J Nucl Cardiol 6:470–471.
5. Germano G, Nichols K, Cullom SJ (2001) Gated perfusion SPECT: technical considerations. In DePuey EG, Garcia EV, Berman DS (eds); Cardiac SPECT Imaging, 2nd edn. Philadelphia, PA Lippincott Williams and Wilkins, pp. 103–115.
6. DePuey EG, Heller G, Taillefer R (2001) Clinical application of gated myocardial perfusion spect. In DePuey EG, Garcia EV, Berman DS (eds), Cardiac SPECT Imaging' 2nd edn. Philadelphia, PA, Lippincott Williams and Wilkins, pp. 211–229.
7. Zaret BL (2005) Cardiac performance. In Zaret BL, Beller GA (eds), Clinical Nuclear Cardiology: State of the Art

and Future Directions, 3rd edn. Philadelphia, PA, Elsevier and Mosby, pp. 175–187.
8. Germano G, Berman DS (2005) Regional and global ventricular function and volumes from single-photon emission computed tomography perfusion imaging. In Zaret BL, Beller GA (eds); Clinical Nuclear Cardiology: State of the Art and Future Directions, 3rd edn. Philadelphia, PA, Elsevier and Mosby, pp. 189–211.
9. Germano G, Berman DS (2003) Gated single photon emission computed tomography. In Iskandrian AE, Verani MS (eds), Nuclear Cardiac Imaging. Principles and Applications, 3rd edn. New York, Oxford University Press, pp.121–136.
10. Lum DP, Coel MN (2003) Comparison of automatic quantification software for the measurement of ventricular volume and ejection fraction in gated myocardial perfusion SPECT. Nucl Med Commun 24:259–266.
11. Cullom SJ, Case JA, Bateman TM (1998) Electrocardiographically gated myocardial perfusion SPECT: technical principles and quality control considerations. J Nucl Cardiol 5:418–425.
12. Smanio PE, Watson DD, Segalla DL et al. (1997) Value of gating of technetium- 99m sestamibi single-photon emission computed tomographic imaging. J Am Coll Cardiol 30:1687–1692.
13. DePuey GE, Garcia VE (eds) (2001). Updated imaging guidelines for nuclear cardiology procedures Part 1. J Nucl Cardiol 8(1):G1–G58.
14. Kumar SP, Brewington SD, O'Brien KF, Movahed A (2005) Clinical correlation between increased lung to heart ratio of technetium –99m sestamibi and multivessel coronary artery disease. Int J Cardiol 101: 219–222.
15. Guang-Uei Hung, Kung-Wei Lee, Ching-Pei Chen, Wan-Yu Lin, Kuang-Tao Yang (2005) Relationship of transient ischemic dilation in dipyridamole myocardial perfusion imaging and stress-induced changes of functional parameters evaluated by Tl-201 gated SPECT . J Nucl Cardiol 12(3):268–275.
16. Germano G, Kiat H, Kavanagh PB et al. (1995) Automatic quantification of ejection fraction from gated myocardial perfusion SPECT. J Nucl Med 36:2138–2147.
17. Sharir T, Germano G, Kang X et al. (2001) Prediction of myocardial infarction versus cardiac death by gated myocardial perfusion SPECT: risk stratification by the amount of stress-induced ischemia and the poststress ejection fraction. J Nucl Med 42:831–837.
18. Sharir T, Germano G, Kavanagh PB et al. (1999) Incremental prognostic value of post-stress left ventricular ejection fraction and volume by gated myocardial perfusion single photon emission computed tomography. Circulation 100:1035–1042.
19. Klocke FJ (2003) ACC/AHA/ASNC Guidelines for the Clinical Use of Cardiac Radionuclide Imaging. J Am Coll Cardiol 42(7): 1318–1333.
20. Nakajima K, Higuchi T, Taki J, Kawano M, Tonami N (2001) Accuracy of ventricular volume and ejection fraction measured by gated myocardial SPECT: comparison of 4 software programs. J Nucl Med 42:1571–1578.
21. Taillefer R, DePuey EG, Udelson JE, Beller GA, Latour Y, Reeves F (1997) Comparative diagnostic accuracy of Tl-201 and Tc-99m sestamibi SPECT imaging (perfusion and ECG-gated SPECT) in detecting coronary artery disease in women. J Am Coll Cardiol 29:69–77.
22. Smanio PE, Watson DD, Segalla DL, Vinson EL, Smith WH, Beller GA (1997) Value of gating of technetium-99m sestamibi single-photon emission computed tomographic imaging. J Am Coll Cardiol 30:1687–1692.
23. Chae SC, Heo J, Iskandrian AS, Wasserleben V, Cave V (1993) Identification of extensive coronary artery disease in women by exercise single-photon emission computed tomographic (SPECT) thallium imaging. J Am Coll Cardiol 21:1305–1311.
24. Sharir T, Bacher-Stier C, Dhar S et al. (1000) Identification of severe and extensive coronary artery disease by postexercise regional wall motion abnormalities in Tc-99m sestamibi gated single-photon emission computed tomography. Am J Cardiol 86:1171–1175.
25. Lima RS, Watson DD, Goode AR et al. (2003) Incremental value of combined perfusion and function over perfusion alone by gated SPECT myocardial perfusion imaging for detection of severe three-vessel coronary artery disease. J Am Coll Cardiol 42:64–70.
26. Danias PG, Ahlberg AW, Clark BA 3rd et al. (1998) Combined assessment of myocardial perfusion and left ventricular function with exercise technetium-99m sestamibi gated single-photon emission computed tomography can differentiate between ischemic and nonischemic dilated cardiomyopathy. Am J Cardiol 82:1253–1258.
27. Sciagra R, Leoncini M (2005) Gated single-photon emission computed tomography. The present-day "one-stop-shop" for cardiac imaging. Q J Nucl Med Mol Imaging 49(1):19–29.
28. Go V, Bhatt MR, Hendel RC (2004) The diagnostic and prognostic value of ECG-gated SPECT myocardial perfusion imaging. J Nucl Med 45(5):912–921.
29. Shaw LJ, Iskandrian AE (2004) Prognostic value of gated myocardial perfusion SPECT. J Nucl Cardiol 11(2):171–185.
30. Berman DS, Germano G (1999) The clinical value of assessing left ventricular function from gated SPECT perfusion studies. Rev Port Cardiol 2000 Feb;19 Suppl 1:I31–7; Mansoor MR, Heller GV (1999) Gated SPECT imaging. Semin Nucl Med 29(3):271–278.
31. Cullom SJ, Case JA, Bateman TM (1998) Electrocardiographically gated myocardial perfusion SPECT: technical principles and quality control considerations. J Nucl Cardiol 5(4):418–425.

32. Abidov A, Berman DS (2005) Transient ischemic dilation associated with poststress myocardial stunning of the left ventricle in vasodilator stress myocardial perfusion SPECT: True marker of severe ischemia? J Nucl Cardiol 12:258–260.
33. Nichols K, DePuey EG, Rozanski A (1996) Automation of gated tomographic left ventricular ejection fraction. J Nucl Cardiol 3:475–482.
34. Rozanski A, Nichols K, Yao SS, Malholtra S, Cohen R, DePuey EG (2000) Development and application of normal limits for left ventricular ejection fraction and volume measurements from 99mTc-sestamibi myocardial perfusion gates SPECT. J Nucl Med 41:1445–1450.
35. Odelson JE, Dilsizian V, Bonow RO (2005) Nuclear cardiology. In Zipes DP, Libby P, Bonow RO, Braunwald E (eds), Braunwald's Heart Disease – a Textbook of Cardiovascular Medicine, 7th edn. Philadelphia, PA, Elsevier Saunders, pp. 287–333.

Myocardial Perfusion Scintigraphy in the Assessment of Post-Revascularization – Current Status and Limitations

Jaffar Ali Raza and Assad Movahed

Contents

24.1 Introduction 275
24.2 To Do or Not to Do Routine Stress Test After Revascularization 276
24.3 Myocardial Perfusion Imaging After Percutaneous Coronary Interventions 276
24.4 Limitations 277
24.5 Myocardial Perfusion Imaging After Coronary Artery Bypass Graft 278
24.6 Transmyocardial Laser Revascularization 281
24.7 Conclusion 282
References 283

24.1 Introduction

Myocardial perfusion imaging (MPI) is widely utilized in the non-invasive diagnosis and management of coronary artery disease (CAD). Radionuclide MPI has been well studied in the evaluation, risk stratification and identification of patients with CAD who will benefit from revascularization. Myocardial revascularization using percutaneous coronary interventions (PCI) and coronary artery bypass graft (CABG) has become a mainstay in the treatment of patients with CAD. The idea of performing a functional study after revascularization is to identify the areas that are not revascularized or to look for restenosis and progression of native vessel disease or disease in the grafts. Patients who have undergone revascularization will continue to have CAD progression that will require further evaluation and testing. Symptoms are an unreliable index of development of restenosis, with only 25% of these patients developing angina on exercise testing [1–4]. Sensitivities of the exercise electrocardiogram (ECG) for detecting restenosis range from 40 to 55%, significantly less than reported with single photon emission computed tomography (SPECT) [5, 6]. Marie and colleagues evaluated the usefulness of SPECT thallium exercise testing at 6 months for detecting asymptomatic restenosis in 62 patients who underwent follow-up angiography. The investigators found that exercise ECG testing detected fewer patients with restenosis than exercise SPECT thallium imaging, especially among asymptomatic patients (25% vs 100%, $p < 0.005$) [3]. Hence, it comes as no surprise to cardiologists and nuclear physicians that MPI studies are being performed with increasing frequency in patients who have undergone revascularization.

24.2 To Do or Not to Do Routine Stress Test After Revascularization

Approximately one million PCIs are performed annually in the USA [7]. If all these patients were given routine MPI after revascularization, it would translate into a significant burden on health expenditure. Hence, whether or not to perform routine stress tests with MPI post-PCI is not only an important clinical question but a major health-care economics issue as well. Eisenberg et al. in a report "Utility of routine functional testing after percutaneous transluminal coronary angioplasty: Results from the ROSETTA Registry" [8], found that there were considerable, but not necessarily unexpected differences between the group of patients who underwent routine stress testing versus those who had selective administration of stress tests based on symptoms. Despite the difference in initial strategy regarding post-PCI stress testing; there was little difference in the rate of follow-up procedures, i.e., repeat angiography, PCI or CABG. However, routine functional stress testing post-PCI was associated with only a decreased frequency of follow-up clinical events. They attributed this decrease in clinical events to the early identification and treatment of patients at risk for follow-up events, and/or due to clinical differences between patients who are referred for routine and selective functional testing. In another study of 61 patients with diabetes enrolled in the Aggressive Diagnosis of Restenosis (ADORE) trial, Saririan et al. found routine post-PCI functional testing to be of little clinical value [9]. Also from the ROSETTA trial, routine functional testing was not found to be significantly beneficial even in patients after multi-lesion PCIs [10]. Thus the American College of Cardiology/American Heart Association exercise testing guidelines suggesting that routine functional testing may benefit patients at high risk of restenosis, such as those undergoing multi-lesion PCI or with diabetes mellitus, needs to be revisited. Ischemic chest pain within the first 24–48 hours after PCI (with or without stenting) usually results from procedural events such as abrupt vessel closure, transient coronary spasm, non-occlusive thrombus, side branch occlusion, or distal embolization. Stress testing is not warranted in such cases and they should undergo repeat cardiac catheterization.

24.3 Myocardial Perfusion Imaging After Percutaneous Coronary Interventions

Stress MPI has proven to be a useful technique in the evaluation and management of post-PCI patients [11, 12]. Abnormal perfusion patterns early after PCI may reflect periprocedural myocardial injury, side-branch compromise due to plaque shift or stent overlap, new disease, or functional significance of angiographically recognized disease in non-revascularized vessels. The measures of the adequacy of myocardial perfusion (post-angioplasty gradient, reduced thallium clearance and transient thallium defects) have been shown to be predictors of adverse events after coronary angioplasty. Individuals with abnormal perfusion after PCI were at a relative risk of having adverse events approximately four times greater than in patients without such defects [13]. MPI is preferred over exercise ECG in patients who already have undergone revascularization. These patients already have baseline ECG changes, having known CAD, making the post-stress ECG difficult to interpret. SPECT imaging is more sensitive in detecting ischemia over time that may happen after coronary interventions. The extent and severity of ischemia identified post-revascularization may dictate the indication for repeat intervention. The incidence of silent ischemia with restenosis in patients who have undergone PCI is high. Briesblatt et al. compared preangioplasty exercise thallium imaging with exercise thallium 2 weeks to 1 month after PCI in patients with multi-vessel disease (MVD) (11). Repeat thallium imaging identified two patient groups: Group one, 47 patients with no evidence of ischemia in a second vascular distribution, and Group two, 38 patients with evidence of ischemia needing further angioplasty. In Group two, 47% of patients had angioplasty of a second vessel and 79% required multivessel angioplasty at 1-year follow-up. In contrast, only six Group one patients (13%) required angioplasty of a second vessel at 1 year suggesting that incomplete revascularization may be an acceptable approach in many patients with MVD. Exercise SPECT ^{201}Tl done after PCI in asymptomatic patients was able to identify restenosis in individual vessels with 90%, 89% and 89% sensitivity, specificity and accuracy; respectively [2]. In a similar study looking at the chance of restenosis, Wijns et al. found thallium scintigraphy performed 4 weeks after PCI to be helpful. Thallium scintigram (presence of a reversible defect) was able to predict the recurrence of angina in 66%, vs. 38% and restenosis in 74% vs. 50% compared with exercise ECG (ST-segment depression or angina at peak workload) [14]. Their results also suggested that restenosis had occurred to some extent at 4 weeks after the PTCA in most patients in whom it was going to occur. However, current exercise and radionuclide imaging guidelines do not recommend routine stress testing in asymptomatic patients after interventional therapy [1, 15].

The limitations of most of the studies that have evaluated the role of stress testing to detect silent restenosis were performed in the pre-stent era, at a time when restenosis was a common problem. The introduction of stents has produced a dramatic decline in acute complication rates after angioplasty, and the ability of stents to limit restenosis was subsequently demonstrated in the various multicenter randomized trials [16, 17]. Nevertheless, the restenosis rate is reported to be 25% to 39% after coronary stent implantation, mainly because of lumen encroachment by intimal hyperplasia within the stent [18, 19]. The availability of drug-eluting stents, such as sirolimus and paclitaxel stents, have markedly reduced the incidence of in-stent restenosis by between 3% and 8% [20, 21]. Cottin et al. performed a study to analyze the long-term prognostic value of ^{201}Tl-SPECT myocardial imaging in 152 patients after coronary artery stenting. SPECT performed 5 months after stenting showed reversible perfusion defects in 47 patients; ischemia was silent in 70%. Adverse events (MI or death) occurred in 28% of patients with ischemia, including death in 15%, but in only 3% of patients without ischemia. Angina was not an independent predictor of adverse events [22]. They also concluded that, after coronary stenting,: (1) the frequency of persistent silent ischemia in the stented patients is high (31%) in daily routine practice; (2) thallium SPECT at 4 to 6 months after the procedure represents a useful tool in risk stratification; (3) the presence of reversible defects is associated with an increased probability of major cardiac events (relative risk, 10.5). In another study, Zellweger et al. prospectively followed 356 patients who underwent coronary stenting and routine SPECT imaging 6 months thereafter for 4 years. Of these, 81 patients had target vessel ischemia, which was silent in 62% [23]. The accuracy of stress MPI in the setting of stenting seems to vary with the definition of angiographic restenosis. Milavetz et al. examined angiographic restenosis using two definitions: total area narrowing ≥50% or ≥70% of the stent site or stented artery [24]. They found that the SPECT and angiographic findings were concordant in 22 of 33 stented vascular territories using the 50% definition of restenosis and in 29 of 33 stented territories using the 70% definition. Use of the 70% definition of restenosis resulted in improved accuracy of SPECT in detecting a significant stenosis in the stented artery. Sensitivity, specificity, positive predictive value, negative predictive value, and accuracy of SPECT were 95%, 73%, 88%, 89%, and 88%, respectively.

24.4
Limitations

MPI is used to help determine the success of revascularization after PTCA. However, neither exercise testing nor radionuclide imaging is indicated in the first month or two after PCI without a specific indication. Manyari et al. in 43 patients who underwent revascularization, performed SPECT thallium MPI and diagnosed myocardial ischemia in 12 of the 43 scans recorded a few days after PTCA, but in none at later stages. They concluded that ^{201}Tl MPI after PTCA often show delayed improvement and, therefore, an abnormal myocardial perfusion scan soon after PTCA does not necessarily reflect residual coronary stenosis or recurrence [25]. Several other investigators have also documented persistently abnormal scans 12 hours to 6 weeks after successful PTCA in patients, without evidence of restenosis during clinical or angiographic follow-up [26–30]. Although myocardial perfusion in the territory of the dilated coronary vessel improved from the pre-PTCA studies, it remained abnormal in 99 (41%) of 242 patients in studies performed early after PTCA. During follow-up myocardial perfusion studies at 3 to 10 months after PTCA, approximately one-half of patients with an abnormal scan early after balloon angioplasty had normal studies [25, 28]. The mechanism for an abnormal stress perfusion scan very early after successful PTCA is unknown. There have been some studies that support the theory of early restenosis. Analysis of the pooled data have shown that 53 (53%) of the 99 patients with an abnormal early perfusion scan developed angiographic restenosis during later follow-up at 6 to 18 months after PTCA. However, only 17 (12%) of the 143 patients with a normal early myocardial perfusion scan subsequently developed angiographic restenosis [25–27, 30]. Such results have led the authors to conclude that an abnormal early post-PTCA perfusion scan was useful in separating groups with high versus low risk for late restenosis [26, 27, 30]. These data, however, do not offer a pathophysiologic explanation of restenosis but suggest that the mechanisms involved in restenosis and the slow resolution of perfusion abnormalities after PTCA may be the same. These studies were performed during the era of PTCA alone, without stent placement and therefore may not apply to patients who have stents. PTCA may cause early post-procedural vasoconstriction resulting in positive tests. In one small published study, the authors found that patients with myocardial perfusion defects early after coronary stent implantation had a high rate of restenosis, similar to patients with PTCA [31]. Studies have shown that early after PCI, absolute coronary flow reserve is diminished [32, 33]. The ability of stress MPI to detect epicardial coronary disease is based on the regional differences in tracer uptake occurring as a consequence of impaired relative coronary flow reserve. Thus, even in the presence of a patent artery, regional perfusion can be impaired by endothelial dysfunction and medial injury at the treated site and/

or abnormal microvascular and resistive vessel function distal to the site [32, 33]. This could result in the early abnormal scans noted in patients without restenosis.

Radionuclide MPI performed with planar imaging has a high incidence of false positive results. SPECT is particularly advantageous over planar imaging because of its ability to differentiate vascular territories and thus evaluate patients with multivessel disease. ^{201}Tl MPI early after angioplasty may show abnormal results caused by transient insufficient coronary flow reserve [34]. However, if studies are performed 6 weeks or more after angioplasty, early restenosis could be accurately diagnosed.

Appropriate use of noninvasive testing following PCI has never been systematically investigated. Physicians practice patterns vary widely from region to region or even within the region. Current guidelines recommend against routine testing of asymptomatic patients because "the prognostic benefit of controlling silent ischemia needs to be proved" and there is "a lack of data that outcomes are affected by this approach" [1, 35]. However, some authors disagree with that, saying all patients should undergo MPI following PCI, citing data demonstrating adverse outcomes in asymptomatic patients with ischemia [36, 37]. A prospective randomized study assessing the efficacy of routine noninvasive testing and directed re-intervention to optimize management of the increasing number of patients undergoing PCI is required to answer this question. According to Giedd and Bergmann [38], the reasonable current practice based on the available information would not recommend the use of MPI early (<3 months) after PCI due to the high false-positive rate (Table 24.1). In patients who develop chest pain within three months of revascularization, coronary angiography should be performed directly (Fig. 24.1).

Between 3 and 6 months, patients with typical angina, ECG changes, or elevated cardiac enzymes should also undergo angiography. Patients with atypical symptoms who have high-risk characteristics (Table 24.2), defined as patients with decreased left ventricular function, multivessel disease, proximal left anterior descending disease, diabetes mellitus, hazardous occupations, and suboptimal PCI results, should also undergo angiography. Patients who are at low risk for restenosis and who develop atypical symptoms should undergo MPI first (Table 24.3). Although the specificity of MPI 3 to 6 months following PCI is diminished, normal perfusion reliably excludes restenosis. If perfusion is abnormal, angiography should be performed. With the accuracy of MPI performed 6 or more months following PCI being excellent, asymptomatic patients should initially be followed clinically and undergo MPI at 6 to 9 months. Patients with a high-risk scan should be referred for angiography and, if appropriate, revascularization, while patients with normal and low to intermediate risk study would be followed medically with repeat testing every 1 to 3 years or when symptoms occur. The current radionuclide imaging guidelines recommend that the weight of evidence supported (class IIa) routine testing in selected high-risk, asymptomatic patients and recommended that stress SPECT MPI be performed at 3 to 5 years after revascularization [39].

24.5
Myocardial Perfusion Imaging After Coronary Artery Bypass Graft

Stress testing after CABG is beneficial to identify graft disease or occlusion as well as progression of native disease in lesions that have not been bypassed. While arterial grafts have a high patency rate (88% and 83% after 5 and 10 years, respectively), venous graft occlusion occurs in approximately 10% of patients during the first year with subsequent 5 and 10 year patency rates of 74% and 41%, respectively [40, 41]. A metanalysis to examine the diagnostic abilities of exercise treadmill testing (ETT), stress MPI and stress echocardiography to predict graft stenosis or progression of disease in the native circulation post-CABG was done by Chin et al. [42]. Their study demonstrated that for the identification of graft stenosis or progression of native disease, ETT alone has a sensitivity of 45% (95% CI 36% to 54%) and a specificity of 82% (95% CI 68% to 95%). The use of stress MPI increased the sensitivity to 68% (95% CI 51% to 86%) and specificity to 84% (95% CI 78% to 91%). In a small study involving 36 patients, CK-MB level was assessed at 0, 4, 8, 12, 24, 36, 48 and 72 hours after surgery and MPI (SPECT using ^{99m}Tc MIBI) and radionuclide angiography were performed 2 weeks before and 3–4 months after surgery [43]. Patients with an increase in the level of CK-MB isoenzyme (>50 IU/mL) after CABG were found to have a higher rate of perfusion abnormalities and functional deterioration.

Graft stenosis can be accurately identified by MPI, which could also effectively localize the stenosis, particularly if gated SPECT is performed [44, 45]. When ^{201}Tl SPECT imaging and coronary angiography was performed in 50 patients with atypical chest pain at 51 months after surgery, SPECT imaging had a sensitivity and specificity of 80 and 87%, respectively [44]. Exercise stress testing is more sensitive than dipyridamole in such patients, most likely due to attenuation artefact from pharmacologic stress [51]. Gated SPECT stress MPI has higher sensitivity in identifying graft patency. With gated SPECT, occluded grafts were identified in 82% for the left anterior descending artery territory, 92% for the right coronary artery territory, and 75% for

Table 24.1 Restenosis following percutaneous coronary intervention. Reprinted from the Journal of American College of Cardiology, Vol 43, Giedd and Bergmann, Perfusion imaging following PCI, P 328–336. Copyright (2004), with permission from American College of Cardiology Foundation

Author (Ref.)	Year	Patients Studied	Intervention Performed	Follow-Up Angiogram	Restenosis Rate	Asymptomatic Re/stenosis
Holmes et al.	1984	557	PTCA	6 months	34%	24%
Nobuyoshi et al.	1988	229	PTCA	6 months	49%	59%
Hecht et al.	1991	116	PTCA	6 months	60%	36%
Hernandez et al.	1992	839	PTCA	6-9 months	33%	48%
Fischmann et al.	1994	159	PTCA	6 months	42%	N/A
		177	Stent	6 months	32%	N/A
Versaci et al.	1997	46	PTCA	12 months	40%	18%
		49	Stent	12 months	19%	36%
Betriu et al.	1999	199	PTCA	6 months	37%	46%
		198	Stent	6 months	22%	30%
Wehinger et al.	1999	1867	Stent	6 months	33%	N/A
Kastrati et al.	2000	163	PTCA	6 months	38%	N/A
		171	Stent	6 months	36%	N/A
Mudra et al.	2001	457	Stent	6 months	24%	N/A
Ruygrok et al.	2001	1221	PTCA	6 months	31%	53%
		1469	Stent	6 months	16%	58%
Overall restenosis rate and rate of asymptomatic restenosis					30%	47%
Restenosis rate and rate of asymptomatic restenosis following PTCA					35%	45%
Restenosis rate and rate of asymptomatic restenosis following coronary stenting					26%	53%

N/A = data not available, PTCA = percutaneous transluminal coronary angioplasty

the left circumflex artery territory, in contrast to only 61% of patients with planar imaging [44, 46].

A significant number of patients develop reversible perfusion defects suggestive of ischemia that occur within one year after CABG although they do not have angina [47, 48]. One study followed 411 patients for up to a median duration of 5.8 years. During the follow-up, 60 deaths from any cause, 53 initial cardiac deaths or nonfatal myocardial infarctions (MIs) and 22 late (>3 months after the ^{201}Tl study) revascularization procedures were reported. The number of abnormal ^{201}Tl segments on the post-exercise image was the only variable in the multivariate analyses to show a significant association with all three outcomes. The 5-year survival rate free of cardiac death or MI was 93% for patients without angina and a normal image or small post-exercise perfusion defect versus 71% for patients with angina and a medium or large defect [47]. In the Emory Angioplasty versus Surgery Trial (EAST), among those who underwent CABG, 19 (11%) reported angina at 1 year after revascularization, but 47 (27%) had a large or moderate-sized reversible defect on MPI. At 2 years, survival free of cardiac death or MI in patients with large or moderate-sized defects was significantly lower than in those without such findings (88% vs. 96%) [54]. However, routine stress imaging for the evaluation of post-CABG patients early (within 2 years) after CABG should depend upon the presence or absence of symptoms. No significant mortality benefits were seen in the BARI trial in asymptomatic patients irrespective of their test results, although other studies have shown benefits from routine stress MPI [49].

In contrast to early MPI in asymptomatic patients, stress MPI done on post-CABG patients who have

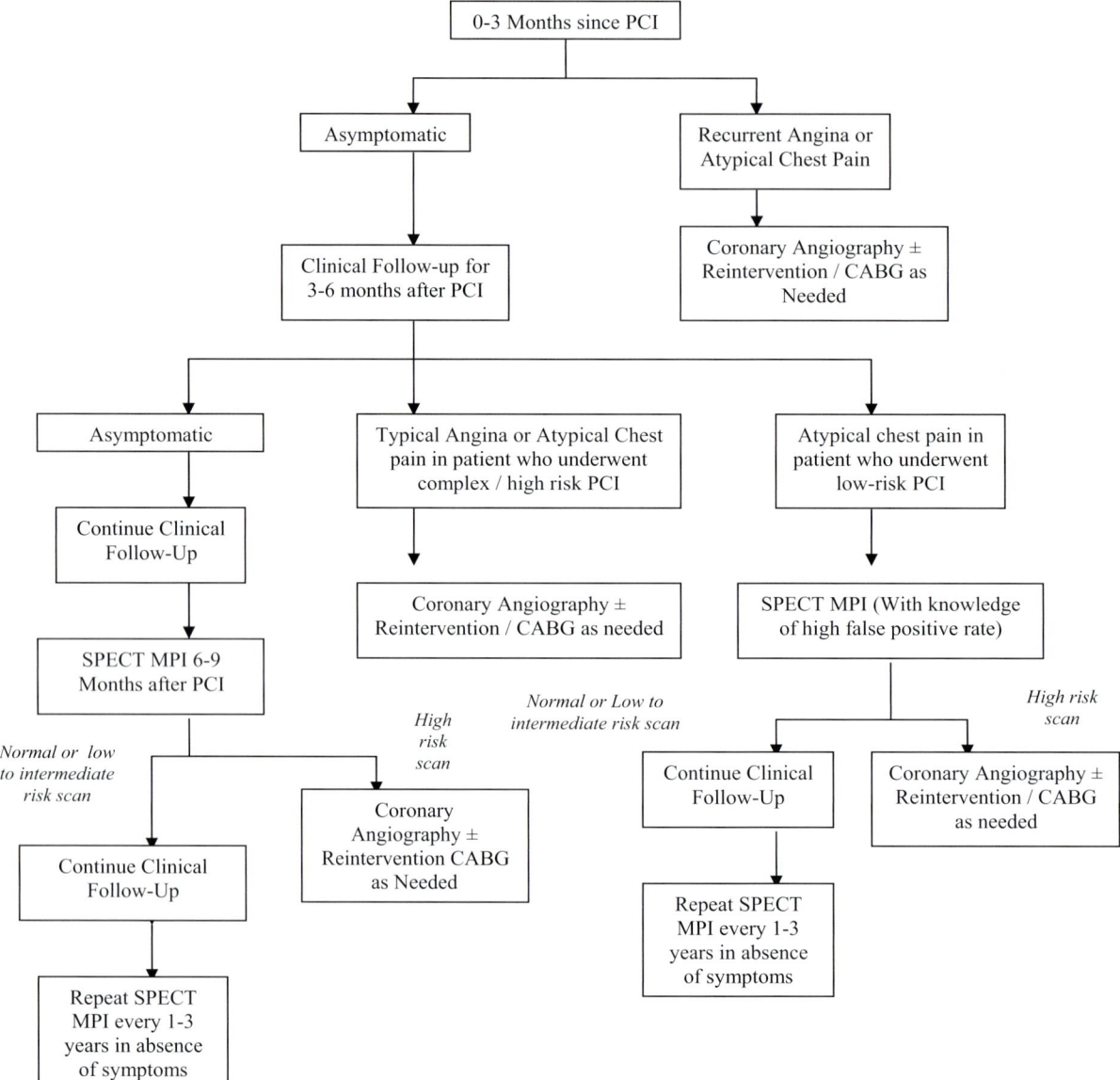

Fig. 24.1 Treatment algorithm following PCI. Reprinted from the Journal of American College of Cardiology, Vol 43, Giedd and Bergmann, Perfusion imaging following PCI, P 328–336., Copyright (2004), with permission from American College of Cardiology Foundation

had saphenous vein grafts more than five years earlier, proved to be an effective method for risk stratification, prognosis, and determination of disease progression [50–53].

Zellweger et al. compared the prognostic significance of SPECT MPI in patients early and late after CABG. They identified 1765 patients, who underwent MPI 7.1 +/- 5.0 years post-CABG. All patients underwent rest T1-201/stress Tc-99m sestamibi MPI and were followed up ≥1 year after testing. Patients with early CABG or PTCA (<60 days after SPECT) were censored. The prognostic population consisted of 1544 patients. A semi-quantitative visual analysis employing a 20-segment model was used to define summed stress score (SSS), summed rest score (SRS), summed difference score (SDS), and the number of nonreversible segments (NRS). During follow-up, 53 cardiac deaths (CD) occurred. There was a significant increase in annual CD

Table 24.2 Factors associated with restenosis. Reprinted from the Journal of American College of Cardiology, Vol 43, Giedd and Bergmann, Perfusion imaging following PCI, P 328-336. Copyright (2004), with permission from American College of Cardiology Foundation

Clinical Factors	Angiographic Factors
Absence of prior myocardial infarction	Branch vessel lesion
Continued smoking	Bypass graft lesion
Diabetes mellitus	Chronic, totally occlusive lesion
Elevated blood insulin levels	Extensive dissection
Male gender	Final translesional gradient ≥ 15–20 mm Hg
Prior restenosis	Greater final diameter stenosis
Severe angina at presentation	Greater length of stented segment
Unstable angina	Greater severity of initial stenosis
Vasospastic angina	Implantation of multiple stents
	Initial translesional gradient ≥40mm Hg
	Left main coronary artery lesion
	Long lesion
	Ostial lesion
	Multiple lesions
	Presence of thrombus
	Proximal anterior descending artery lesion
	Restenotic lesion
	Smaller final minimal lumen diameter
	Smaller reference vessel diameter
	Suboptimal final result

rates as a function of SSS. The annual CD rate was relatively low (1.3%) in patients ≥ 5 years post-CABG. They concluded that MPS is strongly predictive of subsequent CAD in post-CABG patients and adds incremental value over clinical and treadmill test information. They recommend that symptomatic patients ≥ 5 years after CABG and all patients > 5 years post-CABG will benefit from testing [52]. However, the ACC/AHA/ASNC radionuclide imaging guideline concluded that the weight of evidence supports (class IIa) routine stress testing in selected high-risk, asymptomatic patients and recommended that stress SPECT MPI be performed a 3 to 5 years after revascularization [39]. Exercise is the preferred stress, while pharmacological stress is recommended in patients who are unable to exercise.

24.6
Transmyocardial Laser Revascularization

Transmyocardial laser revascularization (TMR) is a new technique for the treatment of refractory angina not amenable to either PCI or CABG [54]. Muxi et al. describe the technique they used and their findings [55]. Standard dipyridamole protocol was used for the pharmacologic stress testing. ^{99m}Tc-Tetrofosmin stress-rest imaging was performed according to the stress-rest protocol. All images were processed according to standard protocols. Areas with normal uptake (> 85%) or absent uptake (< 20%) in the pre-TMR study did not change after the operation. In laser-treated areas a significant decrease in ischemic myocardial uptake was found between the pre-

Table 24.3 Accuracy of myocardial SPECT imaging following percutaneous coronary intervention. Reprinted from the Journal of American College of Cardiology, Vol 43, Giedd and Bergmann, Perfusion imaging following PCI, P 328–336. Copyright (2004), with permission from American College of Cardiology Foundation

Author	Year	No. of Patients	PCI Modality	% With Angina	Mean Time to SPECT	Mean Time to Angiogram	Sens %	Spec %	Acc %
Hect et al.	1991	116	PTCA	65	6 months	1 week	93	77	86
		41		0			96	75	88
		75		100			91	77	85
Marie et al.	1993	62	PTCA	0	6 months	3 days	94	84	87
Milan et al.	1996	37	PTCA	N/A	"late"	1 month	88	78	83
		20					92	67	N/A
Kosa et al.	1998	82 (99)	Stenting	N/A	7 months	1 month	79	78	79
		35 (52)		N/A			100	82	85
Milavetz et al.	1998	33	Stenting	64	3 months	5 days	71	--	67
							95	73	88
Cancer et al.	1998	34 (37)	PTCA	NA	2–48 months	1 month	76	79	78
Beygui et al.	2000	179(208)	PTCA	0	6 months	7 days	63	77	71
		111(138)					56	81	74
Galassi et al.	2000	97 (107)	Stenting	N/A	4 months	2 month	82	84	83
		46 (56)					76	95	89
Overall performance of SPECT MPI							79	79	79

MPI = myocardial perfusion imaging, PCI = percutaneous coronary intervention, SPECT = single-photon emission tomography, Sens = sensitivity, Spec = specificity, PPV = positive predictive value, N/A = data not available

TMR study (8.00 ± 6.45) and the 3-month (1.03±5.65, P<0.001) and 12-month (−0.05±7.05, P<0.001) post-TMR studies. No statistical differences were found in stress or rest perfusion uptake between laser- and non-laser-treated areas during follow-up. However, in the subgroup of patients with ischemic areas before TMR, a significant improvement was also found at stress in treated areas between the pre-TMR study (68.56±15.77) and the 3-month (73.49±14.15, P<0.05) and 12-month (69.52±15.15, P<0.05) post-TMR studies. Verma et al. evaluated the utility of ^{99m}Tc MPI summed stress scores (SSS) and correlation of clinical symptoms in TMR patients (56). Post-operatively, all patients reported an improvement, however, overall SSS was 14 and the TMR segments had higher average SSS per segment 3.2 versus the grafted areas with SSS 1.8. They concluded that symptom improvement may occur with TMR, but ^{99m}Tc MPI might not reveal improvement of ischemia.

24.7
Conclusion

SPECT MPI has evolved to be one of the mainstay diagnostic modalities in the evaluation and prognosis of patients with suspected CAD. Stress MPI should be used in the follow-up of patients who have undergone revascularization to asses the risk of major events and consequently decide whether these patients are better served by medical or repeat interventions. MPI has demonstrated added significant incremental prognostic value to clinical data. The cost of performing these studies in all post revascularization patients could be significant. Routine MPI after revascularization as a measure of therapeutic efficacy or to determine the subsequent risk in asymptomatic patients needs to be determined by future prospective randomized studies.

References

1. Gibbons RJ, Balady GJ, Beasley JW et al. (1997) ACC/AHA Guidelines for Exercise Testing. A report of the American College of Cardiology/American Heart Association Task Force on Practice Guidelines (Committee on Exercise Testing). J Am Coll Cardiol 30:260–311.
2. Hecht HS, Shaw RE, Chin HL, Ryan C, Stertzer SH, Myler RK (1991) Silent ischemia after coronary angioplasty: evaluation of restenosis and extent of ischemia in asymptomatic patients by tomographic thallium-201 exercise imaging and comparison with symptomatic patients. J Am Coll Cardiol 17:670–677.
3. Marie PY, Danchin N, Karcher G et al. (1993) Usefulness of exercise SPECT-thallium to detect asymptomatic restenosis in patients who had angina before coronary angioplasty. Am Heart J 126:571–577.
4. Bengtson JR, Mark DB, Honan MB et al. (1990) Detection of restenosis after elective percutaneous transluminal coronary angioplasty using the exercise treadmill test. Am J Cardiol 65:28–34.
5. Georgoulias P, Demakopoulos N, Kontos A et al. (1998) Tc-99m tetrofosmin myocardial perfusion imaging before and six months after percutaneous transluminal coronary angioplasty. Clin Nucl Med 23:678–682.
6. Garzon PP, Eisenberg MJ (2001) Functional testing for the detection of restenosis after percutaneous transluminal coronary angioplasty: a meta-analysis. Can J Cardiol 17:41–48.
7. AHA (2004) Heart Disease and Stroke Statistics – 2004 Update, Dallas, Texas.
8. Eisenberg et al. (2004) Utility of routine functional testing after percutaneous transluminal coronary angioplasty: Results from the ROSETTA Registry. J Invasive Cardiol 16:318–322.
9. Saririan M, Cugno S, Blankenship J, Huynh T, Sedlis S, Starling M, Pilote L, Wilson B, Eisenberg MJ (2005) Routine versus selective functional testing after percutaneous coronary intervention in patients with diabetes mellitus. J Invasive Cardiol 17:25–29.
10. Goldman LE, Okrainec K, Eisenberg MJ, Schechter D, Lefkovits J, Goudreau E, Deligonul U, Mak KH, Del Core M, Duerr R, Huynh T, Smilovitch M, Sedlis S, Brown DL, Brieger D (2004) ROSETTA Investigators. Six-month outcomes after single- and multi-lesion percutaneous coronary intervention: results from the ROSETTA registry. Can J Cardiol 20:608–612.
11. Breisblatt WM, Barnes JV, Weiland F, Spaccavento LJ (1988) Incomplete revascularization in multivessel percutaneous transluminal coronary angioplasty: the role for stress thallium-201 imaging. J Am Coll Cardiol 11:1183–1190.
12. Zhang X, Liu X, He ZX, Shi R, Yang M, Gao R, Chen J, Yang Y, Fang W (2004) Long-term prognostic value of exercise ^{99m}Tc-MIBI SPET myocardial perfusion imaging in patients after percutaneous coronary intervention. Eur J Nucl Med Mol Imaging 31:655–662.
13. Miller DD, Liu P, Strauss HW, Block PC, Okada RD, Boucher CA (1987) Prognostic value of computer-quantitated exercise thallium imaging early after percutaneous transluminal coronary angioplasty. J Am Coll Cardiol 10:275–283.
14. Wijns W, Serruys PW, Simoons ML, van den Brand M, de Feijter PJ, Reiber JH, Hugenholtz PG (1985) Predictive value of early maximal exercise test and thallium scintigraphy after successful percutaneous transluminal coronary angioplasty. Br Heart J 53:194–200.
15. http://asnc.org/resources/guidelines.cfm
16. Fischman D, Leon M, Baim D et al. (1994) A randomized comparison of coronary-stent placement and balloon angioplasty in the treatment of coronary artery disease. N Engl J Med 331:496–501.
17. Serruys P, De Jaegere P, Kiemeneij F et al. (1994) A comparison of balloon expandable stent implantation with balloon angioplasty in patients with coronary artery disease. N Engl J Med 331:489–495.
18. van Domburg RT, Foley DP, de Jaegere PP et al. (1999) Long term outcome after coronary stent implantation: a 10-year single centre experience of 1000 patients. Heart 82:27–34.
19. Ellis SG, Savage M, Fischman D et al. (1992) Restenosis after placement of Palmaz-Schatz stents in native coronary arteries: initial results of multicenter experience. Circulation 86:1836–1844.
20. Moses JW, Leon MB, Popma JL et al. for SIRIUS Investigators (2003) Sirolimus-eluting stents versus standard stents in patients with stenosis in a native coronary artery. N Engl J Med 349:1315–1323.
21. Stone GW, Ellis SG, Cox DA et al. TAXUS-IV Investigators (2004) A polymer-based, paclitaxel-eluting stent in patients with coronary artery disease. N Engl J Med 350:221–231.
22. Cottin Y, Rezaizadeh K, Touzery C, Barillot I, Zeller M, Prevot S, L'huillier I, Ressencourt O, Andre F, Fraison M, Louis P, Brunotte F, Wolf JE (2001) Long-term prognostic value of 201Tl single-photon emission computed tomographic myocardial perfusion imaging after coronary stenting. Am Heart J 141:999–1006.
23. Zellweger MJ, Weinbacher M, Zutter AW, Jeger RV, Mueller-Brand J, Kaiser C, Buser PT, Pfisterer ME (2003) Long-term outcome of patients with silent versus symptomatic ischemia six months after percutaneous coronary intervention and stenting. J Am Coll Cardiol 42:33–40.
24. Milavetz JJ, Miller TD, Hodge DO, Holmes DR, Gibbons RJ (1998) Accuracy of single-photon emission computed

tomography myocardial perfusion imaging in patients with stents in native coronary arteries. Am J Cardiol 82:857–861.
25. Manyari DE, Knudtson M, Kloiber R, Roth D (1988) Sequential thallium-201 myocardial perfusion studies after successful percutaneous transluminal coronary artery angioplasty: delayed resolution of exercise-induced scintigraphic abnormalities. Circulation 77:86–95.
26. Hardoff R, Shefer A, Gips S et al. (1990) Predicting late restenosis after coronary angioplasty by very early (12 to 24 hours) thallium-201 scintigraphy: implications with regard to mechanisms of late coronary restenosis. J Am Coll Cardiol 15:1486–1492.
27. Jain A, Mahmarian JJ, Borges-Neto S et al. (1988) Clinical significance of perfusion defects by thallium-201 single photon emission computed tomography following oral dipyridamole early after coronary angioplasty. J Am Coll Cardiol 11:970–976.
28. Breisblatt WM, Weiland FL, Spaccavento LJ (1988) Stress thallium-201 imaging after coronary angioplasty predicts restenosis and recurrentsymptoms. J Am Coll Cardiol 12:1199–1204.
29. Carvalho PA, Vekshtein VI, Tumeh SS et al. (1991) Tc-99m MIBI SPECT in the assessment of myocardial reperfusion after percutaneous transluminal coronary angioplasty. Clin Nucl Med16:819–825.
30. Wijns W, Serruys PW, Reiber JHC et al. (1985) Early detection of restenosis after successful percutaneous transluminal angioplasty by exerciseredistribution thallium scintigraphy. Am J Cardiol 55:357–361.
31. Rodes-Cabau J, Candell-Riera J, Domingo E et al. (2001) Frequency and clinical significance of myocardial ischemia detected early after coronary stent implantation. J Nucl Med 42:1768–1772.
32. Wilson RF, Johnson MR, Marcus ML, Aylward PE, Skorton DJ, Collins S, White CW (1988) The effect of coronary angioplasty on coronary flow reserve. Circulation 77:873–885.
33. Uren NG, Crake T, Lefroy DC, de Silva R, Davies GJ, Maseri A (1993) Delayed recovery of coronary resistive vessel function after coronary angioplasty. J Am Coll Cardiol 21:612–621.
34. DePuey EG (1991) Myocardial perfusion imaging with thallium-201 to evaluate patients before and after percutaneous transluminal coronary angioplasty. Circulation 84(3 Suppl):159–165.
35. Ritchie J, Bateman TM, Bonow RO, Crawford MH, Gibbons RJ, Hall RJ, O'Rourke RA, Parisi AF, Verani MS (1995) Guidelines for clinical use of cardiac radionuclide imaging. A report of the American Heart Association/American College of Cardiology Task Force on Assessment of Diagnostic and Therapeutic Cardiovascular Procedures, Committee on Radionuclide Imaging, developed in collaboration with the American Society of Nuclear Cardiology. Circulation 91:1278–1303.
36. Pfisterer M, Rickenbacher P, Kiowski W, Muller-Brand J, Burkart F (1993) Silent ischemia after percutaneous transluminal coronary angioplasty: incidence and prognostic significance. J Am Col Cardiol 22:1446–1454.
37. Alazraki NP, Krawczynska EG (1996) Thallium imaging in management of post-revascularization patients. Q J Nucl Med 40:85–90.
38. Giedd KN, Bergmann SR (2004) Myocardial perfusion imaging following percutaneous coronary intervention: the importance of restenosis, disease progression, and directed reintervention. J Am Coll Cardiol 43:328–336.
39. Klocke FJ, Baird MG, Lorell BH et al. (2003) ACC/AHA/ASNC guidelines for the clinical use of cardiac radionuclide imaging–executive summary: a report of the American College of Cardiology/American Heart Association Task Force on Practice Guidelines (ACC/AHA/ASNC Committee to Revise the 1995 Guidelines for the Clinical Use of Cardiac Radionuclide Imaging). J Am Coll Cardiol 42:1318–1333.
40. Fitzgibbon GM, Kafka HP, Leach AJ, Keon WJ, Hooper GD, Burton JR (1996) Coronary bypass graft fate and patient outcome: angiographic follow-up of 5,065 grafts related to survival and reoperation in 1,388 patients during 25 years. J Am Coll Cardiol 28:616–626.
41. Loop FD, Lytle BW, Cosgrove DM, Stewart RW, Goormastic M, Williams GW, Golding LA, Gill CC, Taylor PC, Sheldon WC et al. (1986) Influence of the internal-mammary-artery graft on 10-year survival and other cardiac events. N Eng J Med 314:1–6.
42. Chin AS, Goldman LE, Eisenberg MJ (2003) Functional testing after coronary artery bypass graft surgery: a meta-analysis. Can J Cardiol 19:802–808.
43. Kwinecki P, Jemielity M, Czepczynski R et al. (2003) Nuclear imaging techniques in the assessment of myocardial perfusion and function after CABG: does it correlate with CK-MB elevation? Nuc Med Rev 6:5–9.
44. Lakkis NM, Mahmarian JJ, Verani MS (1995) Exercise thallium-201 single photon emission computed tomography for evaluation of coronary artery bypass graft patency. Am J Cardiol 76:107–111.
45. Deluca AJ, Cusack E, Aronow WS, Monsen CE (2004) Sensitivity, specificity, positive predictive value, and negative predictive value of the dipyridamole sestamibi stress test in predicting graft occlusion or > or = 50% new native coronary artery disease in men versus women and in patients aged > or = 65 years versus < 65 years who had prior coronary artery bypass grafting. Am J Cardiol 94:625–626.
46. Pfisterer M, Emmenegger H, Schmitt HE et al. (1982) Accuracy of serial myocardial perfusion scintigraphy with thallium-201 for prediction of graft patency early and late

after coronary artery bypass surgery. A controlled prospective study. Circulation 66:1017–1024.
47. Miller TD, Christian TF, Hodge DO, Mullan BP, Gibbons RJ (1998) Prognostic value of exercise thallium-201 imaging performed within 2 years of coronary artery bypass graft surgery. J Am Coll Cardiol 31:848–854.
48. Alazraki NP, Krawczynska EG, Kosinski AS et al. (1999) Prognostic value of thallium-201 single-photon emission computed tomography for patients with multivessel coronary artery disease after revascularization (the Emory Angioplasty versus Surgery Trial [EAST]). Am J Cardiol 84:1369–1374.
49. Krone RJ, Hardison RM, Chaitman BR et al. (2001) Risk stratification after successful coronary revascularization: the lack of a role for routine exercise testing. J Am Coll Cardiol 38:136–142.
50. Palmas W, Bingham S, Diamond GA et al. (1995) Incremental prognostic value of exercise thallium-201 myocardial single-photon emission computed tomography late after coronary artery bypass surgery. J Am Coll Cardiol 25:403–409.
51. Khoury AF, Rivera JM, Mahmarian JJ, Verani MS (1997) Adenosine thallium-201 tomography in evaluation of graft patency late after coronary artery bypass graft surgery. J Am Coll Cardiol 29:1290–1295.
52. Zellweger MJ, Lewin HC, Lai S et al. (2001) When to stress patients after coronary artery bypass surgery? Risk stratification in patients early and late post-CABG using stress myocardial perfusion SPECT: implications of appropriate clinical strategies. J Am Coll Cardiol 37:144–152.
53. Lauer MS, Lytle B, Pashkow F, Snader CE, Marwick TH (1998) Prediction of death and myocardial infarction by screening with exercise-thallium testing after coronary-artery-bypass grafting. Lancet 351:615–622.
54. Hughes GC, Landolfo KP, Lowe JE, Coleman RB, Donovan CL (1999) Perioperative morbidity and mortality after transmyocardial laser revascularization: incidence and risk factors for adverse events. J Am Coll Cardiol 33:1021–1026.
55. Muxi A, Magrina J, Martin F et al. Technetium (2003) 99m-labeled tetrofosmin and iodine 123-labeled metaiodobenzylguanidine scintigraphy in the assessment of transmyocardial laser revascularization. J Thor Cardiovasc Surg 125:1493–1498.
56. Vijayendra KV, Kimberly P, and Elias AI (2004) Utility of technetium-99m myocardial perfusion imaging after transmyocardial laser revascularization. Chest Meeting Abstracts 126:710S.

Nuclear Cardiology in Women

A. Muhammad Umar Khan and John R. Buscombe

Contents

25.1	Introduction	287
25.2	Epidemiology	287
25.3	Racial Differences	288
25.4	Risk Factors and Differences Related to Women	288
25.5	Women, Hormones, and Cardiovascular Morbidity	288
25.6	Diabetes, Women and Cardiac Ischemia	290
25.6.1	Noninvasive Stress Testing in Ischemic Heart Diseases	291
25.6.2	Stress ECG Testing	291
25.6.3	Stress Echocardiography	292
25.6.4	Myocardial Perfusion Scintigraphy	292
25.7	Recent Findings	294
25.8	Conclusions	295
	References	295

25.1 Introduction

Ischemic heart disease (IHD) is considered more common in men than women and most of the initial studies in IHD conducted focused mainly on men. Often women were not included in cardiovascular research programs. The life-time risk of IHD is one in three for women [1], but women themselves consider breast cancer as their major killer rather than IHD [2]. Since the early 1990s some research has concentrated on IHD in women and a better understanding of gender-related differences has been developed; this includes the epidemiology of IHD in women, identifying risk factors, determining the diagnostic problems encountered with IHD, and possible treatment outcomes [3].

Health services research has also shown that although women seek more medical care, use more health care services, and spend more on medications than men, inequalities in care still limit women's access to certain diagnostic procedures and therapies proven to be effective for specific conditions, especially in the developing and underdeveloped world. This is often due to differences in epidemiology, clinical presentation, co-morbidities, hormonal predisposing factors, and gender-related problems encountered in the management (diagnosis and treatment) of IHD.

25.2 Epidemiology

Currently IHD is the leading cause of death and disability in most western industrialized countries, cutting across all ethnic, racial, and gender groups [4]. Approximately 2.5 million women in the USA alone are hospitalized for cardiovascular illness per year, and almost half a million women annually die of their disease, mostly due to IHD. There is a steady rise in the incidence of IHD in women throughout the world, with estimated deaths rising by 80% and disability-adjusted life years lost by 74% by the year 2020 [5, 6]. The current knowledge points out certain gender based-differences in female IHD compared with the male counterpart. Today's women face the same risks and changes in the social and economic environment as their male counterparts, including diet, alcohol, tobacco, sedentary lifestyle and day to day mental stress. However it would appear that the manifestation of IHD in women lags behind men by about 10–15 years. Although women manifest IHD 10 to 15 years later than men, it is now recognized that the overall morbidity and mortality over a lifetime is similar in men and women.

25.3
Racial Differences

The distribution of risk factors in different parts of the world varies considerably, resulting in high and low-risk cultures. Key observations that have led to the identification of classical IHD risk factors have come from international comparisons such as the Seven Countries Study [7]. As the global burden of IHD is great, the burden of risk factors within geographic areas closely matches those disease patterns. In addition to the substantial continuing burden of IHD risk factors in Western industrialized countries, there is an increasing burden of risk in many parts of the world. Lipid and calorie-predominant diets, obesity, sedentary lifestyle, cigarette smoking, hypertension, resulting elevated blood lipids, and diabetes, common in the USA, are increasingly observed in developing nations. These observations undermine the concerns about the coming global epidemic. This study demonstrated that differences in disease rates among the USA, various nations in Europe, and Japan were directly related to blood pressure (BP), eating patterns, blood cholesterol, and cigarette smoking. More recent comparisons with similar findings were found in the Monitoring Trends and Determinants in Cardiovascular Disease (MONICA) Study, which principally included centers not only in Europe but also in North America, Australia, and Asia [8].

Due to the inadequate overall data from different countries about the incidence of IHD in general and women in particular, it has not been possible to find out the true picture in every country. However, studies conducted in the developed world indicate that the south Asian and Afro-Caribbean population in the UK experience significantly raised rates of cardiovascular events. In particular south Asian groups are at a higher risk and have an overall 40% higher death rate from IHD than the white population of the same age group. The rise in mortality rate is irrespective of gender in this group but the males have much earlier cardiovascular events. This group includes Gujarati Hindus, Punjabi Sikhs and Muslims from India and Pakistan. The important causative factors incriminated in this group were higher prevalence of insulin resistance in south Asians, reduced fibrinolytic activity and central obesity and little or no leisure time physical activity. Affecting both genders equally, all these factors may predispose this group to develop IHD. The insulin resistance syndrome is a more commonly implicated factor in the south Asian population for a high incidence of IHD [9]. While smoking is seen as a major risk factor in the south Asian men, in south Asian women, obesity, lack of exercise and subsequent diabetes are the main risk factors. This will affect the way IHD presents in women, and various diagnostic tests best suited to diagnosis.

25.4
Risk Factors and Differences Related to Women

There are other gender-related differences in risk factors for IHD, e.g., mean blood cholesterol levels are higher in women than in men after the sixth decade, and higher in men before that [10]. It is generally only in men that there is an awareness of high cholesterol and a diagnosis is sought and resulting hypercholesterolaemia is treated. Hypertension is seen more commonly in men than in women across the age spectrum, although the differences narrow in the elderly. However, high BP is more likely to be detected, treated, and controlled among women. Smoking tobacco used to be commonly seen in men in most western industrialized nations and the difference between men and women was significant. Now there is a trend of decline in men but an increase in women, especially young women, and the difference has been reduced significantly (Fig. 25.1a and b) [11].

The levels of triglycerides and low density lipoproteins (LDL) tend to be higher in post-menopausal women than men of the same age group, probably due to the lack of oestrogens, which were suppressing the levels prior to menopause.

25.5
Women, Hormones, and Cardiovascular Morbidity

LDL receptors are up-regulated by oestrogens. When the serum levels of endogenous oestrogen fall, LDL receptor activity is reduced. This leads to the elevated serum LDL concentration observed in post-menopausal women [12]. Elevated total cholesterol and LDL levels are major risk factors for IHD in both men and women. Until the appearance of the Heart and Estrogen Replacement Study (HERS) in 1998, it was erroneously believed that menopausal hormone replacement therapy (HRT) provided protection against development of cardiovascular disease. This was supported by data derived from studies conducted on animals and humans [13]. Another set of

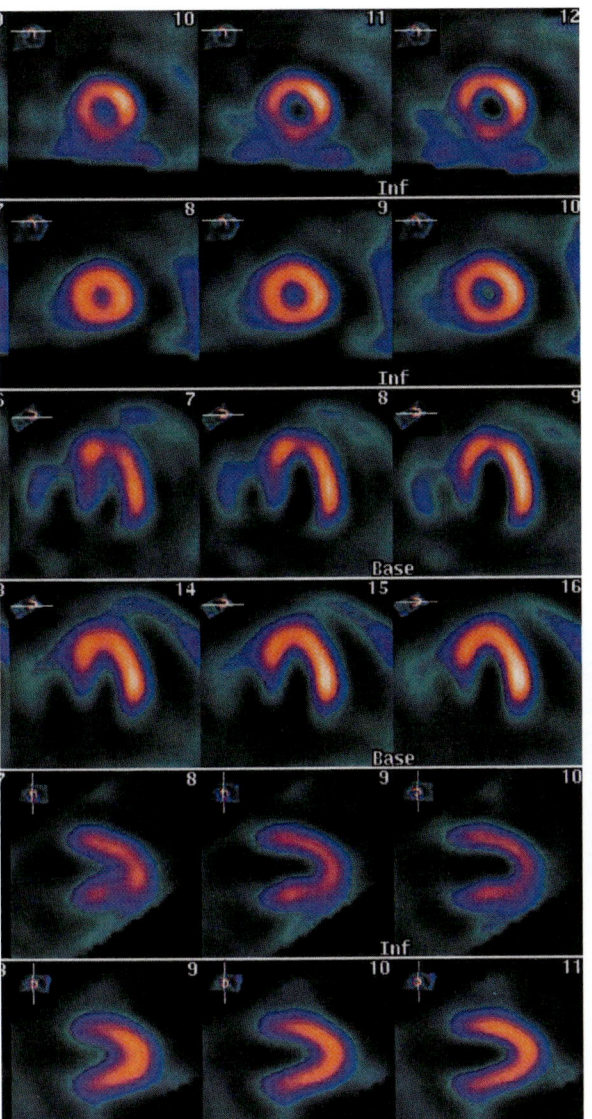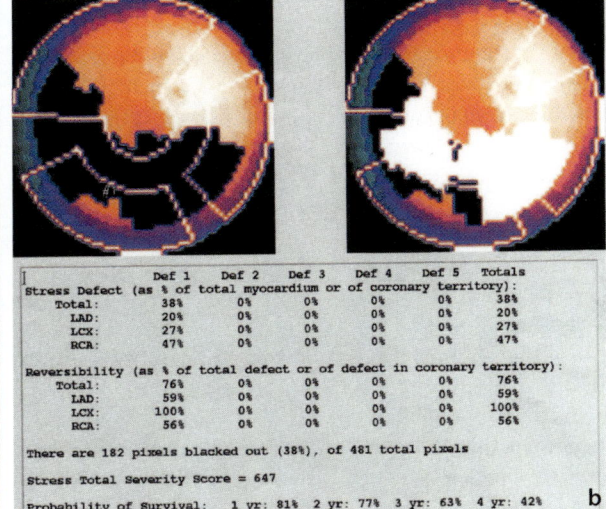

Fig. 25.1 Stress and rest myocardial perfusion scintigraphy in a 28-year-old woman who smokes 30 cigarettes a day. The images (**a**) show poor perfusion in the septum and inferior wall at stress, which improves at rest. The "Emory bulls eye" (**b**) plot confirms extensive ischemia involving 38% of the heart in at least two coronary artery territories. This woman became the youngest recipient of a coronary artery bypass graft

large observational and epidemiological studies also indicated that women taking HRT to avoid the symptoms of menopause in long-term follow-up have a lower incidence of cardiovascular disease than their counterparts who did not have HRT. Due to certain flaws in the sample selection the results of these studies were subject to regular criticism. The HERS was a secondary prevention study to prove the effectiveness of estrogen to reverse or slow the progression of disease in post-menopausal women (mean age 67 years) with a documented history of ischemic heart disease (IHD). Oestrogen treatment did not provide benefit to those women and instead increased IHD events in the initial year of treatment [13]. Another large-scale randomized trial, conducted by the Women's Health Initiative (WHI), which was designed as a primary prevention study, also failed to validate results of initial observational studies indicating the usefulness of oestrogens in IHD prevention, and rather contrary reports were published [14]. The scene was further complicated by multiple concomitant studies from basic sciences indicating a beneficial promise of HRT including increased circulating high-density lipoproteins; increased production of the vasodilator nitric oxide; decreased production of the vasoconstrictor endothelin-1; down regulation of angiotensin-converting enzyme; and decreased migration and proliferation of vascular smooth muscle cells at sites of vascular injury. The discrepancies in all the available data were resolved by observing that the initial observational studies were carried out in women who immediately after meno-

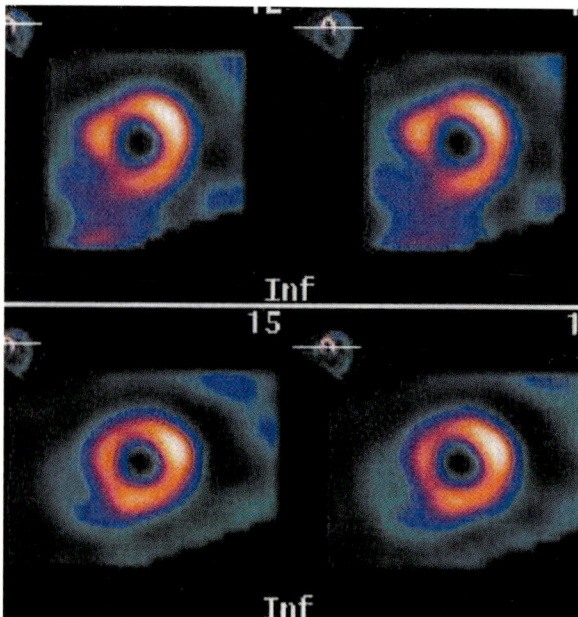

Fig. 25.2 Short axis images showing large vessel disease with inferoseptal ischaemia due to a stenosis in a branch of the left anterior descending artery in a 58-year-old woman with diabetes

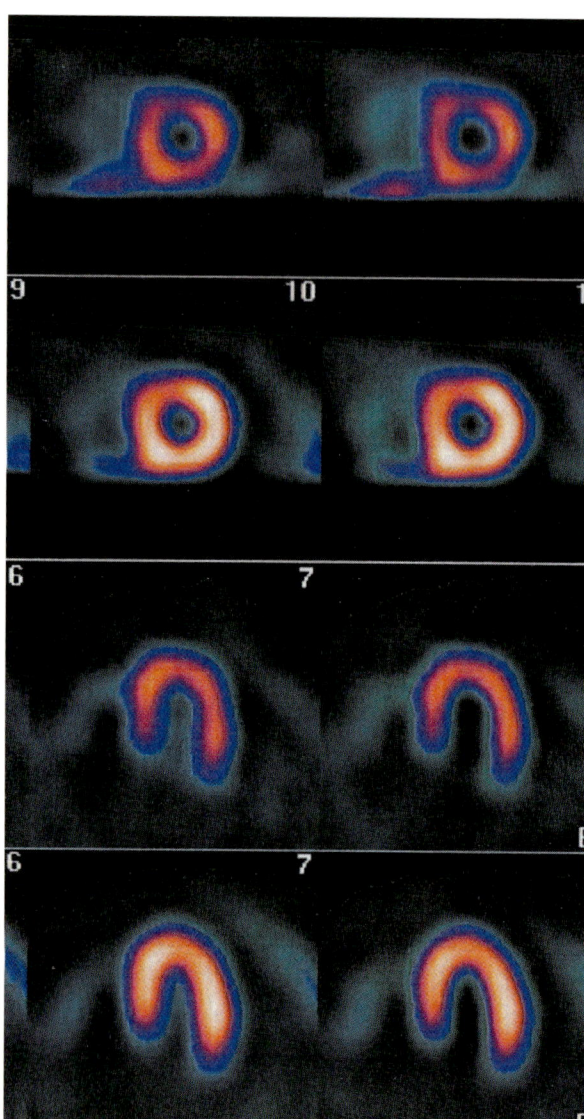

Fig. 25.3 Short and horizontal long axes images of a 74-year-old woman with diabetes and patchy reduction at stress and improvement at rest, suggestive of widespread small vessel disease

pause underwent HRT, while women in the preceding studies of HERS and WHI enrolled women who had been post-menopausal for several years This analysis suggested that the early or peri-menopausal initiation of HRT may be beneficial. The results of the preceding and later animal studies, when analyzed in this scenario, were appearing plausible [15]. Comparison of data acquired from various sources indicated that the type of hormone and administration route are also important variables in the results. Some of these questions may be answered in new research called the Kronos Early Estrogen Prevention Study (KEEPS), designed to see the response of early intervention by HRT and using a uniform weekly transdermal estradiol along with cyclic oral, micronized progesterone, 200 mg for 12 days each month. The results of this group will be compared with a controlled placebo group in terms of carotid intimal medial thickening and prevention of calcium accumulation in coronary arteries. The sample will comprise women in the age range 42–58 years and within 36 months of their final menstrual period. The final results of KEEPS are awaited and may be published by 2011/2012.

25.6
Diabetes, Women and Cardiac Ischemia

Diabetics carry a three times higher risk of developing IHD and the subsequent cardiac events in women compared with men, IHD, is the leading cause of death in patients with diabetes (Figs. 25.2 and 25.3). Diabetes insults myocardium by several mechanisms, the most common of all being ischemia secondary to early atherosclerosis in the coronary vasculature; second is cardiomyopathic disorder (or disorders), which can be characterized by either disorders of both contraction (systolic dysfunction) and filling (diastolic dysfunction) or predominantly by a disorder of filling alone; and last but not least cardiac dysautonomia.

In asymptomatic diabetic women, one out of every five patients has a positive test for ischemia [16]. Once IHD is symptomatic in diabetes, morbidity and mortality are high and are significantly worse than in patients without diabetes. Many physicians already perform screening by stress testing, as suggested by the American Diabetes Association (ADA) consensus guidelines, when two or more additional CAD risk factors are present [17]. However, women may respond less well to formal stress testing than men, especially if overweight, and other forms of cardiac testing, including myocardial perfusion scintigraphy, must be considered. The frequent diabetic silent ischemia, bad prognosis after MI at a younger age than their male counterparts, less favorable outcomes in women after revascularization surgery, and fatal consequences after first cardiac event, demand a special diagnostic strategy for women.

25.6.1
Noninvasive Stress Testing in Ischemic Heart Diseases

Accurate and timely diagnosis of coronary heart disease can significantly reduce the mortality and morbidity in women. In contrast to men, women mostly have non-obstructive IHD and single-vessel disease that leads to an observed decreased diagnostic accuracy and higher false-positive rate for noninvasive exercise stress testing in women versus men. Women sometimes present with a non-specific clinical picture and under-presentation, which further limits the clinical decision making. First, a detailed clinical history and estimation of risk of IHD in women using risk prediction charts should be done to provide the diagnostician with the pretest probability of IHD [18].

The patients to be investigated for noninvasive stress testing can be divided into two broad groups:
- asymptomatic group
- symptomatic group.

In the asymptomatic group the aim is to identify patients at risk of IHD. In this group the pretest probability assessment is important as a low probability group will yield negative results but women with diabetes, known thrombo-occlusive or peripheral vascular disorders and chronic renal failure can benefit from such screening exercises. Recently, a report incorporating the Framingham offspring and cohort revealed that 4%, 13%, and 47% of asymptomatic women aged 50 to 59, 60 to 69, and 70 to 79, respectively, were at intermediate or high risk, with an annual risk of CAD death or MI $\geq 0.6\%$ [19].

In the symptomatic group, imaging is recommended in the intermediate and high probability group by the Consensus Statement From the Cardiac Imaging Committee, Council on Clinical Cardiology, and the Cardiovascular Imaging and Intervention Committee (Council on Cardiovascular Radiology and Intervention, American Heart Association). Women with atypical symptoms but having diabetes, or multiple risk factors (the metabolic syndrome) are at increased CAD risk and should be considered for testing [20]. The results of noninvasive tests should provide the basis for risk-based management plans rather than anatomy based and this will help women having non-obstructive coronary heart disease, which is prevalent in this gender.

25.6.2
Stress ECG Testing

This form of testing is the most commonly used form of stress testing. The results of stress ECG have a reduced sensitivity in women for the following reasons:
- resting ST–T-wave changes;
- lower ECG voltage;
- hormonal factors;
- poor compliance to physical stress.

In some ethnic groups women are quite reluctant or disinclined to undertake such tests because of social, ethnic and religious taboos.

The overall sensitivity of stress ECG for women is 61% versus 72% in men and the specificity is 70% vs. 77% for men [21]. To improve the diagnostic accuracy several additional parameters have been suggested, such as the Duke treadmill score and functional capacity testing, but still practically most physicians and cardiologists prefer to look into ECG changes rather than doing computations and scoring.

In terms of risk assessment, stress ECG proves to be of little help as ST segment changes with stress are considered suboptimal for risk assessment, furthermore the lower work capacity on exercise tests (on average 5 to 7 minutes) due to premature peripheral fatigue, prevents sufficient cardiac workload to cause myocardial ischemia. However, the test still retains its place in the diagnostic workup and evidence to refute its usefulness has not been sufficient to eliminate this test, especially for women. It can be of help in symptomatic women or women with low pretest probability. The clinical validation of newer functional parameters like functional capacity and treadmill scores needs larger and more detailed studies.

25.6.3
Stress Echocardiography

Echocardiography (ECHO) has a proven role in the assessment of haemodynamic changes in the heart and can provide valuable information about the presence of valvular heart disease, wall motion abnormalities and quantification of systolic and diastolic dysfunction. Stress echocardiography (SE) is following the footsteps of stress ECG and looking for stress-induced ischemic changes in comparison with resting ECHO. The preferred mode of stressing the heart for SE is pharmacological stress as it offers prolonged examination time and the convenience of limited movement. However, SE may be performed via treadmill or via supine or upright bicycle exercise according to the liking of the physician.

Dobutamine has proven to have a better sensitivity profile in assessing single vessel disease on SE while adenosine and dipyridmole have proved to be more specific. Data regarding SE in women are not extensive but generally women, due to delayed presentation compared with men, are not fit enough for optimal physical exercise [21, 22].

The diagnostic capabilities of SE are quite gender-neutral and a sensitivity of 80% (89% for triple vessels disease) and specificity of 86% has been reported in women, similar to that for men, and no gross variation in the results of optimally achieved physical stress and pharmacological stress has been presented. There are no significant gender-related differences in the prognostication of the disease process using SE. It has been shown, for example, that women having positive SE for multivessel ischemia are at a ten times higher risk of dying from a cardiac event than women with a normal SE [23]. In conclusion, apart from being operator and experience dependent, the results of SE hold the promise of a cost-efficient tool in diagnosing suspected CAD in women with an intermediate pretest likelihood of IHD.

25.6.4
Myocardial Perfusion Scintigraphy

Myocardial perfusion scintigraphy (MPS) has the highest negative predictive value and can act as a "gatekeeper" deciding who should undergo further management. The best results come from the use of SPECT and additional gating [24].

Gender-specific problems like soft tissue attenuation are encountered in MPS but used to be more pronounced with ^{201}Tl with its lower energy X-rays and lower count densities than ^{99m}Tc labeled agents. The stress-related limitations are the same as those for stress ECG or SE as described in the previous sections.

The following are the causes for reduced specificity of MPS in women, especially using ^{201}Tl:
- breast attenuation artefacts;
- thoracic fat attenuation artefacts;
- smaller heart size.

Among the patient-related artefacts breast attenuation artefact is the forerunner and needs to be identified correctly (Figs. 25.4 and 25.5). Breast attenuation artefacts may appear as fixed defects, reversible defects or may even show signs of reverse redistribution depending on whether the attenuating breast is constant in position or the position with respect to the heart is changed in rest and stress. The more usual form of presentation is a fixed antero-lateral defect, especially with pharmacological stress. It should be kept in mind while interpreting breast attenuation artefacts that the patient is imaged in the supine position, therefore apparently pendulous breasts in the sitting or propped up position not overlying the heart, in a supine posture may partially obscure the heart. The artifact can be produced in the antero-lateral wall in average sized breasts, but large pendulous breasts may cause a lateral wall artifact with homogenously reduced activity in that region. The car-

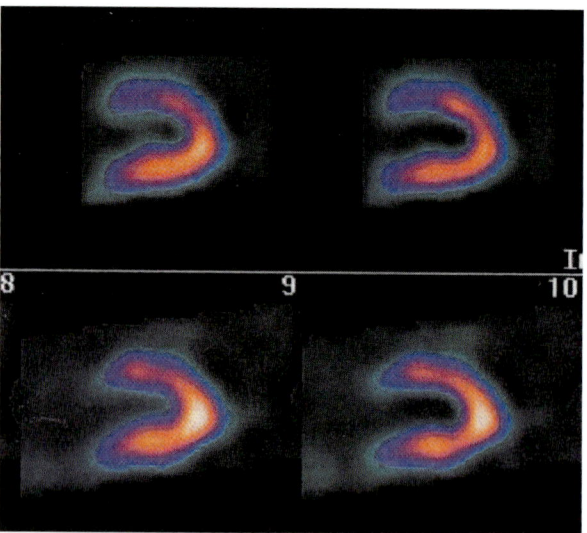

Fig. 25.4 Series of vertical long axes images at stress showing a defect in the basal anterior wall. Could this be attenuation from the breast? The rest images show marked improvement, therefore this is not attenuation but ischemia

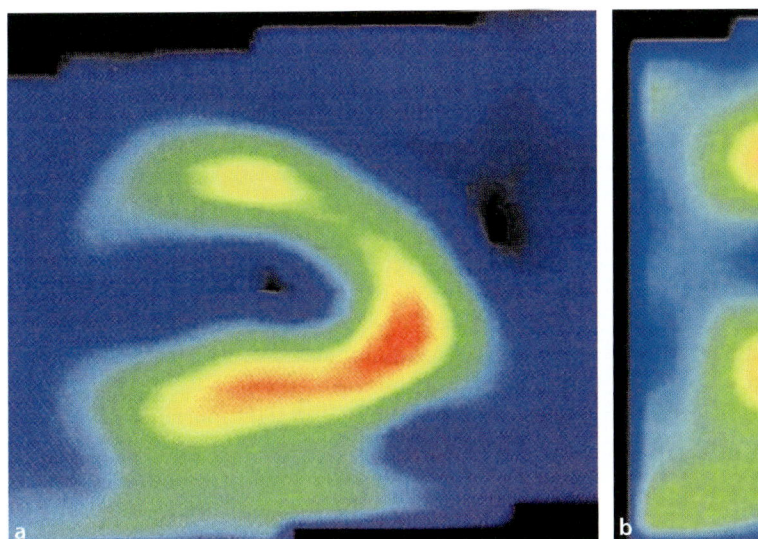
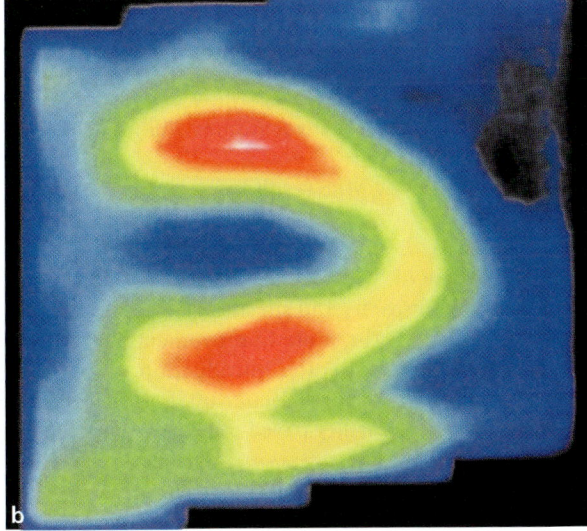

Fig. 25.5 Vertical long axis performed in a woman showing reduction of activity over the anterior wall (**a**). Application of attenuation removes this (**b**) but the sharp eyed will notice it has now caused a defect to appear at the apex

diac axis within the thoracic cage may vary and breast attenuation artifacts may be interpreted in its relation as well. This can be an issue in smokers with some hyperinflation of the lungs and a vertical heart. Breast augmentation implants are usually denser than the normal breast tissues and a plain chest radiograph in the supine position may guide the interpreting physician about the position of the implant. Women who have undergone a mastectomy and wear a breast prosthesis may be instructed to remove them prior to imaging and a note of mastectomy should be made by the attending technologist and physician. The images of women who have undergone a left mastectomy should be processed in a similar way to male patients because if these patients are not processed as male in most of the available software, a breast attenuation correction will be applied and an artifact will be produced in the final output image. Techniques to correct for breast attenuation include use of prone imaging so the breast tissue is "flattened" against the camera couch so reducing the thickness of any attenuating tissue and the use of a calculated "Chang" attenuation correction or a CT or gamma emitter based attenuation map. Interestingly this manipulation often results in an improvement in accuracy in the antero-lateral wall but artifactual defects being seen in the inferoseptal wall. This can mean that one is unclear whether these maneuvers have or have not resulted in another artifact. Some groups therefore prefer not to do any of these changes but "read" the scan in the knowledge that the patient is female. There is no consensus on what, or even if any, method of breast attenuation reduction strategy should be applied.

The second but less gender-specific cause for soft tissue artifacts in SPECT MPS is lateral chest wall attenuation, which is more commonly found in the female population and can further deteriorate the artifact produced by breast attenuation. But it uniformly reduces the photon density in the whole of the myocardium and the artifact is less likely to be really misleading.

To correctly recognize breast and soft tissue attenuation artifacts the following algorithm is suggested by some experts.

- Note the patient's body habitus, chest circumference, breast size, shape, outline and relation to, in supine position.
- If the bra is removed during stress imaging the same positioning should be reproduced for rest images as well.
- History of mastectomy should always be recorded. If a prosthesis is being used it should be removed.
- In a patient having undergone breast augmentation surgery a special note should be made.
- Exact replication of stress and rest imaging positioning.
- Examining the patients study once in rotating cinematic mode may give an idea of breast size and its relation to the heart image, and an artifact may be more clearly appreciated by this simple exercise.
- Processing of the study appropriately in selected software.

- Interpretation of the study should be done in view of all the above observations.
- If gating is added then the artifact will show normal wall motion and thickening while the ischemic or infarcted fragment of myocardium will not move in systole.
- Correlation of the MPS results with stress ECG or SE findings.

The replacement of ^{201}Tl by ^{99m}Tc labeled compounds has improved the sensitivity and specificity of the test, especially in women; furthermore improvements in radiopharmaceutical properties, the introduction of attenuation correction software, and better imaging techniques and equipment has further paved the way for MPS to be a highly recommended test in the demanding field of cardiology [25–28].

Similar to other cardiac stress based modalities myocardial perfusion scintigraphy also faces the problems of suboptimal exercise in women due to advanced age, obesity and social and cultural issues. The ease and safety offered by pharmacological stress agents have encouraged the nuclear cardiologist to induce stress by vasodilators or inotropic agents depending on the respiratory status of the patient. In some institutions physical stress is used in combination with pharmacological stress to reduce the side effect of pharmacological agents. Different centers have tailored their own stress protocol in keeping with resources and limitations. The sensitivity and specificity of adenosine-induced stress, ^{99m}Tc-MIBI MPS, are reported to be 91 and 86%, respectively. As diabetes is more common in women and myocardial ischemia or infarction may not trigger angina in these patients, a physical or inotropic stress may not be free from risks and adenosine stress is suggested in these cases. The adenosine stress MPS has shown to be effective in risk stratification of diabetic women with suspected IHD.

MPS adds valuable prognostic information that significantly modifies the management plans in women. Multiple studies have substantiated the fact that MPS in women can predict subsequent cardiac events like cardiac death and myocardial infarction, and also guide the physician in taking radical steps like coronary revascularization. The very high negative predictive values give MPS the edge over other modalities. A negative myocardial perfusion scan carries a less than 1% annual cardiac event rate; further investigations and intervention in such instances are not warranted. But in women having perfusion defects, their risk of cardiac events are higher than male counterparts having similar perfusion abnormalities [29–31]. To assess the prognostic signs on MPS apart from size and vascular territory of perfusion defects, its reversibility may also be considered an important indicator.

Studies have shown that IHD mortality in diabetic women with normal MPS is 1.6% higher than in women who are non-diabetic and have normal MPS study. In patients for whom the MPS is suggestive of severe abnormality the difference in the annual mortality of diabetic and non-diabetic women is 8.5 and 6.1, respectively. The difference in mortality rates are more pronounced in the insulin-dependent group rather than in the non-insulin-dependent group. The overall cardiac events rate is 50% higher in diabetic women than in non-diabetic women. Gating can provide additional prognostic information when added into the stress MPS protocol.

In conclusion, gated stress MPS SPECT is a useful test, with high negative predictive values and can be used in women with intermediate to high likelihood of IHD or abnormal baseline ECG (Figs. 25.6 and 25.7). Pharmacological stress is safe and can offer convenience in women, who are most of the time incapable of optimum levels of exercise. The final report should stratify the patients into a low to high spectrum of risk associated with the scan findings.

25.7
Recent Findings

Like men, the use of post-stress gating seems to have a significant prognostic value for women. In a study of

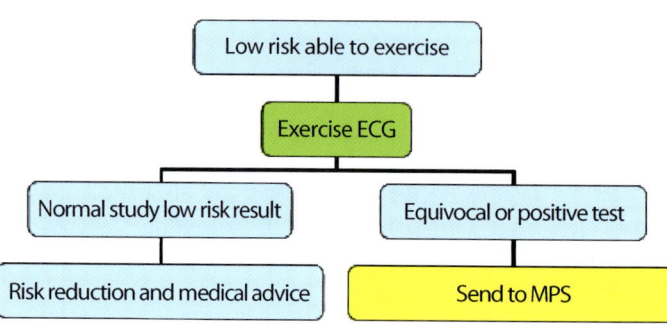

Fig. 25.6 Suggested use of myocardial perfusion scintigraphy in women with low to medium risk of disease who can exercise

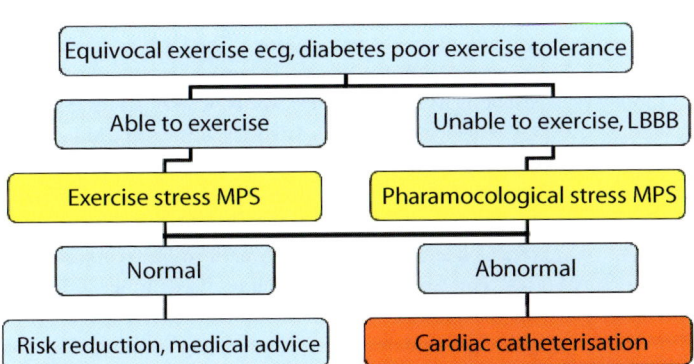

Fig. 25.7 Suggested use of myocardial perfusion scintigraphy in women with low to medium risk of disease who cannot exercise

597 women with low to medium pre-test probability of ischaemic heart disease the women had a higher threshold for a normal ejection fraction. In men any LVEF above 43% had a good prognosis, in women the figure was 51% and a post-stress end systolic volume of 27 mL also led to a poor prognosis for major cardiac events, with over 30% of such women suffering cardiac death or MI within 5 years of the test [32].

In a further retrospective review it was determined that in women there may be a tendency for false positive defects on MPS compared with angiography; this will not only include patients seen as having ischaemia but also changes consistent with infarct, which cannot be confirmed by angiography with a suggestion that as many as 40% of women imaged may appear to have false positive studies if the angiogram is taken as a gold standard. There was no clear prognostic information identified about this patient but care should be taken in reporting positive images in women [33].

A recent multi-centre study in women with suspected heart disease (the Woman's Ischaemic Syndrome Evaluation (WISE) study) confirmed that in women, non-occlusive atherosclerosis where the stenosis in the coronary vessel was less than 50% still had a high rate of admission for chest pain with at least 20% of these women being re-admitted with chest pains in 5 years [34]. The authors confirmed the role of myocardial perfusion scintigraphy and how the prognostic value of MPS was useful in the management and risk stratification of these patients.

A further study has looked at the relationship between female hormones and atherosclerosis in coronary arteries. In pre-menopausal women with polycystic ovaries had similar levels of oestrogens to women with normal ovaries but raised testosterone. These women had a higher rate of diabetes and positive cardiac investigations, suggesting that it is not just the presence of female hormones which protect the heart but the lack of testosterone. This may have a further influence on secondary prevention in women [35].

25.8 Conclusions

The presentation of IHD in women can be atypical; diabetes and hypertension are often risk factors giving a different range of diseases and presentations than men. Ethnic and social variations in women may have a bigger role in both the aetiology and also the method of investigation that can be used when compared to men.

The best results in terms of diagnosis and prognostication come from a combination of pharmacological stress and myocardial perfusion scintigraphy with stress echocardiology being a good second choice.

Several technical factors, including breast attenuation and small vessel disease, may make interpretation of myocardial perfusion studies in women more complex than in men but this can be overcome with a mixture of techniques such as attenuation correction and experience of the reader.

At present, therefore, myocardial perfusion scintigraphy is probably the method of choice for the investigation of women with suspected IHD.

References

1. Lloyd-Jones DM, Larson MG, Beiser A, Levy D (1999) Lifetime risk of developing coronary heart disease. Lancet 353:89–92.
2. Legato MJ, Padus E, Slaughter E (1997) Women's perceptions of their general health, with special reference to their risk of coronary artery disease: results of a national telephone survey. J Womens Health 6:189–198.
3. Kasper AS (2002) Understanding women's health: an overview. Clin Obst Gynecol 45(4):1189–1197.
4. Benjamin E J, Smith SC Jr, Cooper RS, Martha and Luepker RV (2002) Task Force #1—Magnitude of the prevention problem: opportunities and challenges. J Am Coll Cardiol 40(4):588–603.

5. Wenger NK, Speroff L, Packard B (1993) Cardiovascular health and disease in women. N Eng J Med 329(4):247–256.
6. Murray CJL, Lopez AD (1996) The global burden of disease in 1990. In Murray CJL, Lopez AD, Harvard School of Public Health, World Health Organizations and World Bank, Editors, The Global Burden of Disease: A Comprehensive Assessment of Mortality and Disability From Disease, Injuries, and Risk Factors in 1990 and Projected to 2020, Harvard School of Public Health, Cambridge, MA, pp. 247–293.
7. Keys AB (1980) Seven Countries: A Multivariate Analysis of Death and Coronary Heart Disease. Harvard University Press, Cambridge, MA and London, England.
8. Kuulasmaa K, Tunstall-Pedoe H, Dobson A et al. (2000) Estimation of contribution of changes in classic risk factors to trends in coronary event rates across the WHO MONICA Project populations. Lancet 355:675–687.
9. The University of York (1996) Ethnicity and Health: review of literature and guidelines for purchasers in areas of cardiovascular disease, mental health and haemoglobinopathies. NHS Centre for Reviews and Dissemination Social Policy Research Unit. CDR report 5, January, pp. 5–7.
10. McGovern PG, Pankow JS, Shahar E et al. (1996) Recent trends in acute coronary heart disease – mortality, morbidity, medical care, and risk factors. The Minnesota Heart Survey Investigators. N Engl J Med 334:884–890.
11. Giovino GA, Schooley MW et al. (1994) Summer Surveillance for selected tobacco-use behaviors – United States, 1900–1994. Morbidity and Mortality Weekly Report of the Centre for Disease Control Surveillance Summary 43:1–43.
12. Bush TL, Barrett-Connor E, Cowan LD, Criqui MH, Wallace RB, Suchindran CM, Tyroler HA, and Rifkind BM (1987) Cardiovascular mortality and noncontraceptive use of estrogen in women: results from the Lipid Research Clinics Program Follow-up Study. Circulation 75:1102–1109.
13. Hulley S, Grady D, Bush T, Furberg C, Herrington D, Riggs B, Vittinghoff E (1998) Randomized trial of estrogen plus progestin for secondary prevention of coronary heart disease in postmenopausal women. J Am Med Assoc 280:605–613.
14. Stampfer MJ and Colditz GA (1991) Estrogen replacement therapy and coronary heart disease: a quantitative assessment of the epidemiologic evidence. Prev Med 20:47–63.
15. Mikkola TS, Clarkson TB (2002) Estrogen replacement therapy, atherosclerosis, and vascular function. Cardiovasc Res 53:605–619.
16. Wackers FJTh, Young Lh, Inzucchi SE, Chyun DA, Davey JA, Barrett EJ, Taillefer R, Wittlin SD, Heller GV, Filipchuk N, Engel S, Ratner RE, Iskandrian AE (2004) for the Detection of Ischemia in Asymptomatic Diabetics (DIAD) Investigators. Detection of silent myocardial ischemia in asymptomatic diabetic subjects. The DIAD study. Diabetes Care 27:1954–1961.
17. Gibbons RJ, Balady GJ, Bricker JT, Chaitman BR, Fletcher GF, Froelicher VF, Mark DB, McCallister BD, Mooss AN, O'Reilly MG, Winters WL Jr, Gibbons RJ, Antman EM, Alpert JS, Faxon DP, Fuster V, Gregoratos G, Hiratzka LF, Jacobs AK, Russell RO, Smith SC Jr (2002) American College of Cardiology/American Heart Association Task Force on Practice Guidelines (Committee to Update the 1997 Exercise Testing Guidelines). ACC/AHA 2002 guideline update for exercise testing: summary article: a report of the American College of Cardiology/American Heart Association Task Force on Practice Guidelines (Committee to Update the 1997 Exercise Testing Guidelines). Circulation 106:1883–1892.
18. Conroy RM, Pyorala K, Fitzgerald AP, Sans S, Menotti A, De Backer G, De Bacquer D, Ducimetiere P, Jousilahti P, Keil U, Njolstad I, Oganov RG, Thomsen T, Tunstall-Pedoe H, Tverdal A, Wedel H, Whincup P, Wilhelmsen L, Graham IM (2003) SCORE project group. Estimation of ten-year risk of fatal cardiovascular disease in Europe: the SCORE project. Eur Heart J 24:987–1003.
19. Lerner DJ, Kannel WB (1986) Patterns of coronary heart disease morbidity and mortality in the sexes: a 26-year follow-up of the Framingham population. Am Heart J 111:383–390.
20. Mieres JH, Shaw LJ, Arai A, Budoff MJ, Flamm SD, Hundley WG, Marwick TH, Mosca L, Patel AR, Quinones MA, Redberg RF, Taubert KA, Taylor AJ, Thomas GS, Wenger NK (2005) Role of noninvasive testing in the clinical evaluation of women with suspected coronary artery disease. Consensus statement from the cardiac imaging Committee, Council on Clinical Cardiology, and the cardiovascular imaging and intervention Committee, Council on Cardiovascular Radiology and Intervention, American Heart Association. Circulation 111:682–696.
21. Kim C, Kwok YS, Heagerty P, Redberg R (2001) Pharmacologic stress testing for coronary artery disease: a meta-analysis. Am Heart J 142:934–944.
22. Ali Raza J, Reeves WC, Movahed A (2001) Pharmacologic stress agents for evaluation of ischemic heart disease. Int J Cardiol 81:157–67.
23. Arruda-Olson AM, Juracan EM, Mahoney DW, McCully RB, Roger VL, Pellika PA (2002) Prognostic value of exercise echocardiography in 5798 patients: Is there a gender difference? J Am Coll Cardiol 39:625–631.
24. Mieres JH, Shaw LJ, Hendel RC, Miller DD, Bonow RO, Berman DS, Heller GV, Mieres JH, Bairey-Merz CN, Berman DS, Bonow RO, Cacciabaudo JM, Heller GV, Hendel RC, Kiess MC, Miller DD, Polk DM, Shaw LJ, Smanio PE, Walsh MN (2003) Writing Group on Perfusion Imaging in Women. American Society of Nuclear Cardiology con-

sensus statement: Task Force on Women and Coronary Artery Disease – the role of myocardial perfusion imaging in the clinical evaluation of coronary artery disease in women. J Nucl Cardiol 10:95–101.

25. Klocke FJ, Baird MG, Lorell BH, Bateman TM, Messer JV, Berman DS, O'Gara PT, Carabello BA, Russell RO Jr, Cerqueira MD, St John Sutton MG, DeMaria AN, Udelson JE, Kennedy JW, Verani MS, Williams KA, Antman EM, Smith SC Jr, Alpert JS, Gregoratos G, Anderson JL, Hiratzka LF, Faxon DP, Hunt SA, Fuster V, Jacobs AK, Gibbons RJ, Russell RO (2003) American College of Cardiology; American Heart Association Task Force on Practice Guidelines; American Society for Nuclear Cardiology. ACC/AHA/ASNC guidelines for the clinical use of cardiac radionuclide imaging – executive summary: a report of the American College of Cardiology/American Heart Association Task Force on Practice Guidelines (ACC/AHA/ASNC Committee to Revise the 1995 Guidelines for the Clinical Use of Cardiac Radionuclide Imaging). Circulation 108:1404–1418.

26. Taillefer R, DePuey G, Udelson JE, Beller GA, Latour Y, Reeves F (1997) Comparative diagnostic accuracy of Tl-201 and Tc-99m Sestamibi SPECT imaging (perfusion and ECG-gated SPECT) in detecting coronary artery disease in women. J Am Coll Cardiol 29:69–77.

27. Amanullah AM, Berman DS, Hachamovitch R, Kiat H, Kang X, Friedman JD (1997) Identification of severe or extensive coronary artery disease in women by adenosine technetium-99m sestamibi SPECT. Am J Cardiol 80:132–137.

28. Friedman TD, Greene AC, Iskandrian AS, Hakki AH, Kane AS, Segal BL (1982) Exercise thallium 201 myocardial scintigraphy in women: correlation with coronary angiography. Am J Cardiol 49:1632–1637.

29. Hachamovitch R, Berman DS, Kiat H, Bairey CN, Cohen I, Cabico A, Friedman J, Germano G, Van Train KF, Diamond GA (1996) Effective risk stratification using exercise myocardial perfusion SPECT in women: gender-related differences in prognostic nuclear testing. J Am Coll Cardiol 28:34–44.

30. Berman DS, Kang X, Hayes SW, Friedman JD, Cohen I, Abidov A, Shaw LJ, Amanullah AM, Germano G, Hachamovitch R (2003) Adenosine myocardial perfusion single-photon emission computed tomography in women compared with men. Impact of diabetes mellitus on incremental prognostic value and effect on patient management. J Am Coll Cardiol l41:1125–1133.

31. Giri S, Shaw LJ, Murthy DR, Travin MI, Miller DD, Hachamovitch R, Borges-Neto S, Berman DS, Waters DD, Heller GV (2002) Impact of diabetes on the risk stratification using stress single-photon emission computed tomography myocardial perfusion imaging in patients with symptoms suggestive of coronary artery disease. Circulation 105:32–40.

32. Sharir T, Kang X, Germano G, Bax JJ, Shaw LJ, Gransar H, Cohen I, Hayes SW, Friedman JD, Berman DS (2006) Prognostic value of poststress left ventricular volume and ejection fraction by gated myocardial perfusion SPECT in women and men: gender-related differences in normal limits and outcomes. J Nucl Cardiol 13:495–506.

33. Rasulova N, Singh A, Demetriadou O, Georgiou G, Yiannakkaras C, Khodjibekov M, Al-Nahhas A (2008) Clinical significance of myocardial perfusion abnormalities in patients with varying degree of coronary artery stenosis. Nucl Med Commun 29(2):129–136.

34. Johnson BD, Shaw LJ, Pepine CJ, Reis SE, Kelsey SF, Sopko G, Rogers WJ, Mankad S, Sharaf BL, Bittner V, Bairey Merz CN (2006) Persistent chest pain predicts cardiovascular events in women without obstructive coronary artery disease: results from the NIH-NHLBI-sponsored Women's Ischaemia Syndrome Evaluation (WISE) study Eur Heart J 27:1408–1415.

35. Shaw LJ, Merz CN, Azziz R, Stanczyk FZ, Sopko G, Braunstein GD, Kelsey SF, Kip KE, Cooper-Dehoff RM, Johnson BD, Vaccarino V, Reis SE, Bittner V, Hodgson TK, Rogers W, Pepine CJ (2008) Post-Menopausal Women with a History of Irregular Menses and Elevated Androgen Measurements at High Risk for Worsening Cardiovascular Event-Free Survival: Results from the National Institutes of Health National Heart, Lung, and Blood Institute (NHLBI) Sponsored Women's Ischemia Syndrome Evaluation (WISE). J Clin Endocrinol Metab 93:1276–1284.

Myocardial Perfusion Scintigraphy in Acute Chest Pain: Current Status and Limitations

Priya Velappan and Assad Movahed

Contents

26.1 Introduction 299
26.2 History 300
26.3 Diagnostic Value of Acute Rest Myocardial Perfusion Imaging (ARMPI) 300
26.4 Acute Rest Myocardial Perfusion Imaging and Outcome 301
26.5 Timing of Radionuclide Injection 301
26.6 Cost Savings 301
26.7 Conclusions 302
26.8 Future Directions 302
  References 303

26.1 Introduction

Patients with acute chest pain or symptoms suggestive of myocardial ischemia account for a large number of emergency department (ED) visits, approximately 7 million every year in the USA. Over 5 million of these patients are admitted to the hospital [1]. However, only a minority of these patients have symptoms truly due to ischemic heart disease. The remainder does not require admission to the hospital and may cause a tremendous strain on limited economic resources. When the symptoms are classic and accompanied by diagnostic electrocardiographic changes, the diagnosis of acute coronary syndrome is straightforward. However, in patients with non-diagnostic ECG changes and classic or non-classic symptoms, appropriate decision making becomes more difficult. This dilemma has led to the exploration of newer diagnostic methods to appropriately risk-stratify patients in a cost-effective and time-sensitive manner.

Myocardial perfusion imaging (MPI) provides a direct assessment of coronary blood flow and thus appears to be an optimal tool for identifying patients with acute coronary syndromes, who initially appear at low risk based on ECG or clinical characteristics. In acute ischemic syndromes, myocardial hypoperfusion occurs before the onset of left ventricular dysfunction, ECG changes, clinical symptoms and myocardial necrosis. Rest myocardial perfusion imaging becomes abnormal simultaneously with myocardial hypoperfusion. Radionuclide tracer uptake correlates in a linear fashion with blood flow in the range of resting myocardial perfusion and thus provides an accurate estimate of regional myocardial hypoperfusion. As MPI depends on flow abnormalities as well as myocardial necrosis, it can identify patients across the spectrum of acute coronary syndromes, including ischemia and infarction [1].

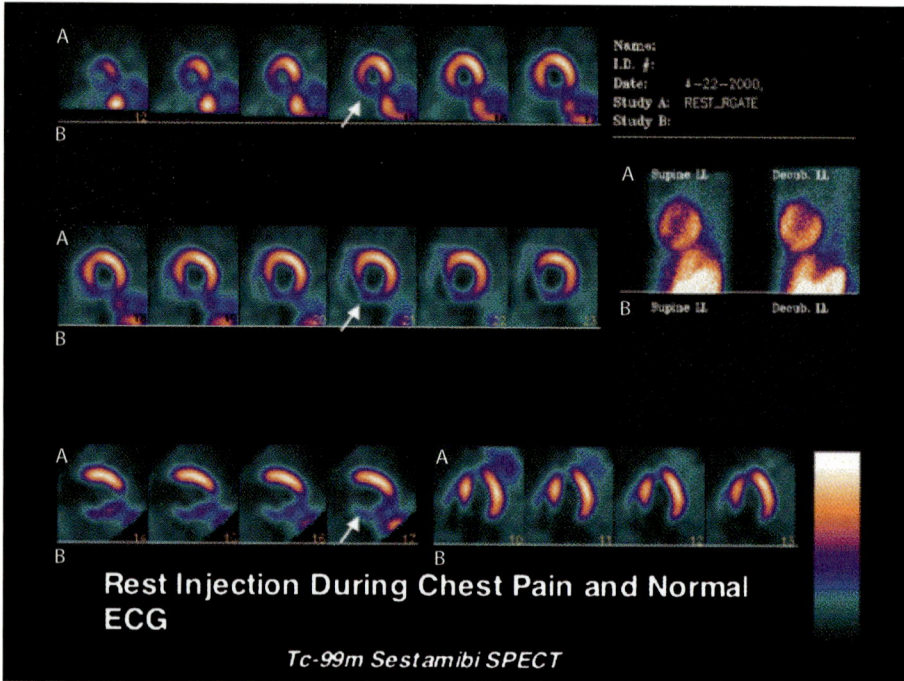

Fig. 26.1 Rest Tc-99m sestamibi images of a 52-year-old man with non-anginal chest pain and non-diagnostic electrocardiographic changes in the chest pain center. A relatively large inferoseptal defect is noted. (Reproduced with permission from [1])

26.2
History

Using rest MPI to identify patients with acute coronary syndromes is not a new concept. Nuclear imaging was first used in the detection of myocardial infarction (MI) more than 30 years ago utilizing various isotopes including rubidium and cesium [2–4]. When Tl-201 came into clinical use, one of its earliest clinical applications was in patients with acute chest pain. Wackers et al. showed that planar Tl-201 imaging has high diagnostic accuracy in patients admitted to hospital for possible acute infarction [5]. Images were abnormal in 100% of patients who had acute MI as well as in 58% of patients who had unstable angina. In contrast, none of the patients diagnosed with stable angina or atypical chest pain had abnormal studies. Several other studies have since reported similar results with Tl-201 [6–8].

However, the routine use of Tl-201 in the ED setting has practical limitations due mainly to its redistribution properties, which require imaging to be completed in a relatively short time after injection. Moreover, it is not readily available for acute imaging. These limitations have been overcome recently by the use of Tc99m myocardial perfusion imaging. Tc99m myocardial perfusion agents are also taken up by the myocardium in proportion to blood flow, but lack significant redistribution [9]. The patients can therefore be injected at the time of chest pain and imaging performed several hours later, with the images representing the blood flow at the time of symptoms. Moreover, their physical characteristics make them better suited to gamma camera imaging, less subject to attenuation and useful with electrocardiographically gated SPECT. They are also readily available for acute imaging (Fig. 26.1).

26.3
Diagnostic Value of Acute Rest Myocardial Perfusion Imaging (ARMPI)

The clinical basis for the use of Tc99m sestamibi SPECT imaging for suspected acute coronary syndrome comes from a study by Bilodeau et al. [10]. This small study with 45 hospitalized patients showed a sensitivity of 96% and a specificity of 79% for the detection of CAD (defined as ≥50% diameter stenosis as detected by coronary angiography performed between 1 and 9 days after admission). In the more common presentation to the ED of patients with chest pain, Varetto et al. demonstrated a sensitivity of 100%, a specificity of 92% and a negative predictive value of 100% for ARMPI [11]. Several subsequent studies including single-center and multi-center observational and randomized studies, involving large numbers and more heterogenous patient populations with acute chest pain, have consistently shown a high sensitivity (96%) for detecting acute MI [12–16]. Those infarcts that are missed are typically small infarcts with an uncomplicated clinical course. It has been shown that in order to visualize an area of myocardial hypoperfusion, it should involve at least 3–5% of the left ventricle [17]. Studies have shown that these patients have significantly lower CKs or have <70% stenosis on coronary angiography [18, 19]. In the study by Kontos et al. investigating rest MPI in patients with elevated troponin levels, more than half of the patients with normal SPECT images had non-significant elevations of CK-MB [19]. ARMPI has only moderate sensitivity for diagnosis of acute MI as regional hypoperfusion also occurs in scar, unstable angina and even in chronic multivessel disease. However, even though these patients do not have an acute MI, they would not be considered low risk enough to be discharged from the ED (Fig. 26.2). Most importantly, as the negative predictive value of ARMPI is very high (99%), patients with negative rest perfusion imaging have a very low probability of an acute coronary syndrome and can be safely discharged from the ED.

26.4
Acute Rest Myocardial Perfusion Imaging and Outcome

In addition to its diagnostic value, ARMPI also provides prognostic information. It can accurately quantify the ischemic area at risk and hence the infarct size. It is well known that the infarct size is an important predictor of outcome in patients with acute MI [20–23]. Similarly the size of myocardial perfusion abnormalities also correlates with long-term prognosis [24, 25]. Myocardial

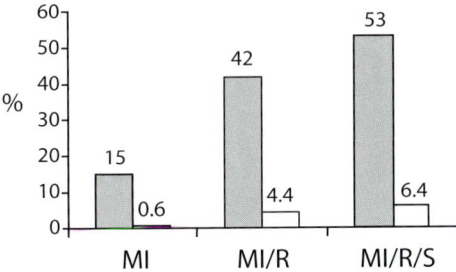

Fig. 26.2 Patients with abnormal rest MPI (gray bars) had significantly ($p < 0.0001$) more cases of MI or revascularization (MI/Revasc), and MI, revascularization or significant coronary artery disease (>70% stenosis) (MI/Sig Dz) than patients with normal rest MPI (white bars). (Reproduced with permission from [14])

perfusion defects noted at discharge have been shown in several studies to correlate with other outcome predictors such as left ventricular ejection fraction, regional wall motion index, end systolic volume and peak CK levels [26–28].

26.5
Timing of Radionuclide Injection

The timing of injection in relation to symptoms is an important issue in ARMPI. It would seem logical that the sensitivity of imaging decreases in the pain-free state. However in most studies involving symptomatic and asymptomatic patients, the sensitivity was not decreased as long as the study was performed within 6 hours of injection [5, 11, 14]. Wackers et al. demonstrated that the incidence of perfusion abnormality was 84%, when Tl-201 injection was performed within 6 hours of anginal symptoms, but decreased to 19% at 12 to 18 hours after the last episode of pain [5]. Kontos et al., in a study with Tc-99m myocardial perfusion agents, found no difference in sensitivity between patients who were and who were not experiencing symptoms at the time of injection [14]. Although the exact time of injection was not reported, none of the patients were injected more than 6 hours after the last episode of pain. In another study by Bilodeau et al. on patients with unstable angina who underwent imaging at presentation and again ≤4 hours after cessation of pain, it was found that the highest sensitivity was at the time of symptoms (96%) [10]. The sensitivity decreased to about 65% with resolution of symptoms, with normalization of perfusion defect in some and decrease in severity of defect in others. The available data is not conclusive about the exact timing of injection. The sensitivity seems to decrease as the time since symptom resolution increases, although it seems to be preserved for at least 4–6 hours.

26.6
Cost Savings

It has been consistently shown by several studies, that when rest MPI is used as an integral part of patient management, patients with acute coronary syndromes are accurately identified, more patients can be discharged from the ED, and overall, more appropriate patients are admitted to hospital. A number of observational studies estimated that significant cost savings would occur as a result of changes in disposition made based on the results from acute MPI [15, 29–31]. Although rest MPI is relatively complex and expensive, its cost maybe offset by the reduced hospitalization rate. Costs might also

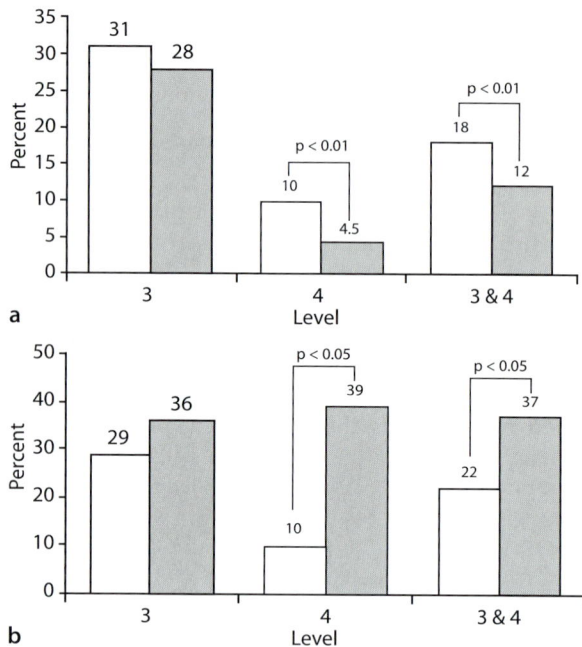

Fig. 26.3 Rate of coronary angiography (a) and revascularization in those who had angiography (b) by triage level for patients who underwent ED perfusion imaging and who had MI excluded (patients were divided into five levels, depending on their likelihood of having CAD, groups 3 and 4 being the ones with possible acute coronary syndromes and having rest MPI as part of their management strategy): control group (*white bars*) and study group (*gray bars*). (Modified from [32])

be reduced by more appropriate selection of diagnostic procedures. The use of rest MPI has been shown to reduce the rate of coronary angiography in low-risk patients (Fig. 26.3) [32].

These observational data have been confirmed in a large randomized trial. The Emergency Room Assessment of Sestamibi for Evaluating Chest Pain (ERASE) study randomized 2475 patients to either routine management or a management strategy that incorporated rest MPI [33]. The use of acute MPI resulted in a significantly lower hospitalization rate and a higher rate of direct discharge from the ED.

26.7
Conclusions

The high negative predictive value of ARMPI and the favorable short- and long-term outcomes of patients with normal rest MPI make it a potentially useful triage tool for patients presenting with acute chest pain. ARMPI can be effectively used in institutions with appropriate resources. Incorporating rest MPI to standard clinical pathways contributes to improved clinical outcomes by decreasing the number of missed myocardial infarcts, reducing unnecessary admissions, and likely lowering overall costs.

26.8
Future Directions

^{123}I-labeled 15-(p-iodophenyl)-3-(R,S)-methylpentadecanoic acid (BMIPP) is a fatty acid analog for SPECT imaging. This radiopharmaceutical has the unique property of detecting abnormalities of fatty acid metabolism resulting from transient ischemia that persist for prolonged periods (ischemic memory) and result in perfusion-metabolism mismatch [34, 35] (Fig. 26.4). The ease of the procedure and the almost 30 hour diagnostic window makes it a potentially useful imaging study for the rapid diagnosis of cardiac ischemia at rest in emergency departments for triage of patients suspected of having acute coronary syndromes.

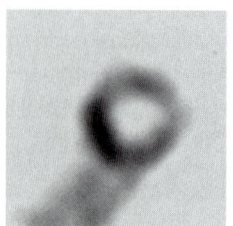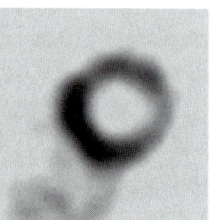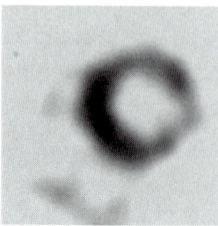

Fig. 26.4 BMIPP myocardial images for three tomographic levels in a 79-year-old man with rest angina and dyspnea. Severely reduced BMIPP uptake was observed in the anterior and lateral regions. Although the patient was treated medically because of chronic renal failure, he died suddenly 1 month later. (Reproduced from [34])

References

1. Kontos MC, Wackers FJ (2004) Acute rest myocardial perfusion imaging for chest pain. J Nucl Cardiol 11(4):470–481.
2. Carr EA Jr, Beierwaltes WH, Wegst AV, Bartlett JD Jr (1962) Myocardial scanning with rubidium-86. J Nucl Med 3:76–82.
3. Carrea JR, Gleason G, Shaw J, Krontz B (1964) The direct diagnosis of myocardial infarction by photoscanning after administration of cesium-131. Am Heart J 68:627–636.
4. Romhilt DW, Adolph RJ, Sodd VJ et al. (1973) Cesium-129 myocardial scintigraphy to detect myocardial infarction. Circulation 48(6):1242–1251.
5. Wackers FJ, Lie KI, Liem KL et al. (1978) Thallium-201 scintigraphy in unstable angina pectoris. Circulation 57(4):738–742.
6. van der Wieken LR, Kan G, Belfer AJ et al. (1983) Thallium-201 scanning to decide CCU admission in patients with non-diagnostic electrocardiograms. Int J Cardiol 4(3):285–299.
7. Mace SE (1989) Thallium myocardial scanning in the emergency department evaluation of chest pain. Am J Emerg Med 7(3):321–328.
8. Henneman PL, Mena IG, Rothstein RJ, Garrett KB, Pleyto AS, French WJ (1992) Evaluation of patients with chest pain and nondiagnostic ECG using thallium-201 myocardial planar imaging and technetium-99m first-pass radionuclide angiography in the emergency department. Ann Emerg Med 21(5):545–550.
9. Okada RD, Glover D, Gaffney T, Williams S (1988) Myocardial kinetics of technetium-99m-hexakis-2-methoxy-2-methylpropyl-isonitrile. Circulation 77(2):491–498.
10. Bilodeau L, Theroux P, Gregoire J, Gagnon D, Arsenault A (1991) Technetium-99m sestamibi tomography in patients with spontaneous chest pain: correlations with clinical, electrocardiographic and angiographic findings. J Am Coll Cardiol 18(7):1684–1691.
11. Varetto T, Cantalupi D, Altieri A, Orlandi C (1993) Emergency room technetium-99m sestamibi imaging to rule out acute myocardial ischemic events in patients with nondiagnostic electrocardiograms. J Am Coll Cardiol 22(7):1804–1808.
12. Hilton TC, Thompson RC, Williams HJ, Saylors R, Fulmer H, Stowers SA (1994) Technetium-99m sestamibi myocardial perfusion imaging in the emergency room evaluation of chest pain. J Am Coll Cardiol 23(5):1016–1022.
13. Tatum JL, Jesse RL, Kontos MC et al. (1997) Comprehensive strategy for the evaluation and triage of the chest pain patient. Ann Emerg Med 29(1):116–125.
14. Kontos MC, Jesse RL, Schmidt KL, Ornato JP, Tatum JL (1997) Value of acute rest sestamibi perfusion imaging for evaluation of patients admitted to the emergency department with chest pain. J Am Coll Cardiol 30(4):976–982.
15. Heller GV, Stowers SA, Hendel RC et al. (1998) Clinical value of acute rest technetium-99m tetrofosmin tomographic myocardial perfusion imaging in patients with acute chest pain and nondiagnostic electrocardiograms. J Am Coll Cardiol 31(5):1011–1017.
16. Kontos MC, Jesse RL, Anderson FP, Schmidt KL, Ornato JP, Tatum JL (1999) Comparison of myocardial perfusion imaging and cardiac troponin I in patients admitted to the emergency department with chest pain. Circulation 99(16):2073–2078.
17. Verani MS, Jeroudi MO, Mahmarian JJ et al. (1988) Quantification of myocardial infarction during coronary occlusion and myocardial salvage after reperfusion using cardiac imaging with technetium-99m hexakis 2-methoxy-isobutyl isonitrile. J Am Coll Cardiol 12(6):1573–1581.
18. Kontos MC, Kurdziel K, McQueen R et al. (2002) Comparison of 2-dimensional echocardiography and myocardial perfusion imaging for diagnosing myocardial infarction in emergency department patients. Am Heart J 143(4):659–667.
19. Kontos MC, Fratkin MJ, Jesse RL, Anderson FP, Ornato JP, Tatum JL (2004) Sensitivity of acute rest myocardial perfusion imaging for identifying patients with myocardial infarction based on a troponin definition. J Nucl Cardiol 11(1):12–19.
20. Lee KL, Woodlief LH, Topol EJ et al. (1995) Predictors of 30-day mortality in the era of reperfusion for acute myocardial infarction. Results from an international trial of 41,021 patients. GUSTO-I Investigators. Circulation 91(6):1659–1668.
21. Fioretti P, Sclavo M, Brower RW, Simoons ML, Hugenholtz PG (1985) Prognosis of patients with different peak serum creatine kinase levels after first myocardial infarction. Eur Heart J 6(6):473–478.
22. White HD, Norris RM, Brown MA, Brandt PW, Whitlock RM, Wild CJ (1987) Left ventricular end-systolic volume as the major determinant of survival after recovery from myocardial infarction. Circulation 76(1):44–51.
23. Sabia P, Afrookteh A, Touchstone DA, Keller MW, Esquivel L, Kaul S (1991) Value of regional wall motion abnormality in the emergency room diagnosis of acute myocardial infarction. A prospective study using two-dimensional echocardiography. Circulation 84(3 Suppl):I85–I92.
24. Miller TD, Christian TF, Hopfenspirger MR, Hodge DO, Gersh BJ, Gibbons RJ (1995) Infarct size after acute myocardial infarction measured by quantitative tomographic ^{99m}Tc sestamibi imaging predicts subsequent mortality. Circulation 92(3):334–341.
25. Miller TD, Hodge DO, Sutton JM et al. (1998) Usefulness of technetium-99m sestamibi infarct size in predicting posthospital mortality following acute myocardial infarction. Am J Cardiol 81(12):1491–1493.
26. Christian TF, Behrenbeck T, Gersh BJ, Gibbons RJ (1991) Relation of left ventricular volume and function over one

year after acute myocardial infarction to infarct size determined by technetium-99m sestamibi. Am J Cardiol 68(1):21–26.
27. Christian TF, Behrenbeck T, Pellikka PA, Huber KC, Chesebro JH, Gibbons RJ (1990) Mismatch of left ventricular function and infarct size demonstrated by technetium-99m isonitrile imaging after reperfusion therapy for acute myocardial infarction: identification of myocardial stunning and hyperkinesia. J Am Coll Cardiol 16(7):1632–1638.
28. Behrenbeck T, Pellikka PA, Huber KC, Bresnahan JF, Gersh BJ, Gibbons RJ (1991) Primary angioplasty in myocardial infarction: assessment of improved myocardial perfusion with technetium-99m isonitrile. J Am Coll Cardiol 17(2):365–372.
29. Weissman IA, Dickinson CZ, Dworkin HJ, O'Neill WW, Juni JE (1996) Cost-effectiveness of myocardial perfusion imaging with SPECT in the emergency department evaluation of patients with unexplained chest pain. Radiology 199(2):353–357.
30. Radensky PW, Hilton TC, Fulmer H, McLaughlin BA, Stowers SA (1997) Potential cost effectiveness of initial myocardial perfusion imaging for assessment of emergency department patients with chest pain. Am J Cardiol 79(5):595–599.
31. Stowers SA, Eisenstein EL, Th Wackers FJ et al. (2000) An economic analysis of an aggressive diagnostic strategy with single photon emission computed tomography myocardial perfusion imaging and early exercise stress testing in emergency department patients who present with chest pain but nondiagnostic electrocardiograms: results from a randomized trial. Ann Emerg Med 35(1):17–25.
32. Kontos MC, Schmidt KL, McCue M et al. (2003) A comprehensive strategy for the evaluation and triage of the chest pain patient: a cost comparison study. J Nucl Cardiol 10(3):284–290.
33. Udelson JE, Beshansky JR, Ballin DS et al. (2002) Myocardial perfusion imaging for evaluation and triage of patients with suspected acute cardiac ischemia: a randomized controlled trial. J Am Med Assoc 288(21):2693–2700.
34. Chikamori T, Fujita H, Nanasato M, Toba M, Nishimura T (2005) Prognostic value of I-123 15-(p-iodophenyl)-3-(R,S) methylpentadecanoic acid myocardial imaging in patients with known or suspected coronary artery disease. J Nucl Cardiol 12(2):172–178.
35. Tamaki N (2005) Role of BMIPP imaging for risk stratification in patients with coronary artery disease. J Nucl Cardiol 12(2):148–150.

Chapter 27

Myocardial Perfusion Scintigraphy in Diabetes: Current Status and Limitations

John O. Prior

Contents

27.1	Introduction	305
27.1.1	CAD and Diabetes	305
27.1.2	Asymptomatic CAD in Diabetes	306
27.1.3	Early Diagnosis of CAD in Patients with Diabetes	307
27.2	Principle	307
27.2.1	Exercise Tolerance Testing	307
27.2.2	Stress Myocardial Perfusion Scintigraphy	307
27.2.3	Stress MPS with ECG-gated SPECT	307
27.2.4	Stress echocardiography	309
27.2.5	Coronary Angiography	309
27.3	Clinical Applications of Stress MPS	311
27.3.1	Diagnosis and Assessment of CAD in DM Patients	311
27.3.2	Risk Stratification of CAD in DM Patients	311
27.3.3	MPS in Symptomatic CAD Patients with Diabetes	312
27.3.4	MPS in Asymptomatic CAD Patients with Diabetes	313
27.3.5	Asymptomatic Patients with Diabetes: Who to Screen?	314
27.4	Discussion	315
27.4.1	Reduced Cardiac Survival in Women with Diabetes	315
27.4.2	Frequency of Stress MPS in Patients with Diabetes	315
27.4.3	Special Considerations for Type 1 Diabetes	316
27.4.4	Emerging Role of Coronary Calcium	316
27.4.5	Management of CAD Patients with Diabetes	316
27.5	Future Trends	317
27.5.1	Screening Asymptomatic Patients with DM for CAD	317
27.5.2	SPECT-CT and Other Noninvasive Cardiac Imaging Modalities	317
27.5.3	Future Challenges for MPS in Diabetic and Prediabetic Patients	318
	References	318

27.1 Introduction

Patients with diabetes have greater cardiovascular disease morbidity and mortality than non-diabetic patients. Since the beginning of clinical nuclear cardiology over two decades ago, myocardial perfusion scintigraphy has become a mature technique for evaluating coronary artery disease and several studies have specifically shown prognostic power in patients with diabetes. Silent ischemia is frequent and associated with a similar or poorer prognosis as non-silent disease. Current opinion is to recommend stress myocardial perfusion scintigraphy in symptomatic or high-risk asymptomatic patients, and the effectiveness of this approach is still under study, but encouraging preliminary results exist. Myocardial perfusion imaging can play an important role in improving clinical management of CAD in patients with diabetes. Important questions remain to be debated regarding who to screen, when to screen, and how to do this in a cost-effective manner.

27.1.1 CAD and Diabetes

There has been a rising prevalence of individuals with diabetes (type I and type II) over the last three decades, with an estimated 170 million patients affected worldwide in 2000, which is expected to reach over 360 million by 2030 [1]. The global public health burden is growing and the human and economic costs of this epidemic are enormous. Diabetes is associated with a two- to four-fold increase in the risk of developing coronary artery disease (CAD) [2]. Moreover, CAD is the leading cause of death among diabetic patients. The risk of major coronary events (myocardial infarct or cardiac death) in patients with diabetes without previous myocardial infarct is comparable with that of non-diabetic patients with previous infarct [3]. This led the American Heart Association to characterize diabetes as a "cardiovascular disease" risk equivalent [4]. Frequently, CAD will be occult in diabetic patients and the first sign may be a myocardial infarct or death [5]. With established CAD, prognosis is worse in diabetic patients than nondiabetic patients; diabetic patients have an increased risk of death at first myocardial infarction with two-fold and three-fold higher short-term mortality in men and women, respectively [5]. In addition, following an acute coronary syndrome, diabetic patients are at increased risk of adverse outcomes (death, cardiogenic shock, heart failure and renal failure), as shown in the large multinational observational GRACE study in 14 countries [6]. Conversely, diabetes or impaired glucose tolerance are common in patients with acute myocardial infarct, with for instance less than 35% of patients having a normal glucose tolerance at 3 months after the infarct [7]. Similarly, abnormal glucose metabolism was also found in one of three patients hospitalized for suspicion of acute coronary syndrome and was strongly associated with confirmation of this diagnosis [8].

27.1.2
Asymptomatic CAD in Diabetes

Patients with diabetes are often affected by occult CAD and have an increased prevalence of silent myocardial infarct and ischemia. The lack of warning symptoms in relation to diabetes is thought to be due to autonomic neuropathy affecting cardiac chest pain perception. Silent myocardial ischemia has been found in about 22–42% of asymptomatic patients, depending on the study population and definition criteria [9–12]. Taken together, these studies show that CAD is frequently occult in the diabetic population, varying from about 20% of truly asymptomatic diabetic patients [12] to >50% in patients with indirect signs of CAD [13]. Prognosis of silent ischemia was examined in the Coronary Artery Surgery Study (CASS), which showed similar risk in those with symptomatic ischemia and poorer risk in those with three-vessel disease [14]. In the subgroup of diabetic patients, Weiner et al. found that silent ischemia had a poorer prognosis in diabetic patients than in nondiabetic patients [15].

Table 27.1 Overview of sensitivity and specificity of noninvasive test for detecting CAD (≥70% stenosis) in patients with diabetes [16–18]

Modality	Sensitivity	Specificity	Remarks
Exercise tolerance testing	47% (68%)*	81% (77%)*	Limited data in diabetes [16]. Unreliable symptoms. Best if 90% of maximum predicted heart rate is reached.
Myocardial perfusion scintigraphy	90% (90%)*	50% (80%)*	Limited data in diabetes [17]. No data in diabetes for ECG-gated SPECT.
Stress echocardiography	82% (88%)*	54% (84%)*	Can be technically challenging to perform; poor images in heavy patients. Specificity can be low in diabetes [18].
Coronary angiography	Gold standard		Unacceptable risk in asymptomatic patient. Costs issues. Cannot assess microvessels.
New methods (general population)			
Electron beam CT	(95%)	(50%)	Low specificity.
CT angiography	(70–91%)	(84%)	Limited use in distal segments.
Magnetic resonance angiography	(50–100%)	(80–90%)	Not for small stenoses, few data. Potential for magnetic resonance of atherosclerotic plaque.
Positron emission tomography	(93%)	(92%)	Better sensitivity and specificity than SPECT. Quantitative myocardial blood flow. Role in detecting endothelial dysfunction.

*Figures in parenthesis are given for the general population.

27.1.3
Early Diagnosis of CAD in Patients with Diabetes

Given the poorer prognosis of CAD in the diabetic population than in the nondiabetic population, an earlier diagnosis has potential benefits in reducing mortality and morbidity such as earlier interventional therapy, heightened patient awareness of atypical signs of myocardial infarct and better compliance with risk-factor modification regimens. It is also expected that early therapeutic intervention may slow disease progression and decrease risk while CAD may be more likely to be modifiable.

27.2
Principle

Several testing modalities are available to clinicians to diagnose CAD. Few data have been specifically validated in diabetic populations. For instance, the exact value of exercise testing is still unknown in diabetic patients. To locate the place of stress MPS among the different modalities available to diagnose CAD in persons with diabetes, a brief overview will be presented. Table 27.1 gives average sensitivities and specificities expected from the different diagnostic tests for CAD in the diabetic population when such studies exist, or in the general population, recognizing that there could be limited applicability to diabetic patients.

27.2.1
Exercise Tolerance Testing

Although exercise tolerance testing occupies a central place in the diagnostic workup of patients with CAD, it has some severe limitations. First, baseline ECG abnormalities (such as the presence of ≥ 1 mm resting ST-segment depression, left bundle branch block or Wolff–Parkinson–White syndrome) or inability to exercise preclude its use to detect stress ischemia. Second, in a substantial proportion of diabetic patients (as much as 50%), tolerance testing is contraindicated or impossible to perform. Third, ST-segment depression cannot localize precisely the diseased coronary territory. Finally, the sensitivity of exercise tolerance testing can be low in diabetic patients generating a high rate of false negative studies, as found by Lee et al. [16] in a retrospective study (Table 27.1).

27.2.2
Stress Myocardial Perfusion Scintigraphy

Stress myocardial perfusion scintigraphy (MPS) is a mature method to determine the presence of CAD by assessing the extent and severity of abnormalities in regional myocardial perfusion reserve with high reproducibility and success rate (≤ 1% of uninterpretable images) [19]. MPS is performed with ^{201}Tl-chloride or ^{99m}Tc-labelled radiopharmaceuticals (the latter producing better image quality and more favourable dosimetry). The stress protocols use either exercise, pharmacological vasodilators or a combination of both (to reduce splanchnic blood flow [20]), as well as positive inotropes (β-receptor agonists), which provide comparable results [21]. Stress MPS has been validated in numerous clinical studies in a wide variety of populations [19]. Figure 27.1 illustrates a typical example of stress MPS in a diabetic patient with known CAD.

27.2.3
Stress MPS with ECG-gated SPECT

ECG-gated SPECT acquisition is currently the state-of-the-art method of performing MPS that attempts to discern attenuation artefacts from true perfusion defects by evaluating the presence or absence of concordant wall motion (Table 27.2). Furthermore, it allows left ventricular systolic and diastolic volumes, as well as ejection fraction (EF) to be determined with excellent correlation with other methods; an abnormal EF < 45% or increased end-systolic volumes add prognostic information over conventional MPS [22, 23]. ECG-gated acquisition improves specificity in areas affected by attenuation artefacts [24], thus achieving better clinical outcome prediction and lower costs [19], as well as avoiding unnecessary admissions to hospital in patients with acute coronary syndromes [23]. The assessment of EF from ECG-gated stress MPS also provided incremental value in predicting cardiac death in diabetic patients [25]. Finally, transient ischemic left ventricular dilation (TID) between rest and post-stress conditions independently is a recognized incremental prognostic marker of cardiovascular events (MI, cardiac death and revascularization) [26]. Figure 27.2 shows the utility of ECG gating in a diabetic patient with microvascular disease.

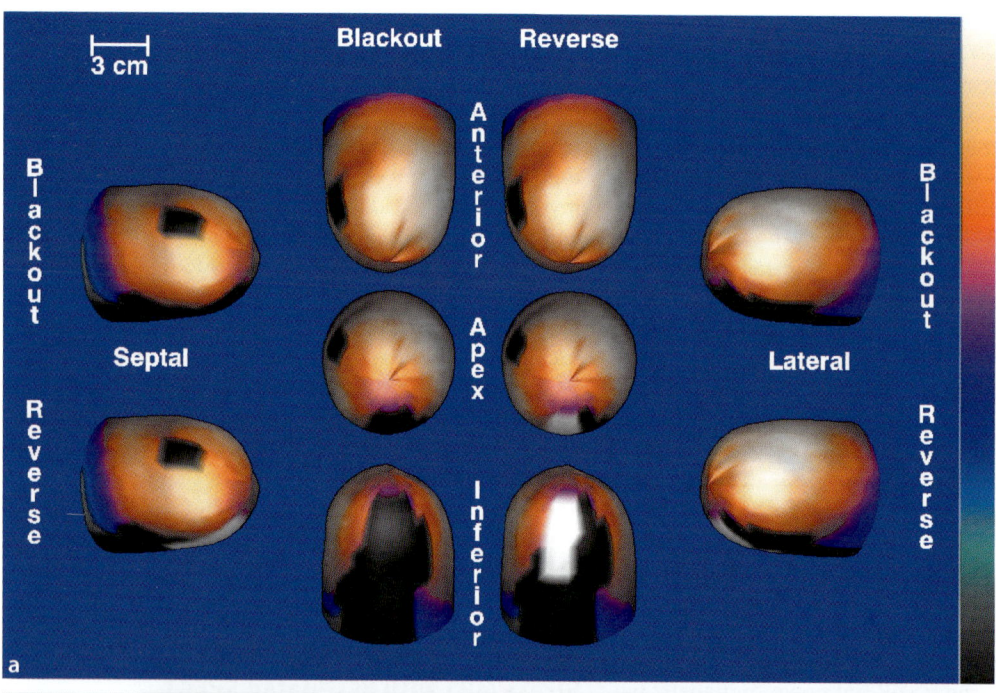
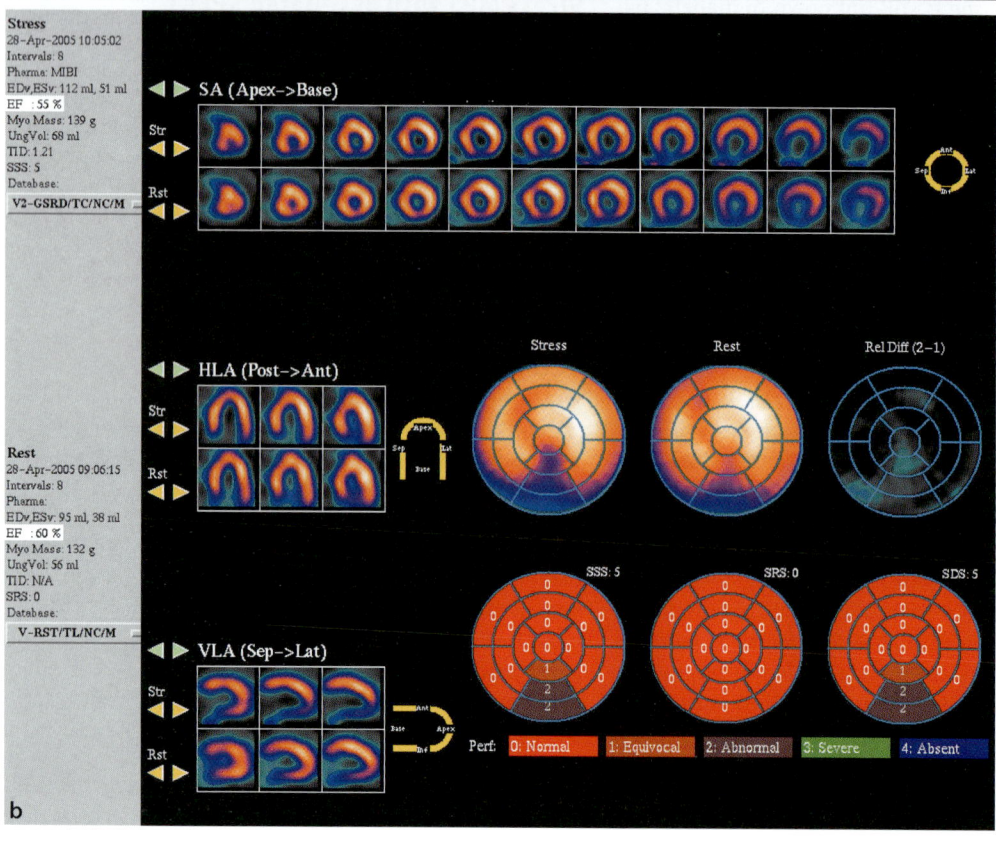

◀ **Fig. 27.1a,b** (**a**) Diabetic patient with two-vessel disease. Myocardial perfusion scintigraphy images during stress and at rest in a 75-year-old male diabetic patient with previous silent myocardial infarct in the right coronary artery territory, who presents with typical chest pain. Stress myocardial perfusion scintigraphy images show a partly reversible stress defect in the inferior territory (Emory Cardiac Toolbox, Atlanta, USA). Black-out areas indicate where perfusion is significantly decreased at stress; white-out area shows where rest perfusion is significantly better than stress perfusion and indicates reversible perfusion defect. (**b**) Stress (*top rows*) and rest (*bottom rows*) slices along the short- (SA), horizontal- (HLA) and vertical long-axes (VLA) and polar plots (4D-MSPECT, University of Michigan, USA). The summed stress score (SSS) was 5, the summed rest score (SRS) 0 and the summed difference score (SDS) 5. ECG-gated SPECT indicated a decrease in left ventricular ejection fraction (60% to 55%) and transient ischemic dilatation (TID = 1.21). Coronary angiography revealed a 90% stenosis of the first marginal branch of the circumflex artery and a total occlusion of the proximal right coronary artery

Table 27.2 Advantages and limitations of ECG-gated stress myocardial perfusion imaging in persons with diabetes

Advantages	Limitations
• Standardized, operator-independent procedure for objective assessment of perfusion and left ventricular function	• Limited data on prognostic information in asymptomatic diabetic patients (DIAD study in progress)
• Higher incremental value than exercise tolerance testing for risk stratification (the larger the MPS defect, the greater the risk); localize ischemia to individual coronary artery territories	• Use of ionizing radiation
• Ability to diagnose residual ischemia within an infarcted area	• Currently no evidence-based guidelines exist to identify asymptomatic diabetic patients to screen. Cost-effectiveness analyses need to be performed
• Higher feasibility (>99%) than stress echocardiography (>50–75%)	• Usefulness for detecting diabetic patients with only microvascular disease may be limited. Further investigations are needed.
• Superior to stress echocardiography for diagnosing one-vessel CAD disease	
• Office-based procedure (availability in nuclear cardiology practice)	

DIAD = Detection of Ischemia in Asymptomatic Diabetes [12, 63].

27.2.4
Stress echocardiography

Stress echocardiography is one of the most effective alternatives to exercise tolerance testing, relying on segmental defects induced by decreased wall motion of ischemic myocardium. Important limitations include high interobserver variability, operator-dependent reproducibility and poor echocardiographic images in overweight or obese persons. Nevertheless, added prognostic value has been verified in diabetic patients [27–29]. The exact role of stress echocardiography in screening asymptomatic patients still remains to be determined, as specificity can be relatively low in persons with diabetes [18] and dobutamine stress echocardiography may be less accurate than stress MPS to detect significant coronary artery stenosis in asymptomatic diabetic patients [30]. However, this technique seems to be best suited to meet the economic costs of large population screening [31].

27.2.5
Coronary Angiography

Traditionally, coronary angiography has been the gold standard to derive sensitivity and specificity estimates for the different noninvasive methods. However, coronary angiography can only detect epicardial, macrovascular disease and there is a complex relationship between risk and severity of coronary artery narrowing

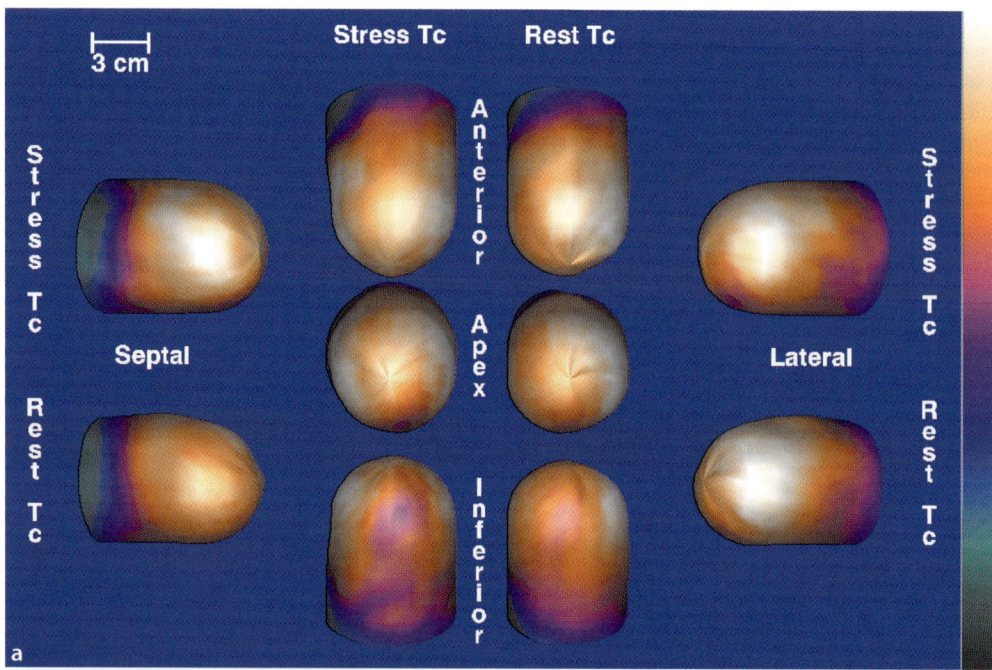
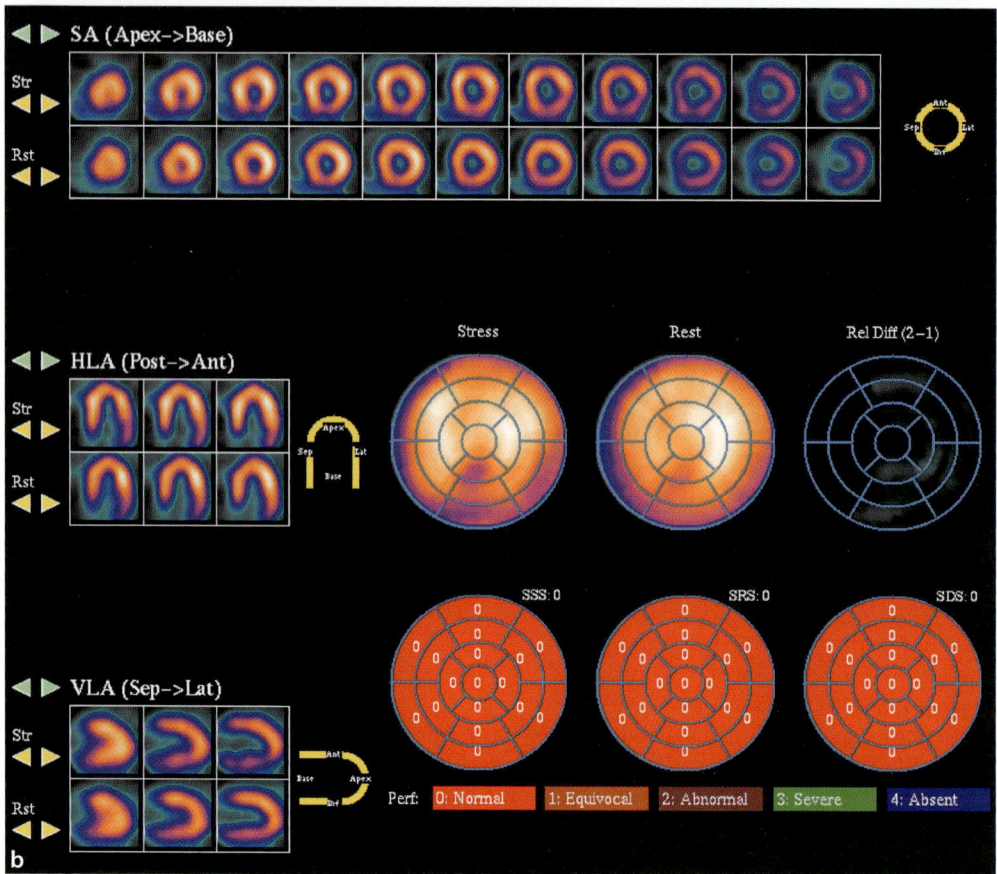

◀ **Fig. 27.2a,b** (a) Diabetic patient with microvascular disease. Myocardial perfusion scintigraphy in a 55–year-old male diabetic patient under insulin scheduled for non-cardiac surgery presenting with cardiovascular risk factors (hypertension, hypercholesterolemia, sedentary and peripheral artery disease). The stress and rest images show two small, minor reversible defects in the mid-inferior and basal-inferior segments (Emory Cardiac Toolbox, Atlanta, USA). (b) The reversible mid-inferior and basal inferior defects did not reach significance on polar maps (4D-MSPECT, University of Michigan, USA), with summed stress, rest and difference scores of 0. ECG-gated analysis showed a significant decrease in ejection fraction in post-stress (from 55% to 44%), with some transient ischemic dilatation (TID = 1.19). Coronary angiography showed only a nonsignificant disease (<50%) in the left circumflex artery compatible with diffuse microvascular disease

[32]. Coronary flow reserve is an integrated measure of blood flow through both the large epicardial coronary arteries and the microcirculation [33]. Thus, a diminution of coronary flow reserve may be due to narrowing of the epicardial coronary vessels, microcirculatory abnormalities, or both. Coronary angiography does not allow the direct visualization of coronary microcirculation in humans in vivo. However, its indirect assessment using the coronary flow reserve is possible with quantitative PET [33]. The fact that stress MPS has been shown to present incremental prognostic value over and above coronary angiography [34] may be due to its ability to indirectly assess microcirculatory abnormalities. Coronary angiography cannot be used for screening as it bears an unacceptable risk in asymptomatic patients.

27.3
Clinical Applications of Stress MPS

The different techniques to diagnose CAD specifically in patients with diabetes have been reviewed recently [35–38], as well as the utility of stress MPS in this population for prognosis and risk stratification [30, 39–42].

27.3.1
Diagnosis and Assessment of CAD in DM Patients

Due to the specific alteration of the microvasculature in relation to CAD and diabetes, it was important to verify if results obtained with stress MPS in the general population were also valid in persons with diabetes. Few studies have specifically investigated this diagnostic accuracy in diabetic patients. Among such studies, Kang et al. have retrospectively shown similar sensitivity, specificity and normalcy (proportion of patients with low CAD likelihood with normal MPS) of stress MPS in a group of 203 diabetic patients compared with 260 nondiabetic patients [17].

When comparing the results of stress MPS with coronary angiography, we and others have found that between 40 and 70% of diabetic patients with abnormal stress MPS had no significant epicardial disease [11, 43–47]. Rather than being all false-positive, these abnormal stress MPS studies are more likely to reflect true myocardial perfusion abnormalities due to a reduced capacity to increase blood flow in relation to diffuse atherosclerosis and/or abnormalities of the microcirculation that is underestimated by coronary angiography [33]. Indeed, dysfunction of the coronary vasodilatory capacity, both in epicardial vessels and resistance coronary vessels has been present in relation to diabetes and before obstructive CAD is present in the epicardial coronary arteries [48, 49]. Furthermore, myocardial blood flow is also influenced by autonomic neuropathy a well known complication of diabetes that can produce perfusion abnormalities [50].

In a large retrospective study of 27,165 patients, Miller et al. established that in 1738 asymptomatic diabetic patients, abnormal stress MPS prevalence was comparable with that in 2998 symptomatic diabetic patients (58.6% vs. 59.5%) and higher in 6215 nondiabetic asymptomatic and 16,214 symptomatic patients (46.2% vs. 44.4%, respectively) [13]. The high prevalence found in this study might have been partly due to the definition of "asymptomatic" by the authors, which meant that the patients no longer had the symptom at the time of stress MPS [40].

27.3.2
Risk Stratification of CAD in DM Patients

Previous studies have shown that stress MPS keeps its ability to provide added prognostic value for risk stratification of CAD in diabetic patients, based on retrospective analyses of patients referred to nuclear cardiology laboratories for a variety of reasons [46, 51–56].

Vanzetto et al. investigated the prognostic value of stress MPS with ^{201}Tl in 158 asymptomatic diabetic patients at high risk of developing cardiovascular events due to age (≥65 years), cardiovascular risk factors (smoking, hypertension), peripheral artery disease, resting ECG changes or microalbuminuria (57). Prognostic information was carried by the extent of MPS defects, the presence of perfusion defects in patients not able to exercise, with good negative predictive value for adverse cardiovascular events in the presence of normal MPS.

Using a 2-day protocol with ^{99m}Tc-stestamibi, De Lorenzo et al. following 180 asymptomatic diabetic patients with no known CAD for 35 ± 18 months demonstrated the prognostic value of stress MPS, with significantly increased rates of myocardial infarct or cardiac death for abnormal MPS [9]. Of note, no clinical or stress parameters could predict cardiovascular events or the type of MPS defects (fixed, reversible).

Zellweger et al., retrospectively studying the prognostic information of symptoms vs. objective evidence of CAD in 1737 patients with diabetes and without known CAD, found a higher prevalence of MPS abnormalities in patients with dyspnea and similar event rates, regardless of the presence or absence of angina [54]. Furthermore, MPS added incremental information to clinical symptoms to predict outcomes. Interestingly, dyspnea had independent predictive power regarding the prediction of myocardial infarct or death, with about a threefold increase in cardiovascular events. Dyspnea was often attributed to previous silent myocardial infarctions.

Finally, using the Mayo Clinic database, Rajagopalan et al. retrospectively showed in 1427 asymptomatic diabetic patients that high-risk findings on stress MPS in asymptomatic diabetic patients (18% prevalence) were associated with higher mortality rate and severe CAD prevalence [46].

27.3.3
MPS in Symptomatic CAD Patients with Diabetes

Kang et al. have shown that the sensitivity, specificity and normalcy rates of ECG-gated SPECT stress MPS in diabetic patients symptomatic for CAD were not different from those observed in nondiabetic patients [17]. The same authors have also confirmed the prognostic value of stress MPS in a study of 1271 diabetic patients and found an annual cardiac event rate (myocardial infarct or death) of 1–2% in the presence of normal MPS scans, 3–4% in those with mildly abnormal scans, up to ≥7% for moderately to severely abnormal scans (Figs. 27.3 and 27.4) [53]. For comparison, a meta-analysis of 14 general population studies of over 12,000 patients referred for stress MPS (^{99m}Tc-sestamibi) has shown that a normal or near-normal stress MPS conferred an annual risk of myocardial event or cardiac death of 0.6%, compared with 7.4% in the case of abnormal findings [58].

In a large multicentre retrospective study of 4755 patients (including 929 diabetic patients with known or suspected CAD) followed for an average of 2.5 years, Giri et al. have shown that abnormal stress MPS was an independent predictor for myocardial infarct and cardiac death and that patients with diabetes had higher event rates than patients without diabetes, the highest being for diabetic patients with ischemia (17.1% infarction rate) and for multivessel fixed defect (13.6% cardiac death rate) [52]. This study also demonstrated the added value of stress MPS compared with clinical parameters (Fig. 27.5).

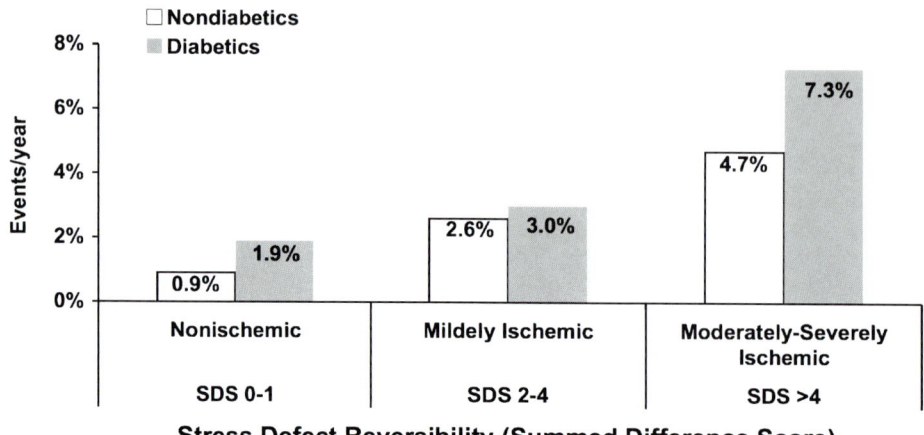

Fig. 27.3 Hard cardiovascular event rates as function of defect reversibility on stress myocardial perfusion scintigraphy. Adapted from [53] with permission from Elsevier

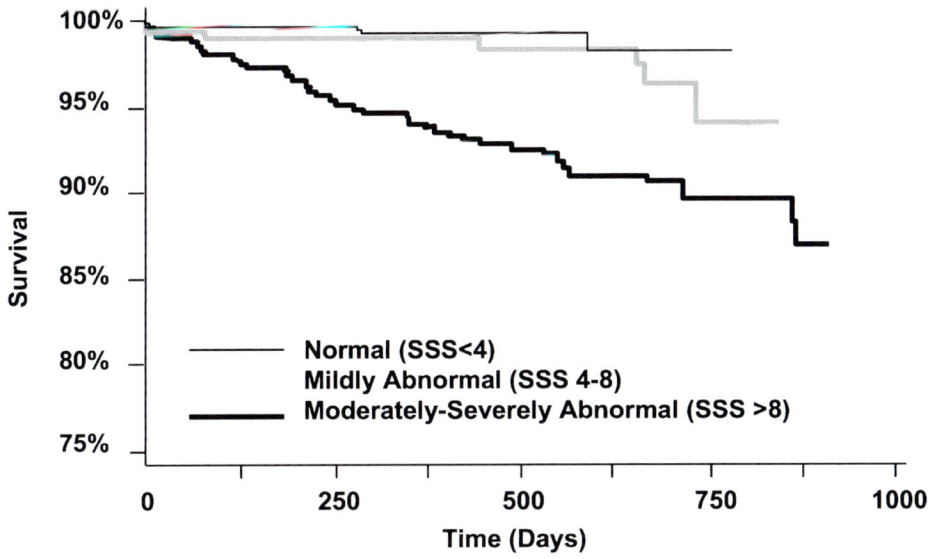

Fig. 27.4 Event-free survival rates in diabetic patients as a function of the severity of stress MPS defects. Adapted from [53] with permission from Elsevier

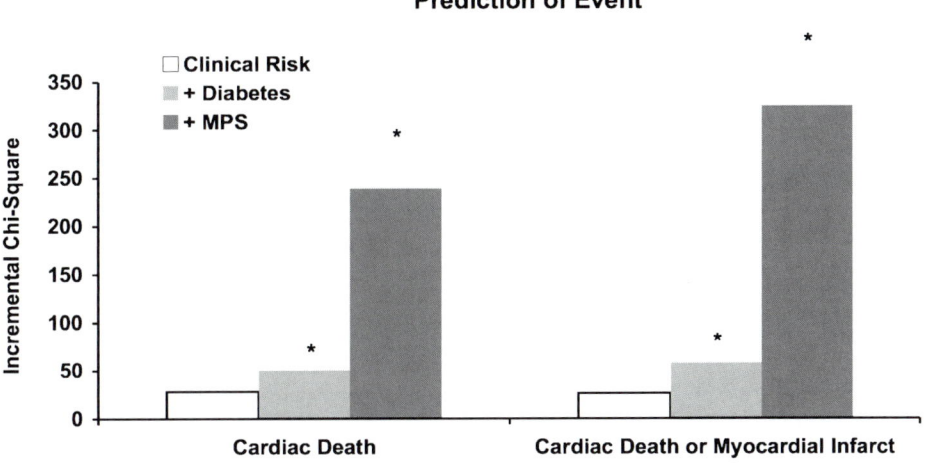

Fig. 27.5 Incremental χ^2 value of nuclear and clinical variables for prediction of cardiovascular events in diabetic patients. $^*p < 0.001$ vs. clinical risk. Adapted from [52] with permission from Lippincott Williams & Wlikins

27.3.4 MPS in Asymptomatic CAD Patients with Diabetes

There is currently a debate centred around which strategy to adopt to screen asymptomatic diabetes for silent CAD, as reflected by the many reviews, viewpoints and editorials in the recent literature [39, 40, 59–62].

The multicentre study on Detection of Ischemia in Asymptomatic Diabetics (DIAD) is a prospective study aimed at defining the prognostic significance of abnormal stress MPS in asymptomatic diabetic patients [63]. In the enrolment phase, 1123 asymptomatic diabetic patients were randomised among a "screening" arm with adenosine ^{99m}Tc-setsamibi stress MPS and a "no screening" arm. Results reveal a 22% prevalence of silent myocardial ischemia, including 5% with severe perfusion abnormalities [12]. Moreover, traditional cardiovascular risk factors or inflammation and thrombotic markers were not predictive; only abnormal Valsalva test, male gender and diabetes duration were. Finally, the authors note that using the American Diabetes Association/American College of Cardiology (ADA/ACC) guidelines [64] for limiting access to screening would have failed to identify 41% of the patients with silent ischemia.

In a recent open-label pilot study, Faglia et al. [65] randomized 141 asymptomatic diabetic patients without known CAD to either screening with exercise tolerance testing and dipyridamole stress echocardiography

Table 27.3 Guidelines to noninvasive screening in asymptomatic patients with diabetes

Guidelines year	Noninvasive screening recommended in presence of:
ADA/ACC [64] 1998	Peripheral artery disease
	Cerebrovascular disease
	Resting ECG abnormalities
	Two or more CVRF (dyslipidémie, hypertension, active smoking, family history of premature CAD, albuminuria)
AHA [72] 2002	No screening recommended in asymptomatic diabetic patients
	As diabetes is a CAD equivalent, aggressive approach to CVRF modification is recommended
SFC/ALFEDIAM [73] 2004 (Revision of the 1995 guidelines [69])	Peripheral artery disease or carotid atheroma
	Microalbuminuria + two traditional CVRF or proteinemia
	> 45 years resuming physical activity
	Type 1 diabetes, duration > 15 years + two or more traditional CVRF
	Type 2 diabetes, > 60 years or duration > 10 years + two or more traditional CVRF
	Age ≥ 65 years

CVRF = cardiovascular risk factors; ADA = American Diabetes Association; ACC = American College of Cardiology; SFC = Société Française de Cardiologie; ALFEDIAM = Association de Langue Française pour l'Etude du Diabète et des Maladies Métaboliques.

($n = 71$) or no screening ($n = 70$). During a 53-month follow-up, significantly less total cardiovascular events occurred in the screening arm compared with the control arm (RR = 0.226, $p = 0.018$) essentially due to a decrease in major coronary events (myocardial infarct). Although it was an open-label study with a small number of patients at high-risk for CAD based on cardiovascular risk factors, this study is the first one to include a control group and to prove the efficacy of screening for preclinical diagnosis of CAD, with the goal to reduce major cardiovascular events in type 2 diabetic patients.

27.3.5
Asymptomatic Patients with Diabetes: Who to Screen?

In truly asymptomatic diabetic patients screened prospectively for CAD, the prevalence of silent ischemia varies between 10 and 30% [12, 43, 47, 66, 67]. As no clear evidence exists about who to screen in asymptomatic diabetic patients, authors [47, 68–70] and expert panels [64, 71–73] have made suggestions regarding who to screen. The three major recommendations are summarized in Table 27.3 and the latest one is illustrated in Fig. 27.6.

Nonetheless, it has been demonstrated that a substantial proportion of diabetic patients with silent myocardial ischemia (about 40%) did not satisfy the ADA/ACC criteria for screening [11, 12, 74]. Indeed, current guidelines may miss potential markers of occult CAD in diabetic patients, such as abnormal autonomic function using a Valsalva test (supine/standing heart rate ratio), which was the strongest predictor in the DIAD study [12].

As the yield of stress MPS in asymptomatic diabetic patients is low (for instance 22% in the DIAD study), the use of stress MPS alone for screening is unlikely to be cost-effective on a large-scale in the absence of macrovascular disease [31]. To achieve better clinical and cost efficiency, strategies are being developed to increase prospective yield of stress MPS by selecting a subgroup of asymptomatic diabetic patients at increased risk of CAD before the use of stress MPS.

No traditional cardiovascular risk factor has been demonstrated to have sufficient sensitivity and specificity to predict silent myocardial ischemia in diabetes [75]. Therefore, a number of additional cardiovascular risk markers have been investigated. Cardiac autonomic dysfunction was associated with ischemia in the prospective DIAD study [12] or in other studies [50, 76] or observations [77]. Erectile dysfunction in men was also associated with MPS abnormalities [11, 78]. New emerging markers such as adhesion molecules, inflammatory parameters, lipoprotein(a) or homocysteine levels, as well as endothelial dysfunction might be of interest and must be evaluated further [75, 79].

Some authors have suggested the use of atherosclerosis burden measurements such as the intima-media thickness ratio [80], the ankle-brachial index or the coronary calcium score [81]. Indeed, sequential use of

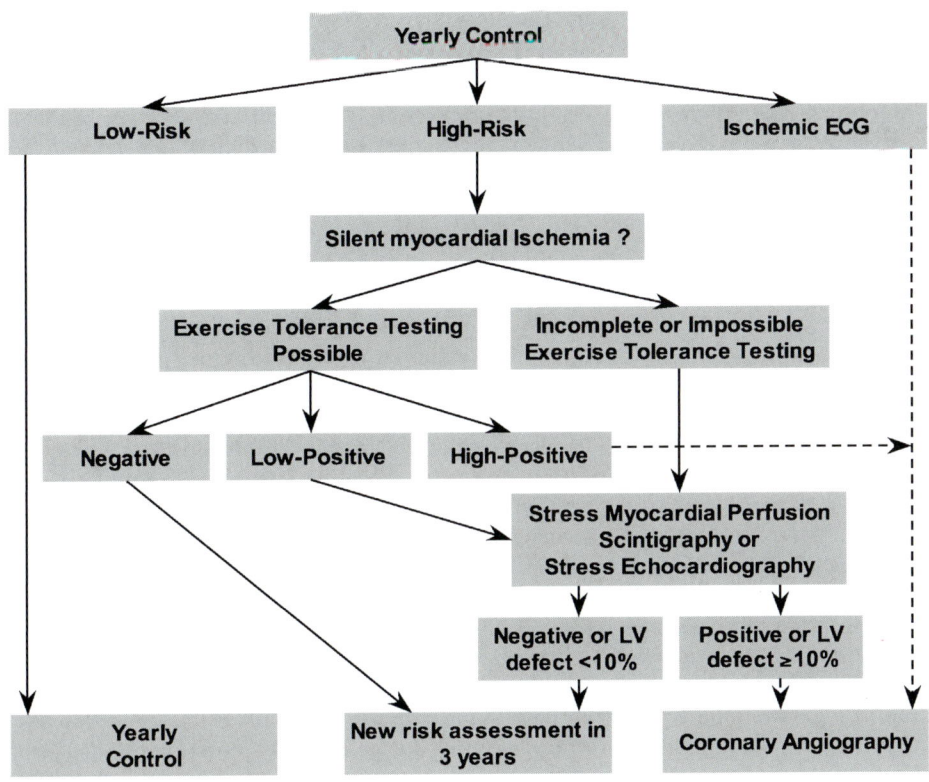

Fig. 27.6 Screening strategy in asymptomatic patients with diabetes (SFC/ALFEDIAM). Ischemic signs on resting ECG are Q-waves (necrosis) or negative T-waves in at least three contiguous leads (subepicardial ischemia) may lead to considering coronary angiography. Adapted from [73] with permission. © Masson, Editeur

low-cost, noninvasive testing followed by stress MPS has been shown to increase the clinical and cost effectiveness of screening in the general [80, 82–84] and diabetic populations [80, 82–84]. Alternatively, the same office-based global risk assessment measures derived from large populations could be used to compute the probability of developing CAD to recommend stress MPS, although some important marker might be missed (i.e. autonomic dysfunction). Others have tried to use composite scores derived from cardiovascular risk factors and markers of atherosclerotic burden in peripheral arteries [85]. The efficacy of such different strategies remains to be determined in larger, multicentre studies.

27.4 Discussion

27.4.1 Reduced Cardiac Survival in Women with Diabetes

Early diagnosis of CAD is crucial in diabetic women, as they tend to have a delayed incidence of CAD compared with that in men, but a greater CAD prevalence and worse prognosis [5]. Previous reports have shown decreased sensitivities and specificities of exercise tolerance testing in the general population of women compared with those in men [86]. However, this was not confirmed when using the latest ECG-gated SPECT stress MPS [62]. Retrospective studies have shown decreased survival in women with diabetes [51, 52], with adjusted event rates exceeding the one observed in diabetic men for similar perfusion defects [51]. Moreover, diabetes seems to cancel the protective premenopausal effect of the female gender in the progression from normal to abnormal stress MPS [87]. If confirmed in prospective studies, these gender differences should be integrated in future guidelines [62].

27.4.2 Frequency of Stress MPS in Patients with Diabetes

The ADA/ACC recommend performing CVRF assessment in asymptomatic diabetic patients on a yearly basis for symptoms that would prompt stress testing. The optimal frequency of stress MPS is currently unknown. A 3–5-year interval would be adequate in asymptomatic diabetic patients without new CVRF and a shorter 1–2-year interval in the case of multiple or new CVRF, as suggested initially by Nesto et al. [88] and confirmed in the study by Giri et al. [52]. Moreover, CAD progression is thought to be accelerated in the presence of diabetes. In preliminary work, Noble et al. have retrospectively analysed patients with an initially normal stress MPS, who had abnormal repeated stress MPS at a later date [87]. Diabetic patients had increased rates of conversion from normal-to-abnormal MPS as compared to nondiabetic patients [32.1% vs. 21.2%].

27.4.3
Special Considerations for Type 1 Diabetes

Although type 1 diabetes affects only 5–10% of the overall diabetic population, its earlier onset age and greater severity of metabolic abnormalities dramatically increases the risk of CAD after age 30. The Writing Group III on risk assessment in persons with diabetes recommended applying the same recommendation for adults with type 2 diabetes to all persons with type 1 diabetes aged ≥16 [89]. Contrasting with type 2 diabetes, patients with type 1 diabetes often develop early microvascular complications. Accordingly, retinopathy, microalbuminuria and nephropathy were found to be important CAD risk factors.

27.4.4
Emerging Role of Coronary Calcium

Coronary calcium burden is a sensitive marker of atherosclerosis, which is known to be more prevalent and more extensive in diabetic patients [90]. Coronary calcium can be measured easily using electron beam computed tomography (EBCT) or multidetector CT (MDCT) and has an excellent sensitivity to detect obstructive CAD, but a low specificity (Table 27.1), well below that desired for a screening test. This does not allow its use to diagnose obstructive CAD alone.

Several authors have made suggestions about the sequential use of coronary calcium scoring to select asymptomatic diabetic patients before MPS [37, 84]. Indeed, diabetic patients with low coronary calcium burden have a low short-term risk of death [91]. This has been prospectively studied by Anand et al. [81], who found greatly enhanced detection of silent ischemia with a 42% prevalence of abnormal stress MPS in asymptomatic patients with coronary calcium > 100. Such an approach remains to be evaluated for clinical- and cost-effectiveness and radiation exposure before widespread use for screening can be recommended.

27.4.5
Management of CAD Patients with Diabetes

To justify screening for silent ischemia in diabetic persons, there must exist an efficient and recognized treatment, which has not been definitively proved yet [60, 61]. Indeed, few trials have compared the different strategies against CAD in diabetic populations.

The efficacy of β-blockers has been shown to reduce the severity and number of silent ischemia episodes [92] and to decrease the mortality risk by 44% [93]. Treatment with angiotensin converting enzyme (ACE) inhibitors provides strong evidence for a cardioprotective effect in diabetic patients regardless of whether they are hypertensive or not, with a 25% relative risk reduction of cardiac death, myocardial infarct and stroke [94]. Statins can also reduce the relative risk of cardiovascular events in diabetic patients by 22–37% [95, 96]. Optimal medical treatment has been shown to reduce the 7-year mortality in diabetic patients with microalbuminuria by 53% (STENO-2 trial) [97].

The superiority of coronary stenting over angioplasty has been established in diabetic patients [98]; other trials have found better results when using abciximab [99] or drug-eluting stents [100]. The question on the use of coronary artery bypass surgery (CABG) vs. stenting in diabetic patients is still unanswered [101]. This decision must be made on individual basis considering age, co-morbidities and analysis of the coronary angiogram [73, 102]. In the Bypass Angioplasty Revascularization Investigation (BARI), the subgroup of diabetic patients with multivessel disease presented with a lower mortality with surgery compared with angioplasty [103]. Today's therapeutic armamentarium of drug-eluting stents and glycoprotein IIb/IIIa receptor inhibitors may actually supersede the earlier mortality advantages seen with CABG compared with normal stents [102]. Although none of the studies conducted so far was in diabetic patients, it is supposed that despite a higher surgical risk, diabetic patients may derive greater benefit from revascularization than do nondiabetic patients, especially in the presence of large amounts of reversible ischemia [104]. A randomized controlled trial is currently under way to compare 5-year mortality of percutaneous coronary interventions and CABG in diabetic patients (BARI-2D) [105] using medical treatment including statins, β-blockers and ACE inhibitors. Another trial (FREEDOM) will start soon to compare drug-eluting stents with adjunctive abciximab vs. CABG in diabetic patients with multivessel CAD.

Evidence to support the rationale for exercise training interventions was presented in a study comparing 12-month exercise training versus standard percutaneous coronary interventions in patients with stable CAD

[106]. This randomized trial showed survival and cost benefit in favour of the exercise training programme with improvement at 12 months of stress radiotracer uptake in areas distal to the target lesion on MPS. Such an approach is certainly worth testing in the diabetic population with optimized medical treatment in larger, multicentre studies.

Although the definite answer about how to treat diabetic patients with silent ischemia is unknown, the clinician has the choice to start aggressive treatment of cardiovascular risk factors and to introduce β-blockers and ACE inhibitors, which have demonstrated efficacy in diabetes [93, 94]. Considering the results of the STENO-2 trial, if a silent ischemia is discovered in an asymptomatic diabetic patient, strict and aggressive control of cardiovascular risk factors may reduce by up to half cardiovascular events when compared with conventional or occasional treatment. The DIAD-2 trial (117) showed that 79% of patients with ischemia on myocardial perfusion scintigraphy resolved on repeat imaging 3 years later. The observed resolution was associated with a greater number of patients taking statins, aspirin and ACE inhibitors than at the time of the original scan. Finally, CABG could be preferred in patients with more than 10% reversible myocardial ischemia, although benefit has not been demonstrated *per se* in diabetic patients, but is strongly suspected [104].

27.5
Future Trends

27.5.1
Screening Asymptomatic Patients with DM for CAD

Clarification of the best clinical and cost efficient screening algorithm in asymptomatic persons with diabetes is awaited. The encouraging preliminary results of Faglia et al. [65] show risk reduction by screening asymptomatic diabetic patients. There are currently insufficient data to support routine angiography or intervention in all asymptomatic diabetic patients with abnormal screening stress MPS; this decision is left to the clinician's judgment.

27.5.2
SPECT-CT and Other Noninvasive Cardiac Imaging Modalities

Several technological developments of noninvasive cardiac imaging are currently underway, such as cardiac magnetic resonance imaging, electron-beam CT and multidetector CT, SPECT-CT and PET-CT. These imaging modalities will be applied to the study of patients with diabetes and are most likely to play an important role, generally in a complementary rather than competitive way.

The latest hybrid SPECT-CT systems integrating a SPECT scanner with a multidetector CT scanner have great potential for improved diagnostic accuracy in overweight or obese patients owing to better attenuation correction, as well as better clinical efficacy by combining anatomic calcium scoring and/or CT-based angiography with stress MPS in the same session [107]. The availability of co-registered anatomic and physiologic processes may be critical for the next developments in nuclear cardiology, notably in the study of molecular targets such as substrates related to angiogenesis, hypoxia, inflammation, necrosis or apoptosis, as well as imaging neurohumoral activity, vulnerable atherosclerotic plaques or the effects of gene therapy.

Measurement of myocardial blood flow with positron emission tomography (PET), initially confined to centres equipped with cyclotrons is becoming a feasible alternative when using generator-based ^{82}Rubidium radioisotope in high-volume nuclear cardiology centres. Cardiac PET is offering superior diagnostic performances to MPS, essentially due to increased resolution, sensitivity and intrinsic attenuation correction and quantitation of absolute myocardial blood flow [23, 108]. This improves CAD detection accuracy, especially in overweight or obese patients more often found among diabetic persons [108]. Furthermore, this modality has can assess coronary circulatory function with the cold pressor test [49]. Abnormally reduced myocardial blood flow response to cold pressor testing has been shown to be a surrogate marker of future cardiovascular events in the general and diabetic population [48, 109].

Magnetic resonance angiography is rapidly evolving and has the potential to become a preferred means to perform noninvasive coronary angiography due to the absence of ionizing radiation or iodine-based contrast products, although actual angiographic performance is lagging behind multidetector CT and is still some way from routine clinical application. Magnetic resonance allows the assessment of cardiac anatomy and physiology (wall motion) with great spatial resolution and offers the promise of characterizing vulnerable plaques to select patients at high risk of cardiac events [110, 111]. However, this technology is not yet widely available, with little data existing on its power to predict future cardiovascular events. Magnetic resonance will not be possible in patients with metallic implants such as cardiac pacemaker or defibrillators.

Table 27.4 Management of CAD in diabetic patients based on risk assessment by myocardial perfusion scintigraphy

	Myocardial perfusion scintigraphy result		
	Normal	Mildly abnormal	Moderately to severely abnormal
Annualized risk of cardiovascular event	1–2%	3–4%	>7%
Management	CVRF modification* Re-test after 1–2 years	Aggressive CVRF modification* Re-test after 1–2 years	Aggressive CVRF modification* Coronary angiography (CT angiography?) Possibly revascularization

CVRF = cardiovascular risk factors.

*For comparison, in the STENO-2 trial [97], the targeted values were: glycosylated haemoglobin HbA1c < 6.5%, blood pressure < 135/80 mmHg, with statins to reach low-density lipoprotein (LDL) cholesterol values < 2.6 mmol/l, with prescription of aspirin, angiotensin-converting enzyme (ACE) inhibitors and folic acid.

27.5.3
Future Challenges for MPS in Diabetic and Prediabetic Patients

Trials on added value of different noninvasive tests and cost-effectiveness analyses are needed before recommendations can be made and policy can be established. However, it is hoped that better use of currently available screening and risk stratification option will be made [39], for instance by the establishment of specific guidelines at the international level to use MPS to classify patients into prognostic groups. For instance, as stress MPS has strong predictive value to identify diabetic patients at higher risk for adverse cardiovascular events, this prognostic information could easily be used for CAD management (Table 27.4).

On the other hand, diabetes is still much under-diagnosed; a recent prospective study of a cohort of patients hospitalized for acute myocardial infarct showed that 57% had dysglycemia, with about 66% who met the criteria for new diabetes not having been diagnosed or treated as such by the managing physician [112]. Although efficient drugs are available to reach targets and to improve outcomes in patients with diabetes, under-treatment is frequent, as revealed by a study in a managed care setting showing that only 72% of diabetic patients were treated for glycemic control, 64% for blood pressure and 28% for dyslipidemia [113]. Of the diabetic patients receiving medication, only 29% were at target for HbA_{1c}, 40% for blood pressure and 32% for LDL cholesterol. More aggressive drug treatment associated with lifestyle changes are necessary to reach desired targets in more patients than is currently achieved [114]. The DIAD-2 trial [117] has shown that in patients with type II diabetes who had inducible ischemia shown by myocardial perfusion scintigraphy, 79% resolved on repeat imaging 3 years later. This improvement was associated with intensification of treatment with cardiac medications.

The link between diabetes and development of CAD is well known. However, abnormalities of the coronary circulation have been evidenced throughout the whole spectrum of insulin resistance, well before the development of overt diabetes [49]. Consequently, more attention will be devoted to prediabetic states such as impaired glucose tolerance or in the metabolic syndrome, which are also associated with excess in mortality risk. In these larger populations, stress MPS has a potential role to play, as already demonstrated by higher likelihood of inducible ischemia on stress MPS in the presence of metabolic syndrome without diabetes [115, 116].

Acknowledgements

The author would like to thank Prof. A. Bischof Delaloye, MD, Prof. R. Darioli, MD, and Dr. J. Ruiz, MD, CHUV University Hospital, Lausanne, Switzerland for their critical comments and suggestions.

References

1. Wild S, Roglic G, Green A, Sicree R, King H (2004) Global prevalence of diabetes: estimates for the year 2000 and projections for 2030. Diabetes Care 27(5):1047–1053.
2. Stamler J, Vaccaro O, Neaton JD, Wentworth D (1993) Diabetes, other risk factors, and 12-yr cardiovascular mortality for men screened in the Multiple Risk Factor Intervention Trial. Diabetes Care 16(2):434–444.

3. Haffner SM, Lehto S, Ronnemaa T, Pyorala K, Laakso M (1998) Mortality from coronary heart disease in subjects with type 2 diabetes and in nondiabetic subjects with and without prior myocardial infarction. N Engl J Med 339(4):229–234.
4. Grundy SM, Benjamin IJ, Burke GL et al. (1999) Diabetes and cardiovascular disease: a statement for healthcare professionals from the American Heart Association. Circulation 100(10):1134–1146.
5. Miettinen H, Lehto S, Salomaa V et al. (1998) Impact of diabetes on mortality after the first myocardial infarction. The FINMONICA Myocardial Infarction Register Study Group. Diabetes Care 21(1):69–75.
6. Franklin K, Goldberg RJ, Spencer F et al. (2004) Implications of diabetes in patients with acute coronary syndromes: The global registry of acute coronary events. Arch Intern Med 164(13):1457–1463.
7. Norhammar A, Tenerz A, Nilsson G et al. (2002) Glucose metabolism in patients with acute myocardial infarction and no previous diagnosis of diabetes mellitus: a prospective study. Lancet 359(9324):2140–2144.
8. Timmer JR, Bilo HJ, Ottervanger JP et al. (2005) Dysglycemia in suspected acute coronary syndromes. Eur J Internal Med 16(1):29–33.
9. De Lorenzo A, Lima RS, Siqueira-Filho AG, Pantoja MR (2002) Prevalence and prognostic value of perfusion defects detected by stress technetium-99m sestamibi myocardial perfusion single-photon emission computed tomography in asymptomatic patients with diabetes mellitus and no known coronary artery disease. Am J Cardiol 90(8):827–832.
10. Inoguchi T, Yamashita T, Umeda F et al. (2000) High incidence of silent myocardial ischemia in elderly patients with non insulin-dependent diabetes mellitus. Diabetes Res Clin Pract 47(1):37–44.
11. Prior JO, Monbaron D, Koehli M, Calcagni ML, Ruiz J, Bischof Delaloye A (2005) Prevalence of symptomatic and silent stress-induced perfusion defects in diabetic patients with suspected coronary artery disease referred for myocardial perfusion scintigraphy. Eur J Nucl Med Mol Imaging 32(1):60–69.
12. Wackers FJ, Young LH, Inzucchi SE et al. (2004) Detection of silent myocardial ischemia in asymptomatic diabetic subjects: the DIAD study. Diabetes Care 27(8):1954–1961.
13. Miller TD, Rajagopalan N, Hodge DO, Frye RL, Gibbons RJ (2004) Yield of stress single-photon emission computed tomography in asymptomatic patients with diabetes. Am Heart J 147(5):890–896.
14. Weiner DA, Ryan TJ, McCabe CH et al. (1988) Risk of developing an acute myocardial infarction or sudden coronary death in patients with exercise-induced silent myocardial ischemia. A report from the Coronary Artery Surgery Study (CASS) registry. Am J Cardiol 62(17):1155–1158.
15. Weiner DA, Ryan TJ, Parsons L et al. (1991) Significance of silent myocardial ischemia during exercise testing in patients with diabetes mellitus: a report from the Coronary Artery Surgery Study (CASS) Registry. Am J Cardiol 68(8):729–734.
16. Lee DP, Fearon WF, Froelicher VF (2001) Clinical utility of the exercise ECG in patients with diabetes and chest pain. Chest 119(5):1576–1581.
17. Kang X, Berman DS, Lewin H et al. (1999) Comparative ability of myocardial perfusion single-photon emission computed tomography to detect coronary artery disease in patients with and without diabetes mellitus. Am Heart J 137(5):949–957.
18. Hennessy TG, Codd MB, Kane G, McCarthy C, McCann HA, Sugrue DD (1997) Evaluation of patients with diabetes mellitus for coronary artery disease using dobutamine stress echocardiography. Coron Artery Dis 8(3–4):171–174.
19. Underwood SR, Anagnostopoulos C, Cerqueira M et al. (2004) Myocardial perfusion scintigraphy: the evidence. Eur J Nucl Med Mol Imaging 31(2):261–291.
20. Updated imaging guidelines for nuclear cardiology procedures, part 1 (2001) J Nucl Cardiol 8(1):G5–G58.
21. Leppo JA (1996) Comparison of pharmacologic stress agents. J Nucl Cardiol 3(6 Pt 2):S22–26.
22. Sharir T, Germano G, Kavanagh PB et al. (1999) Incremental prognostic value of post-stress left ventricular ejection fraction and volume by gated myocardial perfusion single photon emission computed tomography. Circulation 100(10):1035–1042.
23. ACC/AHA/ASNC Guidelines for the clinical use of cardiac radionuclide imaging: a report of the American College of Cardiology/American Heart Association Task Force on Practice Guidelines (ACC/AHA/ASNC Committee to Revise the 1995 Guidelines for the Clinical Use of Cardiac Radionuclide Imaging). 2003. (Accessed July 23, 2005, at http://www.acc.org/clinical/guidelines/radio/rni_fulltext.pdf.)
24. Taillefer R, DePuey EG, Udelson JE, Beller GA, Benjamin C, Gagnon A (1999) Comparison between the end-diastolic images and the summed images of gated ^{99m}Tc-sestamibi SPECT perfusion study in detection of coronary artery disease in women. J Nucl Cardiol 6(2):169–176.
25. Hayes SW, Schisterman EF, Lewin HC et al. (2001) Gated myocardial perfusion SPECT has incremental value for predicting cardiac death in diabetic patients. J Am Coll Cardiol 37(2 Supplement A):381A.
26. Abidov A, Bax JJ, Hayes SW et al. (2003) Transient ischemic dilation ratio of the left ventricle is a significant predictor of future cardiac events in patients with otherwise normal myocardial perfusion SPECT. J Am Coll Cardiol 42(10):1818–1825.

27. Bigi R, Desideri A, Cortigiani L, Bax JJ, Celegon L, Fiorentini C (2001) Stress echocardiography for risk stratification of diabetic patients with known or suspected coronary artery disease. Diabetes Care 24(9):1596–1601.
28. Elhendy A, Arruda AM, Mahoney DW, Pellikka PA (2001) Prognostic stratification of diabetic patients by exercise echocardiography. J Am Coll Cardiol 37(6):1551–1557.
29. Kamalesh M, Matorin R, Sawada S (2002) Prognostic value of a negative stress echocardiographic study in diabetic patients. Am Heart J 143(1):163–168.
30. Le Feuvre CL, Barthelemy O, Dubois-Laforgue D et al. (2005) Stress myocardial scintigraphy and dobutamine echocardiography in the detection of coronary disease in asymptomatic patients with type 2 diabetes. Diabetes Metab 31(2):135–142.
31. Hayashino Y, Nagata-Kobayashi S, Morimoto T, Maeda K, Shimbo T, Fukui T (2004) Cost-effectiveness of screening for coronary artery disease in asymptomatic patients with Type 2 diabetes and additional atherogenic risk factors. J Gen Internal Med 19(12):1181–1191.
32. Topol EJ, Nissen SE (1995) Our preoccupation with coronary luminology. The dissociation between clinical and angiographic findings in ischemic heart disease. Circulation 92(8):2333–2342.
33. Kaufmann PA, Camici PG (2005) Myocardial blood flow measurement by PET: technical aspects and clinical applications. J Nucl Med 46(1):75–88.
34. Hachamovitch R, Berman DS, Shaw LJ et al. (1998) Incremental prognostic value of myocardial perfusion single photon emission computed tomography for the prediction of cardiac death: differential stratification for risk of cardiac death and myocardial infarction. Circulation 97(6):535–543.
35. Antonopoulos A, Vijay Anand D, Lahiri A (2005) Diabetes mellitus: evaluation of patients with known or suspected coronary artery disease and the role played by myocardial perfusion imaging. Nucl Med Commun 26(7):587–591.
36. Ashley EA, Raxwal V, Finlay M, Froelicher V (2002) Diagnosing coronary artery disease in diabetic patients. Diabetes Metab Res Rev 18(3):201–208.
37. Bauduceau B, Le Marec E, Dupuy O et al. (2003) New methods of cardiac imaging: a revolution in the management of diabetics. J Annu Diabetol Hotel Dieu 2003:239–250.
38. Tschoepe D, Burchert W (2004) Non-invasive imaging for coronary artery disease in diabetes. Br J Diabetes Vasc Dis 4(4):245–250.
39. Heller GV (2005) Evaluation of the patient with diabetes mellitus and suspected coronary artery disease. Am J Med 118 Suppl 2:9S-14S.
40. Navare SM, Heller GV (2004) Role of stress single-photon emission computed tomography imaging in asymptomatic patients with diabetes. Am Heart J 147(5):753–755.
41. Noble GL, Heller GV (2005) Single-photon emission computed tomography myocardial perfusion imaging in patients with diabetes. Curr Cardiol Rep 7(2):117–123.
42. Wackers FJ (2005) Diabetes and coronary artery disease: the role of stress myocardial perfusion imaging. Cleve Clin J Med 72(1):21–25, 29–33.
43. Koistinen MJ (1990) Prevalence of asymptomatic myocardial ischaemia in diabetic subjects. Br Med J 301(6743):92–95.
44. Cosson E, Guimfack M, Paries J, Paycha F, Attali JR, Valensi P (2003) Are silent coronary stenoses predictable in diabetic patients and predictive of cardiovascular events? Diabetes Metab 29(5):470–476.
45. Valensi P, Sachs RN, Lormeau B et al. (1997) Silent myocardial ischaemia and left ventricle hypertrophy in diabetic patients. Diabetes Metab 23(5):409–416.
46. Rajagopalan N, Miller TD, Hodge DO, Frye RL, Gibbons RJ (2005) Identifying high-risk asymptomatic diabetic patients who are candidates for screening stress single-photon emission computed tomography imaging. J Am Coll Cardiol 45(1):43–49.
47. Janand-Delenne B, Savin B, Habib G, Bory M, Vague P, Lassmann-Vague V (1999) Silent myocardial ischemia in patients with diabetes: who to screen. Diabetes Care 22(9):1396–1400.
48. Nitenberg A, Ledoux S, Valensi P, Sachs R, Attali JR, Antony I (2001) Impairment of coronary microvascular dilation in response to cold pressor--induced sympathetic stimulation in type 2 diabetic patients with abnormal stress thallium imaging. Diabetes 50(5):1180–1185.
49. Prior JO, Quinones MJ, Hernandez-Pampaloni M et al. (2005) Coronary circulatory dysfunction in insulin resistance, impaired glucose tolerance, and type 2 diabetes mellitus. Circulation 111(18):2291–2298.
50. Di Carli MF, Bianco-Batlles D, Landa ME et al. (1999) Effects of autonomic neuropathy on coronary blood flow in patients with diabetes mellitus. Circulation 100(8):813–819.
51. Berman DS, Kang X, Hayes SW et al. (2003) Adenosine myocardial perfusion single-photon emission computed tomography in women compared with men. Impact of diabetes mellitus on incremental prognostic value and effect on patient management. J Am Coll Cardiol 41(7):1125–1133.
52. Giri S, Shaw LJ, Murthy DR et al. (2002) Impact of diabetes on the risk stratification using stress single-photon emission computed tomography myocardial perfusion imaging in patients with symptoms suggestive of coronary artery disease. Circulation 105(1):32–40.
53. Kang X, Berman DS, Lewin HC et al. (1999) Incremental prognostic value of myocardial perfusion single photon emission computed tomography in patients with diabetes mellitus. Am Heart J 138(6 Pt 1):1025–1032.

54. Zellweger MJ, Hachamovitch R, Kang X et al (2004) Prognostic relevance of symptoms versus objective evidence of coronary artery disease in diabetic patients. Eur Heart J 25(7):543–550.
55. Faglia E, Favales F, Calia P et al. (2002) Cardiac events in 735 type 2 diabetic patients who underwent screening for unknown asymptomatic coronary heart disease: 5-year follow-up report from the Milan Study on Atherosclerosis and Diabetes (MiSAD). Diabetes Care 25(11):2032–2036.
56. Schinkel AF, Elhendy A, van Domburg RT et al. (2002) Prognostic value of dobutamine-atropine stress myocardial perfusion imaging in patients with diabetes. Diabetes Care 25(9):1637–1643.
57. Vanzetto G, Halimi S, Hammoud T et al. (1999) Prediction of cardiovascular events in clinically selected high-risk NIDDM patients. Prognostic value of exercise stress test and thallium-201 single-photon emission computed tomography. Diabetes Care 22(1):19–26.
58. Iskander S, Iskandrian AE (1998) Risk assessment using single-photon emission computed tomographic technetium-99m sestamibi imaging. J Am Coll Cardiol 32(1):57–62.
59. Di Carli MF, Hachamovitch R (2005) Should we screen for occult coronary artery disease among asymptomatic patients with diabetes? J Am Coll Cardiol 45(1):50–53.
60. Miller DD, Shaw LJ (2005) Screening for coronary heart disease: cardiology through the oncology looking glass. J Nucl Cardiol 12(2):158–165.
61. Soman P, Udelson JE (2005) Screening the population for coronary artery disease: is it like screening for cancer? J Nucl Cardiol 12(2):145–147.
62. Mieres JH, Rosman DR, Shaw LJ (2005) The role of myocardial perfusion imaging in special populations: women, diabetics, and heart failure. Semin Nucl Med 35(1):52–61.
63. Wackers FJ, Zaret BL (2002) Detection of myocardial ischemia in patients with diabetes mellitus. Circulation 105(1):5–7.
64. American Diabetes Association (1998) Consensus development conference on the diagnosis of coronary heart disease in people with diabetes: 10–11 February 1998, Miami, Florida. Diabetes Care 21(9):1551–1559.
65. Faglia E, Manuela M, Antonella Q et al. (2005) Risk reduction of cardiac events by screening of unknown asymptomatic coronary artery disease in subjects with type 2 diabetes mellitus at high cardiovascular risk: an open-label randomized pilot study. Am Heart J 149(2):e1–e6.
66. Gerson MC, Khoury JC, Hertzberg VS, Fischer EE, Scott RC (1988) Prediction of coronary artery disease in a population of insulin-requiring diabetic patients: results of an 8-year follow-up study. Am Heart J 116(3):820–826.
67. May O, Arildsen H, Damsgaard EM, Mickley H (1997) Prevalence and prediction of silent ischaemia in diabetes mellitus: a population-based study. Cardiovasc Res 34(1):241–247.
68. Paillole C, Passa P, Paycha F et al. (1992) Non-invasive identification of severe coronary artery disease in patients with long-standing diabetes mellitus. Eur J Med 1(8):464–468.
69. Passa P, Drouin P, Issa-Sayegh M et al. (1995) Coronary disease and diabetes. Diabete Metab 21(6):446–451.
70. Rutter MK, McComb JM, Brady S, Marshall SM (1999) Silent myocardial ischemia and microalbuminuria in asymptomatic subjects with non-insulin-dependent diabetes mellitus. Am J Cardiol 83(1):27–31.
71. Grundy SM, Howard B, Smith S, Jr., Eckel R, Redberg R, Bonow RO (2002) Prevention Conference VI: Diabetes and cardiovascular disease: executive summary: conference proceeding for healthcare professionals from a special writing group of the American Heart Association. Circulation 105(18):2231–2239.
72. Grundy SM, Garber A, Goldberg R et al. (2002) Prevention Conference VI: Diabetes and cardiovascular disease: Writing group IV: lifestyle and medical management of risk factors. Circulation 105(18):e153–e158.
73. Puel J, Valensi P, Vanzetto G et al. (2004) Identification of myocardial ischemia in the diabetic patient. Joint ALFEDIAM and SFC recommendations. Diabetes Metab 30(3 Pt 3):3S3–18.
74. Monbaron D, Jeanrenaud X, Prior J et al. (2003) Effectiveness of guidelines for the screening of coronary artery disease in asymptomatic type 2 diabetic patients. Diabetes 52:A162–A162.
75. Cosson E, Attali JR, Valensi P (2005) Markers for silent myocardial ischemia in diabetes. Are they helpful? Diabetes Metab 31(2):205–213.
76. Lee KH, Jang HJ, Kim YH et al. (2003) Prognostic value of cardiac autonomic neuropathy independent and incremental to perfusion defects in patients with diabetes and suspected coronary artery disease. Am J Cardiol 92(12):1458–1461.
77. Baxter CG, Boon NA, Walker JD (2005) Detection of silent myocardial ischemia in asymptomatic diabetic subjects: the DIAD study. Diabetes Care 28(3):756–757.
78. Gazzaruso C, Giordanetti S, De Amici E et al. (2004) Relationship between erectile dysfunction and silent myocardial ischemia in apparently uncomplicated type 2 diabetic patients. Circulation 110(1):22–26.
79. Gazzaruso C, Garzaniti A, Giordanetti S, Falcone C, Fratino P (2002) Silent coronary artery disease in type 2 diabetes mellitus: the role of Lipoprotein(a), homocysteine and apo(a) polymorphism. Cardiovasc Diabetol 1(1):5.
80. Bernard S, Serusclat A, Targe F et al. (2005) Incremental predictive value of carotid ultrasonography in the assessment of coronary risk in a cohort of asymptomatic type 2 diabetic subjects. Diabetes Care 28(5):1158–1162.

81. Anand DV, Hopkins D, Lim E et al. (2004) Prediction of silent myocardial ischemia in asymptomatic type 2 diabetics without prior coronary artery disease: comparison between traditional risk factors, inflammatory markers and coronary calcium. Circulation 110(17):III-683.
82. Raggi P, Berman DS (2005) Computed tomography coronary calcium screening and myocardial perfusion imaging. J Nucl Cardiol 12(1):96–103.
83. Berman DS, Hachamovitch R, Kiat H et al. (1995) Incremental value of prognostic testing in patients with known or suspected ischemic heart disease: a basis for optimal utilization of exercise technetium-99m sestamibi myocardial perfusion single-photon emission computed tomography. J Am Coll Cardiol 26(3):639–647.
84. Anand DV, Lim E, Raval U, Lipkin D, Lahiri A (2004) Prevalence of silent myocardial ischemia in asymptomatic individuals with subclinical atherosclerosis detected by electron beam tomography. J Nucl Cardiol 11(4):450–457.
85. Perret S, Monbaron D, Haesler E et al. (2005) Coronary artery disease in type 2 diabetic patients: How to improve screening efficiency? Diabetes 54(Suppl. 1):A164.
86. Kwok Y, Kim C, Grady D, Segal M, Redberg R (1999) Meta-analysis of exercise testing to detect coronary artery disease in women. Am J Cardiol 83(5):660–666.
87. Noble GL, Navare SM, Hussain SA et al. (2004) Progression of coronary artery disease in diabetics demonstrated by single isotope rest/stress Tc-99m sestamini myocardial perfusion imaging: more rapid than non-diabetics? J Am Coll Cardiol 43:340A.
88. Nesto RW, Phillips RT, Kett KG et al. (1988) Angina and exertional myocardial ischemia in diabetic and nondiabetic patients: assessment by exercise thallium scintigraphy. Ann Internal Med 108(2):170–175.
89. Redberg RF, Greenland P, Fuster V et al. (2002) Prevention Conference VI: Diabetes and cardiovascular Disease: Writing group III: risk assessment in persons with diabetes. Circulation 105(18):e144–e152.
90. Mielke CH, Shields JP, Broemeling LD (2001) Coronary artery calcium, coronary artery disease, and diabetes. Diabetes Res Clin Pract 53(1):55–61.
91. Raggi P, Shaw LJ, Berman DS, Callister TQ (2004) Prognostic value of coronary artery calcium screening in subjects with and without diabetes. J Am Coll Cardiol 43(9):1663–1669.
92. Davies RF, Goldberg AD, Forman S et al. (1997) Asymptomatic Cardiac Ischemia Pilot (ACIP) study two-year follow-up: outcomes of patients randomized to initial strategies of medical therapy versus revascularization. Circulation 95(8):2037–2043.
93. Jonas M, Reicher-Reiss H, Boyko V et al. (1996) Usefulness of beta-blocker therapy in patients with non-insulin-dependent diabetes mellitus and coronary artery disease. Bezafibrate Infarction Prevention (BIP) Study Group. Am J Cardiol 77(15):1273–1277.
94. Heart Outcomes Prevention Evaluation Study Investigators (2000) Effects of ramipril on cardiovascular and microvascular outcomes in people with diabetes mellitus: results of the HOPE study and MICRO-HOPE substudy. Lancet 355(9200):253–259.
95. Collins R, Armitage J, Parish S, Sleigh P, Peto R (2003) MRC/BHF Heart Protection Study of cholesterol-lowering with simvastatin in 5963 people with diabetes: a randomised placebo-controlled trial. Lancet 361(9374):2005–2016.
96. Colhoun HM, Betteridge DJ, Durrington PN et al. (2004) Primary prevention of cardiovascular disease with atorvastatin in type 2 diabetes in the Collaborative Atorvastatin Diabetes Study (CARDS): multicentre randomised placebo-controlled trial. Lancet 364(9435):685–696.
97. Gaede P, Vedel P, Larsen N, Jensen GV, Parving HH, Pedersen O (2003) Multifactorial intervention and cardiovascular disease in patients with type 2 diabetes. N Engl J Med 348(5):383–393.
98. Van Belle E, Perie M, Braune D et al. (2002) Effects of coronary stenting on vessel patency and long-term clinical outcome after percutaneous coronary revascularization in diabetic patients. J Am Coll Cardiol 40(3):410–417.
99. Marso SP, Lincoff AM, Ellis SG et al. (1999) Optimizing the percutaneous interventional outcomes for patients with diabetes mellitus: results of the EPISTENT (Evaluation of platelet IIb/IIIa inhibitor for stenting trial) diabetic substudy. Circulation 100(25):2477–2484.
100. Morice MC, Serruys PW, Sousa JE et al. (2002) A randomized comparison of a sirolimus-eluting stent with a standard stent for coronary revascularization. N Engl J Med 346(23):1773–1780.
101. Mak KH, Faxon DP (2003) Clinical studies on coronary revascularization in patients with type 2 diabetes. Eur Heart J 24(12):1087–1103.
102. Flaherty JD, Davidson CJ (2005) Diabetes and coronary revascularization. J Am Med Assoc 293(12):1501–1508.
103. 103. BARI (2000) Seven-year outcome in the Bypass Angioplasty Revascularization Investigation (BARI) by treatment and diabetic status. J Am Coll Cardiol 35(5):1122–1129.
104. Hachamovitch R, Hayes SW, Friedman JD, Cohen I, Berman DS (2003) Comparison of the short-term survival benefit associated with revascularization compared with medical therapy in patients with no prior coronary artery disease undergoing stress myocardial perfusion single photon emission computed tomography. Circulation 107(23):2900–2907.
105. Sobel BE, Frye R, Detre KM (2003) Burgeoning dilemmas in the management of diabetes and cardiovascular disease: rationale for the Bypass Angioplasty Revascular-

ization Investigation 2 Diabetes (BARI 2D) Trial. Circulation 107(4):636–642.
106. Hambrecht R, Walther C, Mobius-Winkler S et al. (2004) Percutaneous coronary angioplasty compared with exercise training in patients with stable coronary artery disease: a randomized trial. Circulation 109(11):1371–1378.
107. Computed tomographic imaging within nuclear cardiology (2005) J Nucl Cardiol 12(1):131–142.
108. 108. Machac J (2005) Cardiac positron emission tomography imaging. Semin Nucl Med 35(1):17–36.
109. Nitenberg A, Chemla D, Antony I (2004) Epicardial coronary artery constriction to cold pressor test is predictive of cardiovascular events in hypertensive patients with angiographically normal coronary arteries and without other major coronary risk factor. Atherosclerosis 173(1):115–123.
110. Toussaint JF, LaMuraglia GM, Southern JF, Fuster V, Kantor HL (1996) Magnetic resonance images lipid, fibrous, calcified, hemorrhagic, and thrombotic components of human atherosclerosis in vivo. Circulation 94(5):932–938.
111. Fuster V, Kim RJ (2005) Frontiers in cardiovascular magnetic resonance. Circulation 112(1):135–144.
112. Conaway DG, O'Keefe JH, Reid KJ, Spertus J (2005) Frequency of undiagnosed diabetes mellitus in patients with acute coronary syndrome. Am J Cardiol 96(3):363–365.
113. Beaton SJ, Nag SS, Gunter MJ, Gleeson JM, Sajjan SS, Alexander CM (2004) Adequacy of glycemic, lipid, and blood pressure management for patients with diabetes in a managed care setting. Diabetes Care 27(3):694–698.
114. Skrha J, Ambos A (2005) Can the atherosclerosis prevention targets be achieved in type 2 diabetes? Diabetes Res Clin Pract 68 Suppl 1:S48–S51.
115. Wong ND, Rozanski A, Gransar H et al. (2005) Metabolic syndrome and diabetes are associated with an increased likelihood of inducible myocardial ischemia among patients with subclinical atherosclerosis. Diabetes Care 28(6):1445–1450.
116. Deluca AJ, Saulle LN, Aronow WS, Ravipati G, Weiss MB (2005) Prevalence of silent myocardial ischemia in persons with diabetes mellitus or impaired glucose tolerance and association of hemoglobin a(1c) with prevalence of silent myocardial ischemia. Am J Cardiol 95(12):1472–1474.
117. Wackers F, Chyun D, Young L et al. (2007) Resolution of asymptomatic myocardial ischaemia in patients with type 2 diabetes in the Detection of Ischaemia in Asymptomatic Diabetes (DIAD) study. Diabetes Care 30:2892–2898.

Chapter 28

Artefacts and Pitfalls in Myocardial Perfusion Imaging

Iulia Heinle and Qaisar H. Siraj

Contents

28.1	Introduction	325
28.2	Errors	325
28.3	Before the Patient Arrives – Equipment	326
28.4	The Gamma Camera	326
28.4.1	Uniformity	326
28.4.2	Resolution/Linearity	326
28.4.3	Collimators	326
28.4.4	Centre of Rotation (COR)	326
28.5	Setting up the Acquisition	327
28.5.1	Selection of the Right Type of Orbit	327
28.6	Radiopharmaceutical-Related Artefacts and Pitfalls	327
28.6.1	Tc-99m-labelled Agents	328
28.7	Patient Preparation and Stressing	328
28.8	Radiopharmaceutical Administration	328
28.9	Artefacts Related to Image Timing	329
28.9.1	Tl-201	329
28.9.2	Tc-99m Agents	329
28.9.3	Optimal Imaging Timing	329
28.10	SPECT Image Reconstruction	329
28.10.1	Patient Movement	331
28.10.2	Reconstruction and Filtering	332
28.10.3	Artefacts in Image Orientation and Display	332
28.11	Patient-Related Artefacts	332
28.11.1	Artefacts Caused by Attenuation	332
28.11.2	Breast Attenuation	332
28.11.3	Diaphragmatic Attenuation	334
28.12	Methods to Overcome Attenuation	335
28.12.1	Attenuation Correction	335
28.12.2	Gating SPECT	337
28.13	Left Bundle-Branch Block	337
28.14	Normal Variants Seen on Images	338
28.14.1	Short Septum	338
28.14.2	Papillary Muscles	339
28.14.3	Apical Thinning	339
28.14.4	Alterations of Cardiac Position within the Thorax	339
28.14.5	The 11/7 O'Clock Defect	340
28.15	Changes due to Pathology	340
28.15.1	Hypertrophic Cardiomyopathy	340
28.15.2	Dilated Cardiomyopathy	340
28.15.3	Bland–White–Garland Syndrome	341
28.15.4	Valvular Disease	341
28.15.5	"Balanced" Ischaemia	341
28.16	Conclusions	341
	References	342

28.1 Introduction

Myocardial perfusion imaging (MPI) is a powerful tool in the diagnosis and prognosis of coronary artery disease. Radionuclide cardiac perfusion imaging entails a succession of stages, procedures and operations. The procedure involves a multidisciplinary group of operators and several processes from patient preparation to image interpretation. Any of the stages of the procedure is prone to error. It is therefore important to prospectively identify such errors, minimise their occurrence and take necessary action required to ensure that the effect of these fallibilities on the test result is mitigated.

28.2 Errors

An error in data can occur for a number of reasons. This may be due to technical fault, human error or factors that cannot easily be controlled, such as a patient's weight/body mass index (BMI). Therefore, the prime importance of identifying an error is to reduce its effect. However, a consistent error in: (a) equipment, (b) preparation, (c) reconstruction, and (d) reading or reporting a study must be addressed and corrected. The mechanisms that allow this to happen include the use of robust quality control steps and a clinical audit. Essential to acquiring competency in cardiac image interpretation is the ability of recognising and identifying errors. The knowledge is crucial in minimising, rectifying and correcting. Therefore, it is important to understand the process involved in MPI and the steps within that process where errors, artefacts or pitfalls can be generated and corrected.

28.3 Before the Patient Arrives – Equipment

Before the patient is seen within the department a series of steps need to be taken to ensure the study is obtained with optimal quality. This includes quality assurance of the imaging device PET camera and the preparation and storage of the radiopharmaceutical.

28.4 The Gamma Camera

To ensure good quality images it is important that steps are taken on a regular basis to ensure the gamma camera is performing optimally. Some tests are done on a monthly or weekly basis, but some, such as uniformity, are performed early on the day of the study. If the camera fails this daily test and cannot be corrected, the patient should not be imaged and the test should be cancelled. In many countries regular camera quality control and recording of results is a legal requirement.

28.4.1 Uniformity

Uniformity is a sensitive indicator of a gamma camera system. It is much more important for SPECT than for planar imaging, because of the greater potential to induce artefacts. In general, the non-uniformity should be kept lower than 3% for SPECT [1]. The most common physical causes of non-uniformity are (a) malfunction of one or more of the photomultiplier tubes (PMT) or a crack in the sodium iodide crystal, due to thermal or mechanical factors or to hydration of the crystal by the presence of a cold defect with excess counts at the edge of the defect (Fig. 28.1). Uniformity is normally tested by a Co-57 flood source at the beginning of each day with the appropriate collimators, which will be used for cardiac imaging. Normally the programmes for the daily uniformity flood are automated but at least 5 million counts are needed with a central field of view (CFOV) uniformity of 3% or less (this actually measures the variation, not uniformity, so no area of the central camera face should differ in count rate by more than 3% of the mean). In addition, on a regular basis, normally monthly or after each service the intrinsic uniformity (performed without collimators) from a Tc-99m point source is performed and this is used to provide a uniformity map to correct data for SPECT. In cameras with more than one head, the tests must be done for each head [2].

28.4.2 Resolution/Linearity

This should be tested using a specially designed linear phantom and flood source on a monthly basis. The main error affecting image resolution is spatial distortion, which is apparent as non-uniformities in the flood image. Modern gamma cameras have correction maps incorporated and loss or corruption of the linearity correction map is evident as a significant deterioration in image uniformity and spatial linearity, although system resolution is largely unaffected. Updating the correction map usually rectifies this problem.

28.4.3 Collimators

In general, a low energy general-purpose collimator (LEGP) should be used for ^{201}Tl studies and low energy high-resolution (LEHR) collimation for ^{99m}Tc tracers although many systems now have a hybrid low energy collimator. These collimators are often made of thin lead foil and physical damage will lead to defects on the scan and will be seen on the daily flood. If collimator damage is suspected, if possible, the collimator should be turned 180°, the uniformity re-measured and the defect will move with the collimator. Unfortunately, repair is difficult and replacement of the collimators will be required.

28.4.4 Centre of Rotation (COR)

The correct centring of data reconstruction is essential for an accurate reproduction of anatomical structures

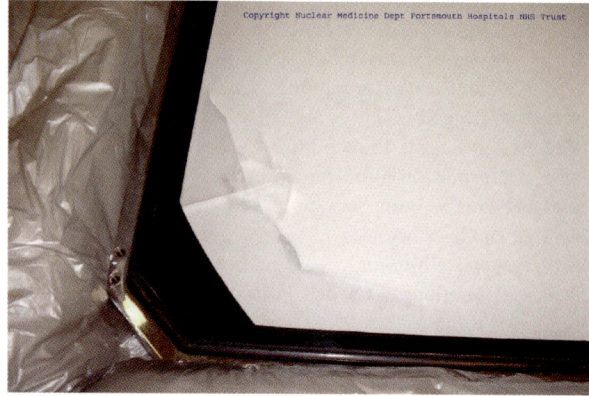

Fig. 28.1 Cracked collimator

and count density distribution [1, 2]. Errors in COR of less than 0.5 pixels (normally about 4 mm) are generally acceptable, but higher values can lead to degradation in image quality and produce possible artefacts [3]. An error in COR often results in image mis-registration of the tomographic data, image blurring and apparent misalignment of the anterior and posterior myocardial walls, with the appearance of an apical defect in the myocardium. This can be worse in multi-head gamma cameras where not only must each head have an accurate COR but also they must all coincide. Testing normally involves rotating the camera in a SPECT acquisition around a linear source (normally a capillary tube filled with Tc-99 m) in the centre of the radius of rotation. This must be done on a regular basis as per the departmental protocol.

28.5
Setting up the Acquisition

It is important that the acquisition is set up in an optimal way, and this includes choice of collimators, photopeak, acquisition matrix and imaging time. The heart should lie as close to the centre of the camera as possible as uniformity there is better than at the edge (Fig. 28.2).

28.5.1
Selection of the Right Type of Orbit

The detector is at variable distances from the heart while orbiting around the patient. Therefore it is essential to select that type of orbit that allows the detector to move as close to the heart as possible, at all angles. The SPECT orbits may be classified as (a) circular, where the detector is at a fixed distance from the COR at all angles, which leads to reduced spatial resolution at all angular projections, and (b) noncircular (elliptical and eccentric), where the detector come closer to the heart in some views, for which the spatial resolution is improved. The variability in spatial resolution is, however, a potential source of artefacts.

A correct photopeak is essential in improving image quality [4]. The peak photopeak is defined by the radionuclide for Tc-99m this is 140 keV. The wider the window the more counts are obtained but the more the scattered photons will be allowed through, reducing image quality; thus, a 10–15% window is a good compromise. However, as scattered photons lose energy they are less energetic than the photopeak, so offsetting the peak by 5% can reduce the number of scattered photons while optimizing the count.

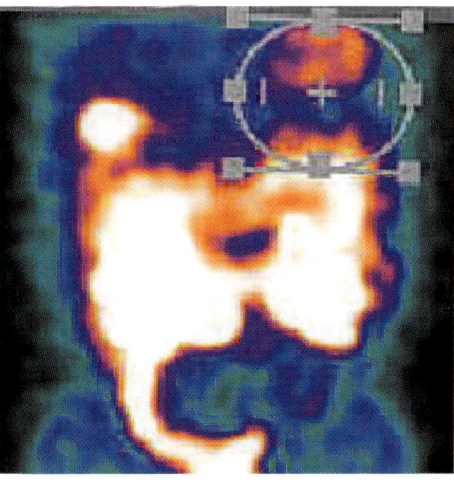

Fig. 28.2 Patient imaged with the heart too close to the top of the gamma camera where uniformity is less. The patient should be re-positioned and re-imaged

Tl-201 offers particular problems in that the 169 keV photopeak is easy to deal with but most counts come from X-rays produced by the energetic Hg-201 daughter of the Tl-201. These have various energies but a window of 70–90 keV catches most of these but will also contain a lot of scattered photons thus reducing the image quality.

28.6
Radiopharmaceutical-Related Artefacts and Pitfalls

Incorrect radiopharmaceutical preparation, handling and storage can induce artefacts in myocardial perfusion imaging (Table 28.1). The preparation of radiopharmaceuticals and their quality assurance is based on international and national legislation. However, a labelling efficiency of at least 95% should be obtained. All radiopharmaceuticals must be prepared in sterile conditions with sufficient shielding to reduce the radiation dose to the person preparing the doses. The dose of the radiopharmaceutical should be appropriately titrated for the individual patient so as to ensure reasonable counting statistics, essential for good imaging. For example, in Europe 5 years ago a total of 1000 MBq for both stress and rest imaging with Tc-99m agents was thought sufficient but now 2000 MBq is thought to be required [5].

Table 28.1 Common causes of artefacts and pitfalls

Radiopharmaceutical preparation, handling and storage
Selection of radiopharmaceutical and dosage
Radiopharmaceutical administration
Artefacts related to the use of multiple radionuclides
Artefacts related to study timing
Common artefacts related to physiological clearance of radioactivity • liver, gallbladder and bowel activity • lung activity • bone marrow activity

28.6.1
Tc-99m-labelled Agents

In general, the presence of free pertechnetate causes increased activity in the stomach, intestinal tract, thyroid and salivary glands. The "age" of Tc-99m eluates can influence the labelling efficiency of Tc99m-sestamibi or Tc-99m tetrofosmin (it is decreased with eluates older than 6–12 hours). Loading the vial with too much Tc-99m pertechnetate results in poor labelling efficiency, as there is only a limited quantity of stannous available for reducing the pertechnetate. In addition Tc-99m MIBI must be heated/boiled at 90°C for 20 minutes and this limits the level of free pertechnetate.

28.7
Patient Preparation and Stressing

Patient preparation is important to ensure optimal imaging, the most common problem being inadequate stress. Patients taking beta blockers will not be able to achieve maximal predicted heart rate with physical stress or dobutamine. Beta-blockade should be stopped for 48 hours prior to the test. If adenosine is used, caffeine-containing substances must be stopped 24 hours prior to the stress. Caffeine is not only present in tea and coffee but in a range of carbonated drinks and over-the-counter drugs. Therefore, these caffeine-containing drinks or drugs should not be taken in the 24 hours prior to the stress. Figure 28.3 shows an example of such an error.

A 2–6 hour fast is advisable for patients to reduce symptoms of nausea and vomiting during stress and this may have to be modified for diabetic patients.

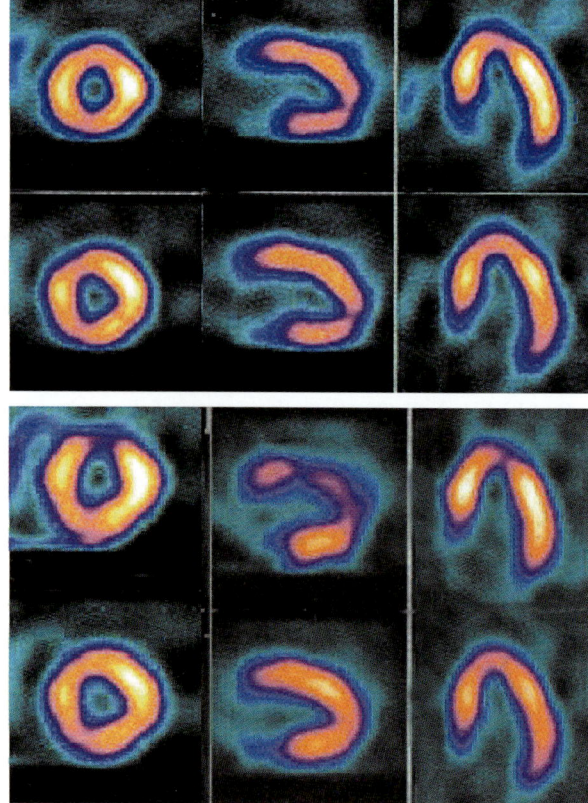

Fig. 28.3 The effect of caffeine. a Negative scan after Dipyridamole stress in a patient who had a cup of tea 4 hours prior to the scan, with repeat study. b Positive scan for LAD ischaemia. Short axis, vertical long axis and horizontal axis stress images at stress (top row) and rest (bottom row)

For the resting scan, these precautions are not required. To ensure correct stressing without compromising patient safety it is important to ensure that the level of stress is sufficient [6]. With adenosine if the patient has not taken caffeine or similar drugs a sufficient stress will be performed with a 4–6 minute infusion and requires minimal patient co-operation. With physical stress the maximal predicted heart rate should be achieved before the tracer is given. Atropine can be given to assist with this, especially with dobutamine which in some patients has a greater inotropic than chronotropic effect.

28.8
Radiopharmaceutical Administration

During stress, the radiotracer is injected at peak exercise, preferably through an intravenous cannula, in an antecubital vein. It is a sensible practice to flush the cannula afterwards with 10–20 mL of saline solution to ensure that the whole dose of radiotracer has been administered. Administration of radiotracers through central and peripheral intravenous lines, tubes and catheters may result in residual radioactivity within the plastic tubing or reservoir because of insufficient saline flushing or adherence to plastic of some radiopharmaceutical products.

Images with very poor count statistics are obtained if the radiotracer is injected extravascularly or when the activity remains in the intravenous line. Inadequate radioactivity administered for the patient weight can also result in poor count statistics.

28.9
Artefacts Related to Image Timing

28.9.1
Tl-201

These tend to be exaggerated post-stress as the patient tends to be in a recovery phase, and depend on the radiopharmaceutical used and the type of stress. With Tl-201, early imaging should be done to reduce the chance of early redistribution and failure to identify ischaemic segments. Therefore, optimally imaging should start by 5 minutes post-stress and no later than 15 minutes. However if the patient had strenuous activity before imaging they will still be in a recovery phase using diaphragmatic breathing. This will result in the heart being pushed up further in inspiration. As the breathing quietens the diaphragmatic movement is reduced and the heart appears to drop in the chest; this process is called creep. It is difficult to predict as patients respond to stress differently but is often dealt with by motion correction software.

28.9.2
Tc-99m Agents

The issues with Tc-99m MIBI and tetrofosmin are different and due to superimposition of visceral activity such as liver, gallbladder and bowel activity over the myocardial walls (Figs. 28.4 and 28.5).

The concentration of ^{99m}Tc-labelled agents in the abdominal viscera is greater than ^{201}Tl. ^{99m}Tc-sestamibi is excreted primarily through the hepatobiliary system, therefore the liver, gallbladder, small bowel and colon are sequentially visualized in these scans, and more often in resting than in stress, since there is no "shunting" of the tracer to the myocardial and skeletal muscles, as happens after exercise. A greater liver uptake of ^{99m}Tc-sestamibi has been observed in pharmacological studies with adenosine/dipyridamole compared with the treadmill test [7]. Some studies showed that ^{99m}Tc-tetrofosmin has a lower hepatic activity and faster clearance than ^{99m}Tc-sestamibi, thus decreasing the potential for artefacts due to superimposed abdominal activity.

Occasionally, the transverse colon has a relatively higher position and its splenic flexure can be adjacent to the inferior and infero-lateral walls of the left ventricle, resulting in artefacts. Duodeno-gastric and enterogastric reflux of ^{99m}Tc-tetrofosmin have been shown to interfere with SPECT processes and result in artefacts of the inferior wall of the left ventricle. This may be seen more commonly in a one-day protocol on the second scan of the imaging day.

Superimposed bowel or liver activity may create artefacts, which makes the interpretation of the study difficult and often ends up as equivocal scans. The common scenarios encountered in day to day practice are (a) underestimating the true defects in the inferior wall, due to the overlapped high activity, (b) over-estimating true defects in the inferior wall, due to over-subtraction of counts during the image processing and (c) misinterpretation of the perfusion in the adjacent or contralateral segments, which appears to have a paucity of counts. These problems are less evident with iterative reconstruction algorithms. To minimize the visceral activity several methods have been advocated, but still the problem persists.

The value of administering a fatty meal between the injection of tracer and imaging is debated but most centres find it useful and recommend a meal such as a cheese sandwich or chocolate, although again this may pose problems for diabetics.

28.9.3
Optimal Imaging Timing

For Tl-201 optimal imaging is at 5 minutes post-injection and for Tc-99m tetrofosmin 45 minutes and for Tc-99m MIBI 60 minutes post-injection of tracer.

28.10
SPECT Image Reconstruction

The image reconstruction is probably the area where most errors can occur. SPECT reconstruction is influenced by a number of factors including previously discussed aspects such as camera uniformity, reconstruction technique, and display.

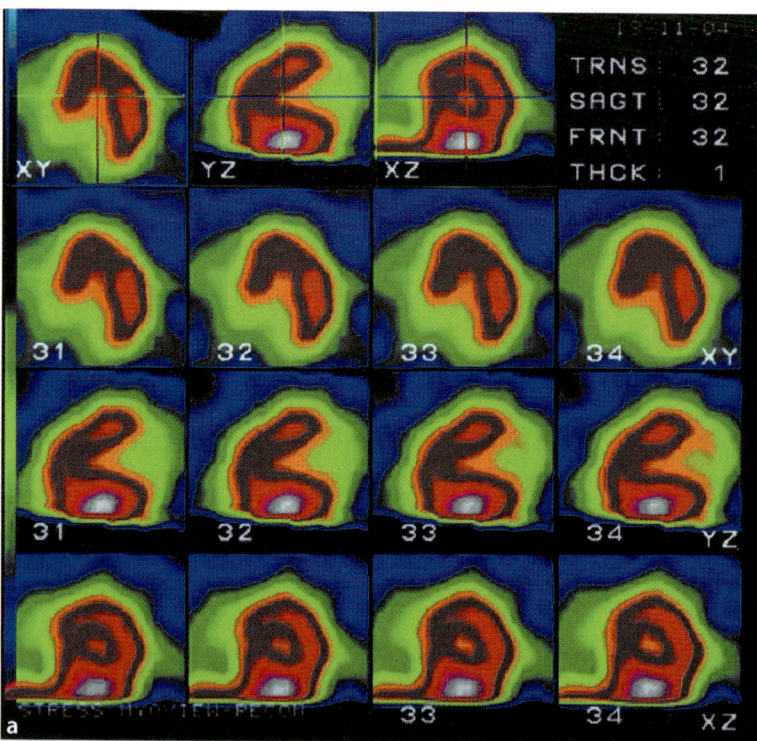
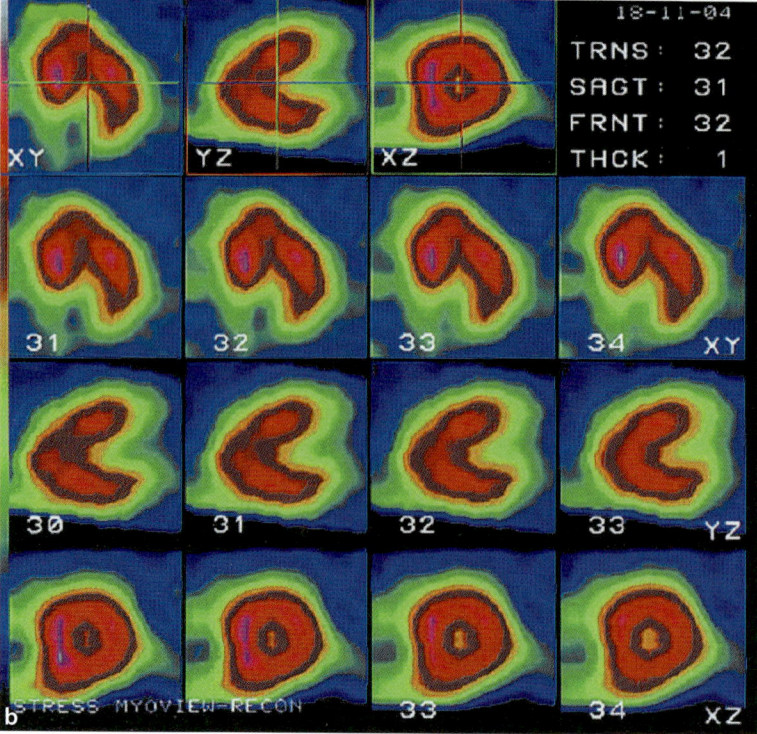

Fig. 28.4a,b a Suboptimal stress study 60 minutes post-injection, due to adjacent gut activity. b Study was repeated 3 hours post-injection and after a large meal was ingested. Normal tracer distribution is seen, with no evidence of reversible ischaemia

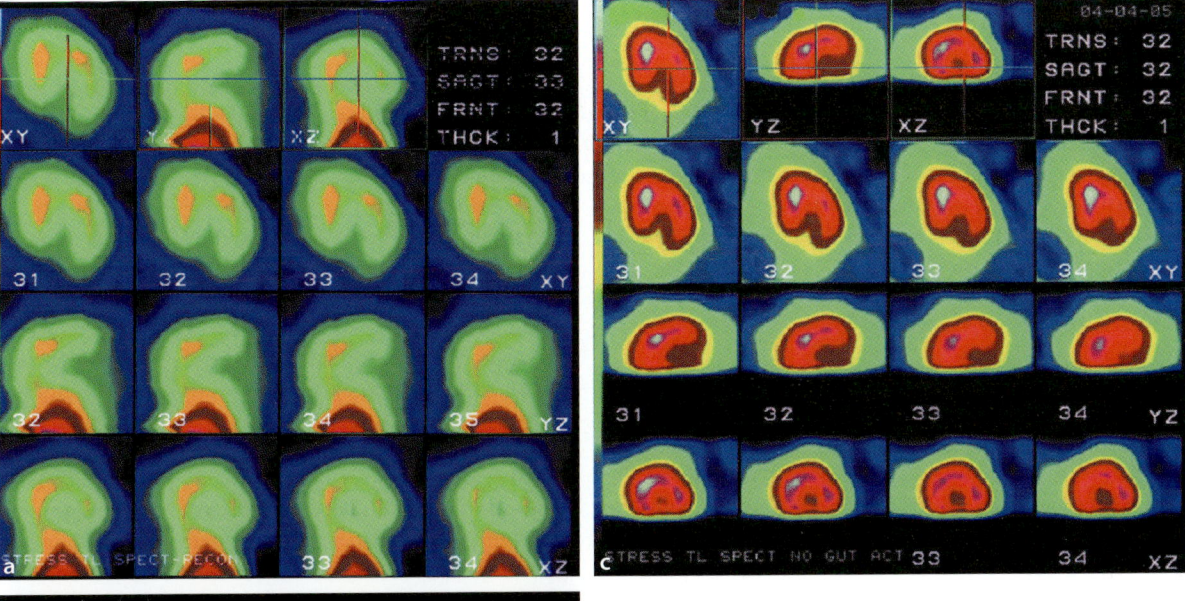

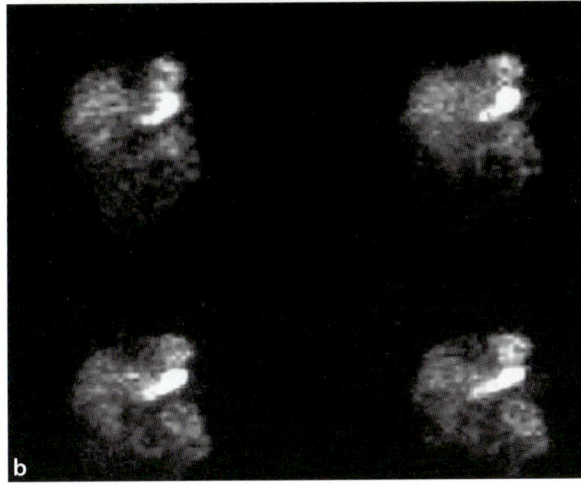

Fig. 28.5a–c Difficult study to interpret due to superimposition of extracardiac activity over the inferior wall, with poor visualization of LV walls on stress: a stress study with ^{201}Tl showing significant gut activity; b review of the raw data; c delayed redistribution scan shows clearance of the extracardiac activity

28.10.1
Patient Movement

While it is possible to reduce movement as much as possible, movement does occur and most gamma camera computers have software to correct for this. Most commonly movement is in the plane across the camera head and the patient slips down during imaging or cardiac creep occurs [8]. Early movement correction software normally corrected only in one plane but modern methods correct movement in all three planes. If possible movement should be restricted to 2 pixels (8 mm) in any direction. Failure to so will result in an image where the septum appears to overshoot the lateral wall and inferior wall counts will not be seen, giving a false positive defect in the scan. Movement can be verified by visual inspection of the raw data normally in "cine" mode looking for movement of the heart in any direction. This can also be seen using the sonogram display where a step in the sonogram detects movement. If correction is unavailable or not possible, great care must be taken in reporting, as any defect may be artefactual.

28.10.2
Reconstruction and Filtering

Most systems now use iterative reconstruction, which can be less affected by high levels of gut activity than back-projection. Although iterative reconstruction can still result in apparent myocardial perfusion defects due to "count stealing" from adjacent tissues – for example, intense stomach uptake can result in an apparent defect in the infero-lateral wall.

Often the best thing to do is to get the patient to eat some food and re-image them 1 hour later when gut activity has cleared away.

Most modern gamma camera systems use automated count-optimized reconstruction filters; if the field of view contains high levels of activity in the GI tract the computer uses this for reconstruction, leading to an over-filtered cardiac image, which will appear to have defects that are artefactual. This can be checked by inspecting the raw data. If there are high activities in the gut and a filtering problem is considered likely the study can be re-reconstructed using a tighter region of interest to try to exclude the GI tract activity, masking out the gut activity or using a different filter.

28.10.3
Artefacts in Image Orientation and Display

It is important to check the size, intensity, formatting and orientation of the images. Alignment is very important for SPECT imaging, particularly when comparing image sets obtained under different physiological conditions (stress and rest, stress and redistribution/reinjection images).

Each series of images (short-axis, vertical and horizontal long axes) must be normalized to the brightest pixel in the entire series. The colour scale is used to provide semiquantitative information about the count distribution throughout the myocardium.

28.11
Patient-Related Artefacts

Even with the best techniques patients come in all sizes and shapes and sometimes the patient themselves will introduce errors. These can often be predicted and taken into account during imaging the most common of these is the problem of attenuation.

28.11.1
Artefacts Caused by Attenuation

Attenuation is by far the most common cause of artefacts in myocardial perfusion imaging.

Photon attenuation in planar imaging can be caused by external non-anatomical structures or internal structures. External non-anatomical structures, such as clothes, jewellery, coins in the pockets or other metallic objects, pens, etc., may be potential sources of error when overlying the heart area. Breast implants may be denser than normal breasts and can also result in artefactual appearances. Intrathoracic structures, such as cardiac pacemakers, previously ingested radiographic contrast material, prosthetic joints, other orthopaedic internal fixation devices, shunt reservoirs, tubing within the thorax, etc. can also cause attenuation. Although pacemakers are implanted above and below the diaphragm, it is not common for a pacemaker to create difficulties in image interpretation. The most common attenuation artefacts in SPECT are caused by breast and diaphragm.

28.11.2
Breast Attenuation

The severity and extent of attenuation caused by breast depend on several factors, such as the size, density, shape and position of the left breast relative to the myocardium, as well as on the chest circumference [9] (Fig. 28.6). The position of the left breast overlying the heart may lead to apparent anterior, apical, anteroseptal or, less commonly, lateral perfusion abnormalities, especially seen in elderly women with pendulous breasts.

It is important to maintain the same position of the breast relative to the left myocardium during the stress and rest acquisitions. This position is dependent on several factors. The position of the patient on the SPECT imaging table is important. It is advisable to acquire the images with the left arm of the patient raised above the head, and this position should be identical for both stress and rest acquisitions [7]. If the position of the breast relative to the left ventricle is the same during the stress and rest acquisition, the attenuation artefact may appear as a fixed defect; conversely, a change in breast position can mimic a reversible defect. Removal of a women's bra may assist as a bra can result in an increase of soft tissue attenuation, by thickening the breast. Those with external breast prosthesis should remove these. The role of prone imaging to crush the breast under the thorax and thus flatten the breast tissue remains unproven [10].

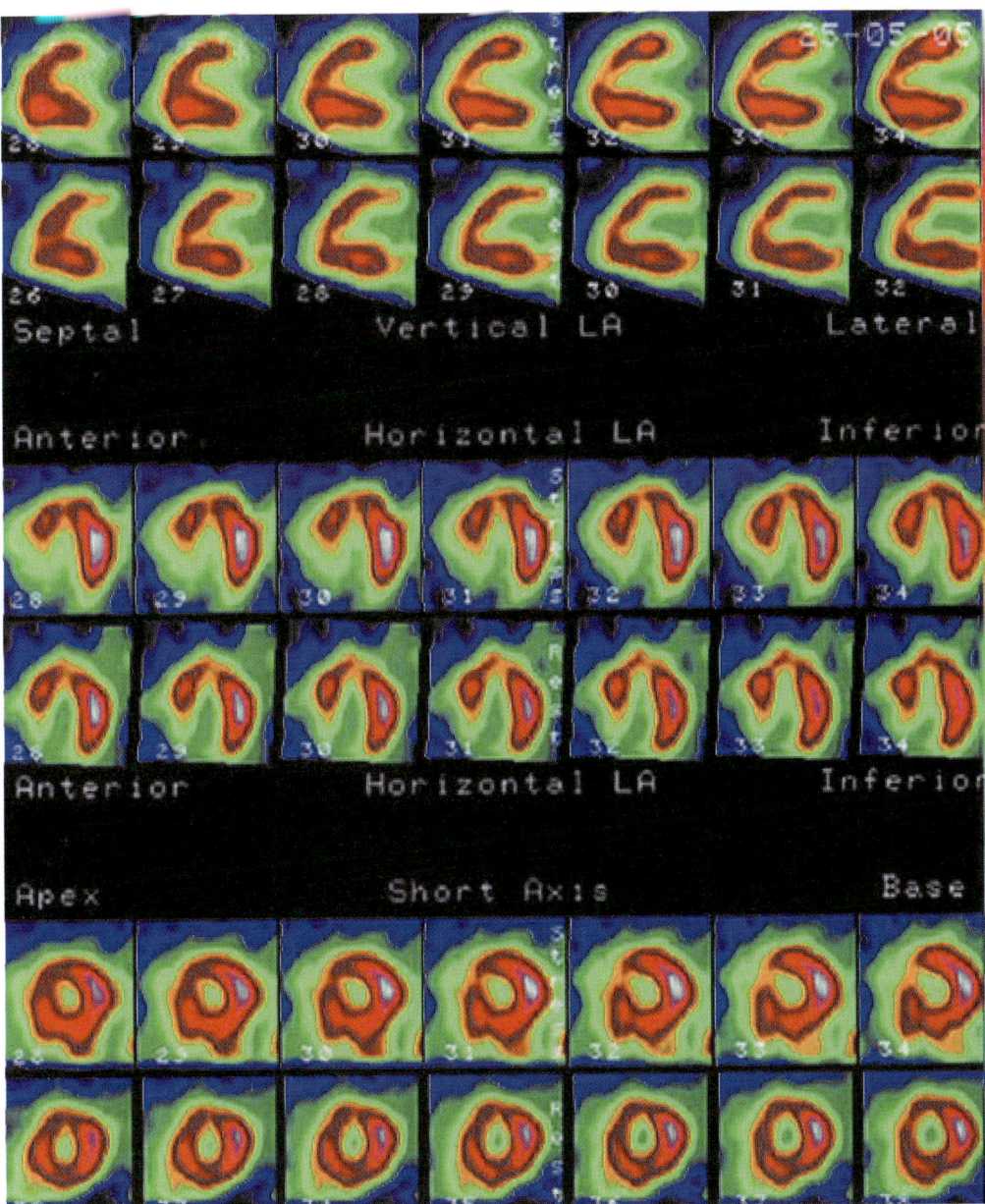

Fig. 28.6 Tomographic images showing reduced uptake in the anterior wall due to breast attenuation

28.11.3
Diaphragmatic Attenuation

While breast attenuation is considered an issue in women; in men the most common form of attenuation is from the left diaphragm which typically affects the inferior wall and has been reported to occur in approximately 25% of patients undergoing myocardial perfusion imaging in the supine position (Figs. 28.7–28.10) [11]. Left hemidiaphragmatic elevation can result in accentuated attenuation and inferior myocardial perfusion artefacts. The most common causes of diaphragmatic elevation include a muscular diaphragm, obesity, pulmonary parenchymal disease, pleural disease, atelectesis, diaphragmatic paralysis after thoracic surgery (i.e. after coronary by-pass surgery), gastric dilation and ascites (due to liver disease or peritoneal dialysis) [7].

The attenuation artefacts caused by diaphragmatic elevation are usually seen as fixed defects on stress and rest images and could be misread as an inferior infarction

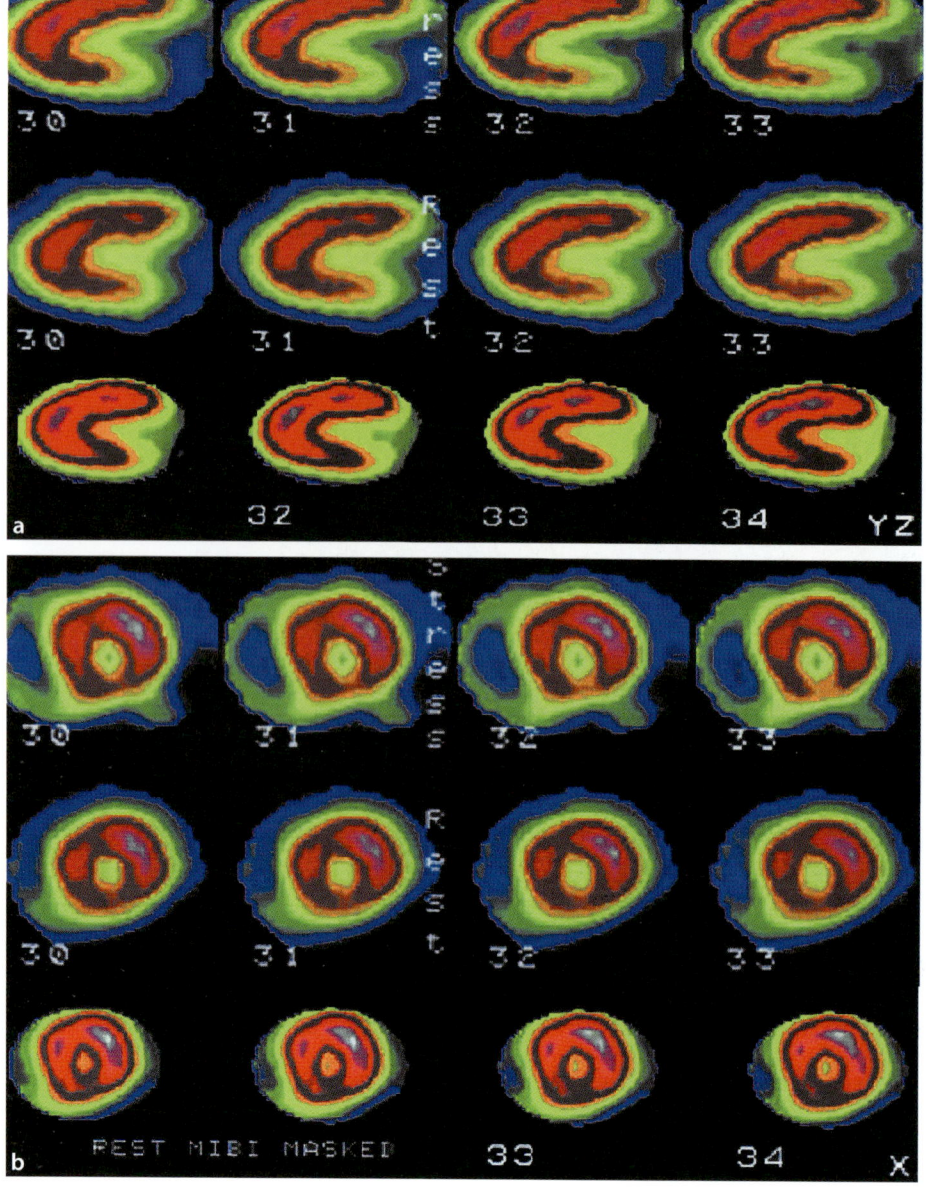

Fig. 28.7 **a** Vertical long axis images; **b** short axis images. First row = stress scan; second row = rest scan; third row = prone. There is symmetrical reduction in uptake in the inferior wall on the stress and the rest scan, with normal uptake in the inferior wall on prone images, confirming diaphragmatic attenuation only

28.12 Methods to Overcome Attenuation

28.12.1 Attenuation Correction

Both the pre-reconstruction method developed by Sorensen and the post-reconstruction Chang method assume uniform body attenuation. However, attenuation within the body is not uniform, therefore accurate attenuation correction requires a precise estimate of the patient specific attenuation distribution. Attenuation maps are generated by sequential or simultaneous acquisition of emission and transmission images, the latter being used for the attenuation correction of the SPECT data [12]. Many of these new techniques for the generation of the attenuation maps do not currently account for scatter in the emission data and may cause an overcorrection of counts in part of the myocardium.

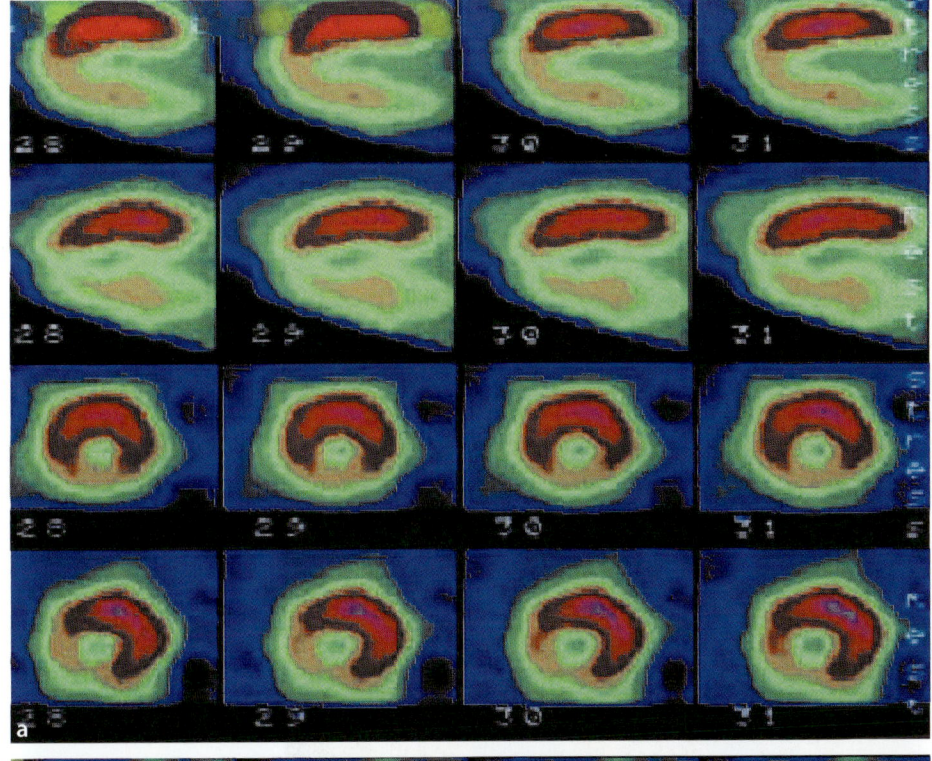

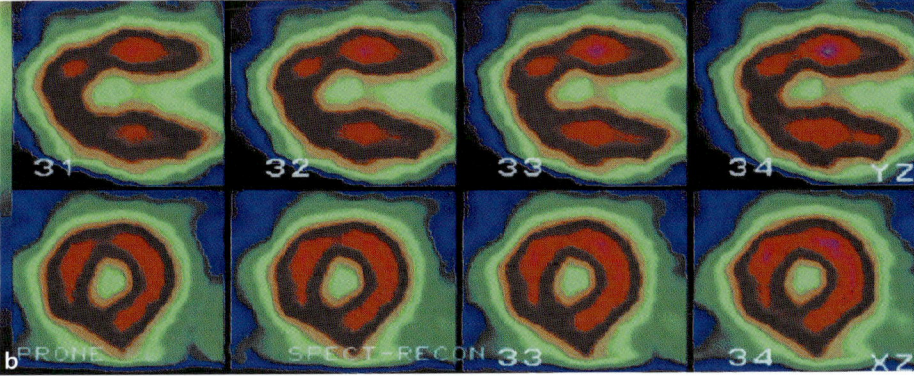

Fig. 28.8 **a** Symmetrical loss of uptake in the inferior wall on stress and rest images. **b** By imaging the patient in the prone posture after stress there was completely normal uptake in the inferior wall. This finding was consistent with diaphragmatic attenuation

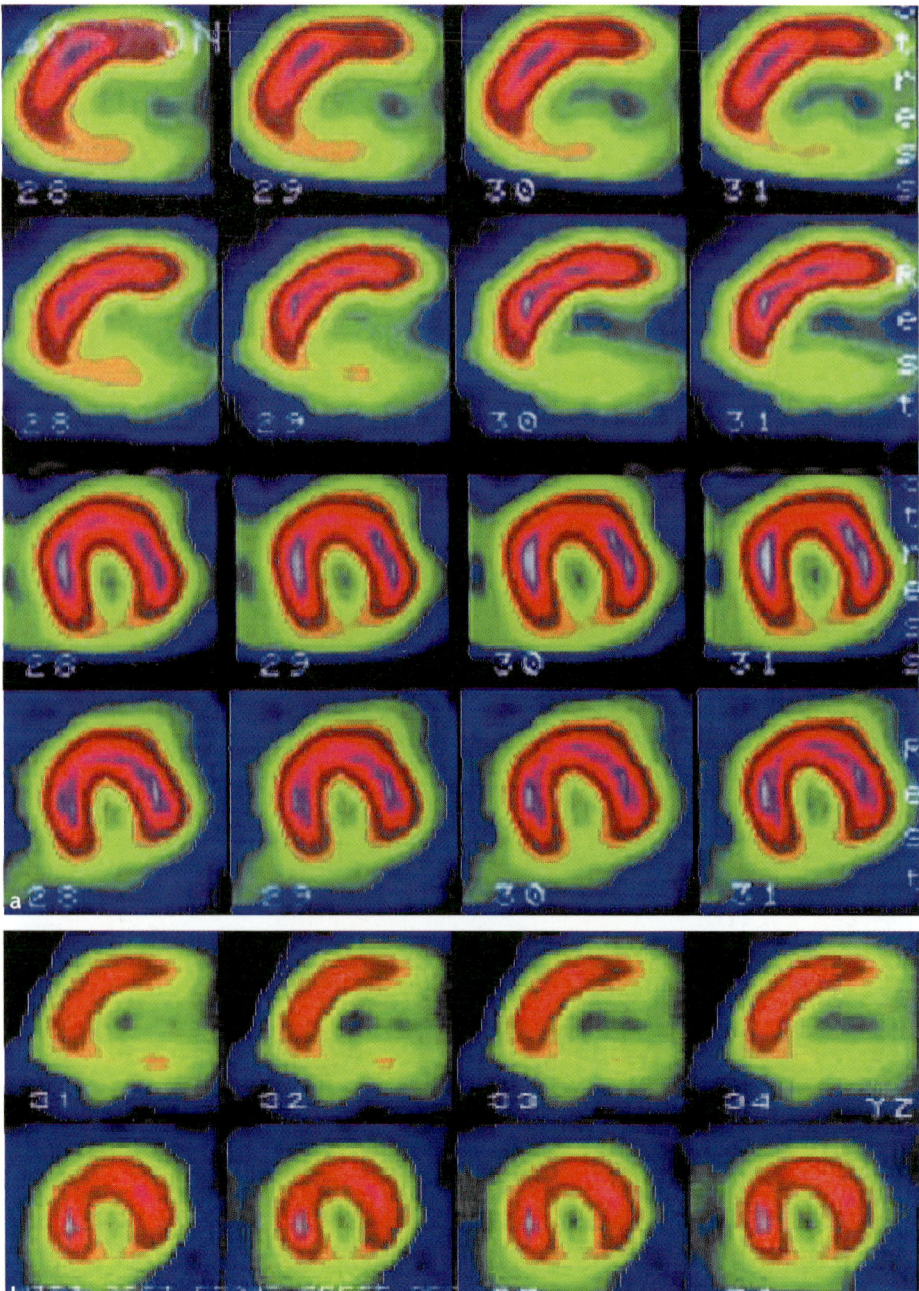

Fig. 28.9 a Symmetrical loss of uptake in the inferior wall on stress and rest images, with **b** no improvement on prone scan images, consistent with inferior myocardial infarction

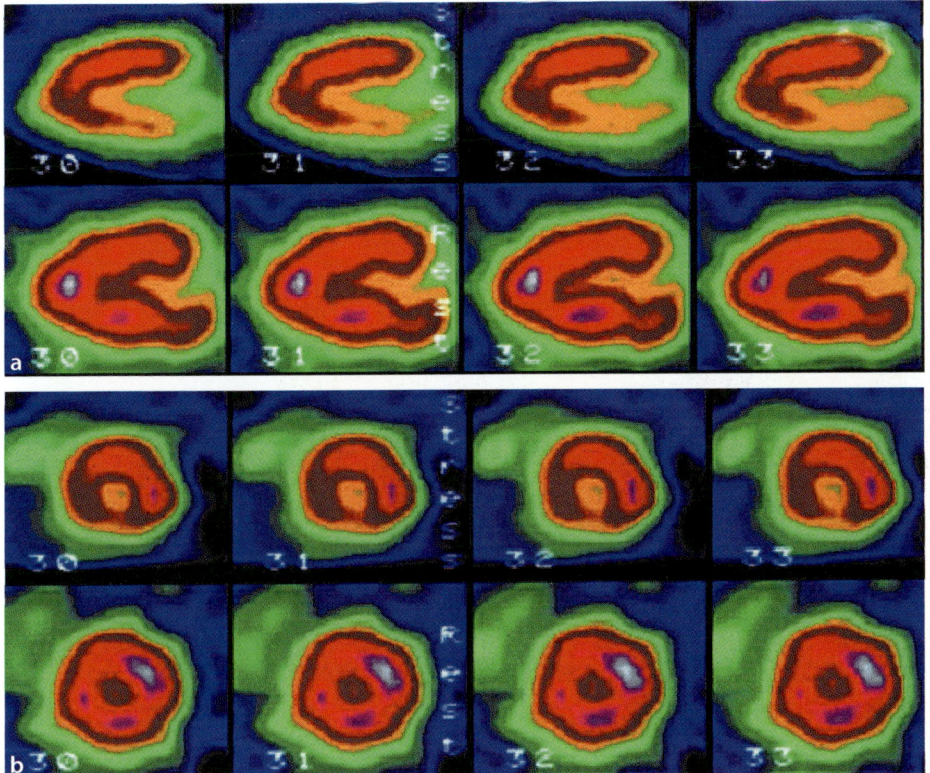

Fig. 28.10 a Vertical long axis images; b short axis images. First row of images represents stress supine, the second stress prone. Stress scan shows inferior wall perfusion defect with normal uptake seen here on prone images, highly suggestive of artefactual diaphragmatic attenuation

Recently, transmission source attenuation correction systems have been developed for SPECT imaging, similar to the systems used in PET. An ideal transmission source for cardiac perfusion SPECT imaging requires that the source should be relatively inexpensive and commercially available, has a long half-life for practical clinical use and has favourable spectral properties for gamma camera imaging. The transmission image is usually obtained using different photon energy compared with the emission image in simultaneous acquisition, the attenuation map must correspond to the photopeak emission energy [9]. ^{153}Gd is a popular choice for transmission imaging, due to its physical characteristics: long half-life (242 days) and energy of 100 keV, which is between ^{201}Tl and ^{99m}Tc photopeak energies. More recently SPECT-CT imaging devices using a CT density map for attenuation correction have been advocated but not yet fully verified.

28.12.2
Gating SPECT

ECG gating is a routine method used in many centres to distinguish between true perfusion defects and artefacts and has an additional role in providing information on left ventricular function. Based on gated SPECT imaging, a fixed perfusion defect with normal myocardial contractility and wall thickening can be characterized as attenuation artefact, whereas a myocardial infarction, if it is transmural and extensive, will demonstrate hypokinesia and decreased wall thickening. However, some caution is essential, since small subendocardial myocardial infarction might be associated with normal contractility and not exhibiting wall thickening abnormalities and therefore the defect can be falsely attributed to soft tissue attenuation. At the same time, hibernating myocardium (which is viable myocardium) might not be able to have normal contractility function [7].

28.13
Left Bundle-Branch Block

Several investigators have reported "false positive" myocardial perfusion images in patients with LBBB (left bundle-branch block), who undergo exercise or dobutamine stress testing [13, 14]. In such patients, the heart rate is significantly increased with exercise and the diastolic perfusion time is decreased, which results in a decreased radiotracer extraction by the interventricular septum relative to the lateral wall. Stress images can therefore show septal or anteroseptal defects that are reversible, mimicking an exercise-induced ischaemia (Fig. 28.11). Gating the studies is helpful in differentiating a true defect from a false positive finding, since the septal wall will usually exhibit paradoxical motion but with preserved thickening in the absence of ischaemic injury. In patients with LBBB without significant coronary artery disease, it has also been observed that the perfusion defects spare the apex.

28.14
Normal Variants Seen on Images

Although the study may be technically perfect or any errors corrected, there is a series of normal variants in cardiac anatomy and physiology. For the inexperienced this may offer some puzzling variants in imaging (Table 28.2). Most of these will be identical on both stress and rest and it is recommended that they are reported on and a statement made that they represent a normal variant.

28.14.1
Short Septum

This is particularly common in women where the basal septum wall is fibrous and will not allow uptake of the radiopharmaceutical, a rarer variant is the short inferior wall (Fig. 28.12).

Table 28.2 Normal variants

Short septum
Papillary muscles
Apical thinning
Alterations of cardiac position within the thorax
The 11/7 o'clock defect

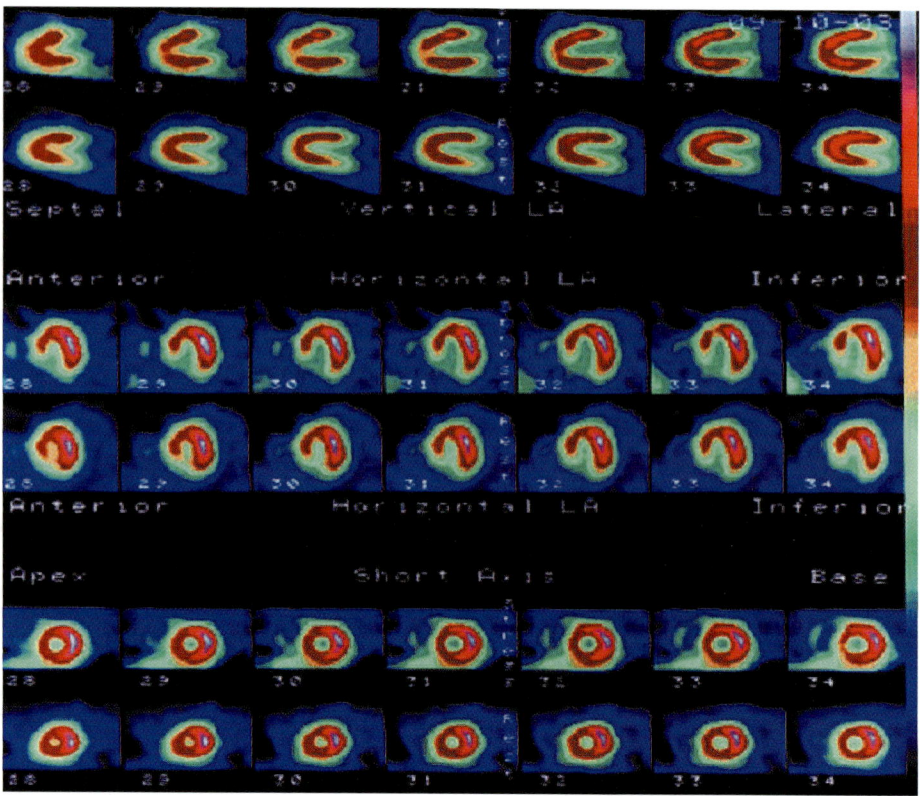

Fig. 28.11 Patient with LBBB post successful ablation for type A WPW syndrome, presenting with some chest discomfort and occasional palpitations. Scan shows mild reduction of uptake in the interventricular septum with essentially same appearance on rest scan images, due to the shortened duration of the diastolic coronary flow caused by delayed relaxation at increased heart rate

28.14.2 Papillary Muscles

The uptake of the tracer is increased in the prominent or hypertrophic papillary muscles, giving the appearance of localized "hot spots" in the anterolateral and posterolateral walls (typically seen at the "2 and 7 o'clock" positions on short axis images) and of perfusion defects in the adjacent areas, particularly in the inferior wall.

28.14.3 Apical Thinning

This can be either a normal variant – the apical myocardium is thinner and the count rate is reduced compared with other myocardial segments – or an artefact produced by varying spatial resolution of the acquired images (higher at the apex because of detector proximity) and some partial volume effect. It usually simulates a fixed defect. However, gating the images is very helpful in differentiating it from an apical scar as scar tissue is hypokinetic or even dyskinetic

28.14.4 Alterations of Cardiac Position within the Thorax

Dextro- and levorotation of the heart within the thorax result in alterations of the position of left ventricular myocardial walls relative to the detector (Fig. 28.13). In patients with dextrorotation of the heart, the anterior and septal walls lie closer to the detector, while the lateral walls lie further from it, thus resulting in an apparent relative increase in count density in septal and anterior walls and a decrease in lateral wall. In contrast, patients with cardiac levorotation have lateral myocardial walls closer to the detector and interventricular septum further from it, resulting in an apparent relative increase of count density in the lateral walls and low count density of the septal walls

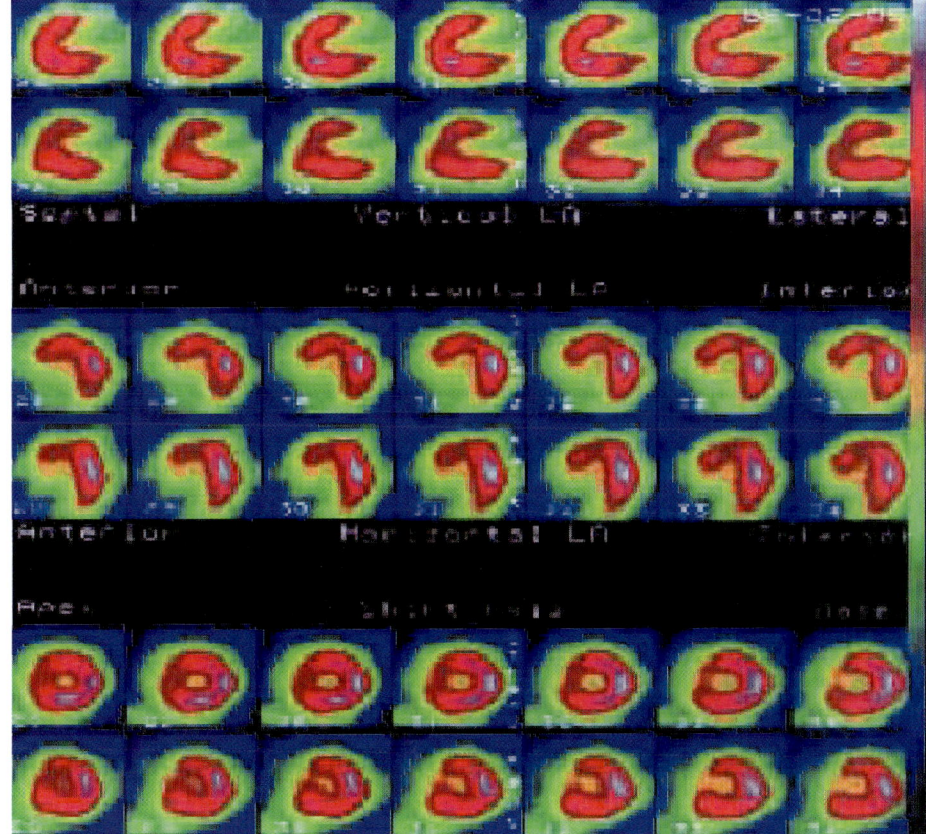

Fig. 28.12 The appearances of a short septum where the basal septum is replaced by fibrous tissue

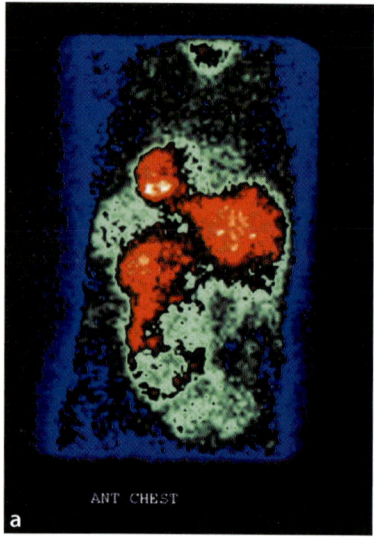
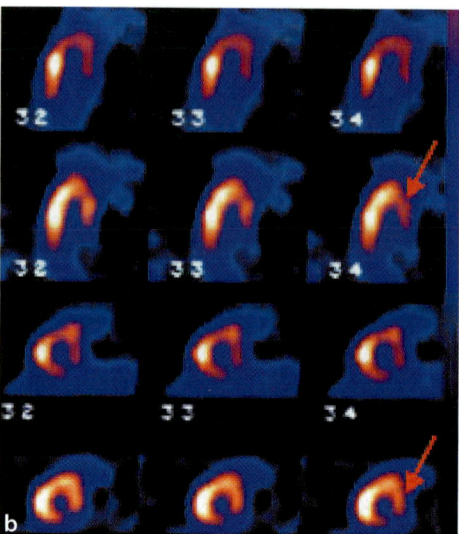

Fig. 28.13 Patient with dextrocardia and situs inversus. **a** Note the "mirrored" position of the interventricular septum and lateral wall. **b** Images show better uptake in the anteroseptal region (arrow) on the rest scan, suggestive of reversible myocardial ischaemia in this region

Table 28.3 Other pathology superimposed on CAD

Cardiomyopathy
- hypertrophic
- dilated

Left bundle branch block

Valvular heart disease
- mitral valve prolapse
- aortic stenosis
- aortic regurgitation

Idiopathic subaortic stenosis

Bland–White–Garland syndrome

Coronary spasm

Syndrome X

Recent post-percutaneous coronary intervention or rotational atherectomy

28.14.5
The 11/7 O'Clock Defect

This pseudodefect, which is usually seen in the anteroseptal region (11 o'clock) in short-axis tomograms, probably represents attenuation by the right ventricle since it usually lies, together with the 7 o'clock defect, close to the insertion points of the right ventricular wall. These are normally seen when count rates are low. A gated study, however, will show normal wall motion in these areas showing them to be viable.

28.15
Changes due to Pathology

There is a range of pathologies that can lead to mis-reading of myocardial perfusion scintigraphies; these are strictly not artefacts but the reporter needs to be aware of their existence (Table 28.3).

28.15.1
Hypertrophic Cardiomyopathy

Regional myocardial hypertrophy will appear as a high-density count region, thus resulting in a wrong normalization of images and false perfusion defects in the adjacent myocardial walls. It is common for hypertensive patients to have a relatively high density of counts in the interventricular septum, on both stress and rest images, which leads to an apparent decrease of count density in the lateral wall [15]. Asymmetric septal hypertrophy may produce a similar artefact.

28.15.2
Dilated Cardiomyopathy

In patients with dilated cardiomyopathy often due to a combination of diabetes and hypertension, patchy perfusion defects are commonly seen on both stress and rest images but may be worse on the rest images due to reduced count rates from the thinner myocardium. This may give rise to the phenomenon of reverse reperfusion where the rest scan is worse than the stress study.

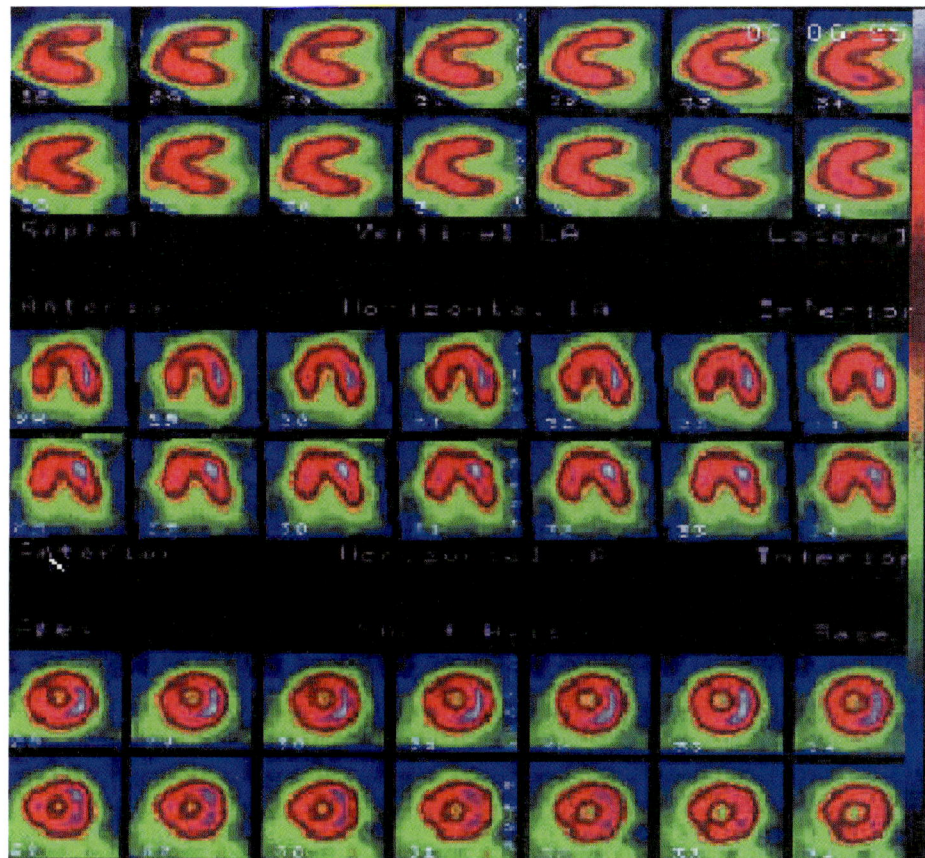

Fig. 28.14 Myocardial images showing a false positive defect in mitral valve stenosis

28.15.3
Bland–White–Garland Syndrome

The syndrome is defined as an anomaly in origin of the left coronary artery from the pulmonary artery. Although the anomaly most commonly results in death during early infancy, survival into adulthood can occur if collateral coronary flow is sufficient. An anterior wall perfusion defect has been reported generally in these patients. An inferior/posterior perfusion defect may also be seen secondary to a right coronary artery to left coronary artery to pulmonary artery shunt.

28.15.4
Valvular Disease

Fixed defects have been noted with various forms of valvular disease for example about 5% of patients appear to have a false positive study (Fig. 28.14) although in many patients the condition is related to previous infarction. Patients with aortic regurgitation and mild aortic stenosis may have apparent fixed apical defects.

28.15.5
"Balanced" Ischaemia

Patients with symmetric three-vessel disease may show a global hypoperfusion that can be misinterpreted as a relatively normal scan, in the absence of absolute quantification. Indirect indicators of multivessel coronary artery disease in myocardial perfusion imaging include left ventricular dilatation post-stress imaging and increased lung uptake on Tl-201 imaging (Fig. 28.15).

28.16
Conclusions

Myocardial perfusion scintigraphy is a multi-step procedure. Problems resulting in poor quality imaging can occur before the patient arrives in the department and due to poor patient preparation, incomplete quality control of the gamma camera or the radiopharmaceutical. There may be problems with acquisition and SPECT reconstruction. The patient may themselves present issues with their body size, BMI, shape, movement dur-

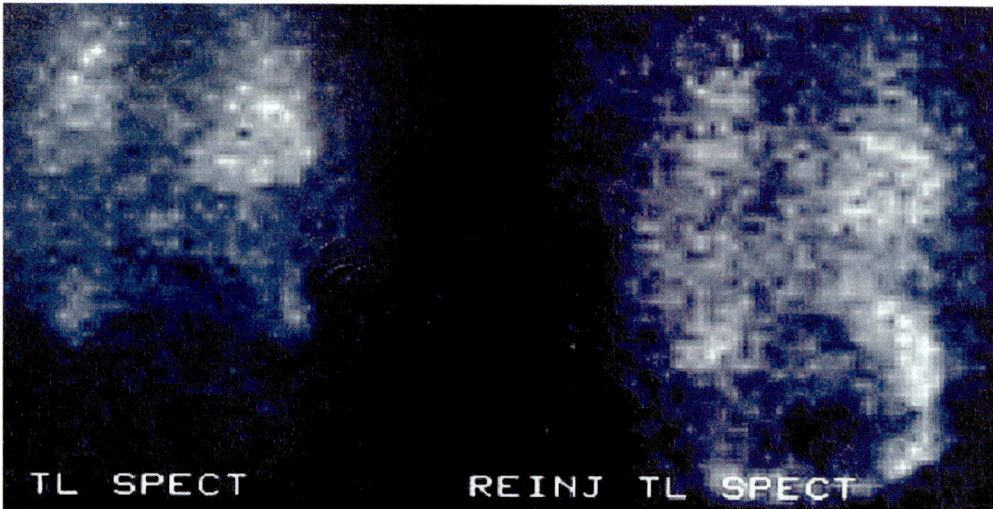

Fig. 28.15 Lung uptake of Tl-201 in balanced ischaemia

ing acquisition, physiological or pathological variants in the heart itself. Knowledge of these possible errors is required to ensure accurate reporting of each cardiac scan.

References

1. Cullom SJ (2001) Cardiac SPECT imaging. Principles of cardiac SPECT. Am J Cardiol 87:3-16.
2. O'Connor MK (1999) Instrument- and computer-related problems and Artefacts in nuclear medicine. Semin Nucl Med 26:256–277.
3. Cerquira MD, Matsuoka D, Ritchie JL et al. (1988) The influence of collimators on SPECT center of rotation measurements: artefact generation and acceptance testing. J Nucl Med 29:1393–1397.
4. Ryo U, Bekerman C, Pinsky S (eds) (1985) Atlas of Nuclear Medicine Artefacts and Variants. Chicago, IL, Year Book Medical.
5. Robinson CN, van Aswegen A, Julious SA, Nunan TO, Thomson WH, Tindale WB, Tout DA, Underwood SR (2008) The relationship between administered radiopharmaceutical activity in myocardial perfusion scintigraphy and imaging outcome Eur J Nucl Med Mol Imaging 35:329–335.
6. Anagnostopoulos C, Harbinson M, Kelion A, Kundley K, Loong CY, Notghi A, Reyes E, Tindale W, Underwood SR (2004) Procedure guidelines for radionuclide myocardial perfusion imaging. Heart 90:i1–i10.
7. DePuey EG (1994) How to detect and avoid myocardial perfusion defects J Nucl Med 35:699–702.
8. Currie Gm, Wheat JM (2004) The impact of acquisition protocol on the incidence of patient motion in ^{99m}Tc based myocardial perfusion SPECT. Nucl Med Commun 25:1191–1195.
9. Galt JR, Cullon SJ, Garcia EV Attenuation and scatter compensation in myocardial perfusion SPECT. Semin Nucl Med, 100(29):204–220.
10. Segall GM, Davis MJ (1989) Prone versus supine thallium myocardial SPECT: a method to decrease artifactual inferior wall defects. J Nucl Med 30:548–555.
11. Wackers FJTh (1992) Artefacts in planar and SPECT myocardial perfusion imaging. Am J Cardiol Imag 6:42–58.
12. Manglos SH, Thomas FD, Gagne GM et al. (1993) Phantom study of breast tissue attenuation in myocardial imaging. J Nucl Med 34:992–996.
13. Campeau RJ, Garcia OM, Colon R, Agusala M, Correa OA (1993) False positive Tc-99m sestamibi SPECT in a patient with left bundle branch block. Clin Nucl Med 18:40–42.
14. Caner B, Rezaghi C, Uysal U et al. (1997) Dobutamine thallium-201 myocardial SPECT in patients with left bundle branch block and normal coronary arteries. J Nucl Med 38:424–427.
15. DePuey EG, Guertler-Krawczynska E, Perkins JV, Robbons WL (1988) Alterations in myocardial thallium-201 distribution in patients with chronic systemic hypertension undergoing single-photon emission computed tomography. Am J Cardiol 62:234–238.

Multiple Gated Equilibrium Blood Pool Imaging (MUGA)

Rakesh Kumar

Contents

29.1	Introduction	343
29.2	Radiopharmaceuticals	343
29.2.1	In Vivo Labeling	344
29.2.2	Modified In Vivo Labeling	344
29.2.3	In Vitro Labeling	344
29.3	Data Acquisition	344
29.3.1	Position	344
29.3.2	ECG Gating	344
29.3.3	R–R Window and Beat Rejection	345
29.3.4	List Mode	345
29.4	Techniques	346
29.4.1	Planar Gated Equilibrium Radionuclide Angiography	346
29.4.2	Gated Tomographic Equilibrium Blood Pool Imaging	346
29.5	Stress Protocols	346
29.5.1	Physical Stress	346
29.5.2	Pharmacological Stress	346
29.6	Data Analysis and Interpretation	346
29.6.1	Qualitative Analysis	346
29.6.2	Ejection Fraction	347
29.6.3	LV Diastolic Filling	349
29.6.4	LV Volumes	349
29.6.5	Phase and Amplitude Images	349
29.7	Clinical Applications	349
29.7.1	Myocardial Infarction	350
29.7.2	Coronary Artery Disease	350
29.7.3	Congestive Heart Failure	351
29.8	Cardiomyopathy	351
29.9	Toxicity of Doxorubicin (Adriamycin)	351
29.10	Congenital Heart Disease (CHD)	351
	References	352

29.1 Introduction

In 1925, Herrmann Blumgart used radioactive indicators in human beings for evaluation of cardiac function. Prinzmetal and colleagues were the first to publish first-pass radionuclide angiography (RNA) results in normal subjects and those with valvular and congenital heart disease, using intravenous injection of Na-24 [1]. With the advent of computers in the 1970s, images were evaluated quantitatively and compared for dynamic changes that occur within a cardiac cycle. In 1971, Strauss and colleagues introduced the concept of using electrocardiography (ECG) to trigger image frame acquisition [2].

Ventricular function can be assessed with radionuclide techniques by two methods. The first involves analysing the initial transit of an intravenously administered radionuclide bolus as it traverses the central circulation. This has been called first-pass radionuclide angiocardiography, and it involves sampling for only the first 15 to 30 seconds after the injection. The second, more widely applied, technique for the radionuclide evaluation of ventricular performance is equilibrium radionuclide angiocardiography (ERNA). Both these methods have certain advantages and disadvantages. The following nomenclature is also used for this technique: Radionuclide ventriculography (RVG), MUGA, and gated blood pool imaging.

29.2 Radiopharmaceuticals

Tc99m remains the most commonly used radioisotope for first-pass and gated equilibrium studies. The first-pass study can be performed with Tc99m-pertecnetate, Tc99m-diethylenetriamine pentaacetic acid (DTPA), or any other Tc99m-labeled compound as the radiotracer. The majority of first-pass studies are performed with the renal imaging agent Tc-99m-DTPA because of the relatively low radiation exposure to patients, particularly with regard to reducing thyroid gland uptake, which was substantial with sodium pertechnetate. However, first-pass can be performed in conjunction with gated equilibrium imaging by injecting stannous pyrophosphate prior to a bolus of Tc-99m pertechnetate for red blood cell labeling.

Gated equilibrium imaging can be performed using a radiotracer that remains within the intravascular space for a longer period of time. Initially Tc99m-human serum albumin (HSA) was used for this purpose with reasonable success [3, 4]. However, Tc99m-HSA was abandoned for the following reasons: the image quality was relatively poor; acquisition periods were long; and labeling was stable for a short time only. In the late 1970s, Tc99m-HSA was replaced by a more efficient method of labeling patients' own RBCs with Tc99m-pertecnetate. The reduced form of technetium is required to bind to the globin chain of hemoglobin in the RBCs. The reduction state of technetium can be achieved by stannous ion (stannous pyrophosphate). However, it is very important to inject the optimal dose of stannous ion as a low dose will result in free technetium and a high dose can reduce technetium before its entry into the RBCs, leading to poor quality labeling. At present there are three efficient methods exist for RBC labeling.

29.2.1
In Vivo Labeling

This is the simplest and most commonly used approach in which RBC labeling takes place within the intravascular compartment [5, 6]. In this technique a stannous pyrophosphate injection of 10–20 μg per kg (approximately 2–3 mg) is given intravenously. The stannous ions diffuse passively through the RBC membrane. After 15–30 minutes, 15-25 mCi of Tc99m-pertechnetate is injected intravenously. Soon after entering the RBCs, the negatively charged Tc99m-pertechnetate is reduced by the positively charged stannous. The reduced Tc99m-pertechnetate binds to the beta chain of hemoglobin. The labeling efficiency of this technique varies from 85–95%.

29.2.2
Modified In Vivo Labeling

This technique is a combination of both in vivo and in vitro techniques. In this method, stannous pyrophosphate is injected intravenously. After 30 minutes, 5 mL of blood is withdrawn in a shielded syringe, which contains 15–25 mCi of Tc99m-pertechnetate and 1 mL of acid-citrate-dextrose solution as an anticoagulant. This blood is reinjected into the patient after 10 minutes incubation. The labeling efficiency of this technique varies from 92–95% [7].

29.2.3
In Vitro Labeling

This is the most complex method of RBC labeling among the three methods. For this, 10–20 mL of the patient's blood is withdrawn in a syringe. Stannous citrate is added to provide stannous ion and anticoagulation of the blood. After 5 minutes of gentle agitation, the blood is centrifuged. Supernant is discarded and packed RBCs are mixed with 15–25 mCi of Tc99m-pertechnetate. Before reinjection of radiolabeled blood, proper mixing is done by gentle agitation. For this technique, a clean and sterile working environment is mandatory. The labeling efficiency of this technique is more than 95% [8].

29.3
Data Acquisition

A small field-of-view (SFOV) gamma camera is best as it provides higher resolution images. In addition, a SFOV gamma camera can be manipulated easily and positioned very close to the chest for all views. The large field-of-view (LFOV) gamma camera provides lower resolution and also requires zoom.

29.3.1
Position

The angle that best separates right and left ventricular tracer activity is the best to calculate LVEF and other parameters. This is called the best septal view and can be obtained with the detector in a 30–60° left anterior oblique (LAO) position for most patients. Since the position of the heart varies among patients, the best results of left ventricular functions are obtained when the data is acquired in multiple views. These additional views are right anterior oblique (RAO), anterior, LAO, and left lateral (Fig. 29.1). However, during physical or pharmacological stress intervention, the data is acquired only in one position, usually LAO as this best separates right and left ventricular blood pool.

29.3.2
ECG Gating

Synchronization of data acquisition based on the cardiac cycle (ECG) is known as gating. ECG gating is required to obtain adequate density images over multiple cardiac cycles, which otherwise would be blurred due to cardiac motion. In this technique, one cardiac cycle is divided into a fixed number of multiple intervals

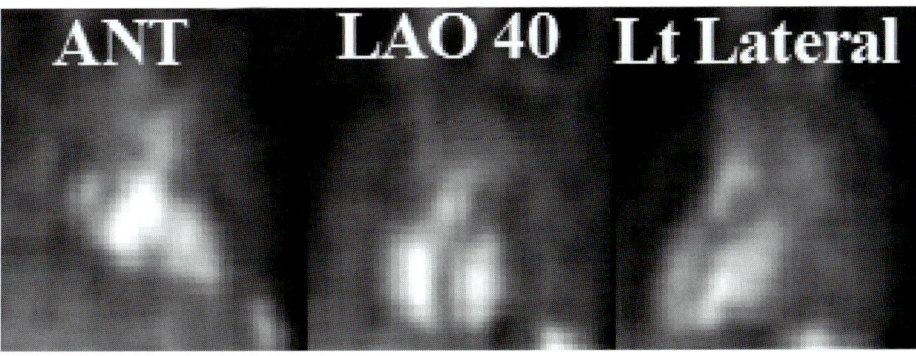

Fig. 29.1 Example of anterior, best septal and left lateral views of a resting equilibrium radionuclide angiogram (ERNA) study

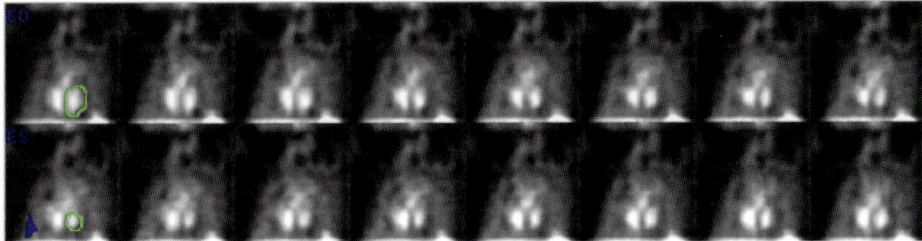

Fig. 29.2 R wave gated radionuclide ventriculogram in best septal view (LAO 40). Semiautomatic regions of interest (ROIs) in end diastole (ED) and end systole (ES) are marked. Note the change in size and count density of the left ventricle during the entire cardiac cycle

(frames). In most gamma camera computer systems a cardiac cycle is divided into 16 to 24 frames. Usually, the R wave acts as the signal for the start of the data acquisition sequence. A separate image is obtained for each interval (frame). The image data corresponding to the first interval is placed into the first frame; image data corresponding to the second interval is placed into the second frame and so on (Fig. 29.2). An adequate study of 250,000 to 400,000 counts per frame requires acquisition of 300 to 400 cardiac cycles.

29.3.3
R–R Window and Beat Rejection

A constant R–R interval during acquisition is important to obtain a good quality study. Any significant irregular R–R interval results in collection of poor quality of data. The optimal R–R window for a given study depends on the rhythm of the cardiac cycle. Generally, for all routine clinical purposes, a 10 to 15% R–R window is used. This means any cardiac cycle that is longer or shorter by 10 to 15% of the predefined interval will not be accepted. A narrower R–R window is better for acquisition of good data, but requires a regular rhythm and longer study duration. If the R–R window is too wide, a large number of undesired premature ventricular contractions (PVCs) will be accepted and these will affect the quality of the image data especially the diastolic portion of the time activity curve.

29.3.4
List Mode

Patients who do not have regular cardiac rhythm have the problem of poor quality image data acquisition. In list mode acquisition, the entire acquired data is stored without any preset framing criteria. The position and time of every count from the gamma camera and ECG signals are also stored. For list mode acquisition a large capacity memory disk is required. After acquisition is complete, various R–R windows can be set to screen the data if there are enough cycles in that window.

29.4 Techniques

29.4.1 Planar Gated Equilibrium Radionuclide Angiography

The most unique application of ERNA is the ability to obtain and rapidly evaluate Fourier transformation phase and amplitude images. The Fourier transformation process fits the changes that occur in each pixel to a cosine wave, which is then characterized by the degree of change throughout the cycle (amplitude) and the relative timing of the fitted cosine wave (phase). The amplitude and phase images are used to detect regional wall motion abnormalities.

29.4.2 Gated Tomographic Equilibrium Blood Pool Imaging

In 1980, Moore et al. described single photon emission tomography equilibrium radionuclide angioventriculographuphy (SPECT ERNA). This technique has advantages over planar ERNA in terms of its ability to evaluate the regional wall motion and the size and shape of the ventricle, without the limitation of overlap of the cardiac chambers 9–11]. Corbett et al. demonstrated that SPECT blood pool imaging could be quantified for EF and analysed for regional wall motion with a degree of accuracy not available from planar ERNA [11]. Similar to the planar technique, SPECT ERNA has been analysed for Fourier amplitude and phase, rendering accurate three-dimensional assessment of the origin of ventricular tachycardias [12].

29.5 Stress Protocols

Evaluation of LV function at stress has higher diagnostic and prognostic value in patients with coronary artery disease.

29.5.1 Physical Stress

The conventional physical exercise using treadmill is not suitable for ERNA due to motion. Bicycle ergometers can be used for exercise stress in both the upright and supine position with continuous ECG and blood pressure monitoring. However, the major problem with bicycle ergometers is that many patients experience leg fatigue before achieving adequate cardiovascular stress. The alternative to bicycle ergometer exercise is handgrip isometric exercise and cold pressure testing.

29.5.2 Pharmacological Stress

A subset of patients who cannot undergo physical stress should undergo pharmacological stress. Catecholamine infusion and coronary vasodilators are commonly used pharmaceuticals. Dobutamine is the most common pharmacological stress agent, and has significant acceptance among clinicians. Dobutamine is a potent stimulator of beta-1 receptors and a mild beta-2 and alpha-1 agonist [13]. The agent has both inotropic and chronotropic action on the heart. Hence, it produces hemodynamic changes that mimic those produced by exercise. The protocol of dobutamine stress is given in Fig. 29.3.

29.6 Data Analysis and Interpretation

29.6.1 Qualitative Analysis

Before the analysis of any data, one should look for cine display of all the views obtained. This will provide a visual assessment of the size of both the ventricles and their relationship to other nearby structures, which is important for marking region of interest (ROI). In addition, a fair idea of wall motion will also be obtained by visual assessment. A normal wall motion is defined as contraction of all ventricular segments at the same time,

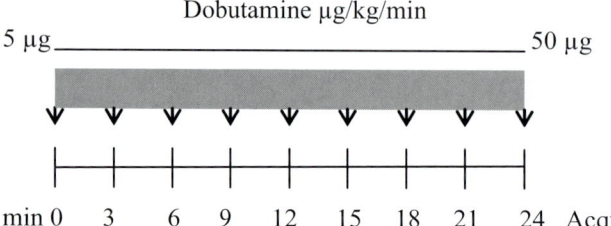

Fig. 29.3 Imaging protocol of dobutamine scintigraphy

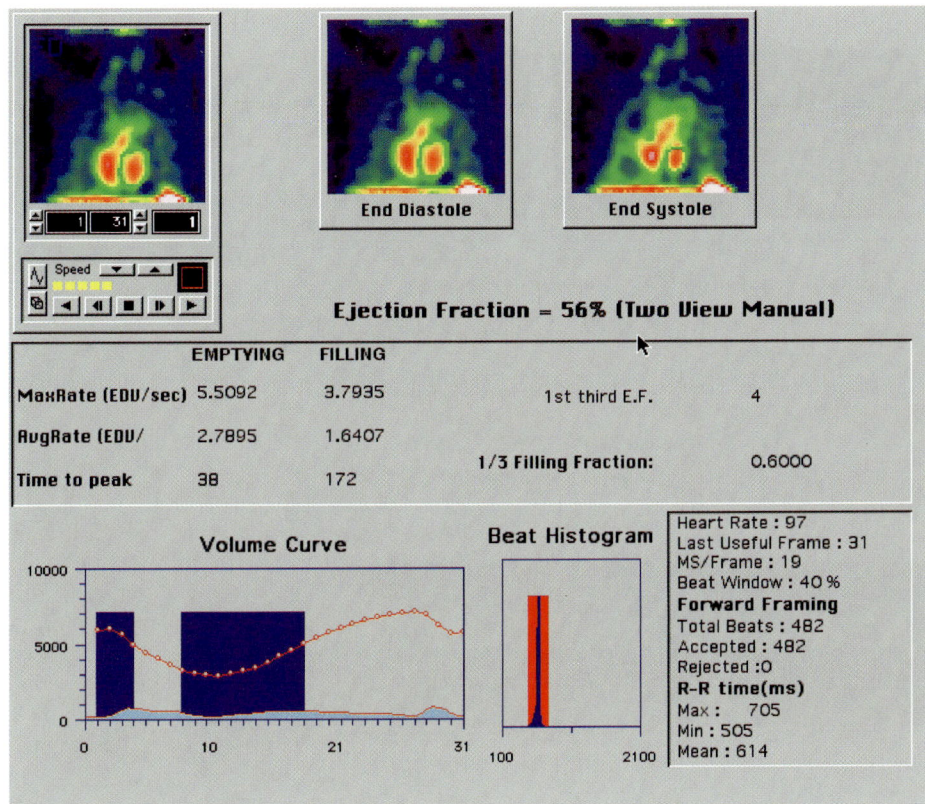

Fig. 29.4 Composite computer generated display of analysis of resting equilibrium radionuclide angiogram. Note the filling and emptying rates of the left ventricle

at the same rate and to the same extent. Abnormal wall motions can be termed as akinetic when there is no motion; hypokinetic when there is diminished contraction; and dykinetic when there is paradoxical wall motion (part of wall bulging out during systole). A ventricular aneurysm is formed by a thin wall of fibrous tissue. An aneurysm is either akinetic or dyskinetic and a neck can be seen during systole, when the surrounding myocardium contracts.

ROI (Fig. 29.4). Left ventricular ED and ES counts are corrected for extra cardiac background activity before a LV time activity curve is generated (Fig. 29.5). The LVEF is calculated as follows:

$$\frac{\text{End-diastolic Counts} - \text{End-systolic Counts}}{\text{End-diastolic Counts}}$$

29.6.2 Ejection Fraction

Estimation of global LVEF is the most important quantitative parameter in ERNA study. This can be estimated by drawing an ROI on the best septal view and generating the time activity curve of the left ventricle. There is a range of computer software provided with commercially available gamma cameras. Despite the difference in software, most of them are based on the calculation of changes in count density in the ROI during the cardiac cycle. The ROI can be generated manually or by semiautomatic and automatic methods. Manual and semiautomatic methods are better and allow the operator to change end diastolic (ED) and end systolic (ES)

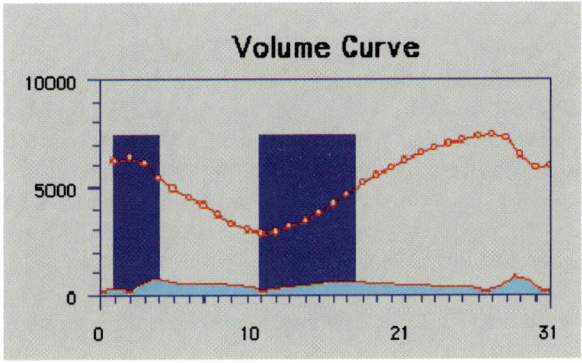

Fig. 29.5 Left ventricular time activity curve

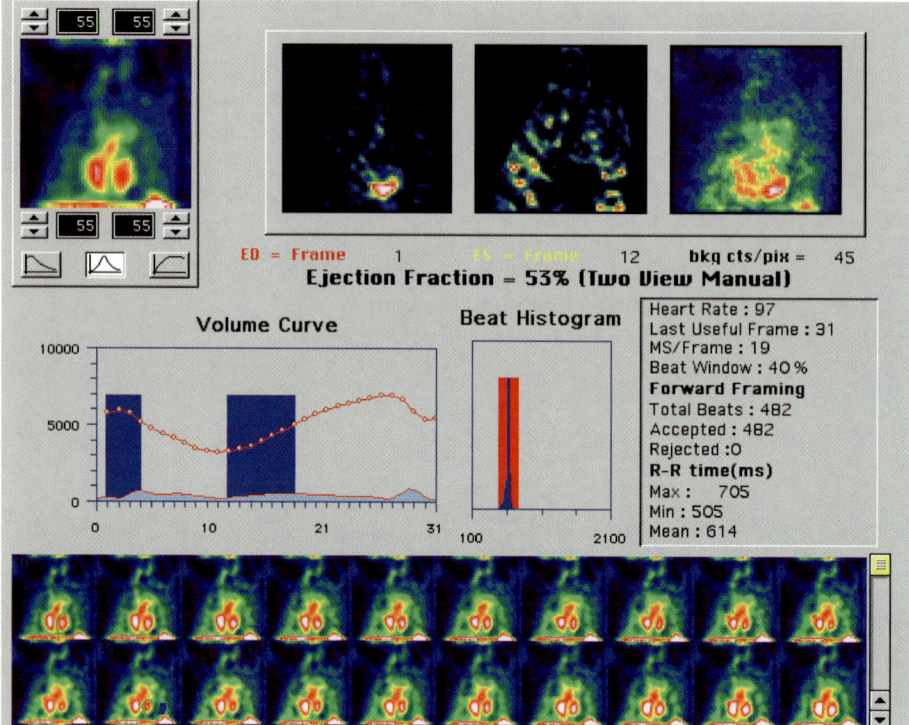

Fig. 29.6 Composite computer generated display of analysis of resting equilibrium radionuclide angiogram. Sequential images showing the changes in left ventricle during cardiac cycle are shown at the bottom

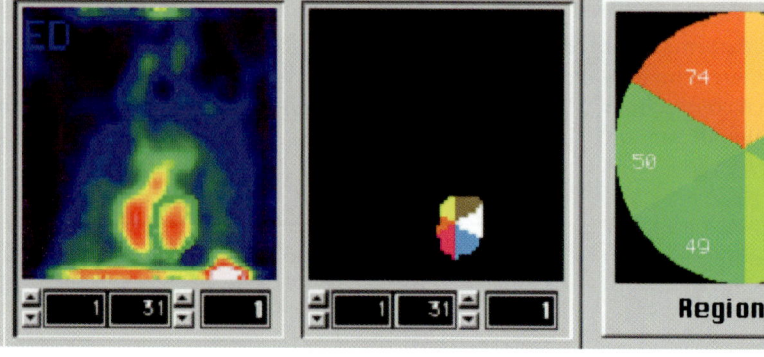

Fig. 29.7 Calculation of regional ejection fraction from six pie-shaped regions centered in the center of left ventricle

By determining the center of the LV and dividing it into different zones the regional left ventricular ejection fractions can be calculated. The normal LVEF varies from 50 to 80% at rest and 56 to 86% at stress (Fig. 29.6). Impaired LV function is termed as mild when LVEF is 40% to 49%; moderate when LVEF is 30% to 39%; and severe when LVEF is less than 30%.

Regional EF represents EF for different segments of the ventricles (Fig. 29.7). Regional EF provides three-dimensional data compared with two-dimensional data provided by wall motion. One should remember that regional EF and wall motion are two different parameters.

Right ventricular ejection fraction (RVEF) is not calculated routinely from the ERNA study because of underestimation of EF due to the overlapping right atrium. The phase images are useful in localizing valve plane and are helpful in drawing correct ROIs. The normal RVEF varies from 45 to 70% [14].

29.6.3
LV Diastolic Filling

ERNA can readily evaluate diastolic function. A variety of different diastolic filling indices can be obtained from the filling portion of the LV time activity curve. The three most important parameters are left ventricular peak filling rate (PFR), time to peak filling rate (tPFR) and filling fraction (FR) (Fig. 29.4). The PFR is the time point in the LV time activity curve at which counts are increasing at their fastest rate. tPFR is the time from the end of systole to the time of peak filling rate. The PFR is expressed in EDV/second, while tPFR is expressed in milliseconds. FR is the calculation of percentage filling at different time points in diastole. It can be expressed as first third (1/3 FF), first half (1/2 FF) and so on.

29.6.4
LV Volumes

Ventricular volume can be determined with relative ease using either geometric or count-based methods with ERNA. The geometric method is based on the same mathematical assumption that applies to contrast angiographic data [15]. The count-based method is based on the principle of equilibrium. Therefore the injected radionuclide is distributed in direct proportion to the blood volume of any given chamber and changes in radioactivity during the cardiac cycle are equivalent to the changes in volume in that chamber. In clinical practice, a small sample of blood is obtained for measurement and calibration using the gamma camera. After applying, a correction factor due to the attenuation of counts by the body, volumes can be derived from the external count rates in a particular region (usually over the left or right ventricle). Many commercially available gamma camera based computers have new count-based software for the measurement of ventricular volume that does not require such a correction [16]. This innovative approach simplifies volume analysis. Count-based methods are better than conventional area–length geometric methods, because they do not depend on geometric assumptions about the shape of the left ventricle.

Normally stroke volume counts are equal for both right and left ventricle. However, in patients with mitral valve or aortic valve insufficency the LV stroke volume counts are more than the RV stroke volume counts.

29.6.5
Phase and Amplitude Images

Phase image analysis is a parametric method of graphic representation of the timing of events in the cardiac cycle. It is based on the first Fourier harmonic fit of the blood pool time versus radioactivity curve. The resultant generated curve is a cosine curve, which mimics the original data of the cardiac cycle. The beginning of the first frame is typically assigned a phase angle of 0° that results in a value of 180° for ES and 360° ED. A phase histogram can be obtained from the data of each phase angle.

The amplitude image is simply the magnitude or depth of the fitted curve and is similar to the stroke volume image (Fig. 29.8). It represents the maximum change in counts between the peak and nadir of the fitted curve. For stroke volume image, ES counts are subtracted from ED counts. These images are helpful in identifying regional ventricular functions and abnormal wall motion.

29.7
Clinical Applications

The clinical application of MUGA techniques to assess ventricular function often competes directly with

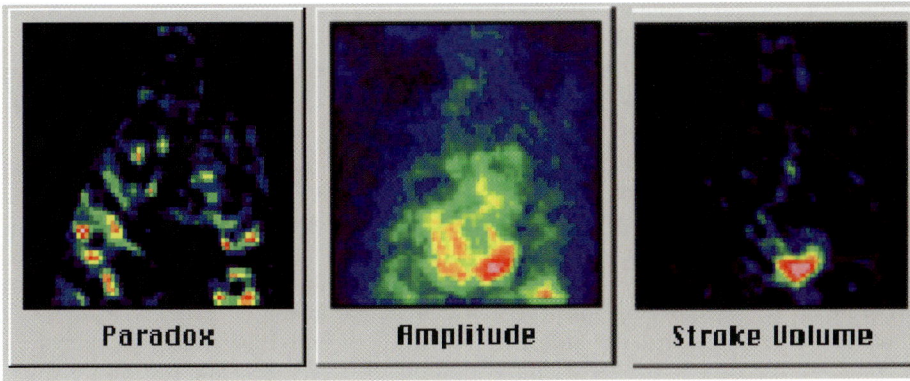

Fig. 29.8 Normal paradox, amplitude and stroke volume images

cardiac echocardiography. Initially, the most common clinical application of MUGA was the assessment of EF. Later on, these applications expanded to include regional wall motion, exercise LV function, RV function, myocardial contraction patterns, absolute ventricular volume measurements, valvular regurgitation, and LV filling and emptying rates [17].

There are number of clinical indications of ERNA, but the prognosis of coronary artery disease and evaluation of cardiotoxicity are two most enduring applications of gated equilibrium imaging. It has a definite role in prognostication of patients with coronary artery disease and valvular heart disease. Serial EFs are useful in the evaluation of the cumulative effects of chemotherapy on ventricular function [18–20].

29.7.1
Myocardial Infarction

29.7.1.1 Diagnosis

Myocardial infarction can be diagnosed on ERNA by detecting abnormal wall motion and decreased global LVEF and regional EF. ERNA not only helps in localizing the site of infarction but also detects the size and severity of the infarction. Greater than 30% of cases inferior wall MI is also associated with right ventricular MI [21]. Therefore, it is always better to acquire a first pass study during the radiotracer injection for RBC labeling. The first pass study helps the accurate detection of LV function and detection of a shunt due to rupture of the septum as a result of MI.

29.7.1.2 Prognosis

The resting LV functions after MI have been used to prognosticate patients. Several reports have documented the importance of the global ejection fraction as a major prognostic index. The measurement of ejection fraction is now standard in patients after a myocardial infarction. The impairment of LV function is directly related to poor prognosis. Impaired right ventricular function is seen in 40% of patients with inferior wall MI. But RV involvement with anterior wall MI is not common. The associated right ventricular infarction has poor prognosis compared with those without RV infarction. After myocardial infarction, assessment for the formation of a ventricular aneurysm, an extreme example of ventricular remodeling, provides further prognostic information [22]. LVEF is considered to be the single most important factor defining the outcome after a myocardial infarction [23–25].

29.7.2
Coronary Artery Disease

29.7.2.1 Diagnosis

In clinical practice stress myocardial perfusion scintigraphy is a more frequently applied technique than ERNA for the diagnosis of ischemia heart disease. Although stress-induced myocardial ischemia can be detected with ERNA, the specificity is very low. Development of new wall motion abnormalities and a failure to increase LVEF by more than 5% or no change in EF or decrease in EF in response to stress are the diagnostic criteria of ischemia on ERNA. The most common non-ischemic conditions that cause abnormal response to stress LVEF are cardiomyopathy, valvular heart disease, pericardial disease, drug toxicity, etc.

29.7.2.2 Prognosis

Resting LVEF is a powerful predictor of the subsequent outcome in patients with CAD. It has been well documented by many authors that LV contractile function has significant prognostic value in CAD patients [26, 27]. The Coronary Artery Surgery Study (CASS) also documented the importance of ejection fraction as a prognostic indicator, particularly in patients with multivessel CAD [27]. Ejection fraction was found to be the single best prognostic factor in determining long-term outcome in survivors of cardiac arrest [28[. LVEF at the peak of exercise was found to be powerful predictor of poor prognosis [29, 30]. It is interesting to note that when ERNA data were combined with clinical information and compared with catheterization data, it was found that stress ERNA data with clinical information has as good a prognostic value as that provided by catheterization [31]. Stress ERNA before an operation has been found to be a major predictor of symptomatic outcome of coronary artery bypass surgery [32]. However, in recent times this role has largely been replaced by myocardial perfusion scintigraphy. If first pass RNA is obtained along with myocardial perfusion scintigraphy, RNA ejection fraction provides prognostic information besides that provided by clinical and myocardial perfusion imaging [33].

29.7.2.3 Assessment of Myocardial Viability

Identification of myocardial viability has an important bearing on the management of patients with CAD. Stunned myocardium and hibernating myocardium are the conditions in which baseline resting LV functions are poor, but myocardium is still alive. However, if these patients are identified and treated in time by restoration of blood supply, there are high chances of improvement in LV function. Identification of viable but non-functional myocardium can be achieved by estimation of LV functions after administration of nitroglycerin or injecting low dose of dobutamine [34, 35]. Change in regional wall motion and or ejection fraction immediately after cessation of exercise, with catecholamine infusion and after nitroglycerin is an indicator of myocardial viability. In recent times, this indication of ERNA has been totally replaced by myocardial perfusion scintigraphy, which not only provides myocardial perfusion but also ventricular ejection fraction.

29.7.3
Congestive Heart Failure

Dyspnea can be due to cardiac or non-cardiac pathology. Therefore it is very important to discriminate these two as these have an important bearing on the management. Resting and stress ERNA may be helpful and provide important information for the assessment of congestive heart failure. From the standpoint of ventricular function, the importance of evaluating systolic compared with diastolic dysfunction can be readily appreciated. Radionuclide studies of myocardial viability and ischemia also provide insight into the appropriate therapy for patients with heart failure and coronary artery disease [36]. ERNA is very useful in differentiating systolic and diastolic causes of CHF.

Analysis of left ventricular volume adds substantially to the evaluation of patients with heart failure and severely depressed systolic function. ERNA can evaluate therapeutic efficacy from changes in ventricular volume without concomitant changes in the LVEF [37]. In addition, evaluating changes in ventricular architecture, expansion of myocardial infarcts, and ventricular remodeling requires an assessment of ventricular shape and volumetric change. The importance of assessing diastolic function has increased with the recognition of the clinical syndrome of congestive heart failure, preserved systolic function, and impaired ventricular filling [38]. Diastolic function can also be assessed by LV volume curve and ventricular filling rates. Abnormal ventricular filling is a characteristic of both hypertrophy and coronary disease [38–40]. Abnormal diastolic functions in patients with CHF have been noted in as many as 30% of patients hospitalized [38]. Clinical recognition of this condition is of the utmost importance, because routine therapy for heart failure with inotropic agents or vasodilators will not improve underlying pathology.

29.8
Cardiomyopathy

Cardiomyopathies are a group of diseases, which are classified as idiopathic, hypertrophic, and restrictive. In idiopathic cardiomyopathy, the LV cavity is dilated with poor LVEF, and wall motion is uniformly diminished. ERNA may be helpful in differentiating idiopathic cardiomyopathy from ischemic cardiomyopathy. Right ventricular involvement is commonly seen in idiopathic cardiomyopathy, where ischemic cardiomyopathy is associated with akinesia or dyskinesia [41]. Improvement of LV function in response to exercise is also suggestive of idiopathic cardiomyopathy [42].

Patients with hypertrophic cardiomyopathy usually have asymmetrical hypertrophy. The size of the left ventricle is small and LV function is higher than normal. Diastolic function is usually abnormal due to poor compliance of the hypertrophied myocardium in the majority of patients. ERNA can demonstrate abnormal diastolic filling, therefore it is helpful in diagnosis and evaluation of treatment response to calcium channel blockers. Restrictive cardiomyopathy is due to abnormal diastolic filling. ERNA has been reported helpful in differentiating restrictive cardiomyopathy from constrictive pericardial disease [43].

29.9
Toxicity of Doxorubicin (Adriamycin)

ERNA has been extensively used in monitoring cardiotoxicity in cancer patients who have received cardiotoxic chemotherapy, particularly doxorubicin [44]. Doxorubicin cardiotoxicity is dose related and rarely seen at cumulative doses less than 400 mg/m^2. However, in patients who receive doses of more than 550 mg/m^2, cardiotoxicity is seen in about 30% of patients. Therefore, it is important to monitor these patients to detect early cardiotoxicity [45]. Appropriate guidelines for treating patients with doxorubicin have been developed on the basis of the ejection fraction at rest. A fall of more than 15% in LVEF detected by ERNA is the indication for cessation of doxorubicin therapy [18, 45–47]. The use of the ejection fraction at rest appears to provide data sufficiently reliable to obviate the need for routine endocardial biopsy in the monitoring of these patients.

29.10
Congenital Heart Disease (CHD)

In the era of CT, MRI and echocardiography, which provide better anatomic details, the role of first pass, ERNA is limited. The best indication of first pass ERNA in patients with CHD is detection and quantitation of left-to-right shunts [48,49]. It can be detected by a mathematical method known as curve-fitting technique (Qp/Qs ratio). This technique can detect shunts as small as 20%. RNA is the investigation of choice for serial measurement of EFs in patients with CHD. In addition, it can evaluate the response to medical or surgical treatments.

References

1. Corday PE, Bergman HC, Schwartz L, Spritzler RJ (1948) Radiocardiography a new method for studying the blood flow through the chambers of the heart in human beings. Science 108:340–341.
2. Strauss HW, Zaret BL, Hurley PJ, Natarajan TK, Pitt B (1971) A scintiphotographic method for measuring left ventricular ejection fraction in man without cardiac catheterization, Am J Cardiol 28:575–580.
3. Secker-Walker RH, Resnick L, Kunz H, Parker JA, Hill RL, Potchen EJ (1973) Measurement of left ventricular ejection fraction. J Nucl Med. 4:798–802.
4. Nishimura T, Hamada S, Hayashida K, Uehara T, Katabuchi T, Hayashi M (1989) Cardiac blood-pool scintigraphy using technetium-99m DTPA-HSA: comparison with in vivo technetium-99m RBC labeling. J Nucl Med 30:1713–1717.
5. Pavel DG, Zimmer M, Patterson VN (1977) In vivo labeling of red blood cells with ^{99m}Tc: a new approach to blood pool visualization. J Nucl Med 18:305–308.
6. Hamilton RG, Alderson PO (1977) A comparative evaluation of techniques for rapid and efficient in vivo labeling of red cells with [^{99m}Tc] pertechnetate. J Nucl Med 18:1010–1013.
7. Callahan RJ, Froelich JW, McKusick KA, Leppo J, Strauss HW (1982) A modified method for the in vivo labeling of red blood cells with Tc-99m: concise communication. J Nucl Med 23:315–318.
8. Hegge FN, Hamilton GW, Larson SM, Ritchie JL, Richards P (1978) Cardiac chamber imaging: a comparison of red blood cells labeled with Tc-99m in vitro and in vivo. J Nucl Med 19:129–134.
9. Tamaki N, Mukai T, Ishii Y et al. (1983) Multiaxial tomography of heart chambers by gated blood-pool emission computed tomography using a rotating gamma camera. Radiology 147:547–554.
10. Barat JL, Brendel AJ, Colle JP et al. (1984) Quantitative analysis of left-ventricular function using gated single photon emission tomography. J Nucl Med 25:1167–1174.
11. Corbett JR, Jansen DE, Lewis SE et al. (1985) Tomographic gated blood pool radionuclide ventriculography analysis of wall motion and left ventricular volumes in patients with coronary artery disease, J Am Coll Cardiol 6:349–358.
12. Casset-Senon D, Babuty D, Alison D et al. (2000) Delayed contraction area responsible for sustained ventricular tachycardia in an arrhythmogenic right ventricular cardiomyopathy demonstration by Fourier analysis of SPECT equilibrium radionuclide angiography. J Nucl Cardiol 7:539–542.
13. Henkin RE (1984) Interventional equilibrium in blood pool studies. Crit Rev Diagn Imaging. 20:261–282.
14. Winzelberg GG, Boucher CA et al. (1981) Right ventricular function in aortic and mitral valve disease. Chest 79:520–528.
15. Sandler H, Dodge HT (1968) The use of single plane angiocardiograms for the calculation of left ventricular volume in man. Am Heart J 75:325–334.
16. Levy WC, Cerqueira MD, Matsuoka DT, Harp GD, Sheehan FH, Stratton JR (1992) Four radionuclide methods for left ventricular volume determination: comparison of a manual and an automated technique. J Nucl Med 33:763–770.
17. Williams KA (2005) A historical perspective on measurement of ventricular function with scintigraphic techniques: Part II – Ventricular function with gated techniques for blood pool and perfusion imaging. J Nucl Cardiol 22:208–215.
18. Agarwala S, Kumar R, Bhatnagar V, Bajpai M, Gupta DK, Mitra DK (2000) High incidence of adriamycin cardiotoxicity in children even at low cumulative doses: role of radionuclide cardiac angiography. J Pediatr Surg 35:1786–1789.
19. Palmeri ST, Bonow RO, Myers CE et al. (1986) Prospective evaluation of doxorubicin cardiotoxicity by rest and exercise radionuclide angiography. Am J Cardiol 58:607–613.
20. Schwartz RG, McKenzie WB, Alexander J et al. (1987) Congestive heart failure and left ventricular dysfunction complicating doxorubicin therapy. Seven-year experience using serial radionuclide angiocardiography. Am J Med 82:1109–1118.
21. Isner JM, Roberts WC (1978) Right ventricular infarction complicating left ventricular infarction secondary to coronary heart disease. Frequency, location, associated findings and significance from analysis of 236 necropsy patients with acute or healed myocardial infarction. Am J Cardiol 42:885–894.
22. Meizlish JL, Berger HJ, Plankey M, Errico D, Levy W, Zaret BL (1984) Functional left ventricular aneurysm formation after acute anterior transmural myocardial infarction: incidence, natural history, and prognostic implications. N Engl J Med 311:1001–1006.
23. The Multicenter Postinfarction Research Group (1983) Risk stratification and survival after myocardial infarction. N Engl J Med 309:331–336.
24. Ahnve S, Gilpin E, Henning H, Curtis G, Collins D, Ross J Jr (1986) Limitations and advantages of the ejection fraction for defining high risk after acute myocardial infarction. Am J Cardiol 58:872–878.

25. de Chillou C, Sadoul N, Bizeau O et al. (1997) Prognostic value of thrombolysis, coronary artery patency, signal-averaged electrocardiography, left ventricular ejection fraction, and Holter electrocardiographic monitoring for life-threatening ventricular arrhythmias after a first acute myocardial infarction. Am J Cardiol 80:852–858.
26. Harris PJ, Harrell FE Jr, Lee KL, Rosati RA (1980) Non-fatal myocardial infarction in medically treated patients with coronary artery disease. Am J Cardiol 46:937–942.
27. Coronary Artery Surgery Study (CASS): a randomized trial of coronary bypass surgery: survival data (1983) Circulation 68:939–950.
28. Ritchie JL, Hallstrom AP, Troubaugh GB, Caldwell JH, Cobb LA (1985) Out-of-hospital sudden coronary death: rest and exercise radionuclide left ventricular function in survivors. Am J Cardiol 55:645–651.
29. Lee KL, Pryor DB, Pieper KS et al. (1990) Prognostic value of radionuclide angiography in medically treated patients with coronary artery disease. A comparison with clinical and catheterization variables. Circulation 82:1705–1717.
30. Shaw LJ, Heinle SK, Borges-Neto S, Kesler K, Coleman RE, Jones RH (1998) Prognosis by measurements of left ventricular function during exercise. Duke Noninvasive Research Working Group. J Nucl Med 39:140–146.
31. Taliercio CP, Clements IP, Zinsmeister AR, Gibbons RJ (1988) Prognostic value and limitations of exercise radionuclide angiography in medically treated coronary artery disease. Mayo Clin Proc 63:573–582.
32. Jones RH, Floyd RD, Austin EH et al. (1983) The role of radionuclide angiocardiography in the preoperative prediction of pain relief and prolonged survival following coronary artery bypass grafting. Ann Surg 197:743–754.
33. Mast ST, Shaw LK, Ravizzini GC et al. (2001) Incremental prognostic value of RNA ejection fraction measurements during pharmacologic stress testing: a comparison with clinical and perfusion variables. J Nucl Med 42:871–877.
34. Takeuchi M, Fujitani K, Kurogane K et al. (1985) Effects of diltiazem and nitroglycerin on left ventricular diastolic properties in patients with coronary artery disease. Jpn Heart J 26:509–520.
35. Barilla F, Gheorghiade M, Alam M, Khaja F, Goldstein S (1991) Low-dose dobutamine in patients with acute myocardial infarction identifies viable but not contractile myocardium and predicts the magnitude of improvement in wall motion abnormalities in response to coronary revascularisation. Am Heart J 122:1522–1531.
36. Bonow RO, Dilsizian V, Cuocolo A, Bacharach SL (1991) Identification of viable myocardium in patients with chronic coronary artery disease and left ventricular dysfunction: comparison of thallium scintigraphy with reinjection and PET imaging with ^{18}F-Fluorodeoxyglucose. Circulation 83:26–37.
37. Firth BG, Dehmer GJ, Markham RV, Willerson JT, Hillis LD (1982) Assessment of vasodilator therapy in patients with severe congestive heart failure: limitations of measurements of left ventricular ejection fraction and volumes. Am J Cardiol 50:954–959.
38. Soufer R, Wohlgelernter D, Vita NA et al. (1985) Intact systolic left ventricular function in clinical congestive heart failure. Am J Cardiol 55:1032–1036.
39. Bonow RO, Vitale DF, Maron BJ, Bacharach SL, Frederick TM, Green MV (1987) Regional left ventricular asynchrony and impaired global left ventricular filling in hypertrophic cardiomyopathy: effect of Verapamil. J Am Coll Cardiol 9:1108–1116.
40. Fouad FM, Slominski JM, Tarazi RC (1984) Left ventricular diastolic function in hypertension: relation to left ventricular mass and systolic function. J Am Coll Cardiol 3:1500–1506.
41. Iskandrian AS, Helfeld H, Lemlek J, Lee J, Iskandrian B, Heo J (1992) Differentiation between primary dilated cardiomyopathy and ischemic cardiomyopathy based on right ventricular performance. Am Heart J 123:768–773.
42. Schoolmeester WL, Simpson AG, Sauerbrunn BJ, Fletcher RD (1981) Radionuclide angiographic assessment of left ventricular function during exercise in patients with a severely reduced ejection fraction. Am J Cardiol 47:804–809.
43. Bonow RO, Rosing DR, Bacharach SL et al. (1981) Effects of Verapamil on left ventricular systolic function and diastolic filling in patients with hypertrophic cardiomyopathy. Circulation 64:787–796.
44. Schwartz RG, McKenzie WB, Alexander J et al. (1987) Congestive heart failure and left ventricular dysfunction complicating doxorubicin therapy: seven-year experience using serial radionuclide angiocardiography. Am J Med 82:1109–1118.
45. Mitani I, Jain D, Joska TM, Burtness B, Zaret BL (2003) Doxorubicin cardiotoxicity: prevention of congestive heart failure with serial cardiac function monitoring with equilibrium radionuclide angiocardiography in the current era. J Nucl Cardiol 10:132–139.
46. Alexander J, Dainiak N, Berger HJ et al. (1979) Serial assessment of doxorubicin cardiotoxicity with quantitative radionuclide angiocardiography. N Engl J Med 300:278–283.
47. Nousiainen T, Jantunen E, Vanninen E, Hartikainen J (2002) Early decline in left ventricular ejection fraction predicts doxorubicin cardiotoxicity in lymphoma patients. Br J Cancer 86:1697–1700.
48. Kriss JP, Enright LP, Hayden WG, Wexler L, Shumway NE (1972) Radioisotopic angiocardiography: findings in congenital heart disease. J Nucl Med 13:31–40.
49. Gal R, Port SC (1987) Radionuclide angiography in congenitally corrected transposition of the great vessels in an adult. J Nucl Med 28:116–118.

Chapter 30

First Pass Studies – Current Status and Limitations

Radhakrishnan Jayan and Linda Smith

Contents

30.1	Introduction	355
30.2	Physiology	355
30.3	Procedure	355
30.4	Radiopharmaceuticals	356
30.5	Acquisition	356
30.6	Quality Control	357
30.7	Clinical Roles	357
30.7.1	Determination of Ventricular Function	357
30.7.2	Determination of Left to Right Shunts	357
30.7.3	Determination of Right to Left Shunts	360
30.8	Conclusion	360
	References	360

30.1 Introduction

First pass radionuclide studies provide a useful non-invasive tool for evaluating cardio-pulmonary circulation and the pathologies that affect these systems. The first pass of a bolus of radioactivity can provide functional information about ventricular function, abnormalities such as cardiac shunts and abnormalities affecting the pulmonary circulation. Quantification of the severity of the abnormality is also possible, helping in decisions regarding patient management.

The first attempt to evaluate congenital heart disease using radioactive tracers was reported by Prinzmetal in 1949 [1]. Although the number of first pass radionuclide studies has fallen in recent years due to the advances in echocardiography and invasive cardiac catheterisation, these studies still can be a useful adjunct yielding helpful information in selected patients.

30.2 Physiology

First pass angiocardiography studies are dynamic studies that trace the passage of a bolus of a radiopharmaceutical through the heart and pulmonary circulation. The radiopharmaceutical flows sequentially through the superior venacava (SVC), right atrium (RA), right ventricle (RV), pulmonary arteries (PA) and lungs, left atrium (LA), left ventricle (LV), aorta and great vessels (Fig. 30.1a)

A sequence of short duration images is acquired to demonstrate tracer transit and this helps identify anomalies in the normal circulation described above.

30.3 Procedure

A large proximal vein ideally in the right ante-cubital fossa should be cannulated with a large gauge cannula. It is a very important requisite of a first pass study that a tight bolus of radioactivity is delivered to the heart. This is particularly important in studies to determine the

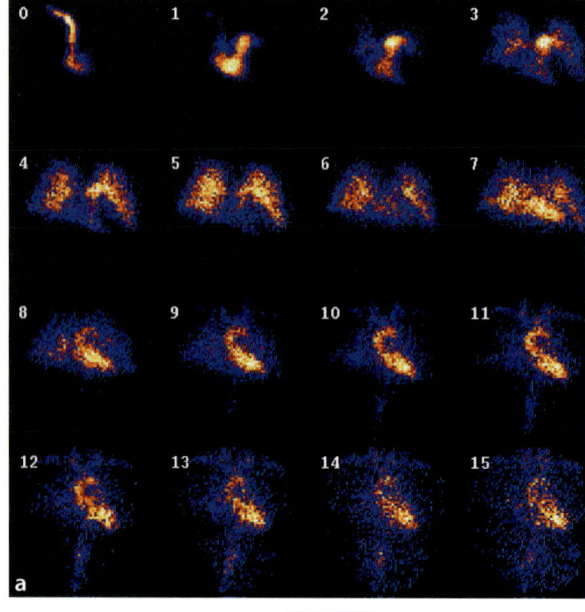
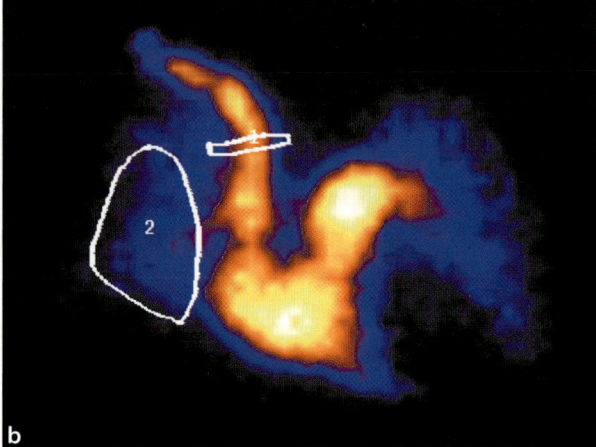
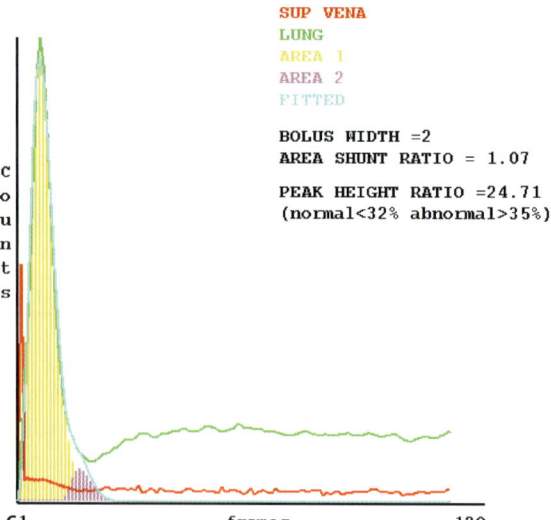

Fig. 30.1a,b,c (a) Normal first pass of a radioactive bolus through the central circulation. The SVC and RA are seen in Frame 0, RV in frame 1, PA in Frame 2 and 3, pulmonary circulation with normal clearance in frames 4–7, LV from Frame 7 and systemic circulation from Frame 9 onwards. The pulmonary clearance is normally rapid and the lung fields, RA and RV do not have tracer during the LV phase. (b) Analysis of the study: Regions of interest drawn over SVC and the lungs. (c) Region of interest drawn through the SVC indicates a satisfactory bolus width of 2 seconds (*red line*). The lung curve (*green*) overlaps with the fitted gamma function, is symmetrical and shows a crisp rapid downslope, indicating no early recirculation through the lungs. Qp/Qs value is 1.07, indicating that there is no left to right shunt

presence of left to right shunts. Fragmentation of the bolus can lead to difficulty in temporal separation of events and may lead to the wrong or misleading results. Hence operator experience in rapid injection of a tight bolus is very essential. Some centres have tried to achieve a good bolus by injecting in the early reactive hyperemic phase induced after inflating a blood-pressure cuff to a pressure above the arterial pressure for 3 minutes.

30.4
Radiopharmaceuticals

Technetium-99m Diethylenetriamine pentaacetic acid is widely used for first pass studies although any Technetium-99m labelled radiopharmaceutical can be used. The specific activity of the radiopharmaceutical should be high to ensure a small sized bolus.

30.5
Acquisition

Most modern gamma cameras are capable of acquiring at high-count rates, which are required to perform first pass studies. Images are usually acquired at 2 frames per second for 60 seconds on a 64×64 matrix. Electrocardiography (ECG) gated list mode acquisition is ideal for first pass imaging as it provides the flexibility of data review, re-binning and analysis [2]. Acquisition should be started a few seconds before the injection as the first few frames may otherwise be missed. Acquisition is generally performed in a single anterior or right anterior oblique view. Simultaneous biplanar acquisition with a double-headed camera has been tried to improve assessment of wall motion [3].

30.6
Quality Control

It is essential to assess the quality of the bolus before processing a first pass study. This can be done by drawing a region of interest through the superior venacava. The width of the time activity curve should be 3 seconds or less to ensure a good quality non-fragmented bolus. If the bolus is shown to be fragmented then further analysis may not be possible (Fig. 30.1b,c).

30.7
Clinical Roles

First pass radionuclide studies provide a simple method of assessing biventricular function, valvular regurgitation and left to right shunts without invasive pulmonary arterial catheterisation.

30.7.1
Determination of Ventricular Function

For determination of LV function the bolus of tracer is imaged as it passes through the cardiac chambers. Either left or right ventricular function can be determined although there is more experience with determination of left ventricular function.

A region of interest (ROI) is drawn over the left ventricle or right ventricle which can be separated from activity elsewhere by the temporal sequence of events. Ejection fraction can then be determined in the same way as for gated blood pool imaging (MUGA) using background-corrected end-diastolic and end-systolic images. Good correlation has been observed between ejection fraction and wall motion abnormalities observed on first pass studies and gated blood pool imaging [4].

This technique needs to be used with care in hearts with very abnormal anatomy, since it requires the acquisition of views of the ventricles that exclude counts from other chambers. In practice this can usually be achieved for the left ventricle, but often not satisfactorily with the right ventricle. In either case, the projection used for analysis of ventricular function needs to be chosen carefully, taking into account the abnormal anatomy [5].

30.7.2
Determination of Left to Right Shunts

Determination of the severity of the shunt is important for the management of patients with left to right shunts. Folse and Braunwald showed that left to right shunts could be diagnosed using pulmonary vascular curves using the peak counts of the initial and recirculation curves (C2/C1) [6]. However, further studies showed that this ratio cannot adequately differentiate between patients with shunts and valvular heart disease [7].

Treves et al. described a method of detecting left to right shunts and determining their severity by determination of pulmonary to systemic flow ratios using a first pass radionuclide study [8] This ratio is obtained after injection of a bolus of radioactivity intravenously and by fitting a gamma variate curve to time-activity curves generated drawing a manual region of interest in the lung. A newer method using factor analysis to provide automatic curve generation, which is less operator-dependent, was described by Mena et al. [9].

In a normal individual with no left to right shunting there is an initial rapid peak as the bolus passes through the lungs. This is followed by a late broad second peak, which is due to the tracer recirculating through the lungs after passing through the systemic circulation (Fig. 30.1c).

In the presence of a shunt, early recirculation is seen due to the tracer passing from the left heart to the right heart before systemic circulation occurs. This causes a second peak, usually on the downslope of the first (Fig. 30.2c). The area under the first peak ($A1$) is proportional to pulmonary blood flow (Qp). The area under the second peak ($A2$) is proportional to the shunt. The systemic blood flow (Qs) is equal to the difference between the pulmonary flow and the shunt ($A1-A2$).

The pulmonary to systemic flow ratio Qp/Qs can thus be calculated as

$A1/(A1-A2)$.

In the absence of a shunt $A2$ is 0 and the ratio is 1, i.e., systemic and pulmonary flow are equal. In practice, values less than 1.2 are considered normal taking into account statistical variations. The higher the ratio, the more severe the shunt.

The results obtained by Treves et al. show that this method can accurately quantitate the shunts when Qp/Qs is greater than 1.2 and less than 3.0 in patients with intracardiac left to right shunts, assuming that there is no bidirectional shunt. In patients with patent ductus arteriosus different shunt ratios may be obtained if the regions of interest are drawn over each lung. This is likely to reflect true haemodynamics due to differential shunting to each lung through the patent ductus.

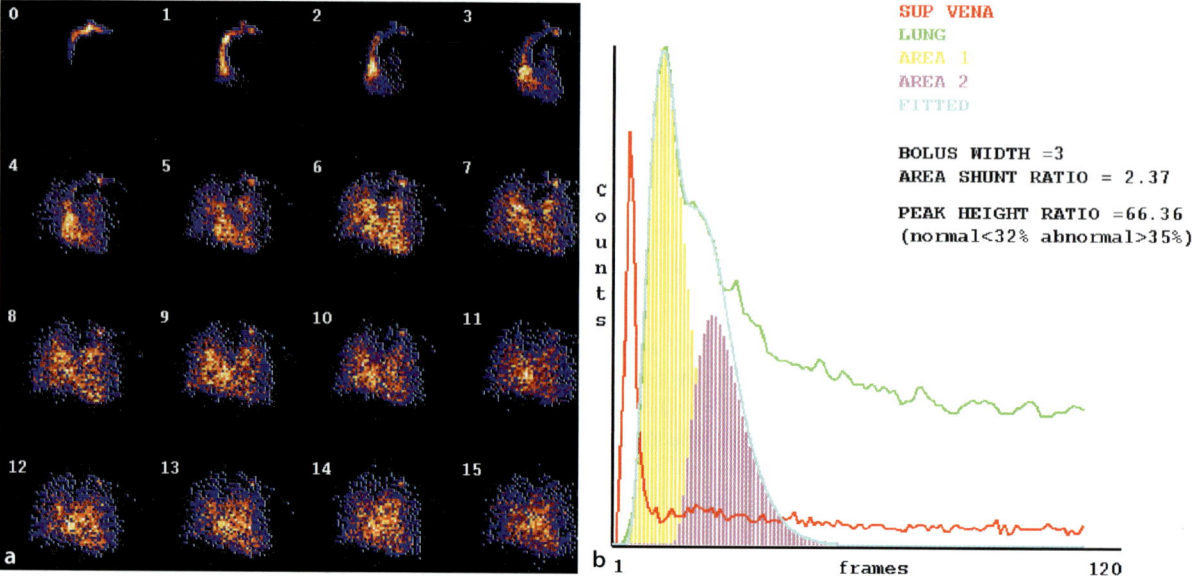

Fig. 30.2a,b Left to right shunt. (**a**) The first pass study shows RV in Frame 4, pulmonary circulation from Frame 5 onwards, and LV from Frame 6. Abnormal persistence of lung activity is seen even after LV is visualised due to the early pulmonary recirculation through the left to right shunt. (**b**) Satisfactory bolus is indicated by the SVC curve (*red*). The lung curve (*green*) is interrupted on its downslope by a second peak, which represents early recirculation through the lung through the left to right shunt. The Qp/Qs value is 2.37, indicating a significant shunt

It is very important to ensure that the bolus is not fragmented using the quality control method described above. In the original series by Treves et al. 15% of studies were not analysed due to fragmentation of the bolus. Deconvolution techniques have been tried to correct for the effect of fragmented bolus injections, but generally have not been very widely used [10, 11].

Factors other than the injection technique may cause spreading out of the bolus and affect the accuracy of the study. These include regurgitant tricuspid valve or pulmonary valve lesions or a dilated right ventricle (Fig. 30.3). Care should be taken to ensure that these factors are not present before undertaking the study. Other limitations of first pass studies include patients with bidirectional shunts.

Madsen et al. investigated a modified technique for quantifying Qp/Qs in left-to-right cardiac shunts. In this method, the gamma variate, which is fitted to the first pass portion of the lung curve, is used to generate a curve, which simulates the response of a normal lung curve with systemic recirculation. The difference between this curve and the observed lung curve is then used to calculate Qp/Qs. They claimed that this method was more accurate than the Maltz–Treves method and had less interobserver variability [12].

Rigo et al. described another method of measuring left to right shunts using gated equilibrium angiocardiography. In this method, Qp/Qs was measured as the right ventricular stroke counts divided by the left ventricular stroke counts and as the LV stroke counts divided by the RV stroke counts in patients with RV and LV diastolic volume overload, respectively [13]. The gamma variate method was found to be superior in the detection and estimation of small shunts, whereas the stroke count method yielded closer agreement with oximetry data when Qp/Qs was 2 or larger [14].

Table 30.1 Limitations of radionuclide first pass study in evaluation of left to right shunt

Tricuspid/pulmonary regurgitation
Right heart failure
Bidirectional shunt
Patent ductus arteriosus
Assessment of large shunts ($Qp/Qs > 3$)
Need for good venous access
Good injection technique

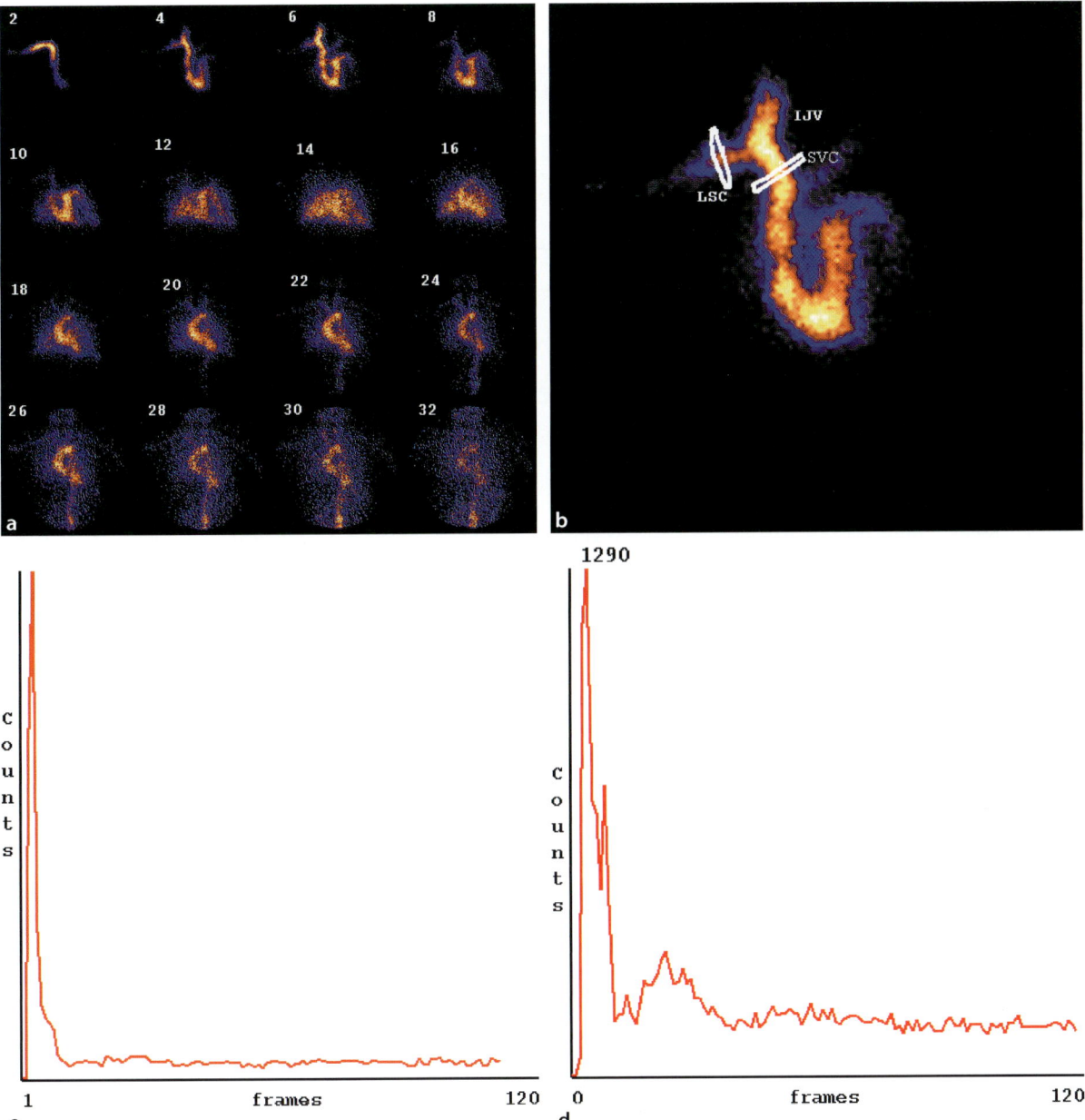

Fig. 30.3a,b Tricuspid valve regurgitation affecting first pass study. (**a**) The tracer is seen to pass normally through the left subclavian vein; subsequent frames show regurgitation of tracer from the RV into the SVC, left subclavian and internal jugular veins (IJV). (**b**) ROIs over left subclavian vein and superior venacava and regurgitant jet into the internal jugular vein (*arrow*). (**c**) ROI 1 over subclavian vein shows a tight bolus indicating good injection technique. (**d**) ROI 2 over the SVC demonstrates fragmentation of the bolus due to tracer regurgitation from the RV. Retrospective review revealed that the patient had tricuspid valve regurgitation, which affected analysis of the study yielding an inconclusive result

The other methods of determining Qp/Qs ratios are oximetry and Doppler echocardiography. Phase contrast MRI (PC MRI) has also been tried in this regard [15].

Baker et al. compared the ratio of pulmonary to systemic flow measured both by oximetry and first pass radionuclide angiography using the area under the curve method in 100 children with suspected left to right shunts. They concluded that although there are important limitations to the radionuclide method, it is the more precise and less invasive of the two, and is to be preferred when the accurate measurement of left to right shunts is required [16]. As all the above techniques have their limitations there is no single gold standard and often, clinical decisions may have to be based on a combination of these studies [17].

30.7.3
Determination of Right to Left Shunts

First pass studies are not useful in assessment of right to left shunts.

Tc-99m macroaggregates of albumin (MAA), which is extensively used for demonstration of pulmonary perfusion, can also be used to demonstrate right to left cardiac shunts. About 100,000 particles per dose is generally used for this application, which is half the number used in perfusion (V/Q) scanning.

Tc-99m-labelled nanocolloid can also be used for evaluating right to left shunts. In normal individuals without a right to left shunt the Tc-99m MAA particles are trapped in the pulmonary vasculature. In patients with right to left shunts a portion of the injected material bypasses the pulmonary circulation and lodges in the systemic capillaries and this can be used for shunt quantification. Appearance of Tc-99m MAA particles in the brain is more specific for a shunt than the kidneys.

A moderately large study comparing pulse oximetry and radioisotope measurement of right-to-left (R-L) shunt for the early detection of pulmonary arteriovenous malformations causing right to left shunt with digital subtraction angiography as gold standard showed that the radio-isotope method was superior, with sensitivity and specificity of 87 and 67%, respectively compared with corresponding values of 73 and 35% for the oximetry method [18].

30.8
Conclusion

There is a limited but useful role for first pass studies in assessment of patients with congenital heart disease. These studies provide useful functional information in patients for initial assessment and also for follow-up for long-term survivors of surgery for congenital heart disease.

References

1. Prinzmetal M, Corday E, Spritzler RJ, Flieg W (1949) Radiocardiography and its clinical applications. J Am Med Assoc 139:617.
2. Nichols K DePuey EG Rozanski A (1997) First-pass radionuclide angiocardiography with single crystal cameras. J Nucl Cardiol 4:61–73.
3. DePuey EG, Salensky H, Melancon S, Nichols KJ (1994) Simultaneous biplane first- pass radionuclide angiocardiography using a scintillation camera with two perpendicular detectors. J Nucl Med 35(10):1593–601.
4. Esquerre JP, Coca FJ, Gantet P, Ouhayoun E (1995) Feasibility of first pass radionuclide angiocardiography with a single crystal digital gamma camera. Eur J Nucl Med 22(6):521–527.
5. Baker E (2000) Radionuclide investigation of congenital heart disease. Heart 84:467–468.
6. Maltz DL, Treves S (1973) Quantitative radionuclide angiocardiography. Determination of Qp:Qs in children. Circulation XLVII(May):1049–1056.
7. Folse R, Braunwald E (1962) Pulmonary vascular dilution curves recorded by external detection in the diagnosis of left-to-right shunts. Br Heart J 24:166–167.
8. Stocker FP, Kinser J, Weber JW, Rosler H (1973) Paediatric radioangiocardiography: shunt diagnosis. Circulation 47:819.
9. Villanueva-Meyer J, Philippe L, Cordero S, Marcus CS and Mena I (1986) Use of factor analysis in the evaluation of left to right cardiac shunts. J Nucl Med 27(9):1442–1448.
10. Kuruc A, Treves S, Parker JA, Cheng C, Sawan A (1983) Radionuclide angiocardiography: an improved deconvolution technique after suboptimal bolus injection. Radiology 148(1):233–238.
11. Brendel AJ, Commenges D, Salamon R, Ducassou D, Blanquet P (1983) Decovolution analysis of radionuclide angiocardiography curves: problems arising from fragmented bolus injections. Eur J Nucl Med 8(3):93–98.
12. Madsen MT, Argenyi E, Preslar J, Grover-McKay J, Kirchner PT (1991) An improved method for the quantification of left-to-right cardiac shunts. J Nucl Med 32(9):1808–1812.
13. Rigo P, Chevigne M (1982) Measurement of left-to-right shunts by gated radionuclide angiography. J Nucl Med 23(12):1070–1075.
14. Eterovic D, Dujic Z, Popovis S, Miric D Gated versus first pass radioangiography in the valuation of left to right shunts. Clin Nucl Med 20(6):534–537.
15. Beerbaum P, Körperich H, Barth P, Esdorn H, Meyer H (2001) Noninvasive quantification of left-to-right shunt in pediatric patients. Circulation 103:2476.

16. Baker EJ, Ellam SV, Lorber A, Jones OD, Maisey MN (1985) Superiority of radionuclide over oximetric measurement of left to right shunts. Br Heart J 53(5):535–540.
17. Evangelista A, Aguade S, Candell-Riera J, Angel J, Soler-Soler J et al. (1998) Quantification of left to right shunt in atrial septal defect using oximetry, isotopes and Doppler echocardiography. Rev Esp Cardiol 51Suppl 1: 2–9.
18. Thompson RD, Jackson JA. Peters M, Doré CJ, Hughes JMB (1999) Sensitivity and specificity of radioisotope right-left shunt measurements and pulse oximetry for the early detection of pulmonary arteriovenous malformations. Chest 115:109–113.

Cardiac PET: Physics and Methodology

Lefteris Livieratos

Contents

31.1	Introduction	363
31.2	Basic Principles of PET Imaging	364
31.2.1	Positron Emission and Positron Annihilation	364
31.2.2	PET Detection Systems	365
31.3	Data Acquisition	367
31.3.1	Performance Characteristics of PET Systems	368
31.4	Data Processing and Corrections	370
31.4.1	The Attenuation Problem	371
31.4.2	Detector Normalisation	372
31.4.3	Randoms Correction	373
31.4.4	Scatter Correction	373
31.4.5	Image Reconstruction	374
31.4.6	Gated and Dynamic Data Acquisition	374
31.4.7	Tracer Kinetic Modelling	374
31.5	Recent Trends in Cardiac PET Imaging	374
	References	375

31.1 Introduction

Positron emission tomography (PET) is an imaging modality that uses positron emitting radioisotopes to provide measurements of regional tissue function in vivo. Its advantages include the ability to utilise isotopes of elements naturally occurring in biological molecules and its unique property to provide an exact solution to the problem of photon attenuation, thus allowing accurate representation of tracer concentrations in the images. Clinical applications of PET are found in Oncology, Cardiology, Neurology and Psychiatry. Examples of positron emitting isotopes used in PET imaging are shown in Table 31.1. In the field of Cardiology, measurements of tracer concentrations in vivo provide an invaluable tool for the diagnosis and study of cardiac physiology and disease. Positron emission tomography has found application in Cardiology in studies of regional myocardial blood flow, metabolism and pharmacology.

Single photon imaging techniques, such as ^{201}Tl or ^{99m}Tc imaging with either planar scintigraphy or SPECT, used for the assessment of tissue perfusion, only allow the detection of directional changes of regional myocardial blood flow. Advances in PET methodology and tracer kinetic modelling make it possible to use the inherent quantitative ability of PET to measure myocardial blood flow (MBF) in absolute terms (e.g., in mL/min/100g of tissue). A number of tracers have been employed to measure MBF with PET, including ^{15}O-labelled water ($H_2^{15}O$) [1–3], ^{13}N-labelled ammonia ($^{13}NH_3$) [4, 5], and ^{82}Rb [6]. Although there is still a discussion about the ideal MBF tracer [7], $H_2^{15}O$ and $^{13}NH_3$ are most widely used, with the former considered theoretically superior as it is metabolically inert, freely diffusable and independent of myocardial flow rate and metabolism, and the latter providing better image quality. Quantification of MBF with PET made it possible to study cardiac function at rest and stress at the level of the coronary microvasculature, previously restricted to investigations of epicardial coronary arteries with other technique [8].

In the area of myocardial metabolism, PET found application in studies of oxidative metabolism and glucose

Table 31.1 Properties of the most commonly used radioisotopes in PET

Nuclide	E_{max} (MeV)	E_{mode} (MeV)	$t_{½}$ (min)	Range in water (mm)		Examples of labelled compounds
				Max	Mean (FWHM)	
^{11}C	0.959	0.326	20.4	4.1	1.1	Precursor for organic molecules ^{11}C-HED and ^{11}C-CGP – pre- and post-synaptic autonomic function ^{11}C-MQNB muscarinic receptors
^{13}N	1.197	0.432	9.96	5.1	1.5	^{13}NH$_3$
^{15}O	1.738	0.696	2.03	7.3	2.5	^{15}O$_2$, H$_2$^{15}O, C^{15}O, C^{15}O$_2$
^{18}F	0.633	0.202	109.8	2.4	0.6	[^{18}F]-DG, ^{18}F-
^{68}Ga	1.898	0.783	68.3	8.2	2.9	[^{68}Ga]-EDTA
^{82}Rb	3.40	1.385	1.25	14.1	5.9	^{82}RbCl

utilisation. Glucose utilisation by the myocardium can be assessed with [^{18}F]-2-fluoro-2-deoxyglucose (FDG) [9] although absolute quantification is restricted to measurements under standardised dietary conditions, e.g., during insulin clamp [8]. PET measurements with FDG have been used to study myocardial viability [10], to assess the condition of patients undergoing revascularisation [11] and, in conjunction with MBF measurements, to study hibernating myocardium [8].

A number of tracers have been used to study myocardial oxidative metabolism. Palmitate labelled with ^{11}C has been used to study fatty acid metabolism in acute myocardial ischaemia [12], and ^{11}C-labelled acetate was used as an indirect marker of myocardial oxygen consumption [13]. However, due to the complexity of tissue kinetics, no appropriate models were established to allow absolute quantification [8]. Use of ^{15}O-labelled molecular oxygen to quantify myocardial oxygen consumption has been more successful [14].

In the area of myocardial pharmacology, a number of ligands have been labelled and used in PET Cardiology [8, 15] and include studies with the β-adrenoceptor antagonist ^{11}C-labelled CGP12177, and pre-synaptic sympathetic receptor studies with ^{18}F-fluorometaraminol, ^{18}F-fluorodopamine and ^{11}C-hydroxyephedrine.

31.2 Basic Principles of PET Imaging

31.2.1 Positron Emission and Positron Annihilation

Positrons are positively charged electrons emitted from a proton-rich nucleus as part of its radioactive disintegration. The energy spectrum of the emitted beta particles is continuous up to a maximum energy E_{max}, which is characteristic for the nucleus (Table 31.1). The general form of the positron emission scheme is:

$$^{A}_{Z}X \longrightarrow\ ^{A}_{Z-1}Y + ^{0}_{+1}\beta^{+} + ^{0}_{0}\nu + E$$

The excess energy E released during decay is shared between the particles produced. In many cases, the daughter nucleus Y returns to its stable state and an orbital electron is ejected from the atom, producing the characteristic X-rays that may be observed superimposed on the continuous spectrum of the positrons.

After emission from the nucleus, the positron continuously loses kinetic energy by interactions with surrounding atoms as it passes through matter. In this process the positron is continuously deflected from its original path. The finite range that positrons have to travel before annihilation, contributes uncertainty to the localisation of the originating nucleus and imposes a lower limit on the spatial resolution of the technique. Positron range, and consequently the uncertainty in

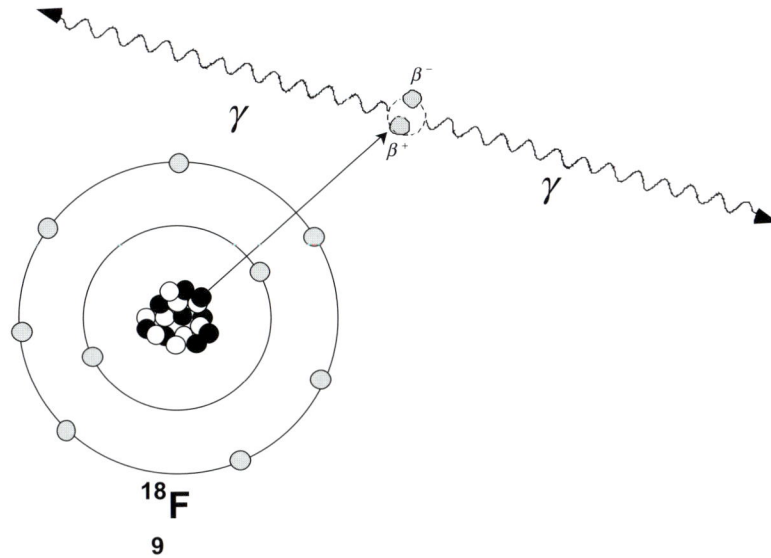

Fig. 31.1 Schematic diagram of positron annihilation

spatial localisation associated with it, increases with increasing initial energy of the positron (Table 31.1).

The positron eventually combines with an electron when both are essentially at rest. The metastable intermediate hydrogen-like element positronium (mean life ~10^{-7} s) may be formed by the positron and electron combining. Formation of positronium has a low probability in water or tissue where direct annihilation of the electron and the positron is more favourable. The positron and electron eventually combine and annihilate, emitting two photons of 511 keV (the rest-mass equivalent of each particle). The two photons are emitted at 180° to each other in order to conserve momentum (Fig. 31.1). The emission of three photons has also a small probability (<1%) to occur.

In many cases a non-zero momentum before the annihilation results in the photon pair not being emitted strictly at 180°. This contributes a further uncertainty to the localisation of the nuclear decay event of ~0.5° FWHM from strictly 180°, which can degrade resolution by a further 1.5 mm (dependent on the distance between the two coincidence detectors).

31.2.2
PET Detection Systems

31.2.2.1 Annihilation Coincidence Detection

The fundamental measurement in PET is the detection of the two photons that emerge from a positron annihilation event. This relies on the principle of "annihilation coincidence detection" (ACD) (Fig. 31.2). ACD takes advantage of the fact that the two annihilation photons are emitted in opposite directions and emerge simultaneously from the same event. Therefore, if two photons are detected by two opposing detectors simultaneously (i.e., within a narrow time interval), their originating positron annihilation event is registered along the volume defined by the two detectors, which is referred to as a line of response (LOR).

Since ACD defines the annihilation event within a specific LOR without the use of physical collimation, it is often described as an "electronic collimation" technique. Unlike single-photon detection where physical collimation is used to provide positional information, electronic collimation allows the detection of events for each detector in coincidence with multiple opposing detectors. This results in a significant increase in sensitivity of up to 10–20 times in 2D mode and ~150 times in 3D, compared with single-photon detection such as in SPECT [16, 17]. Since, with electronic collimation, the position of the annihilation event is confined within the LOR between the two detectors, another consequence of ACD is the uniform spatial response in PET. This is demonstrated by the "point spread function" (PSF), the spatial profile of a point source as a function of position, which remains fairly constant within the field of view of the two detectors, unlike single-photon detection where the PSF is significantly depth-dependent [18].

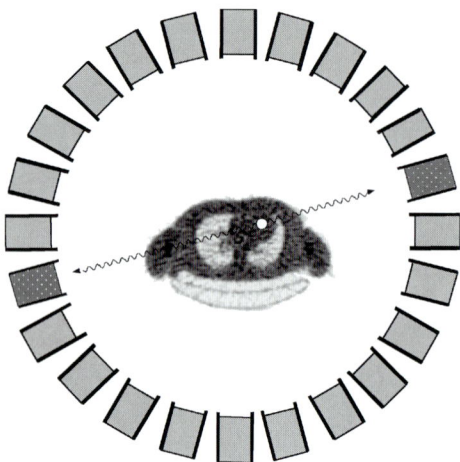

Fig. 31.2 Schematic diagram of PET scanner indicating detection of annihilation photons by two opposing detectors in coincidence

31.2.2.2 Types of Coincidence Events

The detection of events in PET relies on the two photons being detected within a coincidence timing window and subsequently being both within a defined energy window and forming a line within acceptable geometry. Those events that satisfy the above criteria are usually referred to as prompt events. The aim of PET is to record true coincidence events, formed by the two photons of an annihilation, which are detected within the coincidence timing window without having undergone any interaction with matter. However, in reality not all prompt events are true coincidence events; they may also correspond to scattered, random or multiple coincidences (Fig. 31.3).

Scattered coincidences occur when one or both of the photons have undergone at least one Compton scattering prior to being detected within the coincidence timing window. Since the direction of the photon is changed after Compton scattering, the detected coincidence will result in the event being wrongly registered outside the originating LOR. This also includes the assignment of a false LOR due to a photon originating from outside the field of view of the tomograph. Due to the low energy loss in forward scattering and the relatively poor energy resolution of most detectors used in PET, scattered events cannot easily be distinguished electronically on the basis of their energy. Scattered coincidences contribute a low frequency background to the final image, resulting in decreased contrast and compromised quantification. The distribution of scatter, for specific scanner geometry, depends on the distribution of activity, shape and size of the object. In order to improve signal-to-noise and recover accurate quantification, corrections for scattered coincidences must be applied, often at the expense of increased noise in the images.

Random coincidences occur when two photons from different annihilation events are accidentally detected within the same coincidence timing window. Since the detected photons originate from spatially unrelated annihilation events, the corresponding LOR will be wrongly assigned to the acquired data. This may also include the assignment of a false LOR due to one or both of the photons originating from outside the field of view of the scanner. The detection of random coincidences contributes a fairly uniform background to the final image, resulting in decreased contrast and overestimation

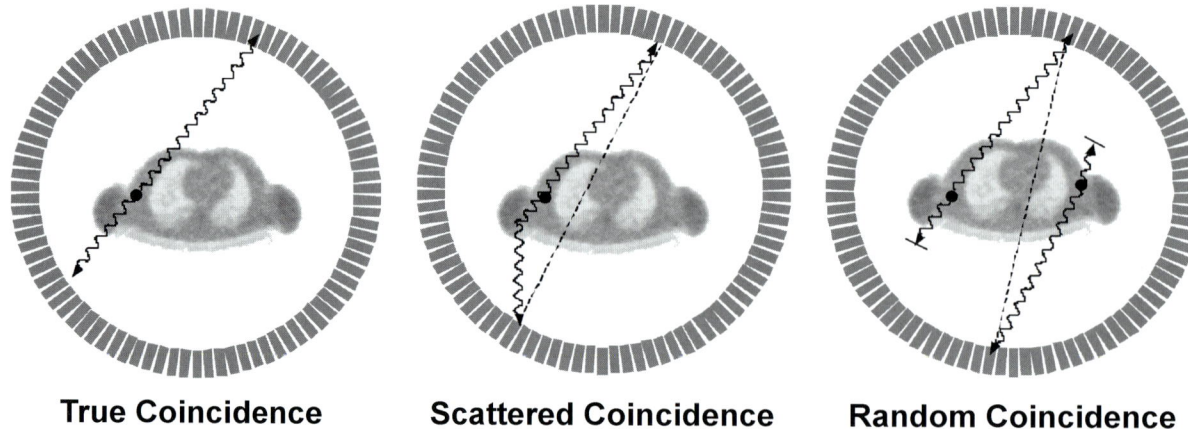

Fig. 31.3 Types of coincidence events

of activity concentrations. Random coincidences can be corrected by subtracting an estimate from the prompt events for each LOR (at the expense of added noise). Estimates of random events are often obtained during acquisition using a delayed window or calculated from the single photon or prompt event rates.

Multiple coincidences occur when three photons from different annihilation events are detected within the coincidence timing window. Due to the ambiguity in assigning a LOR, multiple coincidences are simply discarded.

removing the septa and acquiring all available data (an acquisition mode referred to as 3D mode), even at the expense of increased acceptance of scatter and random coincidences, this was not realised until the 1980s when reconstruction algorithms capable of handling these data became available [19–21]. The significant sensitivity improvement in 3D mode, realised initially in brain imaging, led to the development of the first commercial scanner with mechanically retractable septa [22] and the feature became available in subsequent commercial multi-ring systems.

31.3
Data Acquisition

Although various geometries and types of detectors have been employed in the development of PET systems, the ring geometry remains until now the predominant design for commercial PET systems. Such systems utilise a large number of crystal detector elements arranged as a stack of rings surrounding the object (typically >500 crystals per ring, >20 detector rings). Large area detectors have also been used in a number of designs; however, these are associated with the problem of increased detector dead-time and consequently restricted count rate performance as a larger individual detector encounters a higher number of photons.

The detection of photons in PET is similar to the scintillation process in a gamma-camera. Incident photons interact with the detector producing ionisation of the crystal lattice consequently resulting in de-excitation of the crystal via the emission of visible light (Fig. 31.4). Single detector elements are often coupled together, with their light shared by a number of photomultiplier tubes (PMTs), although one-to-one coupling has also been employed in a number of PET designs. Visible light produced by the scintillation process is converted into an electron by the photocathode of the PMT and consequently amplified by the anodes of the PMT to produce current detectable by the front-end electronics of the system. Simultaneous (i.e., within a finite time window) detection of two photons in opposing detector elements is registered by the system as a prompt coincidence event.

Annular shielding (septa) may be permanently or temporarily retracted between detector rings in order to restrict detection of annihilation photons only within the cross-section of the object defined by a detector ring (Fig. 31.5). The presence of septa dramatically reduces the detection of scatter coincidences however at the expense of overall reduction in sensitivity. This mode of acquisition with inter-plane septa is often referred to as 2D mode. Despite the obvious benefit in sensitivity by

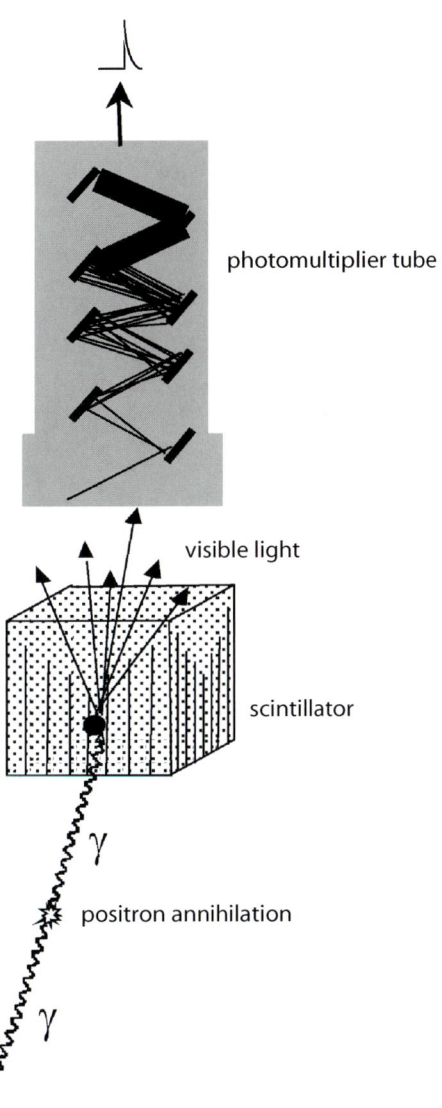

Fig. 31.4 Schematic diagram of the scintillation process in PET

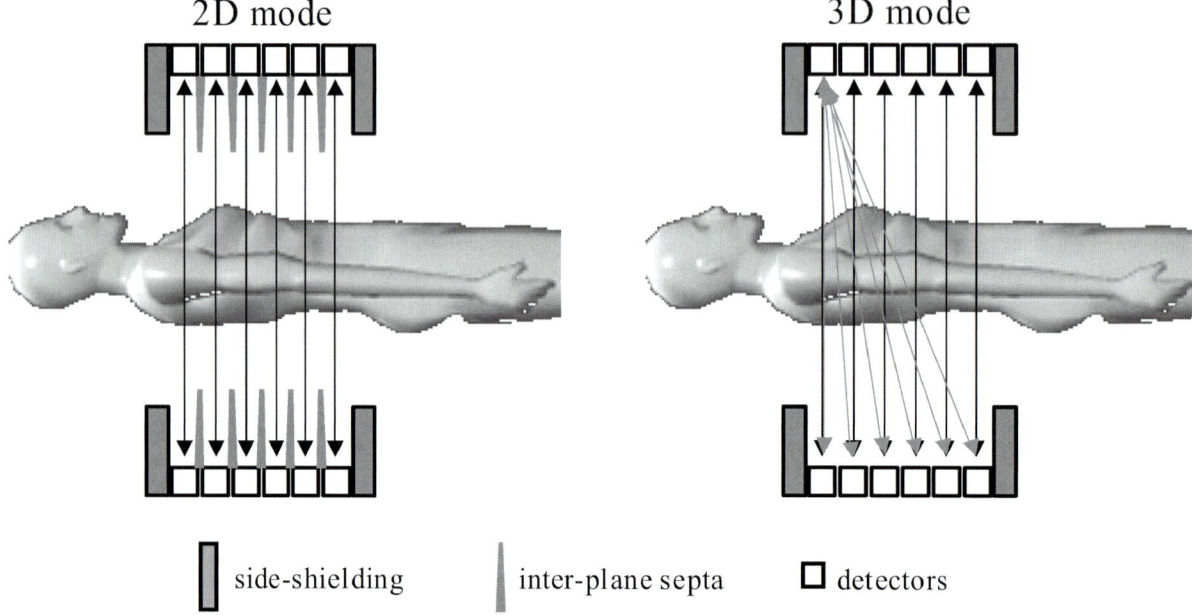

Fig. 31.5 Schematic diagram of scanner cross-section through detector rings demonstrating 2D and 3D PET acquisition modes

31.3.1
Performance Characteristics of PET Systems

A number of fundamental properties define the performance of a tomograph for PET imaging. Standard protocols for characterising a PET system have been defined [23–25] and are periodically amended [26]. Generally, a PET system with high spatial resolution, a low contribution from scatter or mechanisms to account for it and high true coincidences detection sensitivity over a wide dynamic range of count rates is desirable. However, depending on clinical application, different priorities might be set or additional features may be required. In cardiac imaging, and specifically for tracers with rapid presence in the field-of-view of the scanner during the first-pass through the heart, the count rate performance of the PET system becomes important. In this section we look at the main performance characteristics of PET systems.

31.3.1.1 Spatial Resolution

Spatial resolution, expressed in terms of the full width at half maximum (FWHM) and full width at tenth maximum (FWTM) of the point spread function, is usually measured at a number of axial and transaxial positions using a point or line source of activity. Current PET systems capable of cardiac imaging have intrinsic spatial resolution of 4–6 mm.

Factors affecting the spatial resolution of a PET system include [27, 28]:
- the inherent properties of positron range and non-collinearity of the annihilation photons;
- the dimensions of the detector elements;
- the light output of the detectors;
- the distance between the detector elements and the geometry of septa if present;
- the stopping power of the detector material;
- the incident angle of the photons in the detectors, affected by the detection geometry;
- the data sampling pattern and potentially, any data reduction schemes applied to the data after acquisition [29, 30].

In addition to the inherent properties of the PET system, the image reconstruction parameters, such as noise-reduction filters, will affect the resolution of the final image. Spatial resolution on the reconstructed transverse images of current PET scanners is typically around 6 mm.

Good spatial resolution is desirable in order to avoid partial volume effects. However, improvements in resolution should be accompanied by approximately a cubic improvement in sensitivity in order to maintain signal-to-noise levels [31].

31.3.1.2 Energy Resolution

The energy resolution of a system depends on the properties of the detector elements. Increasing the effective atomic number of the detector material increases the probability of incident photons depositing all their energy within the detector element, improving the definition of the photopeak. Increasing the size of the detector elements will have a similar effect, but at the expense of spatial resolution. Typically, energy resolution between 10% and 20% (FWHM) at 511 keV is observed in most systems [28].

Good energy resolution is desirable for better discrimination of scattered photons, especially for 3D PET where scatter presence is higher. However, due to the poor energy resolution of most PET systems, direct elimination of scatter is not feasible and a broad acquisition energy window is defined around the photopeak, typically between 350 and 850 keV.

31.3.1.3 Scatter Fraction

Scatter fraction is a measure of the relative sensitivity of the PET system to photons scattered in the object or off the components of the tomograph such as side-shielding and the detectors. Generally, the scatter fraction is expressed as the ratio of scattered to total coincidences (scattered plus unscattered) for a given object and activity distribution. For a given object, scatter fraction depends upon the acquisition energy window, the scanner geometry, the presence of septa and side-shielding. Typically, scatter fraction is around 10% in 2D while in 3D, due to the increased acceptance of scatter in the absence of septa, it increases to around 35%. Although numerous scatter correction schemes have been developed (Sect. 31.4.4), a low contribution from scatter into the raw data, demonstrated by a low scatter fraction, is always more desirable for a PET system.

31.3.1.4 Count-Rate Performance

Detector dead-time refers to the system's inability to respond to a new event for a short time after the detection and processing of a proceeding event. It is ascribed to both limitations of the scintillation crystal and the pulse-processing electronics. The resulting dead-time losses become significant at higher count rates and it is therefore important to assess them as a function of activity levels. However, count-rate measurements cannot be directly related to signal-to-noise in the final image. Furthermore, comparison of performance for different scanners, or different acquisition conditions on the same scanner, are difficult to make due to the strong dependence of count rates on the physical parameters of the system. For these reasons, the concept of noise equivalent counts (NEC) [32] is often used as a more objective means for performance evaluation related to image quality. Noise equivalent counts express the count rate after the influence of scatter and random events has been taken into account.

Count-rate performance, influenced by random and scattered coincidences and dead-time, is strongly dependent on scanner geometry. Due to the removal of interplane septa in 3D PET and the trend for larger axial FOV, the influence from activity from outside the scanner's direct FOV may also become significant through an extended exposure to single events. As a result of increased single photon flux, detectors may experience increased dead-time, random coincidence rate and scatter from outside the FOV degrading image quality. It is important to take these effects into consideration when optimising the acquisition parameters for a scanning protocol, especially for studies such as cardiac blood flow, which involve a rapid uptake of the tracer through the heart before it is distributed through the body, requiring a wide count-rate dynamic range.

31.3.1.5 Sensitivity

The sensitivity of a PET scanner, expressed as the unscattered true coincidence count rate per unit activity concentration, depends on a number of parameters [25, 33] such as the detector material, size and packing fraction, the geometry of the detector ring and interplane septa, the energy window and acquisition mode (2D/3D). Scanner sensitivity may be quoted as either the count rate per unit activity concentration for a 20 cm diameter cylinder after subtraction of scatter at low randoms and dead-time [24, 25] or as absolute sensitivity in air [26, 34], which provides a sensitivity measure free of the influence of scatter and attenuation. High sensitivity is generally desirable in order to achieve acquisition of data with sufficient signal-to-noise within the dose and scanning time constrains. Scanner sensitivity after scatter subtraction is in the range of 200–300 kcps/μCi/mL in 2D and 500–1300 kcps/μCi/mL in 3D mode [35]. Absolute sensitivity varies between 0.004 cps/Bq in 2D mode and 0.058 cps/Bq in 3D.

31.3.1.6 Detector Scintillators

The performance characteristics of a PET system will ultimately be defined by its geometry and the physical properties of the detectors. The characteristics of an ideal scintillator include [35, 36]:

- high detection efficiency, which requires high effective atomic number and high density for large cross-section of interaction;
- short decay constant, for good coincidence timing accuracy, low dead-time and high count-rate capabilities;
- high light output, for high spatial resolution and packing ratio of the detector elements with PMTs or other photodetectors;
- good energy resolution, for the discrimination of scattered events;
- refraction index similar to that of the optical coupling of the photodetector for optimal transmission of the scintillation light;
- good mechanical and physical properties such as radiation hardness, non-hydroscopic properties and ruggedness to allow fabrication of small crystals.

The physical properties of some of the scintillator materials used in PET are listed in Table 31.2. Despite the investigation of a large number of scintillators for PET, BGO and NaI(Tl) have been predominately used. BGO became the dominant detector for commercial PET systems, mainly due to its high detection efficiency, however, new materials with shorter decay times, like LSO and GSO, have recently been introduced with the aim to improve count-rate performance of current PET systems.

31.4
Data Processing and Corrections

Apart from the biological affinity of PET tracers to physiological processes, the main advantage of PET is its potential to provide images where counts are related to activity concentrations in the body with no dependence of the position of each voxel within the object. In order to achieve this, a number of corrections need to be applied to the data. Attenuation correction is of major importance for cardiac PET due to the high attenuation encountered by photons transmitted through the body and the non-uniform attenuation in the thorax. Corrections for detector efficiency variations and for random and scatter coincidences, which are generally high in the body, are also important in order to restore accurate representation of activity concentrations and avoid artefacts. After initial corrections projection data are reconstructed to form the final image. Further analysis such as region-of-interest analysis and tracer kinetic modelling may be employed in order to extract physiological measures such as myocardial blood flow.

Table 31.2 Physical properties of some of the detector materials used in PET (collated from [28, 36, 73])

	Sodium Iodide (NaI(Tl))	Bismuth Germanate (BGO)	Cerium-doped Lutetium Orthosilicate (LSO)	Cerium-doped Gadolinium Orthosilicate (GSO)	Cesium Fluoride (CsF)	Barium Fluoride (BaF$_2$)
Effective atomic number	51	75	65	59	52	53
Density (g/cc)	3.7	7.1	7.4	6.71	4.64	4.88
Scintillation efficiency (% of NaI(Tl))	100	15	75	25	5	5
Peak wavelength (nm)	410	480	420	440	390	225,310
Scintillation decay time (nsec)	230	300	40	56,600	5	0.8,620
Hygroscopic?	yes	no	no	no	yes	no

31.4.1
The Attenuation Problem

For the 511 keV photons produced by positron annihilation, Compton scattering is the dominant mechanism of interaction in human tissue. As a photon beam passes through matter, each of the interactions that take place removes photons from the beam. For a well-collimated geometry (narrow-beam geometry) the attenuation of a mono-energetic photon beam through matter is described by an exponential function:

$$I(x) = I_0 e^{-\mu x} \quad (31.1)$$

where I_0 is the intensity of the unattenuated photon beam and $I(x)$ is the intensity of the photon beam measured at a thickness x through an absorber of linear attenuation coefficient $\mu = \mu(Z,E)$ at the energy E. The linear attenuation coefficient of an absorber expresses a macroscopic measure of the probability of interaction of photons with matter per unit distance through the absorber. The linear attenuation coefficient is expressed in units of (length)$^{-1}$ and it is a function of the atomic number Z of the absorber and the energy E of the incident photons. The linear attenuation coefficient at the photon energy of 511 keV for water/soft-tissue is $^{\text{soft-tissue}}\mu_{(511\text{kev})} = 0.096$ cm^{-1} while for bone and lead is $^{\text{bone}}\mu_{(511\text{kev})} = 0.173$ cm^{-1} and $^{\text{lead}}\mu_{(511\text{kev})} = 1.83$ cm^{-1}, respectively [16, 28, 37].

The effect of attenuation is that the number of coincidence events detected along a line of response will be reduced by an exponential factor (similar to that in Eq. (31.1)) compared with the number of events originally emerging along the line. The advantage of PET is that this exponential factor describing the loss of counts due to photon attenuation (also referred to as attenuation raysum) is independent of the exact emission site of the two annihilation photons along the line of response. Figure 31.6 demonstrates that the attenuation raysum through a LOR is independent of the position of the source along the LOR. The attenuation along the measured LOR through the object will be:

$$e^{-\int_{-\infty}^{+\infty} dy_r \mu(x,y)} = e^{-\mu x} e^{-\mu(D-x)} = e^{-\mu D} \quad (31.2)$$

assuming constant linear attenuation coefficient μ within the object (Fig. 31.6a). (For non-uniform distribution of attenuation coefficients the local value $\mu(x,y)$ at each point along the LOR will be taken into account in the calculation of the raysum.) Thus, the integral is independent of the position of annihilation along the detected LOR. This property is utilised to correct for photon attenuation in PET by transmission measurements with sources outside the body (Fig. 31.6b). The analytical solution to the problem of attenuation is unique in PET and it is one of the fundamental advantages of the modality, unlike in SPECT, where attenuation depends on the exact depth of the origin of the photons (which is generally not known).

The attenuation raysums can be derived either by calculations, assuming a distribution of $\mu(x,y)$ [38] when this is fairly uniform across the object, or, most commonly, by transmission measurements. In transmission measurements with external sources the attenuation raysums are obtained according to Eq. (31.2) as the ratio of the un-attenuated counts measured with no object in the field of view (often referred to as blank scan), to the counts transmitted through the object.

Early PET tomographs used a positron emitting rod source of ^{68}Ge-^{68}Ga (half-life of parent ^{68}Ge, $t_{1/2} = 270.8$d) that was extended in front of the detectors during transmission scanning [18]. Annihilation events are recorded in coincidence mode between the detectors close to the source and the opposing detectors (Fig. 31.7a). In later designs the ring source was replaced by a rotating rod source [39] (Fig. 31.7b) in a geometry which remained common through to later generations of PET tomographs. This geometry allowed the electronic masking or windowing of the data to restrict acceptance of those events that were collinear with the position of the source. This technique reduced the acceptance of scatter and random events and al-

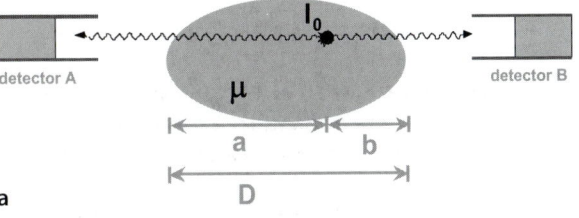

a

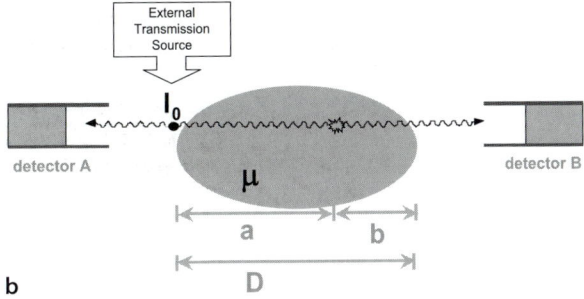

b

Fig. 31.6 Attenuation through an object in coincidence detection, notation as in Eq. (2)

lowed post-injection transmission and simultaneous emission-transmission scanning [40] for increased patient throughput. The use of single photon detection for transmission measurements was later implemented in a number of systems [41–43] mainly because of the dramatic increase in count rate compared to coincidence transmission measurements and advantages related to the half-life, cost and availability of radioisotopes suitable for single photon transmission sources (e.g., ^{137}Cs, $t_{1/2} = 30.2$ years, $E_\gamma = 662$ keV).

More recently with the introduction of combined PET/CT scanners the use of X-ray CT data for attenuation correction of the PET data became possible [44, 45]. The complex dependence of attenuation coefficients by both the photon energy and the effective atomic number of the absorbing material requires some treatment of the CT data prior to use for correction of the 511 keV photons. This often involves image segmentation of the CT data into classes (bone, soft-tissue) and independent scaling of values for each class of voxels. One major implication of the introduction of combined PET/CT systems is the reduction of the transmission scan duration, and consequently overall study duration. This reduction in transmission scan duration may be more beneficial in oncology studies that involve the acquisition of several bed positions to cover most of the body.

Accurate attenuation correction is of major importance for cardiac imaging [46] especially due to the magnitude of attenuation correction factors in the thorax that can reach values in the range 60–100 for certain projections through the body. Furthermore, the attenuation encountered by photons transmitted through the thorax is highly non-uniform due to differences in the attenuation coefficients in lung, bone and soft-tissue. An example of the effect of attenuation correction on reconstructed cardiac ^{18}FDG data is shown in Fig. 31.7. Tracer uptake across the myocardium can be severely affected by the effects of photon attenuation as demonstrated by the comparison of the attenuation corrected and non-corrected images.

31.4.2
Detector Normalisation

Lines-of-response acquired within a data set have different efficiency due to a number of reasons, including: detector efficiency variations, i.e., due to the position

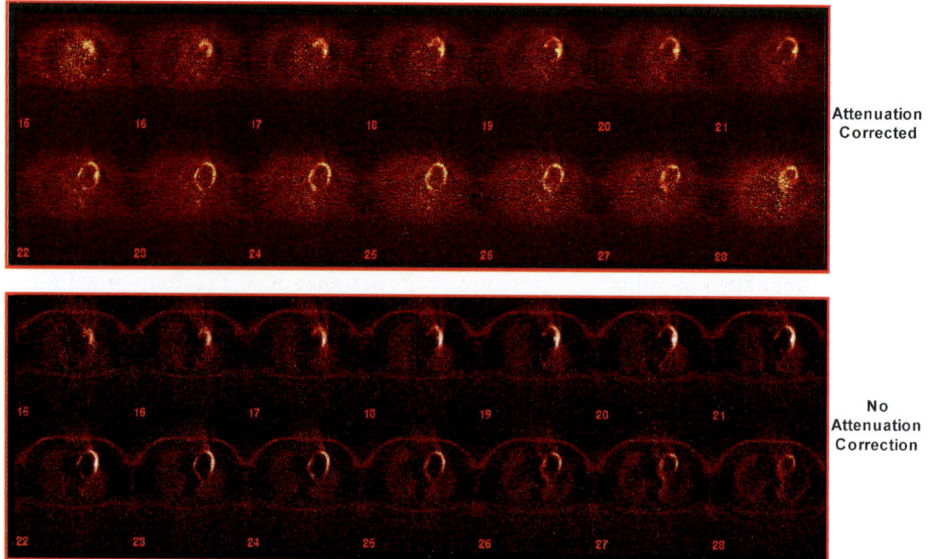

Cardiac FDG: 40-50 mins post injection; 5mm transverse slices; ECAT EXACT 3D

Fig. 31.7 Example of cardiac FDG scan demonstrating the effect of attenuation correction to myocardial activity distribution

of detector elements within the scanner, physical variations in crystal and variations in PMT gains, geometric effects, such as variations in spacing and width of LORs, detection solid angle and incident angle of photons and sampling pattern due to merging of LORs for data compression. Other effects, such as structural alignment of the detectors or shadowing from the septa, may also cause variations in the efficiency of the LORs. Correction for these effects is important in order to avoid image artefacts and inaccuracies in quantification. The process of correcting for these differences in the efficiency of the LORs is called normalisation. Generally, detector efficiencies are calculated from the inverse of the counts from uniform irradiation with a planar, ring or rotating line source [47]. Typically several hours are required to acquire data of adequate statistical quality since low activity levels must be used to avoid dead-time effects. In an attempt to improve the statistical properties of normalisation, hence reducing acquisition times to practical levels, methods based on modelling normalisation coefficients into a series of individual components, each reflecting a particular source of detector non-uniformities, have also been employed [48].

31.4.3
Randoms Correction

Random coincidences occur because of the finite width of the time window used in coincidence detection. Narrowing the coincidence time window would reduce the number of detected random events, however, at the expense of detected true coincidences unless a faster detector is used. Random coincidences contribute a fairly uniform background, resulting in decreased contrast and overestimation of activity concentrations, and therefore it is necessary to estimate and remove them from the data. A number of schemes have been used for randoms correction. The most commonly used method estimates randoms using a delayed coincidence circuit [49]. A second circuit, parallel to the coincidence detection, is employed with a delay well beyond the coincidence resolving time (typically, coincidence resolving time for a BGO system of ~12 ns, delay window of 50–100 ns) thus no true coincidences will be registered. The randoms are then estimated by the coincidence rate at this delayed circuit and can be subtracted on-line from the prompt events or stored separately for later processing. The method of the delayed coincidence circuit has the advantage of detecting accurately the randoms at the same count-rate/dead-time conditions as for the prompts. However, the statistical noise in the randoms estimate is added back to the data through the subtraction from the prompts, effectively doubling the noise related to random events.

Randoms rates can also be calculated from the single event rates of the individual detectors, S_A and S_B and the resolving time 2τ, as:

$$R_{AB} = 2\tau S_A S_B$$

The advantage of this method is a better statistical quality as the singles count rates are generally two orders of magnitude higher than the randoms rate. However, for the same reason, detector dead-time due to singles is higher and differences with random event rates may need to be accounted for.

31.4.4
Scatter Correction

While in 2D PET scatter in the thorax is typically less than 15%, scattered coincidences in 3D PET may contribute up to approximately 50% to the total detected events [50]. For accurate quantification of tracer concentrations, scattered events must be estimated and subtracted from the recorded data. Due to the generally poor energy resolution of PET systems, scattered photons cannot be directly discriminated on the basis of their energy. A number of scatter correction schemes have been proposed for use in 3D PET, including:

- energy window manipulation methods, such as the dual energy window scatter correction [51], where scatter in the photopeak is estimated by the relative countrate in an auxiliary energy window;
- pre-reconstruction filtering and/or subtraction operations, such as the convolution-subtraction method [52], where scatter is estimated by convolution of the emission projection data with a scatter spread function;
- model-based scatter correction, where the contribution of scatter is calculated from analytical formulae from the emission and transmission data [53, 54];
- methods based on Monte Carlo calculations to estimate scatter [55].

Although the first two methods might be limited to less complex activity distributions, such as in brain imaging, the model-based method has been also found to provide accurate estimates of scatter in the thorax [56, 57]. Although model-based correction is computationally intensive, faster implementations have been shown to provide a more practical and efficient approach [58].

31.4.5
Image Reconstruction

The problem of image reconstruction from projections has received much attention parallel to the development of transmission and emission tomography and its application to PET has been extensively reviewed [59–61]. In 2D PET, filtered back-projection (FBP) is commonly used, while iterative methods, such as the maximum likehood – expectation maximisation (ML-EM) [62] and the ordered subsets – expectation maximisation (OSEM) [63], have increasingly drawn interest due to their superior properties in terms of signal-to-noise.

FBP can be extended to 3D if all the projections, over all azimuthal and polar angles, are available. However, in the case of 3D PET, measurements of projections are constrained within the physical limits of the scanner and some of the measured 2D projections are bound to be partially truncated. As a result, the requirement of FBP for shift invariant response does no longer hold. A solution to the problem is provided by the reprojection algorithm [20] by completing the unmeasured projections from estimates from 2D reconstructions of a subset of the 3D data. Other approaches include the reduction of the problem from 3D to 2D by rebinning techniques such as single slice rebinning [29], multi-slice rebinning [64] and Fourier rebinning [65]. The implementation of iterative methods directly in 3D PET remains limited due to the computer memory requirements to store a large transition matrix. However, attempts have been made to implement 3D iterative techniques in parallel processor systems [66].

31.4.6
Gated and Dynamic Data Acquisition

In addition to measurements of regional myocardial metabolism, it is also possible to assess global function using gated PET acquisition to measure left-ventricular ejection fraction and volumes [67, 68]. During cardiac gating electrocardiographic (ECG) signal is used to trigger data acquisition so that events detected within pre-defined segments of the cardiac cycle are stored separately for independent reconstruction into images [69]. Dynamic data acquisition is employed for studies that require following the time course of the tracer in the body, such as myocardial blood flow studies with $H_2^{15}O$, where pre-set time segments of the scan are saved as individual frames for reconstruction as separate images. Some of the limitations of pre-setting parameters for gating and dynamic acquisition may be overcome by list mode acquisition where individual coincidence events are stored serially for retrospective processing (sorting of data event-by-event into projections) prior to reconstruction.

31.4.7
Tracer Kinetic Modelling

Tracer kinetic modelling has been employed with dynamic PET in order to derive parameters of physiological function such as myocardial blood flow, for example in terms of mL/min/100 g of tissue measured with MBF studies. Tracer kinetic modelling is a vast topic in PET [1–15] and its details are beyond the scope of this review. Briefly, implementations of a single tissue compartment model have been used in myocardial blood flow studies while a two-tissue compartment model has found application in myocardial metabolism studies with FDG. Automated voxel classification methods such as factor analysis and cluster analysis have often been employed [70, 71] in order to assist the definition of myocardial and ventricular ROIs on dynamic images which may otherwise be a challenging process due to the poor image signal-to-noise of individual time frames.

31.5
Recent Trends in Cardiac PET Imaging

Current developments in PET are strongly driven by applications in oncology, which account for the majority of clinical investigations in PET. There are two major implications from the recent developments in PET instrumentation: the introduction of combined PET/CT scanners and the wider use of 3D acquisition mode. Both have the advantage of reducing overall scanning time for FDG whole-body oncology studies. CT-based attenuation correction can be implemented on ultra-fast X-ray CT data acquired over a fraction of the conventional PET transmission scans. Similarly, increased sensitivity in 3D mode results in reduced overall emission scan times, which is important for oncology whole-body studies, which require typically 4–8 bed positions. However, the benefits of these methodological developments for cardiac PET currently remain under discussion [72, 74]. The increase in sensitivity due to the absence of septa in 3D PET comes inevitably with increased random and scattered events. The practical implications are a large number of unwanted events (which may be in the range of 50% of the detected events) and a long dead time. Although current scatter correction schemes seem to be sufficient in dealing with scatter in 3D PET, long dead time remains an issue especially for cardiac studies that may involve a rapid uptake of the tracer through the scanner field-of-view. The use of detector materials with improved count rate capabilities has been employed in various systems, however, improvements in PET systems currently remain to be fully exploited for clinical applications requiring wide range of count rates.

The advantage of fast acquisition times with CT-based transmission measurements does not have the same impact in cardiac imaging as in whole-body oncology imaging where multiple bed positions are required. Post-acquisition processing of the X-ray transmission data (normally acquired at photon energies of <80 keV) is required in order to derive equivalent attenuation correction factors for the 511 keV emission photons, a process which may potentially add extra complexity. Furthermore, an area of increasing interest, mainly due to the rapid development of combined PET/CT, focuses on the effects of respiratory motion. Respiratory motion may affect quantification accuracy or introduce artefacts, for example due to mis-alignment of PET and CT data acquired at different breathing conditions. A number of schemes have been proposed for limiting respiratory motion effects, however, further investigation is required to assess their impact in clinical studies.

Despite the fact that a number of methodological issues may currently require further development, the recent introduction of multi-slice helical CT scanners available in hybrid PET/CT systems opens up new possibilities of clinical applications such as image fusion of PET with CT angiography or ECG-gated CT that may provide a more integrated approach to cardiac imaging.

References

1. Bergmann SR, Fox KA, Rand AL, D. MK, Welch MJ, Karkham J, Sobel BE (1984) Quantification of regional myocardial blood flow in vivo with $H_2^{15}O$. Circulation 70:724–733.
2. Iida H, Kanno I, Takahashi A, Miura S, Murakami M, Takahashi K, Ono Y, Shishido F, Inugami A, Tomura N et al. (1988) Measurement of absolute myocardial blood flow with $H_2^{15}O$ and dynamic positron-emission tomography. Strategy for quantification in relation to the partial-volume effect. Circulation 78:104–115.
3. Araujo LI, Lammertsma AA, Rhodes CG, McFalls EO, Iida H, Rechavia E, Galassi A, De Silva R, Jones T, Maseri A (1991) Noninvasive quantification of regional myocardial blood flow in coronary artery disease with oxygen-15-labeled carbon dioxide inhalation and positron emission tomography. Circulation 83:875–885.
4. Schelbert HR, Phelps ME, Hoffman EJ, Huang SC, Selin CE, Kuhl DE (1979) Regional myocardial perfusion assessed with N-13 labeled ammonia and positron emission computerized axial tomography. Am J Cardiol 43:209–218.
5. Krivokapich J, Smith GT, Huang SC, Hoffman EJ, Ratib O, Phelps ME, Schelbert HR (1980) 13N ammonia myocardial imaging at rest and with exercise in normal volunteers. Quantification of absolute myocardial perfusion with dynamic positron emission tomography. Circulation 80:1328–1337.
6. Herrero P, Markham J, Shelton ME, Weinheimer CJ, Bergmann SR (1990) Noninvasive quantification of regional myocardial perfusion with rubidium-82 and positron emission tomography. Exploration of a mathematical model. Circulation 82:1377–1386.
7. Hutchins GD (2001) What is the best approach to quantify myocardial blood flow with PET? (Invited Commentary). J Nucl Med 42:1183–1184.
8. Camici P, Spinks T (2000) Advanced Imaging – PET. In de Bono D, Sobel BE (eds). Acute Coronary Syndromes, pp.148–172.
9. Huang S-C, Phelps ME (1986) Principles of tracer kinetic modelling in positron emission tomography and autoradiography. In Phelps ME, Mazziotta JC, Schelbert HR (eds). Positron Emission Tomography And Autoradiography. Principles and Applications for the Brain and Heart. New York, Raven Press, pp. 287–346.
10. Marinho NV, Keogh BE, Costa DC, Lammerstma AA, Ell PJ, Camici PG (1996) Pathophysiology of chronic left ventricular dysfunction. New insights from the measurement of absolute myocardial blood flow and glucose utilization. Circulation 93:737–744.
11. Fath-Ordoubadi F, Beatt KJ, Spyrou N, Camici PG (1999) Efficacy of coronary angioplasty for the treatment of hibernating myocardium. Heart 82:210–216.
12. Schelbert HR, Henze E, Keen R, Schon HR, Hansen H, Selin C, Huang SC, Barrio JR, Phelps ME (1983) C-11 palmitate for the noninvasive evaluation of regional myocardial fatty acid metabolism with positron-computed tomography. IV. In vivo evaluation of acute demand-induced ischemia in dogs. Am Heart J 106:736–750.
13. Armbrecht JJ, Buxton DB, Brunken RC, Phelps ME, Schelbert HR (1989) Regional myocardial oxygen consumption determined noninvasively in humans with [1-11C] acetate and dynamic positron tomography. Circulation 80:863–872.
14. Iida H, Rhodes CG, Araujo LI, Yamamoto Y, de Silva R, Maseri A, Jones T (1996) Noninvasive quantification of regional myocardial metabolic rate for oxygen by use of 15O2 inhalation and positron emission tomography. Theory, error analysis, and application in humans. Circulation 94:792–807.
15. Syrota A. Positron emission tomography: Evaluation of cardiac receptors. In Marcus M, Schelbert H, Skorton D, Wolf G (eds). Cardiac Imaging. Philadelphia, WB Saunders Company, pp. 1256–1270.
16. Sorenson JA, Phelps ME (1987) Physics in Nuclear Medicine. Orlando, Florida, Grune & Straton.

17. Bailey DL, Zito F, Gilardi MC, Savi AR, Fazio F, Jones T (1994) Performance comparison of a state-of-the-art neuro-SPET scanner and a dedicated neuro-PET scanner. Eur J Nucl Med 21:381–387.
18. Phelps ME, Hoffman EJ, Mullani NA, Ter-Pogossian MM (1975) Application of annihilation coincidence detection to transaxial reconstruction tomography. J Nucl Med 16:210–224.
19. Colsher JG (1980) Fully-three-dimensional positron emission tomography. Phys Med Biol 25:103–115.
20. Kinahan PE, Rogers JG (1989) Analytic 3D image reconstruction using all detected events. IEEE Trans Nucl Sci 36:964–968.
21. Townsend DW, Spinks T, Jones T, Geissbuhler A, Defrise M, Gilardi MC, Heather J (1989) Three dimensional reconstruction of PET data from a multi-ring camera. IEEE Trans Nucl Sci 36:1056–1065.
22. Spinks TJ, Jones T, Bailey DL, Townsend DW, Grootoonk S, Bloomfield PM, Gilardi MC, Casey ME, Sipe B, Reed J (1992) Physical performance of a positron tomograph for brain imaging with retractable septa. Phys Med Biol 37:1637–1655.
23. NEMA (1993) Performance Measurements of Positron Emission Tomographs. Washington, National Electrical Manufacturers Association.
24. Karp JS, Daube-Witherspoon ME, Hoffman EJ, Lewellen TK, Links JM, Wong WH, Hichwa RD, Casey ME, Colsher JG, Hitchens RE et al. (1991) Performance standards in positron emission tomography. J Nucl Med 32:2342–2350.
25. Guzzardi R, Bellina CR, Knoop B, Jordan K, Ostertag H, Reist HW, Spinks TJ, Vacher J (1991) Methodologies for performance evaluation of positron emission tomographs. Nucl Med Biol 35:141–157.
26. NEMA (2000) Performance Measurements of Positron Emission Tomographs. Washington, National Electrical Manufacturers Association.
27. Phelps ME, Mazziotta JC, Shelbert HR (1986) Positron Emission Tomography and Autoradiography. Principles and Applications for the Brain and Heart. New York, Raven Press.
28. Bailey DL, Karp JS, Surti S (2003) Physics and instrumentation in PET, in Valk PE et al. (eds). Positron Emission Tomography: Basic Science and Clinical Practic. Springer-Verlag, London, pp. 69–90.
29. Sossi V, Stazyk M, Kinahan P, Ruth TJ (1994) The performance of the single-slice rebinning technique for imaging the human striatum as evaluated by phantom studies. Phys Med Biol 39:369–380.
30. Matej S, Karp JS, Lewitt RM, Becher AJ (1998) Performance of the Fourier rebinning algorithm for PET with large acceptance angles. Phys Med Biol 43:787–795.
31. Hoffman EJ, Huang SC, Phelps ME (1979) Quantitation in positron emission computed tomography: 1. Effect of object size. J Comput Assist Tomogr 3:299–308.
32. Strother SC, Casey ME, Hoffman EJ (1990) Measuring PET scanner sensitivity: relating countrates to image signal-to-noise ratios using noise equivalent counts. IEEE Trans Nucl Sci 37:783–788.
33. Bailey DL (2003) Data acquisition and performance characterization in PET, in Valk PE, Bailey DL, Townsend DW, Maisey MN (eds). Positron Emission Tomography: Basic Science and Clinical Practice. Springer-Verlag, London, pp. 41–67.
34. Bailey DL, Jones T, Spinks TJ (1991) A method for measuring the absolute sensitivity of positron emission tomographic scanners. Eur J Nucl Med 18:374–379.
35. Humm JL, Rosenfeld A, Del Guerra A (2003) From PET detectors to PET scanners. Eur J Nuc Med Mol Imaging 30:1574–1597.
36. Melcher CL (2000) Scintillation crystals for PET. J Nucl Med 41:1051–1055.
37. Hubbell JH (1969) Photon Cross Sections, Attenuation Coefficients, and Energy Absorption Coefficients From 10 keV to 100 GeV, National Bureau of Standards, US Dept of Commerce.
38. Huang SC, Carson RE, Phelps ME, Hoffman EJ, Schelbert HR, Kuhl DE (1981) A boundary method for attenuation correction in positron computed tomography. J Nucl Med 22:627–637.
39. Derenzo SE, Budinger TF, Huesman RH, Cahoon JL, Vuletich T (1981) Imaging properties of a positron tomograph with 280 BGO crystals. IEEE Trans Nucl Sci 28:81–89.
40. Thompson CJ, Ranger N, Evans AC, Gjedde A (1991) Validation of simultaneous PET emission and transmission scans. J Nucl Med 32:154–160.
41. deKemp RA, Nahmias C (1994) Attenuation correction in PET using single photon transmission measurement. Med Phys 21:771–778.
42. Karp JS, Muehllehner G, Qu H, Yan XH (1995) Singles transmission in volume-imaging PET with a 137Cs source. Phys Med Biol 40:929–944.
43. Yu SK, Nahmias C (1995) Single-photon transmission measurements in positron tomography using 137Cs. Phys Med Biol 40:1255–1266.
44. Kinahan PE, Hasegawa BH, Beyer T (2003) X-ray-based attenuation correction for positron emission tomography/computed tomography scanners. Semin Nucl Med 33(3):166–179.
45. Kinahan PE, Townsend DW, Beyer T, Sashin D (1998) Attenuation correction for a combined 3D PET/CT scanner. Med Phys 25:2046–2053.
46. Bailey DL (1998) Transmission scanning in emission tomography. Eur J Nucl Med 25:774–787.
47. Hoffman, EJ, Phelps ME (1986) Positron emission tomography: principles and quantitation, in Phelps ME, Mazziotta JC, Schelbert HR (eds). Positron Emission Tomography and Autoradiography. Principles and Applica-

tions for the Brain and Heart. New York, Raven Press, pp. 237–286.
48. Casey ME, Gadagkar H, Newport D (1995) A component based method for normalization in volume PET, in Grangeat P, Amans J-L (eds). 3rd International Conference on Three-Dimensional Image Reconstruction in Radiology and Nuclear Medicine, Aix-les-Bains, pp. 67–71.
49. Dyson NA (1960) The annihilation coincidence method of localizing positron-emitting isotopes, and a comparison with parallel counting. Phys Med Biol 4:376–390.
50. Bailey DL (1998) Quantitative procedures in 3D PET, in Bendriem B, Townsend DW (eds). The Theory and Practice of 3D PET 1. Dordrecht, Kluwer Academic, pp. 55–109.
51. Grootoonk S, Spinks TJ, Sashin D, Spyrou NM, Jones T (1996) Correction for scatter in 3D brain PET using a dual energy window method. Phys Med Biol 41:2757–2774.
52. Bailey DL, Meikle SR (1994) A convolution-subtraction scatter correction method for 3D PET. Phys Med Biol 39:411–424.
53. Ollinger JM (1996) Model-based scatter correction for fully 3D PET. Phys Med Biol 41:153–176.
54. Watson CC, Newport D, Casey ME (1996) A single scatter simulation technique for scatter correction in 3D PET, in Grangeat P, Amans J-L (eds). Three-Dimensional Image Reconstruction in Radiology and Nuclear Medicine 4. Dordrecht, Kluwer Academic, 255–268.
55. Levin CS, Dahlbom M, Hoffman EJ (1995) A Monte Carlo Correction for the Effect of Compton Scattering in 3-D PET Brain Imaging. IEEE Trans Nucl Sci NS-42:1181–1185.
56. Watson CC, Newport D, Casey ME, deKemp RA, Beanlands RS, Schmand M (1997) Evaluation of simulation-based scatter correction for 3-D PET cardiac imaging. IEEE Trans Nucl Sci 44:90–97.
57. Spinks TJ, Jones T, Bloomfield PM, Bailey DL, Miller M, Hogg D, Jones WF, Vaigneur K, Reed J, Young J, Newport D, Moyers C, Casey ME, Nutt R (2000) Physical characteristics of the ECAT EXACT3D positron tomograph. Phys Med Biol 45:2601–2618.
58. Watson CC (2000) New, faster, image-based scatter correction for 3D PET. IEEE Trans Nucl Sci 47:1587–1594.
59. Herman, GT, Lewitt RM, Rowland SW, Bracewell RN, Altschuler MD, Budinger TF, Gullberg GT, Huesman RH, Wood EH et al. (1979) Image Reconstruction from Projections. Springer-Verlag.
60. Defrise M (2001) A short reader's guide to 3D tomographic reconstruction. Comput Med Imaging Graph 25(2):113–116
61. Defrise M, Kinahan PE (1998) Data acquisition and image reconstruction for 3D PET, in Bendriem B, Townsend DW (eds). The Theory and Practice of 3D PET. Dordrecht, The Netherlands, Kluwer Academic.
62. Shepp LA, Vardi Y (1982) Maximum likelihood reconstruction for emission tomography. IEEE Trans Med Imag MI-1:113–122.
63. Hudson HM, Larkin RS (1994) Accelerated image reconstruction using ordered subsets of projection data. IEEE Trans Med Imag MI-13:601–609.
64. Lewitt RM, Muehllehner G, Karp JS (1994) Three-dimensional image reconstruction for PET by multi-slice rebinning and axial image filtering. Phys Med Biol 39:321–339.
65. Defrise M, Kinahan PE, Townsend DW, Michel C, Sibomana M, Newport DF (1997) Exact and approximate rebinning algorithms for 3-D PET data. IEEE Trans Med Imaging 16:145–158.
66. Labbé C, Thielemans K, Zaidi H, Morel C (1999) An object-oriented library incorporating efficient projection/backprojection operators for volume reconstruction in 3D PET. Proc. of 3D99 Conference, Egmond aan Zee, The Netherlands
67. Rajappan K, Livieratos L, Camici PG, Pennell DJ (2002) Measurement of ventricular volumes and function – a comparison of gated positron emission tomography and cardiovascular magnetic resonance. J Nucl Med 43:806–810.
68. Schaefer WM et al. (2003) Validation of an evaluation routine for left ventricular volumes, ejection fraction and wall motion from gated cardiac FDG PET: a comparison with cardiac magnetic resonance imaging. Eur J Nucl Med Mol Imaging 30(4):545–553.
69. Hoffman EJ, Phelps ME, Wisenberg G, Schelbert HR, Kuhl DE (1979) Electrocardiographic gating in positron emission computed tomography. J Comput Assist Tomogr 3:733–739.
70. Hermansen F, Ashburner J, Spinks TJ, Kooner JS, Camici PG, Lammertsma AA (1998) Generation of myocardial factor images directly from the dynamic oxygen-15-water scan without use of an oxygen-15-carbon monoxide blood-pool scan. J Nucl Med 39(10):1696–1702.
71. Schäfers KP, Spinks TJ, Camici PG, Bloomfield PM, Rhodes CG, Law MP, Baker CSR, Rimoldi O (2002) Absolute quantification of myocardial blood flow with $H(2)(15)O$ and 3-dimensional PET: an experimental validation. J Nucl Med 43(8):1031–1040.
72. Bacharach SL (2004) The new-generation PET/CT scanners: implications for cardiac imaging. J Nucl Cardiol 11(4):388–92
73. Moses WW, Derenzo SE, Budinger TF (1994) PET detector modules based on novel detector technologies. Nucl Instr Meth Phys Res A353:189–194.
74. Schwaiger M, Ziegler S, Nekolla SG (2005) PET/CT: challenge for nuclear cardiology. J Nucl Med 46(10):1664–1678

PET Radiopharmaceuticals in Nuclear Cardiology: Current Status and Limitations

James R. Ballinger

Contents

32.1 Introduction 379
32.2 PET Radiopharmaceuticals in Current Use 379
32.2.1 Myocardial Perfusion Imaging 379
32.2.2 Myocardial Metabolism/Viability 381
32.3 Characteristics of Selected PET Radiopharmaceuticals 382
32.3.1 ^{82}Rb-Rubidium chloride [1, 5] 382
32.3.2 ^{13}N-Ammonia [6, 7, 15–17] 382
32.3.3 ^{15}O-Water [9, 16–18] 382
32.3.4 ^{18}F-FDG [16, 17, 19, 20] 382
32.3.5 ^{11}C-Acetate [16, 21] 383
32.4 Future Trends 383
32.4.1 Alternative Perfusion Tracers 383
32.4.2 Neurotransmitters/Receptors 383
32.4.3 Other Targets 383
32.5 Concluding Remarks 384
References 384

32.1 Introduction

PET was developed in the 1970s primarily for studies of the brain. However, interest in cardiac PET grew in the 1980s, leading to more widespread availability of whole body PET scanners. This in turn contributed to the application of PET in oncology, which mushroomed in the 1990s. Growth in cardiac PET has, however, been more modest and shows great variation among countries. Many cardiac PET studies are performed using radiopharmaceuticals developed for other purposes, primarily ^{18}F-fluorodeoxyglucose and ^{15}O-water, although a significant fraction of studies use the strontium-82/rubidium-82 generator developed specifically for cardiac PET. The properties of PET radiopharmaceuticals currently in clinical use for myocardial perfusion and metabolism will be reviewed (Tables 32.1 and 32.2), followed by discussion of agents which may become more widely used in the future.

32.2 PET Radiopharmaceuticals in Current Use

32.2.1 Myocardial Perfusion Imaging

The field of nuclear cardiology developed with the introduction of myocardial perfusion imaging using ^{201}Tl thallous chloride and ejection fraction determination using ^{99m}Tc-labelled red blood cells in the late 1970s. ^{201}Tl is an analogue of potassium and is taken up actively via the Na$^+$/K$^+$ ATPase system, resulting in high extraction from the circulation into myocytes, and an initial distribution in the myocardium which reflects regional perfusion. This led to the search for a positron-emitting analogue of potassium that could be used in the same way, resulting in the introduction of rubidium-82 (^{82}Rb), which has a half-life of 75 seconds and is obtained from its parent radionuclide strontium-82 (^{82}Sr) via a generator system. The half-life of ^{82}Sr is 25 days, meaning that

Table 32.1 Selected characteristics of radiopharmaceuticals commonly used in cardiac PET studies

Radiopharmaceutical	Indication	Half-life (minutes)	Means of production
^{82}Rb-Rubidium chloride	Perfusion	1.25	generator, parent half-life 25 days
^{13}N-Ammonia	Perfusion	10	on-site cyclotron
^{15}O-Water	Perfusion	2	on-site cyclotron
^{18}F-Fluorodeoxyglucose	Glucose metabolism	110	on-site or remote cyclotron
^{11}C-Acetate	Oxidative metabolism	20	on-site cyclotron

Table 32.2 Advantages and disadvantages of some radiopharmaceuticals commonly used in cardiac PET studies

Radiopharmaceutical	Advantages	Disadvantages
^{82}Rb-Rubidium chloride	convenient availability from generator generator is commercially available and licensed in USA virtually unlimited number of patients short rest/stress protocol due to half-life	requires high workload for generator to be cost-effective high positron energy degrades spatial resolution
^{13}N-Ammonia	convenient for small number of patient studies	short half-life cyclotron-produced cyclotron time must be scheduled
^{15}O-Water	convenient for small number of patient studies short rest/stress protocol due to half-life	very short half-life cyclotron-produced correction for blood pool activity required cyclotron time must be scheduled
^{18}F-Fluorodeoxyglucose	widely available can be obtained from remote cyclotron	sensitive to plasma glucose level
^{11}C-Acetate	convenient for small number of patient studies	short half-life cyclotron-produced

the useful life of the generator is about 1 month. Because of the short half-life of the daughter radionuclide, the generator can be re-eluted at 10-minute intervals with full yield. The generator is eluted with saline and infused directly into the patient [1–3].

To differentiate between ischemia and infarction, separate studies are performed at rest and following exercise or, more commonly, pharmacological stress, as is used with SPECT myocardial perfusion imaging. The short half-life of ^{82}Rb permits the entire rest/stress protocol to be completed within 45 minutes, which is very convenient for the patient [4]. In general, the results are semi-quantitative, rather than giving absolute quantification in perfusion units of mL/min/g tissue. A disadvantage of the short half-life of ^{82}Rb is that counting statistics can be relatively poor. The ^{82}Sr/^{82}Rb generator is commercially available in the USA as Cardio-Gen-82® from Bracco Diagnostics Inc. [1]. The generator is expensive but a high throughput (e.g., 6–10 patients per day) makes the cost per study comparable with that incurred with SPECT myocardial perfusion imaging. The design and validation of an in-house generator has been published [5].

^{13}N-Ammonia was initially evaluated for myocardial perfusion imaging using planar scintillation cameras [6] but applied to PET when the technology became available [7]. ^{13}N has a half-life of 10 minutes and must be obtained from an on-site cyclotron. Initial uptake in the lung clears rapidly allowing visualisation of the heart, though lung clearance may be delayed in smokers. A complete rest/stress protocol requires about 2 hours to allow for decay of ^{13}N between studies [4]. ^{13}N-Ammonia is a widely used alternative in centres which do not have a high enough volume of studies to make use of the ^{82}Sr/^{82}Rb generator cost-effective. Absolute quantification of myocardial perfusion can be performed with ^{13}N-ammonia [8].

^{15}O-Water is widely used for measurement of regional cerebral perfusion, but can also be used in the heart [9]. ^{15}O has a half-life of 2 minutes and must be obtained from an on-site cyclotron. Delivery of ^{15}O-water to myocardial (and other) cells is efficient but rapid washout occurs, which necessitates dynamic imaging or subtraction of blood pool activity. The short half-life allows a conveniently short rest/stress imaging protocol but can result in poor counting statistics. Absolute quantification can be performed [9].

A recent analysis of three studies which directly compared myocardial perfusion imaging with PET and SPECT in a total of 264 patients showed that PET outperformed SPECT significantly in terms of senstivity, specificity, and diagnostic accuracy [4]. An important application of quantitative studies with PET is the assessment of coronary flow reserve (CFR), which in normal individuals is >2. Determination of CFR has been shown to be useful in verification of efficacy of pharmacological vasodilation, detection of global/diffuse disease, evaluation of extent of multivessel disease, evaluation of significance of individual vessel lesions, detection of collateral coronary steal syndrome, evaluation of endothelial function, and in monitoring therapy [4]. CFR is also useful for detecting early coronary artery disease, before there is significant obstruction.

32.2.2
Myocardial Metabolism/Viability

Although myocardial perfusion imaging has earned an important place in the management of heart disease, it cannot demonstrate viability. It is important to be able to detect viable myocardium which may benefit from revascularisation. For this purpose, ^{18}F-fluorodeoxyglucose (FDG), the work-horse of clinical PET, has proved useful, and this study is normally performed in conjunction with myocardial perfusion imaging. ^{18}F has a half-life of 110 minutes and is produced in a cyclotron, but it can be distributed to centres at quite some distance. Supply and distribution networks have been established in many countries because of the importance of ^{18}F-FDG imaging in oncology. ^{18}F-FDG is an analogue of glucose, which is transported into cells by glucose transporters and phosphorylated to ^{18}F-FDG-6-PO$_4$ by hexokinase but not further metabolised. Dephosphorylation and washout are negligible, so ^{18}F-FDG-6-PO$_4$ is trapped and accumulates as an integral of glucose transport and metabolism [10].

The major sources of energy for the heart under normal conditions are glucose and free fatty acids. When there is less oxygen available under acute ischemia, utilisation of fatty acids for oxidative metabolism is decreased and glucose becomes the preferred substrate for energy production via anaerobic glycolysis [10]. However, the heart also adapts to the availability of substrates. In the fasting state, fatty acids are the preferred substrate, whereas increased plasma glucose and insulin levels lead to glucose becoming the prime source of energy [11]. In fasting individuals, low cardiac uptake of ^{18}F-FDG may result in inadequate image quality, therefore the glucose-loaded state is preferred for viability imaging. This presents a challenge in patients with diabetes, many of whom suffer coronary artery disease. In this situation, adequate images can be obtained using the hyperinsulinemic-euglycemic glucose clamp technique or small intravenous doses of insulin [12]. In many centres it is routine to measure plasma glucose levels in all patients prior to an ^{18}F-FDG study.

Because glucose uptake and metabolism can only take place in viable cells, ^{18}F-FDG imaging provides complementary information to perfusion scanning. As a result, three scenarios can occur: normal perfusion with normal metabolism; reduced perfusion with reduced metabolism (perfusion–metabolism match, representing irreversibly damaged, non-viable myocardium); and reduced perfusion with normal or near-normal metabolism (perfusion–metabolism mismatch, indicating reversibly damaged, viable myocardium). The predictive value of metabolic imaging was demonstrated almost 20 years ago [13] and the combination of perfusion and glucose metabolic imaging has become a standard and widely used technique for determining myocardial viability [10].

Carbon-11 (^{11}C) labelled acetate is a tracer of citric acid flux and thus indirectly of oxidative metabolism. ^{11}C has a half-life of 20 minutes and is obtained from an on-site cylotron. ^{11}C-Acetate is predominantly metabolised to ^{11}C-carbon dioxide, which clears from the heart and the efflux rate closely correlates with myocardial oxygen consumption over a wide range of flow, substrate use, and metabolic conditions. Estimates of myocardial oxygen consumption are clinically useful in assessing tissue viability after acute myocardial infarction or in chronic coronary artery disease. It may also provide measurement of cardiac efficiency and be useful for monitoring therapy [14].

32.3
Characteristics of Selected PET Radiopharmaceuticals

32.3.1
^{82}Rb-Rubidium chloride [1, 5]

Chemistry and constituents: ^{82}Rb-Rubidium chloride in saline. Half-life 75 seconds. Maximum β$^+$ energy 3.3 MeV.

Physiological characteristics: Behaves as an analogue of potassium, taken up into the heart actively by Na$^+$/K$^+$ ATPase pump.

Biodistribution: Rapidly cleared from blood. Taken up to a variable degree by all tissues and organs except the brain.

Dosimetry: Effective dose equivalent 4.8 μSv/MBq or 7.2 mSv per standard 1500-MBq dose. Highest absorbed doses: thyroid, 38; adrenals, 20; kidneys, 18 μGy/MBq.

Preparation: Available from ^{82}Sr/^{82}Rb generator with hydrous stannic oxide column. Parent half-life 25 days. Useful life of generator approximately 1 month. Generator is eluted with saline, which is infused directly into patient. Commercially available, licensed in USA.

Quality control: Test for breakthrough of ^{82}Sr and ^{85}Sr using high resolution gamma spectrometry or an ionisation chamber; limit of 0.02 kBq ^{82}Sr and 0.2 kBq ^{85}Sr per MBq ^{82}Rb. Not more than 1 μg tin per mL eluate.

32.3.2
^{13}N-Ammonia [6, 7, 15–17]

Chemistry and constituents: ^{13}N-Ammonia in saline. Half-life 10 minutes. Maximum β$^+$ energy 1.2 MeV.

Physiological characteristics: Ammonia equilibrates with ammonium ion in the bloodstream. It is the neutral ammonia species, which diffuses across biological membranes into cells and is enzymatically converted into glutamine. First pass extraction is 80% at normal flow but falls off at high flow rates.

Biodistribution: Rapidly cleared from circulation, extracted by liver (15%), lungs, myocardium (2–4%), brain, kidney, and bladder.

Dosimetry: Effective dose equivalent 2.2 μSv/MBq or 1.7 mSv per standard 740-MBq dose. Highest absorbed doses: bladder, 7 μGy/MBq.

Preparation: Proton irradiation of water target in cyclotron followed by reduction, distillation, and trapping in a slightly acidic solution.

Quality control: HPLC on cation exchange resin eluted with dilute nitric acid. Colour test for aluminium (limit 2 ppm).

32.3.3
^{15}O-Water [9, 16–18]

Chemistry and constituents: ^{15}O-Water in saline. Half-life 2 minutes. Maximum β$^+$ energy 1.7 MeV.

Physiological characteristics: Diffuses freely across membranes.

Biodistribution: Enters total body water space. Rapidly diffuses into myocardial cells but also washes out, necessitating subtraction of blood pool activity.

Dosimetry: Effective dose equivalent 1.16 μSv/MBq or 2.6 mSv per standard 2200-MBq dose. Highest absorbed doses: ovaries, 1.8; lower large intestine, 1.5; red marrow, 1.5; upper large intestine, 1.3 μGy/MBq.

Preparation: Molecular oxygen reacts with small amount of hydrogen.

Quality control: Test for ammonium and nitrates. HPLC on aminopropylsilyl silica gel eluted with phosphate buffer.

32.3.4
^{18}F-FDG [16, 17, 19, 20]

Chemistry and constituents: ^{18}F-2-Fluoro-2-deoxy-D-glucose (FDG) in saline. Half-life 110 minutes. Maximum β$^+$ energy 0.63 MeV.

Physiological characteristics: Behaves as an analogue of glucose. Uptake via glucose transporter and phosphorylated by hexokinase, but no further metabolism.

Biodistribution: Rapidly cleared from circulation, half-time <1 minute. Three phases can be identified with half-lives of 0.2–0.3 min, 10–13 min, and 80–95 min. About 30% excreted via kidneys. Tissues of highest retention are the heart and brain.

Dosimetry: Effective dose equivalent 29 μSv/MBq or 11 mSv per standard 370-MBq dose. Highest absorbed doses: bladder wall, 120; heart, 45 μGy/MBq.

Preparation: Usually prepared from ^{18}F-fluoride by nucleophilic reaction with tetra-acetylated mannose triflate, followed by deprotection and purification. Automatic synthesis units widely available. Commercially available.

Quality control: Testing for radiochemical purity (% of activity present as ^{18}F-FDG) and chemical purity (limits for chlorodeoxyglucose, precursor Kryptofix, acetonitrile solvent). HPLC on strongly basic anion exchange resin eluted with dilute sodium hydroxide and thin-layer chromatography on silica gel developed with 95% acetonitrile.

32.3.5
^{11}C-Acetate [16, 21]

Chemistry and constituents: ^{11}C-Sodium acctate in saline. Half-life 20 minutes. Maximum β$^+$ energy 0.96 MeV.

Physiological characteristics: Metabolised to ^{11}C-CO$_2$ in the heart and exhaled through the lungs. Trapped in lipids in some tumours.

Biodistribution: Rapid accumulation in the heart, lungs (3.5%), kidneys, liver (7.5%), pancreas, spleen, stomach, bowel (9%), and bone marrow, followed by washout from all organs though most rapidly from heart. It is not excreted via the kidneys.

Dosimetry: Effective dose equivalent 6.2 μSv/MBq or 4.6 mSv per standard 740-MBq dose. Highest absorbed doses: pancreas, 17; bowel, 11; kidneys, 9.2; spleen, 9.2 μGy/MBq.

Preparation: ^{11}C-Carbon dioxide reacts with ethylmagnesium bromide followed by hydrolysis and purification.

Quality control: HPLC on strongly basic anion exchange resin eluted with dilute sodium hydroxide. Residual solvents.

32.4
Future Trends

32.4.1
Alternative Perfusion Tracers

The available perfusion tracers either require an expensive generator or an on-site cyclotron. A perfusion tracer labelled with ^{18}F could be supplied from a remote cyclotron to allow myocardial perfusion imaging in a centre with a low volume of patients. Studenov and Berridge developed a series of ^{18}F-labelled quaternary ammonium salts (essentially "fluoro-ammonia") but have not yet found a compound with optimal properties [22].

The ^{82}Rb generator is limited to cardiac studies. There are two other generator systems that may be applicable to a wider variety of studies. Copper-62 (^{62}Cu) PTSM can be prepared from a zinc-62 (^{62}Zn)/^{62}Cu generator and has been used for myocardial perfusion imaging [23]. However, half-life of ^{62}Zn is 9 hours, which means that the generator has a useful life of only one day. Another alternative is a gallium-68 (^{68}Ga) chelate, available from a long-lived germanium-68 (^{68}Ge)/^{68}Ga generator [24]. Neither the ^{62}Cu nor the ^{68}Ga generator is widely available at present but may become so in the future due to the variety of tracers that can be prepared using these radiolabels, particularly for use in oncology [25, 26].

32.4.2
Neurotransmitters/Receptors

Although there was early interest in mapping the cholinergic system in the heart [27], the majority of tracers under evaluation currently are radiolabelled catecholamines, such as 6-^{18}F-fluorodopamine, (-)-6-^{18}F-fluoronorepinephrine, and (-)-^{11}C-epinephrine, and radiolabelled catecholamine analogues, such as ^{11}C-meta-hydroxyephedrine, ^{18}F-fluorometaraminol, and ^{11}C-phenylephrine [28]. Using serial studies with ^{18}F-fluorodopamine, Fallen et al. were able to demonstrate sympathetic reinnervation following acute myocardial infarction [29]. In parallel, there has been interest in imaging beta adrenergic receptor density, which may be useful in evaluation of ischemia, dilated cardiomyopathy, and heart failure [30].

32.4.3
Other Targets

Hypoxia: It is important to detect hypoxic but viable tissue following myocardial infarction and chronically ischemic "hibernating" myocardium in order to optimise therapy. Hypoxia tracers such as ^{18}F-fluoromisonidazole and ^{62}Cu-ATSM are selectively trapped in hypoxic tissue by a bioreductive mechanism and result in hot spot images [31, 32]. Moreover, this single scan would be more convenient than a combination of perfusion and metabolic imaging.

Apoptosis: Apoptosis is an indicator of a variety of conditions within the heart, including ischemia/reperfusion injury, autoimmune myocarditis, areas at risk following acute myocardial infarction, and in transplant rejection [33]. The protein annexin V, which binds to phosphatidyl choline externalised by cells undergoing apoptosis, has been labelled with ^{18}F and ^{124}I for PET imaging [34, 35].

Angiogenesis: Angiogenesis is an essential feature of treatment of and/or recovery from atherosclerotic coronary artery disease, heart failure, revascularisation, and cardiac transplantation [36, 37]. The main targets of imaging have been αvβ3 integrin and vascular endothelial growth factor (VEGF). Arginine-glycine-aspartate (RGD) is a peptide sequence which binds integrin, and derivatives labelled with ^{18}F and ^{64}Cu have been evaluated in patients with cancer [38, 39]. An antibody which binds to VEGF has been labelled with ^{124}I [40].

Endothelial factors: Endothelin-1, a peptide synthesised by vascular endothelial cells, is a potent vasoconstrictor and has mitogenic properties [41]. It is believed to play a role in the failure of saphenous vein coronary artery bypass grafts. Johnstrom et al. studied an ^{18}F-labelled analogue of endothelin-1 and found unexpected low uptake in the heart due to high binding in the lung and kidney; pretreatment with an endothelin-B subtype receptor antagonist blocked this non-target uptake and allowed the heart to be visualised [42].

Gene therapy: Gene therapy is an emerging area for treatment of heart disease [36]. PET is well suited to monitor gene therapy in the heart, as well as in cancer, using probes for the herpes simplex virus type 1 thymidine kinase reporter gene (HSV1-tk) such as ^{18}F-FHBG and ^{124}I-FIAU [43, 44].

32.5
Concluding Remarks

PET has assumed an important role in nuclear cardiology, although access and utilisation rates vary widely around the world. Myocardial perfusion and metabolic imaging provide unique information, which is important clinically. More widespread availability of alternative generator systems could provide a more convenient source of tracers for myocardial perfusion imaging. Radiopharmaceuticals are under development for a variety of specific cardiac indications and their eventual clinical role remains to be seen. The technology of PET is robust and well established. The future of cardiac PET depends upon the interplay between the development of tracers and elucidation of their role in clinical care.

References

1. Anonymous (2000) CardioGen-82® Rubidium Rb 82 Generator product monograph. Bracco Diagnostics Inc., Princeton NJ.
2. Selwyn AP, Allan RM, L'Abbate A et al. (1982) Relation between regional myocardial uptake of rubidium-82 and perfusion: Absolute reduction of cation uptake in ischemia. Am J Cardiol 50:112–121.
3. Goldstein RA, Mullani NA, Marani SK, Fisher DJ, O'Brien HA Jr, Loberg MD (1983) Myocardial perfusion with rubidium-82. II. Effects of metabolic and pharmacological interventions. J Nucl Med 24:907–915.
4. Machac J (2005) Cardiac positron emission tomography imaging. Semin Nucl Med 35:17–36.
5. Alvarez-Diez TM, deKemp R, Beanlands R, Vincent J (1999) Manufacture of strontium-82/rubidium-82 generators and quality control of rubidium-82 chloride for myocardial perfusion imaging in patients using positron emission tomography. Appl Radiat Isot 50:1015–1023.
6. Walsh WF, Fill HR, Harper PV (1977) Nitrogen-13-labeled ammonia for myocardial imaging. Semin Nucl Med 7:59–66.
7. Schelbert HR, Phelps ME, Hoffman EJ, Huang SC, Selin CE, Kuhl DE (1979) Regional myocardial perfusion assessed with N-13 labeled ammonia and positron emission computerized axial tomography. Am J Cardiol 43:209–218.
8. Hutchins GD (1997) Quantitative evaluation of myocardial blood flow with [^{13}N]ammonia. Cardiology 88:106–115.
9. Bergmann SR, Herrero P, Markham J, Weinheimer CJ, Walsh MN (1989) Noninvasive quantitation of myocardial blood flow in human subjects with oxygen-15-labeled water and positron emission tomography. J Am Coll Cardiol 14:639–652.
10. Visser FC (2001) Imaging of cardiac metabolism using radiolabelled glucose, fatty acids and acetate. Coron Artery Dis 12:S12–S18.
11. Choi Y, Brunken RC, Hawkins RA et al. (1993) Factors affecting myocardial 2-[F-18]fluoro-2-deoxy-D-glucose uptake in positron emission tomography studies of normal humans. Eur J Nucl Med 20:308–318.
12. Schoder H, Campisi R, Ohtake T et al. (1999) Blood flow-metabolism imaging with positron emission tomography in patients with diabetes mellitus for the assessment of reversible left ventricular contractile dysfunction. J Am Coll Cardiol 33:1328–1337.
13. Tillisch J, Brunken R, Marshall R et al. (1986) Reversibility of cardiac wall motion abnormalities predicted by positron emission tomography. N Engl J Med 314:884–888.
14. Melin JA, Vanoverschelde JL, Bol A, Heyndrickx G, Wijns W (1994) The use of carbon 11-labeled acetate for assessment of aerobic metabolism. J Nucl Cardiol 1:S48–S57.
15. Schelbert HR, Phelps ME, Huang SC et al. (1981) N-13 ammonia as an indicator of myocardial blood flow. Circulation 63:1259–1272.
16. European Directorate for the Quality of Medicines (2002) European Pharmacopoeia, 4th edn.
17. Meyer GJ, Waters SL, Coenen HH, Luxen A, Maziere B, Langstrom B (1995) PET radiopharmaceuticals in Europe: Current use and data relevant for the formulation of summaries of product characteristics (SPCs). Eur J Nucl Med 22:1420–1432.
18. Brihaye C, Depresseux JC, Comar D (1995) Radiation dosimetry for bolus administration of oxygen-15-water. J Nucl Med 36:651–656.
19. Jones SC, Alavi A, Christman D, Montanez I, Wolf AP, Reivich M (1982) The radiation dosimetry of 2[F-18]fluoro-2-deoxy-D-glucose in man. J Nucl Med 23:613–617.
20. Mejia AA, Nakamura T, Masatoshi I, Hatazawa J, Masaki M, Watanuki S (1991) Estimation of absorbed doses in humans due to intravenous administration of fluorine-

18-fluorodeoxyglucose in PET studies. J Nucl Med 32:699–706.
21. Seltzer MA, Jahan SA, Sparks R et al. (2004) Radiation dose estimates in humans for ^{11}C-acetate whole-body PET. J Nucl Med 45:1233–1236.
22. Studenov AR, Berridge MS (2001) Synthesis and properties of ^{18}F-labeled potential myocardial blood flow tracers. Nucl Med Biol 28:683–693.
23. Wallhaus TR, Lacy J, Stewart R et al. (2001) Copper-62-pyruvaldehyde bis(N-methyl-thiosemicarbazone) PET imaging in the detection of coronary artery disease in humans. J Nucl Cardiol 8:67–74.
24. Tsang BW, Mathias CJ, Green MA (1993) A gallium-68 radiopharmaceutical that is retained in myocardium: ^{68}Ga[(4,6-MeO$_2$sal)$_2$BAPEN]$^+$. J Nucl Med 34:1127–1131.
25. Fujibayashi Y, Taniuchi H, Yonekura Y, Ohtani H, Konishi J, Yokoyama A (1997) Copper-62-ATSM: a new hypoxia imaging agent with high membrane permeability and low redox potential. J Nucl Med 38:1155–1160.
26. Hofmann M, Maecke H, Borner R et al. (2001) Biokinetics and imaging with the somatostatin receptor PET radioligand ^{68}Ga-DOTATOC: Preliminary data. Eur J Nucl Med 28:1751–1757.
27. Maziere M, Comar D, Godot JM, Collard P, Cepeda C, Naquet R (1981) In vivo characterization of myocardium muscarinic receptors by positron emission tomography. Life Sci 29:2391–2397.
28. Langer O, Halldin C (2002) PET and SPET tracers for mapping the cardiac nervous system. Eur J Nucl Med Mol Imaging 29:416–434.
29. Fallen EL, Coates G, Nahmias C et al. (1999) Recovery rates of regional sympathetic reinnervation and myocardial blood flow after acute myocardial infarction. Am Heart J 137:863–869.
30. de Jong RM, Blanksma PK, van Waarde A, van Veldhuisen DJ (2002) Measurement of myocardial β-adrenoreceptor density in clinical studies: a role for positron emission tomography? Eur J Nucl Med 29:88–97.
31. Sinusas AJ (1999) The potential for myocardial imaging with hypoxia markers. Semin Nucl Med 29:330–338.
32. Takahashi N, Fujibayashi Y, Yonekura Y et al. (2001) Copper-62 ATSM as a hypoxic tissue tracer in myocardial ischemia. Ann Nucl Med 15:293–296.
33. Blankenberg FG, Strauss HW (2001) Noninvasive strategies to image cardiovascular apoptosis. Cardiol Clin 19:165–172.
34. Zijlstra S, Gunawan J, Burchert W (2003) Synthesis and evaluation of a ^{18}F-labelled recombinant annexin-V derivative, for identification and quantification of apoptotic cells with PET. Appl Radiat Isot 58:201–207.
35. Glaser M, Collingridge DR, Aboagye EO et al. (2003) Iodine-124 labelled Annexin-V as a potential radiotracer to study apoptosis using positron emission tomography. Appl Radiat Isot 58:55–62.
36. Mukherjee D (2004) Current clinical perspectives on myocardial angiogenesis. Mol Cell Biochem 264:157–167.
37. McDonald DM, Choyke PL (2003) Imaging of angiogenesis: From microscope to clinic. Nat Med 9:713–725.
38. Chen X, Sievers E, Hou Y et al. (2005) Integrin αvβ3-targeted imaging of lung cancer. Neoplasia 7:271–279.
39. Haubner R, Weber WA, Beer AJ et al. (2005) Noninvasive visualisation of the activated αvβ3 integrin in cancer patients by positron emission tomography and [^{18}F]galacto-RGD. PLoS Med 2:e70.
40. Collingridge DR, Carroll VA, Glaser M et al. (2002) The development of [^{124}I]iodinated-VG76e: A novel tracer for imaging vascular endothelial growth factor in vivo using positron emission tomography. Cancer Res 62:5912–5919.
41. Davenport AP, Maguire JJ (2001) The endothelin system in human saphenous vein graft disease. Curr Opin Pharmacol 1:176–182.
42. Johnstrom P, Fryer TD, Richards HK et al. (2005) Positron emission tomography using ^{18}F-labelled endothelin-1 reveals prevention of binding to cardiac receptors owing to tissue-specific clearance by ETB receptors in vivo. Br J Pharmacol 144:115–122.
43. Wu JC, Chen IY, Wang Y et al. (2004) Molecular imaging of the kinetics of vascular endothelial growth factor gene expression in ischemic myocardium. Circulation 110:685–691.
44. Simoes MV, Miyagawa M, Reder S et al. (2005) Myocardial kinetics of reporter probe ^{124}I-FIAU in isolated perfused rat hearts after in vivo adenoviral transfer of herpes simplex virus type 1 thymidine kinase reporter gene. J Nucl Med 46:98–105.

Cardiac PET Imaging: Current Status and Limitations

33

Ishtiaque H Mohiuddin and Assad Movahed

Contents

33.1	Introduction	387
33.2	Principle	388
33.3	Clinical Applications	388
33.4	Positron Emission Tomography in Assessment of Viability	389
33.5	FDG-SPECT Imaging	390
33.6	Fatty Acid Imaging	391
33.7	Comparison with Non-nuclear Techniques	392
33.8	Implications of Detecting Viable Myocardium	392
33.9	Cardiac Neurotransmission Imaging	393
33.10.	Recommendations	393
33.11	Role of Metabolic PET Imaging in the Study of Specific Disease Processes	394
33.11.1	Coronary Artery Disease	394
33.11.2	Left Ventricular Hypertrophy	394
33.11.3	Dilated Cardiomyopathy (DCM)/Heart Failure	394
33.11.4	Obesity-Insulin Resistance	395
33.11.5	Diabetes Mellitus	395
33.12	Future Trends	395
	References	395

33.1 Introduction

Since the birth of the first commercial Positron Emission Tomography (PET) scanner in 1975, PET scan technology has come a long way, and entered the era of clinical applications in the late 1980s. Various clinical applications continue to evolve. Currently, PET imaging plays an important role in the clinical evaluation of patients with known or suspected ischemic heart disease. It produces images of molecular-level physiological function, which can be used to measure many vital processes, including glucose metabolism, blood flow and perfusion, and oxygen utilization. This exciting technology extends the capabilities of other advanced imaging modalities such as echocardiogram, MRI and CT. For example, it uses proven tomographic algorithms to display data as cross-sectional images in any plane. These images represent the distribution of internal radiotracers (Fig. 33.1). Unlike anatomical imaging modalities such as CT and MRI, PET permits the assessment of chemical and physiological changes related to metabolism. This is important because a functional change often predates structural changes in tissues. PET images may therefore demonstrate pathological changes long before they would be revealed by CT and MRI.

Unlike traditional nuclear medicine, PET uses unique radiopharmaceuticals, or "tracers," labeled with isotopes, which are the basic elements of biological substrates. The positron-emitting radionuclides of the biologically ubiquitous elements oxygen (O^{15}), carbon (C^{11}), and nitrogen (N^{13}), as well as fluorine (F^{18}) substituting for hydrogen, can be incorporated into a wide variety of substrates or substrate analogs that participate in diverse metabolic pathways without altering the biochemical properties of the substrate of interest. These isotopes mimic natural substrates such as sugars, water, proteins, and oxygen. As a result, PET will often reveal more about the cellular-level metabolic status of a disease than other types of imaging modalities. By combining the knowledge of the metabolic pathways of interest with kinetic models that faithfully describe the fate of the tracer in tissue, an accurate interpretation of the tracer kinetics as they relate to the metabolic process of

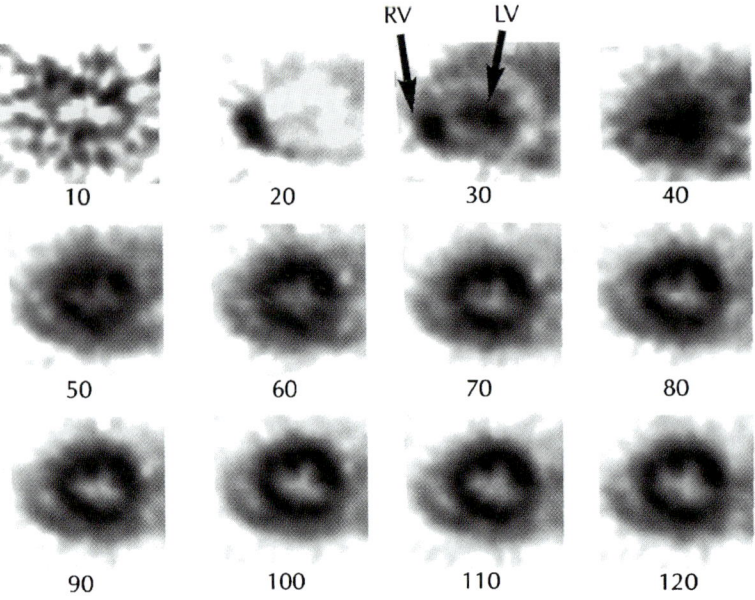

Fig. 33.1 Serially acquired 10-second images illustrating transit of intravenous radiotracer bolus through central circulation. The early images depict tracer activity predominantly in the right heart, followed by dispersion of the tracer into the lungs, return into LV, and subsequent clearance of tracer activity from arterial blood into myocardium. The late static image depicts the tracer activity retained in the LV myocardium after the radiotracer has disappeared from the blood pool. (From Atlas of Nuclear Cardiology by Vasken Dilsizian and Jagat Narula, Current Medicine, Inc., Philadelphia)

interest can be achieved. Indeed, using this approach, measurements of myocardial blood flow, myocardial oxygen consumption (VO_2), glucose utilization, fatty acid fractional uptake, myocardial total utilization, oxidation, and fractional oxidation in the same subject can be measured.

PET also stands out in its ability to quantify physiological and biochemical measurements in vivo. Although a simplified qualitative mode is available, PET images can be acquired quantitatively to reflect the actual amounts of tracer in the regions of interest. The availability of PET/CT scanners allows the integration of structure and function of the heart in ways that were never possible before.

33.2
Principle

PET is based on the detection of coincidence of two 511-keV annihilation radiations that originate from β^+-emitting sources (e.g., the patient). Positrons are annihilated in body tissue and produce two 511-keV annihilation photons that are emitted in opposite directions. Two photons are detected by two detectors connected in coincidence, and data collected over 360° around the body axis of the patient are used to reconstruct the image of the activity distribution in the slice of interest. A schematic diagram of a PET system using four pairs of detectors is illustrated in Fig. 33.2.

33.3
Clinical Applications

PET has the unique ability to cross the boundaries of specialties, adding new dimensions to a physician's ability to:

- Diagnose disease before structural changes become detectable potentially improving the prognosis;
- Detect endothelial dysfunction, an early event in atherosclerosis that precedes the structural changes in coronary arteries and causes coronary vasoreactivity disturbances;
- Manage patient therapy by monitoring the response to a given regimen and providing early feedback on its efficacy. This can help reduce or avoid the cost of ineffective treatments or unnecessary hospitalization;

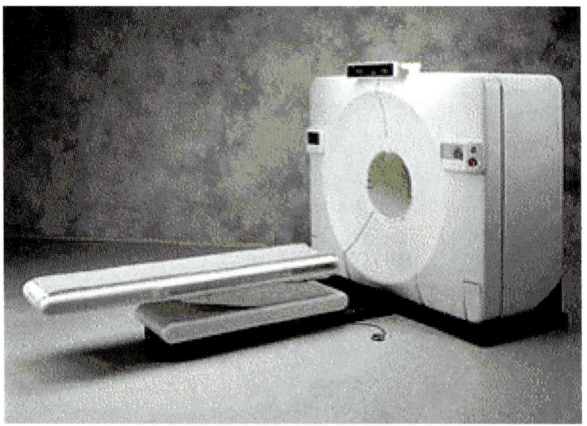

Fig. 33.2 A PET-CT scanner V (Courtesy, GE)

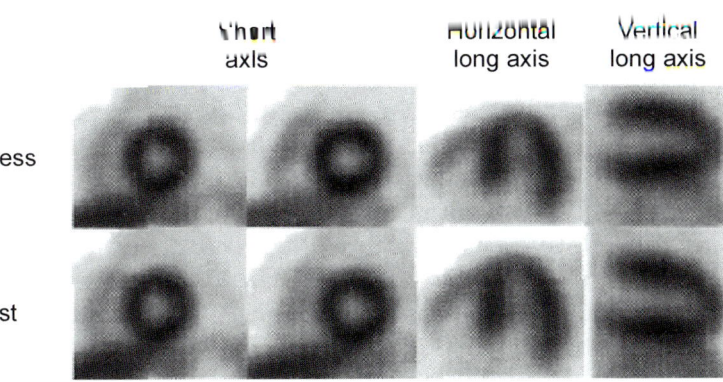

Fig. 33.3 Relatively homogenous distribution of myocardial blood flow in normal human heart after injection of N^{13} NH$_3$, shown in short axis, horizontal long axis and vertical long axis tomographic views. (From Atlas of Nuclear Cardiology by Vasken Dilsizian and Jagat Narula, Current Medicine, Inc., Philadelphia)

- In some cases, replace multiple diagnostic procedures with a single examination;
- Help predict the prognosis for surgical procedures, to eliminating those that won't benefit the patient, thus significantly reducing the cost of healthcare delivery.

PET is already making critical contributions to more cost-effective patient management in three primary medical disciplines: oncology, cardiology and neurology. As researchers use PET to explore the basic physiology underlying disease processes, additional clinical applications are likely to evolve. Our discussion in this chapter will be limited to applications of PET imaging in cardiology

- Myocardial perfusion
- Myocardial metabolism
- Myocardial viability in coronary artery disease
- Use of PET in noninvasive diagnostic testing of patients with vascular disease prior to major cardiac surgery
- Hypertrophic cardiomyopathy

33.4 Positron Emission Tomography in Assessment of Viability

Myocardial viability has been defined as the temporal improvement in contractile function of a dysfunctional region after restoration of blood flow. PET is an established noninvasive method of evaluating myocardial perfusion and viability [1]. This technique has the advantage of being able to assess perfusion and metabolism simultaneously. PET scanning involves the use of positron-emitting isotopes such as oxygen-15 (O^{15}), carbon-11 (C^{11}), nitrogen-13 (N^{13}), and fluorine-18 (F^{18}), which are incorporated into physiologically active molecules.

Under normal circumstances myocyte metabolism depends primarily on fatty acids. Ischemia shifts myocyte metabolism preferentially from fatty acids to glucose. Thus, uptake of a glucose analog, fluorine-18 labeled deoxyglucose (FDG) by myocytes in an area of dysfunctional myocardium indicates metabolic activity and thus, viability. Regional perfusion can be simultaneously assessed with an agent that remains in the vascular space and thus demonstrates the distribution of blood flow (such as N^{13} ammonia or Rb^{82}). Hence, PET imaging has the potential to differentiate between normal, stunned, hibernating, and scarred myocardium (Figs. 33.3, 33.4, 33.5). The presence of enhanced FDG uptake in regions of decreased blood flow (known as a "PET metabolism-perfusion mismatch") defines hibernating myocardium by PET imaging, while a concordant reduction in both metabolism and flow ("PET match") is thought to represent predominantly scarred myocardium. Regional dysfunction in the presence of normal perfusion is indicative of stunning.

Myocardial segments with significant reductions in both blood flow and FDG uptake have only a 20% chance of functional improvement following revascularization. In comparison, dysfunctional territories deemed to be hibernating by PET have approximately an 80 to 85% chance of functional improvement following revascularization [2–9]. A study by Hass et al. [12] showed that the determination of myocardial viability evaluation in patients with coronary artery disease and severe left ventricular dysfunction before referral to coronary artery revascularization affects clinical outcome with respect to both in-hospital mortality and 1-year survival rate. In this retrospective study, the perioperative and postoperative event-free survival rate was significantly lower in patients who were referred for revascularization on the basis of clinical presentation and angiographic data but without viability testing (group A) compared with those who were selected according to the extent of viable tissue determined by PET (group B) in addition to clinical presentation and angiographic data. There were four in-hospital deaths (11.4%) in group A and none in group B ($P=0.04$).

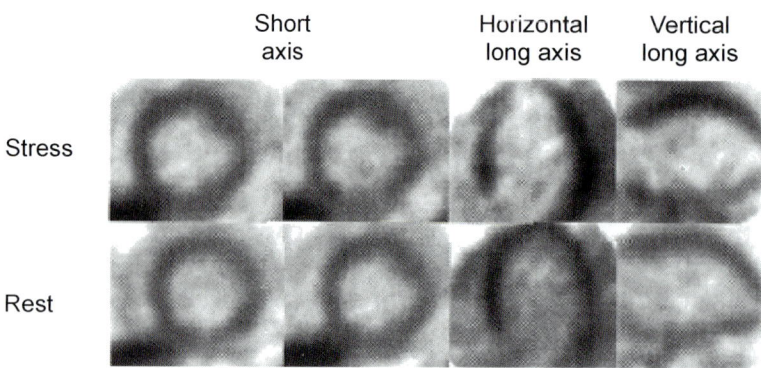

Fig. 33.4 Relative distribution of myocardial blood flow in a patient with coronary artery disease (CAD) after injection of $N^{13}NH_3$, shown in short axis, horizontal long axis and vertical long axis tomographic views. The diminished tracer concentrations in the anterior and septum of the LV reflect a flow defect resulting from an 85% diameter stenosis of the left anterior descending (LAD) coronary artery. Relative myocardial perfusion appears best preserved in the lateral wall. However, a 50% diameter stenosis of the left circumflex (LCX) artery remains unidentified on the perfusion images. (From Atlas of Nuclear Cardiology by Vasken Dilsizian and Jagat Narula, Current Medicine, Inc., Philadelphia)

Moreover, after 12 months, the survival rate was 79% in group A and 97% in group B ($P=0.01$)

Another study examined 43 patients with regional asynergy and a mean left ventricular (LV) ejection fraction of 41% who were evaluated by PET imaging [9]. The positive and negative predictive values of PET imaging for improvement in asynergy and wall motion score after revascularization were 76 and 96%, respectively. Other studies have shown that the extent of myocardium that demonstrates enhanced FDG uptake in patients with ischemic cardiomyopathy may predict the magnitude of improvement in ejection fraction, exercise tolerance and heart failure symptoms after surgical revascularization [50].

Another analysis reported that scar size on FDG PET was an independent predictor of improvement in ejection fraction after revascularization. In 70 patients with a mean resting EF of 26%, scars were divided into territories graded as small, moderate, or large (0 to 16%, 16 to 27.5%, and 27.5 to 47% of total myocardium, respectively) [55]. The change in EF after revascularization was significantly greater for patients with smaller scars (change of 9.0, 3.7, and 1.3% for small, moderate, or large scars, respectively).

The outcome after coronary artery bypass grafting may be improved by incorporating PET derived viability information, in addition to clinical and angiographic data, when selecting patients with impaired LV function for revascularization [12, 13]. As an example, one study evaluated the prognostic significance of the presence of viable myocardium, and its interaction with myocardial revascularization, in patients with LV dysfunction after MI [13]. Nonfatal ischemic events occurred in 48% of medically-treated FDG (+) patients compared with only 8% of FDG (+) revascularized patients and 5% of patients with FDG (−) myocardium; however, mortality was similar among FDG (+) and FDG (−) patients.

It remains unclear if PET is more useful than SPECT for viability assessment [14–16]. Some studies, including one randomized trial, found that the ability to detect myocardial viability with PET or SPECT imaging was the same and that there was no difference in patient outcome when management decisions were based upon the results of either technique [14, 15]. Patients in this study had generally moderate LV dysfunction (LV EF approximately 30%). PET has theoretical advantages over SPECT in the setting of very severe LV dysfunction.

33.5 FDG-SPECT Imaging

The use of specialized collimators has allowed the adaptation of widely available SPECT imaging cameras to capture the 511 keV positrons emanating from F^{18} FDG [17–19]. Preliminary data from some studies of patients revascularized for CAD-related LV dysfunction have demonstrated superior predictive values for functional recovery with FDG-SPECT compared with other techniques (particularly thallium-201 SPECT with reinjection and low dose dobutamine echocardiography) [5, 11, 20].

As an example, one study of patients with LV dysfunction reported that significant improvement of global LV function occurred in those with three or more viable segments on FDG-SPECT [20]. Another study found that the combined use of FDG-SPECT and dobutamine echocardiography derived data resulted in the most accurate prediction of functional recovery in hypokinetic segments [11]. On the other hand, one study comparing FDG-SPECT with PET and thallium-201[21] SPECT did report that although FDG-SPECT significantly increased the sensitivity for detecting viable myocardium, 27% of segments were falsely identified as viable when judged nonviable by both PET and thallium-201 [22].

Therefore, the relative merits of FDG-SPECT and the more conventional techniques for viability assessment need to be assessed in further clinical trials. Analogous to PET, obtaining simultaneous perfusion data during FDG SPECT imaging may improve accuracy for viability detection [23, 24]. Future studies will determine whether the physical problems associated with gamma camera imaging of this agent, as well as technical issues such as the need for attenuation correction, can be overcome to a degree that this technique can provide superior information, rather than just similar information, to conventional (and less expensive) SPECT approaches.

33.6
Fatty Acid Imaging

Ischemia shifts myocardial metabolism from long-chain fatty acids, which is the predominant substrate

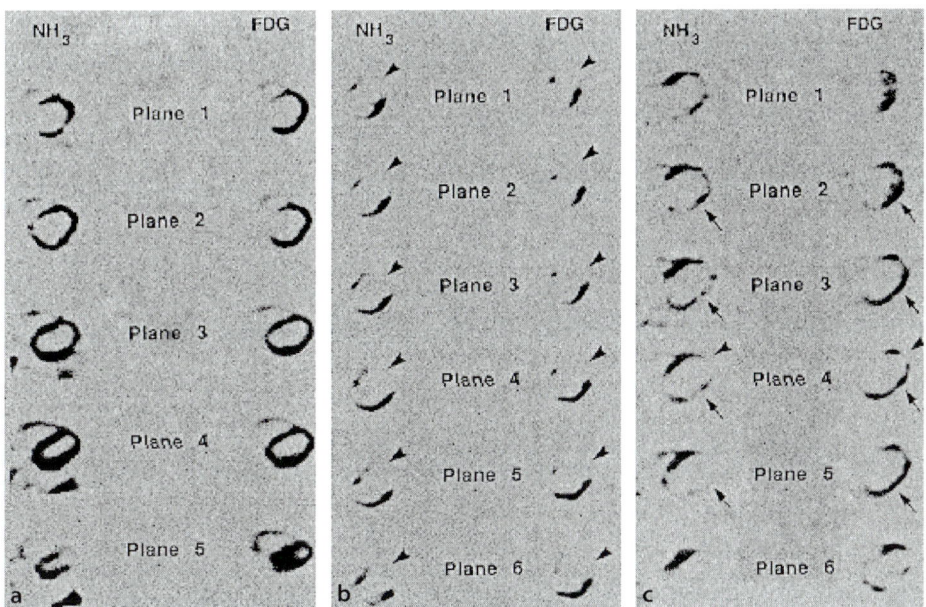

Fig. 33.5a–c Examples of N^{13} ammonia (NH^3) and F^{18} 2 deoxyglucose (FDG) tomographic images. (**a**) A subject with non-ischemic dilated cardiomyopathy, blood flow (N^{13} ammonia) and glucose metabolism (F^{18} deoxyglucose) imaging is homogeneous without any defect in uptake. (**b**) A subject with ischemic cardiomyopathy as shown by concordant decrease in both tracer images (arrowheads). (**c**) A subject with coronary artery disease. Concordant decrease in both tracers (arrowheads) reveals apical and inferior infarction. A mismatch in blood flow (NH_3) (decreased) and glucose metabolism (FDG) (increased) is seen in an extensive area of the posterolateral and true lateral wall representing ischemia (*arrows*). (From Mody et al. J Am Coll Cardiol 17(2) Feb 1991:373–383. Elsevier Inc, New York 10000-1710)

under aerobic conditions, to glucose [26]. This finding prompted the investigation of several radionuclide-labeled fatty acid compounds for use in myocardial imaging. The uptake and washout kinetics of these agents are reflective of distinct pathways of myocardial fatty acid metabolism that are altered in acute ischemia, chronic ischemia and the different states of dysfunctional but viable myocardium. Initial studies used C^{11} palmitate and PET imaging with encouraging results [26, 27]. Subsequent efforts were directed towards adapting these tracers and protocols for the more widely available SPECT cameras, and obviating the need for cyclotron production, thus resulting in the introduction of I-123 labeled agents.

123 I-iodophenylpentadecanoic acid (IPPA) is a straight chain fatty acid that is taken up by the myocardium in proportion to regional perfusion. Under non-ischemic conditions this tracer is rapidly metabolized and released, resulting in rapid washout kinetics [28]. Suppressed metabolism in the presence of ischemia results in longer myocardial retention and a "redistribution" pattern on serial imaging [29]. Qualitative and semi-quantitative analysis of IPPA uptake and washout have been used in various clinical trials to successfully diagnose coronary stenosis [28], detect myocardial ischemia [30], determine myocardial viability [31–33], and predict recovery of regional LV dysfunction following revascularization [34]. One study, for example, demonstrated superiority of this agent over rest-redistribution thallium-201 imaging for viability detection [33]. However, the rapid dynamics of straight chain fatty acid uptake and metabolism is a critical problem for SPECT imaging.

Methyl-branching of the fatty acid chain protects against beta oxidation and considerably slows down washout from the myocardium (metabolic trapping) [35]. Of the methyl-branched fatty acid tracers, 123 I-(p-iodophenyl)-3-(R,S)-methypentadecanoic acid (BMIPP) [36] has been extensively studied in Japan and Europe, and more recently in the USA. Excellent quality images with high heart to background ratios can be obtained 15 to 30 minutes after tracer administration [37]. Because of the metabolic modulation, however, separate imaging with thallium-201 or one of the Tc-99m ligands is required for perfusion assessment.

The clinical utility of BMIPP imaging stems from the fact that abnormalities of fatty acid metabolism resulting from transient ischemia persist for prolonged periods [37]. Therefore, a defect on BMIPP imaging is indicative of recent ischemia, even when perfusion has returned to normal (ischemic memory). Detection of ischemic memory has potential utility in many clinical situations including assessment of chest pain in the emergency department, diagnosis of CAD without stress testing, and vasospastic angina. In dysfunctional myocardium, a disproportionately greater decrease in BMIPP compared with a perfusion trace uptake probably represents ongoing ischemia with recurrent stunning, and has been shown to correlate with preserved inotropic reserve [38], histological evidence of viability [39], and predict post-revascularization recovery of function [40–43]. On the other hand a concordant, severe reduction in both BMIPP uptake and perfusions indicates scar tissue.

33.7
Comparison with Non-nuclear Techniques

Dobutamine echocardiography is an established technique for viability detection. More recently, cardiovascular magnetic resonance (CMR) [44] and myocardial contrast echocardiography (MCE) [45] have also been tested in clinical trials.

Comparative data on viability detection methods are limited. A pooled analysis of clinical trials using radionuclide perfusion imaging, PET and dobutamine echocardiography showed radionuclide perfusion techniques to be more sensitive, dobutamine echocardiography to be more specific and PET to have slightly higher overall accuracy for detecting viability, defined as functional recovery after revascularization [46]. In another meta-analysis [56] the presence of viable myocardium conferred a survival benefit on patients with LV dysfunction who were revascularized irrespective of the technique used to detect viability. The only randomized comparative study showed similar results for Tc-99m sestamibi SPECT imaging and PET. Therefore, it appears that even if small differences in predictive values between the agents or the techniques exist on a region-by-region basis, there may still be no overall difference in impact on decision making for catheterization or revascularization.

33.8
Implications of Detecting Viable Myocardium

A substantial body of observational data has established a relationship between the presence and extent of viability in dysfunctional myocardium, and improved outcome after revascularization. Outcome measures have included regional and global LV function [2, 51, 52], heart failure symptoms [10, 47], and survival [48, 49, 53, 54]. In a pooled analysis of 3088 patients in 24 observational studies, patients with LV dysfunction and preserved myocardial viability were at high risk with an annual mortality of 16%. This was reduced to 3.2% with

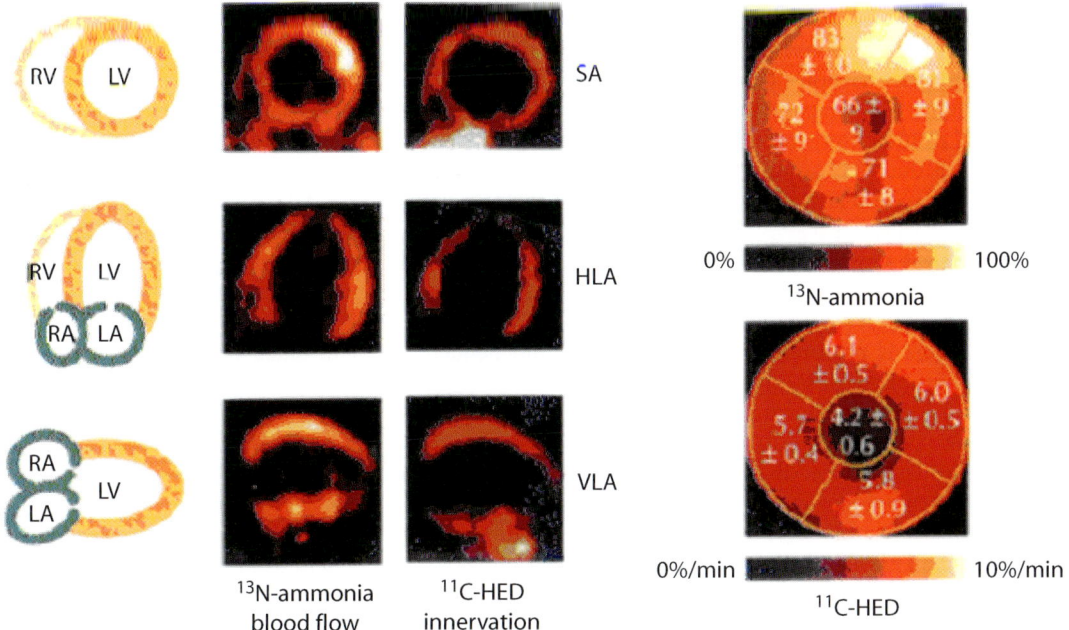

Fig. 33.6 Neuronal imaging in cardiomyopathy. PET images obtained in a patient with DCM and reduced LVEF following injection of N^{13} ammonia and 40 minutes after the injection of C^{11} hydroxyephedrine (C^{11} HED). There is relatively homogenous distribution of N^{13} ammonia, indicating intact myocardial perfusion. However, there is markedly reduced retention of C^{11} HED, indicating partial denervation of the LV in this patient with DCM. (From Atlas of Nuclear Cardiology by Vasken Dilsizian and Jagat Narula, Current Medicine, Inc., Philadelphia)

revascularization. Patients with predominantly nonviable myocardium had a high mortality irrespective of whether they received revascularization (7.7%) or medical management (6.2%).

These data suggest that the presence of viable myocardium, as defined by noninvasive imaging in patients with heart failure, is a marker for very high risk without revascularization. That risk appears to be significantly reduced by revascularization. These conclusions must be noted in the context of the limitations of pooling observational cohort studies, which may bring into play selection biases that cannot be evaluated in the meta-analyzing published literature. More definitive conclusions await results from ongoing trials randomizing heart failure patients without angina to revascularization or no revascularization.

33.9
Cardiac Neurotransmission Imaging

PET can be used to visualize and quantify the pathophysiologic processes that take place in the nerve terminals, synaptic clefts and postsynaptic sites in the heart. In many clinical circumstances, evaluation of abnormalities of the cardiac nerves and ganglia and the neurotransmission process may be of clinical value. PET imaging with F^{18} Flurodopamine can be used to examine cardiac sympathetic innervation in patients with different types of dysautonomia. Scintigraphic uptake of I^{123} MIBG and C^{11} Hydroxyephedrine can identify spontaneous reinnervation taking place after cardiac transplantation (Fig. 33.6). Alterations of cardiac sympathetic innervations in dilated cardiomyopathy with I^{123} MIBG imaging have a potential prognostic value.

33.10.
Recommendations

In patients with stable symptoms of heart failure and/or angina in the setting of LV dysfunction, an exercise or pharmacologic stress SPECT study with thallium-201 or Tc-99m sestamibi (with an accompanying redistribution/reinjection or rest study) will provide comprehensive information regarding functional capacity (treadmill time and workload), the extent of stress-induced ischemia (read as the degree of stress defect reversibility), and the extent of myocardial viability (read as the isotope content within dysfunctional territories). The data related to ischemia and viability permits an estimation of the probability and magnitude of recovery of regional and global dysfunction after bypass surgery or angioplasty; they can thus play an important role in decision making regarding catheterization and revascularization.

In patients with known severe coronary artery disease and known significant regional and global LV dysfunction, the extent of myocardial viability should be considered, even if angina is not present, since revascularization may be appropriate in some cases. Clinical studies have thus far failed to demonstrate superiority of one perfusion tracer (i.e., thallium-201, Tc-99m sestamibi or Tc-99m tetrofosmin) over the others for viability assessment, and individual centers should use standard site protocols.

When the presence and extent of preserved myocardial viability is the only question of concern, a resting perfusion scan should be performed first. The administration of intravenous nitrate or sublingual nitroglycerine 5 minutes before tracer injection at rest may slightly improve sensitivity for viability detection. When the amount of resting tracer uptake clearly establishes the presence (or absence) of viability, stress testing is not generally required. However, in cases of "indeterminate" resting scans, the demonstration of perfusion defect reversibility on stress testing provides additional information indicative of viability. Stress testing is also necessary in patients who may have areas of ischemia as well as viability.

While PET has contributed to our understanding of the physiology of stunning and hibernation and can assess the potential for functional recovery with reasonable accuracy, it is not in routine use for clinical evaluation at most institutions. Referral to a PET center may provide important incremental information in patients in whom questions of viability and revascularization remain after more widely available SPECT imaging. In the few centers where cardiac PET is available on site and is performed frequently, this might be the initial approach to viability assessment.

33.11
Role of Metabolic PET Imaging in the Study of Specific Disease Processes

33.11.1
Coronary Artery Disease

The role of PET imaging in determining myocardial perfusion and viability has been discussed above.

33.11.2
Left Ventricular Hypertrophy

There are several lines of evidence suggesting a link between myocardial fatty acid metabolism and left ventricular hypertrophy (LVH). Observations have shown that in children with genetic defects in enzymatic pathways of myocardial fatty acid oxidation (MFAO) caused LVH [57]. Measurements of myocardial fatty acid metabolism by PET and C-11 palmitate demonstrated that MFAO was the only measurement of fatty acid metabolism that was an independent predictor of left ventricular mass [58].

33.11.3
Dilated Cardiomyopathy (DCM)/Heart Failure

Alterations in myocardial substrate metabolism have been implicated in the pathogenesis of contractile dysfunction and heart failure [59–61]. Early studies of myocardial metabolism assessed patients with heart failure by using PET to estimate the clearance rates of long-chain fatty acid tracers such as C^{11} palmitate [62–64]. The initial uptake of C^{11} palmitate represents primarily MBF; it then clears the myocardium in a biexponential pattern, with the early rapid phase reflecting MFAO and the slow clearance representing incorporation of the tracer into the lipid storage pools. By use of this method, decreased rates of MFAO were shown in patients with myocardial long-chain acyl-coenzyme A (CoA) dehydrogenase genetic defects [65]. Furthermore, the extent of decreased clearance of C-11 palmitate was shown to correlate with the clinical severity. In patients with dilated cardiomyopathy, SPECT with BMIPP also showed impaired myocardial fatty acid uptake [65].

Metabolic imaging has also been used to assess the response to therapy. The efficacy of β-blocker therapy in the treatment of the cardiomyopathic patient is well established. Another unique application of metabolic imaging has been in the measurement of energy transduction in normal and diseased myocardium. By combining measurements of left ventricular myocardial external work (by either echocardiography or right heart catheterization) with measurements of MVO_2 performed by PET and C^{11} acetate, it is possible to estimate cardiac efficiency [67]. With the use of this technique, myocardial efficiency has been shown to be improved in patients with heart failure with both exercise training and cardiac resynchronization therapy, implicating improved myocardial energetics as a potential mechanism [68, 69]. A study with PET and FDG in patients with dilated cardiomyopathy and left bundle branch block demonstrated a septal reduction in myocardial glucose utilization (MGU) that is not matched by a regional reduction in perfusion. Moreover, treatment with cardiac resynchronization therapy resulted in homogenization of this unbalanced glucose metabolism [70]. Treatment with the selective β-blocker metoprolol also leads to a reduction in oxidative metabolism and an improvement in cardiac efficiency in patients with left ventricular dysfunction [71]. PET measurements of F-18 fluoro-6-thia-heptadecanoic acid and FDG kinetics before and during treatment with the β-blocker carvedilol in patients with ischemic cardiomyopathy demonstrated a decrease in MFAU but no change in MGU, potentially providing a mechanism for the improved energy efficiency [66]. Moreover, in patients with dilated cardiomyopathy, the percentage glucose uptake, as measured by PET and FDG, was a predictor for the effectiveness of β-blocker therapy [72].

33.11.4
Obesity-Insulin Resistance

There is a burgeoning body of compelling evidence to suggest that obesity induces marked increases in myocardial fatty acid metabolism. In either dietary-induced or transgenic models of obesity, myocardial fatty acid uptake and oxidation are significantly increased [73–76]. An increase in body mass index is associated with a shift in myocardial substrate metabolism toward greater fatty acid use. Moreover, this dependence on myocardial fatty acid metabolism increased with worsening insulin resistance [77]. This metabolic shift was associated with an increase in MVO_2 and a decline in left ventricular energy transduction.

33.11.5
Diabetes Mellitus

Diabetes mellitus is a well-recognized major risk factor for cardiovascular disease in general and coronary artery disease in particular [78–80]. In addition, cardiomyopathy occurs commonly in diabetic patients independent of known risk factors such as coronary artery disease or hypertension [81]. Evidence is emerging that diabetic cardiomyopathy may be related to derangements in myocardial energy metabolism [82, 83]. In patients with diabetes, glucose utilization is markedly reduced and fatty acids account for 90% to 99% of MVO_2, as opposed to 50% to 70% as observed in nondiabetic subjects [82, 84]. Furthermore, the heart's capacity to switch energy substrates becomes constrained. This dependence on fatty acid metabolism can be attributed to multiple mechanisms including (1) the presence of high plasma levels of fatty acids and triglycerides enhancing both myocardial fatty acid utilization and triacylglycerol formation, (2) the presence of hypoinsulinemia causing subcellular (microsomal) localization of the glucose transporter GLUT-4 and decreased acetyl-CoA carboxylase activity, and (3) the combined effects of high plasma fatty acids and hypoinsulinemia reducing the activity of the pyruvate dehydrogenase complex [85, 86]. With the increase in myocardial fatty acid metabolism, there is an overall decline in glucose metabolism.

33.12
Future Trends

With advancement in instrumentation design, accurate tracer quantifications and attenuation corrections are possible. Improved detector design and electronics will assure more accurate complex compartmental modeling and better characterization of the metabolism of a given substrate. Hybrid PET/CT scanners hold a greater promise for attenuation correction and will permit near-simultaneous assessment of anatomic perfusion, function and metabolism by using a single piece of equipment.

References

1. Schelbert HR (1994) Metabolic imaging to assess myocardial viability. J Nucl Med 35:8S.
2. Tillisch J, Brunken R, Marshall R, Schwaiger M, Mandelkern M, Phelps M, Schelbert H (1986) Reversibility of cardiac wall-motion abnormalities predicted by positron tomography. N Engl J Med 314:884.
3. Tamaki N, Ohtani H, Yamashita K, Magata Y, Yonekura Y, Nohara R, Kambara H, Kawai C, Hirata K, Ban T et al. (1991) Metabolic activity in the areas of new fill-in after thallium-201 reinjection: comparison with positron emission tomography using fluorine-18-deoxyglucose. J Nucl Med 32:673.
4. Lucignani G, Paolini G, Landoni C, Zuccari M, Paganelli G, Galli L, Di C, Vanoli G, Rossetti C, Mariani MA et al. (1992) Presurgical identification of hibernating myocardium by combined use of technetium-99m hexakis 2- methoxyisobutylisonitrile single photon emission tomography and fluorine-18 fluoro-2-deoxy-D-glucose positron emission tomography in patients with coronary artery disease. Eur J Nucl Med 19:874.
5. Tamaki, N, Yonekura Y, Yamashita K, Saji H, Magata Y, Senda M, Konishi Y, Hirata K, Ban T, Konishi J (1989) Positron emission tomography using fluorine-18 deoxyglucose in evaluation of coronary artery bypass grafting. Am J Cardiol 64:860.

6. Marwick TH, MacIntyre WJ, Lafont A, Nemec JJ, Salcedo, EE (1992) Metabolic responses of hibernating and infarcted myocardium to revascularization. A follow-up study of regional perfusion, function, and metabolism. Circulation 85:1347.
7. Carrel T, Jenni R, Haubold-Reuter S, von S, Pasic M, Turina M (1992) Improvement of severely reduced left ventricular function after surgical revascularization in patients with preoperative myocardial infarction. Eur J Cardiothorac Surg 6:479.
8. Gropler RJ, Geltman EM, Sampathkumaran K, Perez JE, Moerlein SM, Sobel BE, Bergmann SR, Siegel BA (1992) Functional recovery after coronary revascularization for chronic coronary artery disease is dependent on maintenance of oxidative metabolism. J Am Coll Cardiol 20:569.
9. Tamaki N, Kawamoto M, Tadamura E, Magata Y, Yonekura Y, Nohara R, Sasayama S, Nishimura K, Ban T, Konishi J (1995) Prediction of reversible ischemia after revascularization. Perfusion and metabolic studies with positron emission tomography. Circulation 91:1697.
10. Di Carli MF, Asgarzadie F, Schelbert HR, Brunken RC, Laks H, Phelps ME, Maddahi J (1995) Quantitative relation between myocardial viability and improvement in heart failure symptoms after revascularization in patients with ischemic cardiomyopathy. Circulation 92:3436.
11. Bax JJ, Cornel JH, Visser FC, Fioretti PM, Van L, Reijs AE, Boersma E, Teule GJ, Visser CA (1996) Prediction of recovery of myocardial dysfunction after revascularization. Comparison of fluorine-18 fluorodeoxyglucose/thallium-201 SPECT, thallium-201 stress-reinjection SPECT and dobutamine echocardiography. J Am Coll Cardiol 28:558.
12. Haas F, Haehnel CJ, Picker W, Nekolla S, Martinoff S, Meisner H, Schwaiger M (1997) Preoperative positron emission tomographic viability assessment and perioperative and postoperative risk in patients with advanced ischemic heart disease. J Am Coll Cardiol 30:1693-1700.
13. Lee KS, Marwick TH, Cook SA, Go RT, Fix JS, James KB, Sapp SK, MacIntyre WJ, Thomas JD (1994) Prognosis of patients with left ventricular dysfunction, with and without viable myocardium after myocardial infarction. Relative efficacy of medical therapy and revascularization. Circulation 90:2687.
14. Siebelink HM, Blanksma PK, Crijns HJ, Bax JJ, van B, Kingma T, Piers DA, Pruim J, Jager PL, Vaalburg W, Van d (2001) No difference in cardiac event-free survival between positron emission tomography-guided and single-photon emission computed tomography-guided patient management: a prospective, randomized comparison of patients with suspicion of jeopardized myocardium. J Am Coll Cardiol 37:81.
15. Marin-Neto, JA, Dilsizian V, Arrighi JA, Perrone-Filardi P, Bacharach SL, Bonow RO (1998) Thallium scintigraphy compared with 18F-fluorodeoxyglucose positron emission tomography for assessing myocardial viability in patients with moderate versus severe left ventricular dysfunction. Am J Cardiol 82:1001.
16. Rohatgi R, Epstein S, Henriquez J, Ababneh AA, Hickey KT, Pinsky D, Akinboboye O, Bergmann SR (2001) Utility of positron emission tomography in predicting cardiac events and survival in patients with coronary artery disease and severe left ventricular dysfunction. Am J Cardiol 87:1096.
17. Kerrou K, Toussaint, JF, Froissart, M, Talbot, JN (2000) Myocardial viability assessment with FDG imaging: comparison of PET, SPECT, and gamma-camera coincidence detection. J Nucl Med 41:2099.
18. Mabuchi M, Kubo, N, Morita, K et al. (2002) Value and limitation of myocardial fluorodeoxyglucose single photon emission computed tomography using ultra-high energy collimators for assessing myocardial viability. Nucl Med Commun 23:879.
19. Fitzgerald J, Parker JA, Danias PG (2000) F-18 fluoro deoxyglucose SPECT for assessment of myocardial viability. J Nucl Cardiol 7:382.
20. Bax JJ, Cornel JH, Visser FC, Fioretti PM, Van L, Huitink JM, Kamp O, Nijland F, Roelandt JR, Visser CA (1997) Prediction of improvement of contractile function in patients with ischemic ventricular dysfunction after revascularization by fluorine-18 fluorodeoxyglucose single-photon emission computed tomography. J Am Coll Cardiol 30:377.
21. Sato H, Iwasaki T, Toyama T et al. (2000) Prediction of functional recovery after revascularization in coronary artery disease using (18)F-FDG and (123)I-BMIPP SPECT. Chest 117:65.
22. Srinivasan G, Kitsiou AN, Bacharach SL, Bartlett ML, Miller-Davis C, Dilsizian V (1998) Fluorodeoxyglucose single photon emission computed tomography: can it replace PET and thallium SPECT for the assessment of myocardial viability? Circulation 97:843.
23. De Boer J, Slart RH, Blanksma PK et al. (2003) Comparison of 99mTc-sestamibi-18F-fluorodeoxyglucose dual isotope simultaneous acquisition and rest-stress 99mTc-sestamibi single photon emission computed tomography for the assessment of myocardial viability. Nucl Med Commun 24:251.
24. Fukuchi K, Katafuchi T, Fukushima K et al. (2000) Estimation of myocardial perfusion and viability using simultaneous 99mTc-tetrofosmin--FDG collimated SPECT. J Nucl Med 41:1318.
25. Neely JR, Rovetto MJ, Oram JF (1972) Myocardial utilization of carbohydrate and lipids. Prog Cardiovasc Dis 15:289.
26. Goldstein RA, Klein MS, Welch MJ, Sobel BE (1980) External assessment of myocardial metabolism with C-11 palmitate in vivo. J Nucl Med 21:342.

27. Schon HR, Schelbert HR, Robinson G et al. (1982) C-11 labeled palmitic acid for the noninvasive evaluation of regional myocardial fatty acid metabolism with positron-computed tomography. I. Kinetics of C-11 palmitic acid in normal myocardium. Am Heart J 103:532.
28. Reske SN, Biersack HJ, Lackner K et al. (1982) Assessment of regional myocardial uptake and metabolism of omega-(p-123I-phenyl) pentadecanoic acid with serial single-photon emission tomography. Nuklearmedizin 21:249.
29. Yang JY, Ruiz M, Calnon DA et al. (1999) Assessment of myocardial viability using 123I-labeled iodophenylpentadecanoic acid at sustained low flow or after acute infarction and reperfusion. J Nucl Med 40:821.
30. Caldwell JH, Martin GV, Link JM et al. (1990) Iodophenylpentadecanoic acid-myocardial blood flow relationship during maximal exercise with coronary occlusion. J Nucl Med 31:99.
31. Murray G, Schad N, Ladd W et al. (1992) Metabolic cardiac imaging in severe coronary disease: assessment of viability with iodine-123-iodophenylpentadecanoic acid and multicrystal gamma camera, and correlation with biopsy. J Nucl Med 33:1269.
32. Hansen CL, Heo J, Oliner C et al. (1995) Prediction of improvement in left ventricular function with iodine-123-IPPA after coronary revascularization. J Nucl Med 36:1987.
33. Iskandrian AS, Powers J, Cave V, Wasserleben V, Cassell D, Heo J (1995) Assessment of myocardial viability by dynamic tomographic iodine 123 iodophenylpentadecanoic acid imaging: comparison with rest-redistribution thallium 201 imaging. J Nucl Cardiol 2:101.
34. Verani MS, Taillefer R, Iskandrian AE et al. (200) 123I-IPPA SPECT for the prediction of enhanced left ventricular function after coronary bypass graft surgery. Multicenter IPPA Viability Trial Investigators. 123I-iodophenylpentadecanoic acid. J Nucl Med 41:1299.
35. Tamaki N, Tadamura E, Kawamoto M et al. (1995) Decreased uptake of iodinated branched fatty acid analog indicates metabolic alterations in ischemic myocardium. J Nucl Med 36:1974.
36. Knapp FF Jr, Goodman MM, Callahan AP, Kirsch G (1986) Radioiodinated 15-(p-iodophenyl)-3,3-dimethylpentadecanoic acid: a useful new agent to evaluate myocardial fatty acid uptake. J Nucl Med 27:521.
37. Tamaki N, Kawamoto M, Yonekura Y et al. (1992) Regional metabolic abnormality in relation to perfusion and wall motion in patients with myocardial infarction: assessment with emission tomography using an iodinated branched fatty acid analog. J Nucl Med 33:659.
38. Hambye AS, Vaerenberg MM, Dobbeleir AA et al. (1998) Abnormal BMIPP uptake in chronically dysfunctional myocardial segments: correlation with contractile response to low-dose dobutamine. J Nucl Med 39:1845.
39. Kudoh T, Tadamura E, Tamaki N et al. (2000) Iodinated free fatty acid and 201Tl uptake in chronically hypoperfused myocardium: histologic correlation study. J Nucl Med 41:293.
40. Franken PR, Dendale P, De Geeter F et al. (1996) Prediction of functional outcome after myocardial infarction using BMIPP and sestamibi scintigraphy. J Nucl Med 37:718.
41. Ito T, Tanouchi J, Kato J et al. (1996) Recovery of impaired left ventricular function in patients with acute myocardial infarction is predicted by the discordance in defect size on 123I-BMIPP and 201Tl SPET images. Eur J Nucl Med 23:917.
42. Hashimoto A, Nakata T, Tsuchihashi K et al. (1996) Postischemic functional recovery and BMIPP uptake after primary percutaneous transluminal coronary angioplasty in acute myocardial infarction. Am J Cardiol 77:25.
43. Naruse H, Arii T, Kondo T et al. (1998) Clinical usefulness of iodine 123-labeled fatty acid imaging in patients with acute myocardial infarction. J Nucl Cardiol 5:275.
44. Kim RJ, Wu E, Rafael A, Chen EL, Parker MA, Simonetti O, Klocke FJ, Bonow RO, Judd RM (2000) The use of contrast-enhanced magnetic resonance imaging to identify reversible myocardial dysfunction. N Engl J Med 343:1445.
45. Kim RJ, Wu E, Rafael A, Chen EL, Parker MA, Simonetti O, Klocke FJ, Bonow RO, Judd RM (2000) The use of contrast-enhanced magnetic resonance imaging to identify reversible myocardial dysfunction. N Engl J Med 343:1445.
46. Bax JJ, Wijns W, Cornel JH, Visser FC, Boersma E, Fioretti PM (1997) Accuracy of currently available techniques for prediction of functional recovery after revascularization in patients with left ventricular dysfunction due to chronic coronary artery disease: comparison of pooled data. J Am Coll Cardiol 30:1451.
47. Marwick TH, Zuchowski C, Lauer MS et al. (1999) Functional status and quality of life in patients with heart failure undergoing coronary bypass surgery after assessment of myocardial viability. J Am Coll Cardiol 33:750.
48. Senior R, Kaul S, Raval U, Lahiri A (2002) Impact of revascularization and myocardial viability determined by nitrate-enhanced Tc-99m sestamibi and Tl-201 imaging on mortality and functional outcome in ischemic cardiomyopathy. J Nucl Cardiol 9:454.
49. Di Carli MF, Maddahi J, Rokhsar S et al. (1998) Long-term survival of patients with coronary artery disease and left ventricular dysfunction: implications for the role of myocardial viability assessment in management decisions. J Thorac Cardiovasc Surg 116:997.
50. Gerber BL, Ordoubadi FF, Wijns W, Vanoverschelde JL, Knuuti MJ, Janier M, Melon P, Blanksma PK, Bol A, Bax JJ, Melin JA, Camici PG (2001) Positron emission tomography using(18)F-fluoro-deoxyglucose and euglycaemic

51. Ragosta M, Beller GA, Watson DD, Kaul S, Gimple LW (1993) Quantitative planar rest-redistribution 201Tl imaging in detection of myocardial viability and prediction of improvement in left ventricular function after coronary bypass surgery in patients with severely depressed left ventricular function. Circulation 87:1630.

52. Bax JJ, Cornel JH, Visser FC, Fioretti PM, Van L, Huitink JM, Kamp O, Nijland F, Roelandt JR, Visser CA (1997) Prediction of improvement of contractile function in patients with ischemic ventricular dysfunction after revascularization by fluorine-18 fluorodeoxyglucose single-photon emission computed tomography. J Am Coll Cardiol 30:377.

53. Senior R, Kaul S, Raval U, Lahiri A (2002) Impact of revascularization and myocardial viability determined by nitrate-enhanced Tc-99m sestamibi and Tl-201 imaging on mortality and functional outcome in ischemic cardiomyopathy. J Nucl Cardiol 9:454.

54. Di Carli MF, Maddahi J, Rokhsar S et al. (1998) Long-term survival of patients with coronary artery disease and left ventricular dysfunction: implications for the role of myocardial viability assessment in management decisions. J Thorac Cardiovasc Surg 116:997.

55. Beanlands RS, Ruddy TD, deKemp RA et al. (2002) Positron emission tomography and recovery following revascularization (PARR-1): the importance of scar and the development of a prediction rule for the degree of recovery of left ventricular function. J Am Coll Cardiol 40:1735.

56. Allman KC, Shaw LJ, Hachamovitch R, Udelson JE (2002) Myocardial viability testing and impact of revascularization on prognosis in patients with coronary artery disease and left ventricular dysfunction: a meta-analysis. J Am Coll Cardiol 39:1151.

57. Roe CR, Coates PM (1995) Mitochondrial fatty acid oxidation disorders. In The metabolic and molecular bases of inherited disease, Scriver CR, Beaudet AI, Sly WS, Valle D (eds). New York, McGraw-Hill, pp. 1501–1533.

58. De las Fuentes L, Herrero P, Peterson LR, Kelly DP, Gropler RJ, Davila-Roman VG (2003) Myocardial fatty acid metabolism: independent predictor of left ventricular mass in hypertension and in left ventricular dysfunction. Hypertension 41:82.

59. Massie BM, Schaefer S, Garcia J, McKirnan MD, Schwartz GG, Wisneski JA (1995) Myocardial high-energy phosphate and substrate metabolism in swine with moderate left ventricular hypertrophy. Circulation 91:1814.

60. Liao R, Nascimben L, Friedrich J, Gwathmey JK, Ingwall JS (1996) Decreased energy reserve in an animal model of dilated cardiomyopathy. Relationship to contractile performance. Circulation Res 78:893.

61. Neubauer S, Horn M, Cramer M, Harre K, Newell JB, Peters W (1997) Myocardial phosphocreatinine-to-ATP ratio is a predictor of mortality in patients with dilated cardiomyopathy. Circulation 96:2190.

62. Goldstein RA, Klein MS, Welch MJ, Sobel BE (1980) External assessment of myocardial metabolism with C-11 palmitate in vivo. J Nucl Med 21:342.

63. Eisenberg JD, Sobel BE, Geltman EM (1987) Differentiation of ischemic from nonischemic cardiomyopathy with positron emission tomography. Am J Cardiol 59:1410.

64. Kelly DP, Mendelsohn NJ, Sobel BE, Bergmann SR (1993) Detection and assessment by positron emission tomography of a genetically determined defect in myocardial fatty acid utilization (long-chain Acyl-CoA dehydrogenase deficiency). Am J Cardiol 71:738.

65. Yazaki Y, Isobe M, Takahashi W, Nishiyama O, Sekiguchi M, Takemura T (1999) Assessment of myocardial fatty acid metabolic abnormalities in patients with idiopathic dilated cardiomyopathy using ^{123}I BMIPP SPECT: correlation with clinicopathological findings and clinical course. Heart 81:153.

66. Wallhaus TR, Taylor M, DeGrado TR, Russell DC, Stanko P, Nickles RJ (2001) Myocardial free fatty acid and glucose use after carvedilol treatment in patients with congestive heart failure. Circulation 103:2441.

67. Beanlands RS, Armstrong WF, Hicks RJ, Nicklas J, Moore C, Hutchins GD (1994) The effects of afterload reduction on myocardial carbon 11-labeled acetate kinetics and noninvasively estimated mechanical efficiency in patients with dilated cardiomyopathy. J Nucl Cardiol 1:3.

68. Stolen KQ, Kemppainen J, Ukkonen H, Kalliokoski KK, Luotolahti M, Lehikoinen P (2003) Exercise training improves biventricular oxidative metabolism and left ventricular efficiency in patients with dilated cardiomyopathy. J Am Coll Cardiol 41:460.

69. Sundell J, Engblom E, Koistinen J, Ylitalo A, Naum A, Stolen KQ (2004) The effects of cardiac resynchronization therapy on left ventricular function, myocardial energetics, and metabolic reserve in patients with dilated cardiomyopathy and heart failure. J Am Coll Cardiol 43:1027.

70. Nowak B, Sinha AM, Schaefer WM, Koch KC, Kaiser HJ, Hanrath P (2003) Cardiac resynchronization therapy homogenizes myocardial glucose metabolism and perfusion in dilated cardiomyopathy and left bundle branch block. J Am Coll Cardiol 41:1523.

71. Beanlands RSB, Nahmias C, Gordon E, Coates G, deKemp R, Firnau G (2000) The effects of β_1-blockade on oxidative metabolism and the metabolic cost of ventricular work in patients with left ventricular dysfunction: a double-blind, placebo-controlled, positron-emission tomography study. Circulation 102:2070.

72. Hasegawa S, Kusuoka H, Maruyama K, Nishimura T, Hori M, Hatazawa J (2004) Myocardial positron emission computed tomographic images obtained with fluorine-18 fluoro-2-deoxyglucose predict the response of idiopathic dilated cardiomyopathy patients to beta-blockers. J Am Coll Cardiol 43:224.
73. Zhou YT, Grayburn P, Karim A, Shimabukuro M, Higa M, Baetens D (2000) Lipotoxic heart disease in obese rats: implications for human obesity. Proc Natl Acad Sci USA 97:1784.
74. Berk PD, Zhou SL, Kiang CL, Stump D, Bradbury M, Isola LM (1997) Uptake of long chain free fatty acids is selectively up-regulated in adipocytes of Zucker rats with genetic obesity and non-insulin-dependent diabetes mellitus. J Biol Chem 272:8830.
75. Luiken JJ, Arumugam Y, Dyck DJ, Bell RC, Pelsers MM, Turcotte LP (2001) Increased rates of fatty acid uptake and plasmalemmal fatty acid transporters in obese Zucker rats. J Biol Chem 276:40567.
76. Commerford SR, Pagliassotti MJ, Melby CL, Wei Y, Gayles EC, Hill JO (2000) Fat oxidation, lipolysis, and free fatty acid cycling in obesity-prone and obesity-resistant rats. Am J Physiol Endocrinol Metab 279:E875.
77. Peterson LR, Herrero P, Schechtman KB, Racette SB, Waggoner AD, Kisrieva-Ware Z (2004) Effect of obesity and insulin resistance on myocardial substrate metabolism and efficiency in young women. Circulation 109:2191.
78. Kannel WB, McGee DL (1979) Diabetes and cardiovascular disease: the Framingham study. J Am Med Assoc 241:2035.
79. Koskinen P, Manttari M, Manninen V, Huttunen JK, Heinonen OP, Frick MH (1992) Coronary heart disease incidence in NIDDM patients in the Helsinki Heart Study. Diabetes Care 15:820.
80. Abbott RD, Donahue RP, Kannel WB, Wilson PW (1988) The impact of diabetes on survival following myocardial infarction in men vs women. The Framingham Study. J Am Med Assoc 260:3456.
81. Rubler S, Dlugash J, Yuceoglu YZ, Kumral T, Branwood AW, Grishman A (1972) New type of cardiomyopathy associated with diabetic glomerulosclerosis. Am J Cardiol 30:595.
82. Stanley WC, Lopaschuck GD, McCormack JG (1997) Regulation of energy substrate metabolism in the diabetic heart. Cardiovasc Res 34:25.
83. Rodrigues B, Cam MC, McNeill JH (1995) Myocardial substrate metabolism: implications for diabetic cardiomyopathy. J Mol Cell Cardiol 27:169.
84. Avogaro A, Nosadini R, Doria A, Fioretto P, Velussi M, Vigorito C (1990) Myocardial metabolism in insulin-deficient diabetic humans without coronary artery disease. Am J Physiol 258:E606.
85. Randle PJ, Priestman DA, Mistry S, Halsall A (1994) Mechanisms modifying glucose oxidation in diabetes mellitus. Diabetologia 37:S155.
86. Kerbey AL, Vary TC, Randle PJ (1985) Molecular mechanisms regulating myocardial glucose oxidation. Basic Res Cardiol 80:93.

Paediatric Nuclear Cardiology

Pietro Zucchetta

Contents

34.1 Introduction 401
34.2 Myocardial Perfusion Imaging 402
34.2.1 Clinical Applications 403
34.2.2 Myocardial PET Scan 403
34.2.3 Lung Perfusion Scan 404
References 405

34.1 Introduction

In recent decades a number of radionuclide cardiac procedures have greatly contributed to the pathophysiologic understanding and clinical diagnosis of congenital and acquired paediatric heart disease.

The dramatic improvement in high-resolution morphological imaging (echocardiography, cardiac catheterization, MRI) has reduced the role of scintigraphic studies in this field, particularly in shunt evaluation. Nonetheless, nuclear medicine continues to make major contributions to the management of these patients, evaluating pulmonary blood flow distribution, myocardial perfusion or ventricular function.

Nuclear medicine studies applied to paediatric cardiology require a specialized approach, even if radiopharmaceuticals and acquisition techniques largely overlap those in adult practice. A completely different disease spectrum (congenital heart disease vs. atherosclerotic coronary artery disease) and the particular needs of patients throughout childhood require significant modifications of adult protocols and a different mind set to obtain high quality, informative studies [1]. Modifications encompass the need to adequately inform and reassure the child and parents, the adapting of acquisition protocols to single patient characteristics (height, weight, cooperation level), the use of sedation, and modified hardware (from smaller ECG electrodes to special acquisition cradles).

Radiation protection is a highly sensitive topic in paediatric imaging, considering the higher radiation sensitivity of children, and every measure must be taken to minimize radiation exposure. Nevertheless radiation protection cannot be reduced to extreme dose reduction [2], which often leads to sub-optimal studies, requiring repeated radiopharmaceuticals administrations or the use of invasive diagnostic techniques. Therefore much effort has been directed towards identification of the most appropriate radiopharmaceutical schedule in children and methods based on weight or body surface area are the most accepted choices (Table 34.1) [3].

Study tailoring to the single patient represents the best way to optimize radiation exposure and should

Table 34.1 Paediatric dose schedule following the suggestion of the Paediatric Task Group of the European Association of Nuclear Medicine [5]

Body weight kg	Fraction of administered activity %	Body weight kg	Fraction of administered activity %	Body weight kg	Fraction of administered activity %
3	10	22	50	42	78
4	14	24	53	44	80
6	19	26	56	46	82
8	23	28	58	48	85
10	27	30	62	50	88
12	32	32	65	52–54	90
14	36	34	68	56–58	95
16	40	36	71	60–70	100
18	44	38	73		
20	48	40	76		

be pursued in cooperation with the referring physician, outlining a clear clinical question and clarifying the pathophysiological setting, which is often quite complex.

34.2
Myocardial Perfusion Imaging

The most frequent indications for myocardial perfusion imaging in paediatric patients are transposition of the great arteries (arterial switch operation), congenital anomalies of the coronary arteries and Kawasaki disease. The relatively low prevalence of such disorders and the difficulties of myocardial SPET studies in children have limited the use of this technique. Nevertheless it maintains in paediatrics the same characteristics of reproducibility and non-invasivity that made it popular in adult cardiology.

At present technetium tracers represent the best choice for myocardial SPET in children. Both ^{99m}Tc-metoxyisobutilisonitrile (^{99m}Tc-MIBI) and ^{99m}Tc-tetrofosmin have no significant redistribution over time [4], allowing image acquisition without the time constraints of ^{201}Thallium (^{201}Tl), which often forced the use of sedation even in older patients. Moreover the emission of ^{201}Tl results in a much higher absorbed dose, and is less than optimal for gamma camera imaging when compared with ^{99m}Tc, particularly for tomographic acquisition.

Dose scaling is usually based on body weight or body surface area [3, 5], with a minimum dose of 100 MBq. Hypoperfused areas detected after rest injection are usually secondary to prior necrosis, whereas stress–rest protocols evaluate "fixed" and reversible ischemia.

Fasting (2–3 hours) is usually advisable before radiopharmaceutical injection, particularly if sedation is foreseen as possible. Physical exercise (preferably treadmill) can be used as stressor, starting from 5–6 years of age, depending on the patient's characteristics (height for bicycle testing, cooperation, muscolo-skeletal development). In infants and younger children pharmacologic testing is more reproducible and requires less compliance from patient and parents. Adenosine and dypiridamole are well known drugs, widely used in adult nuclear cardiology [6–12]. Adenosine has some advantages in paediatrics, namely a shorter duration of action (less than 30 seconds). Therefore side effects, usually mild and self-limiting (flushing, vague abdominal discomfort) vanish promptly after stopping the infusion, avoiding the need for pharmacologic intervention with antagonist drugs (aminophylline). In addition to fasting, patient preparation requires abstention from caffeine-containing food (soft drinks, tea ...) for 24 hours (better 48 hours) [13], and from theophylline and similar drugs. Asthma or a history of significant wheezing is a contraindication to the use of adenosine.

Quick and safe injection of radiopharmaceutical, at peak exercise or when the calculated drug dose has been administered, requires an intravenous line. Adenosine should be infused continuously (140 µg/kg/min) through a second venous access, using a pump. Considering the little volume of tracer dose and the relatively long distribution time of ^{99m}Tc-MIBI and ^{99m}Tc-tetrofosmin, it is possible, when venepuncture is overly difficult, to inject the radiotracer via a three-way stopcock in the same line as the drug infusion, which will be interrupted only for a few seconds.

Imaging is performed 45–90 minutes after radiopharmaceutical injection. Sedation is usually required in neonates, infants and in children aged less than 5–6 years. As in adults, tomographic images (128 × 128 matrix) are acquired on a 180° orbit, with appropriate magnification, depending on the patient's heart size, using high-resolution or ultra-high-resolution collimators. Fan-beam collimators can be of some advantage, particularly in younger patients.

Dual-head systems are highly preferable in paediatric SPET imaging, because the acquisition time can be significantly reduced, maintaining the required image quality. A frame time of 25–30 seconds gives high counts projections in 15–20 minutes.

Gated SPET (G-SPET) is possible, using at least 10–12 intervals sampling to take into account high cardiac frequency. However, it should be remembered that significant inaccuracies in volume determination and ejection fraction calculation could result from the small heart size [14] in the younger age groups.

Processing does not differ significantly from adult studies but iterative reconstruction should be adopted, when feasible, to best preserve finer details in reconstructed images. Defect size in paediatric patients is proportionately smaller than in adults; therefore overfiltering can completely obliterate hypoperfused areas.

34.2.1
Clinical Applications

Anomalous origin of the left coronary artery may induce myocardial ischemia leading to myocardial dysfunction and death, particularly if the origin is in the pulmonary trunk. In this case early surgical correction is needed and scintigraphic imaging has been used to evaluate myocardial perfusion before and after intervention [15, 16]. After reimplantation of the coronary in the aorta it has been possible to document a marked improvement of severe hypoperfusion seen in the pre-op studies.

Myocardial perfusion imaging has frequently been employed [17, 19] in the follow-up of patients operated on for transposition of the great arteries (TGA). Fixed or reversible perfusion defects, usually small in extension and severity, are frequently encountered in these patients [20] and are frequently without effects on ventricular function at rest and during exercise. The most severe lesions, generally associated with perioperatory infarction and/or coronary artery anomalies, bring a poorer prognosis.

The visualization of the right ventricle, hardly detectable in adults, is not uncommon in congenital heart disease and is frequently related to right ventricular hypertrophy determined by ventricular overload. This can be a finding in tetralogy of Fallot or following Senning or Mustard repair in TGA [19]. In these cases it is often necessary to manually correct the heart orientation proposed by commercial software, in order to obtain the correct cutting planes for image display. Some researchers [21] have proposed myocardial perfusion imaging as a complementary method to study the evolution of right ventricular hypertrophy in selected patients.

Many studies have demonstrated the value of perfusion SPET in Kawasaki disease [22–27] and the role of nuclear medicine techniques has been confirmed in the recent Scientific Statement published by the American Heart Association [28]. Scintigraphy has a limited role in the acute phase, when management relies on clinical data and echocardiography. Stress–rest perfusion scanning is most useful during follow-up, evaluating the extension of ischemic areas and disease progression in patients with coronary aneurysms. In these subjects, fixed and reversible perfusion defects are frequently observed.

The demand for myocardial perfusion scintigraphy in paediatric patients operated on for congenital heart disease will probably grow in the future, as early surgical correction becomes more and more effective. Scintigraphic techniques can be successfully employed, even in younger patients, to obtain a reproducible non-invasive functional evaluation of coronary artery circulation, which often plays a critical role, as in the case of prescriptions for physical activities.

34.2.2
Myocardial PET Scan

Myocardial PET scanning, using both ^{18}FDG and ^{13}NH, has been increasingly used in children to assess myocardial viability and to quantify myocardial blood flow and coronary flow reserve. Interesting data have been collected after surgical correction of congenital heart disease (TGA, coronary artery anomalies) [29–35] and during the follow-up of Kawasaki disease [36]. The expanding number of PET facilities should lead to a larger diffusion of such a technique, but more studies are needed to define its role in research and in the clinical work-flow [37, 38].

34.2.3
Lung Perfusion Scan

Pulmonary embolism is uncommon in infants and children, whereas asymmetric pulmonary blood flow is a frequent feature of congenital heart disease, which represents the most common malformation at birth.

Lung perfusion scintigraphy (LPS), using ^{99m}Tc-MAA or ^{99m}Tc-microspheres, was introduced into clinical practice many years ago to assess the distribution of pulmonary blood flow in a quick and safe way [39, 40].

The standard adult radioactivity dose must be reduced according to local radiation protection regulations. Dose scaling is usually based on body surface area or body weight, as previously stated [5]. A similar reduction in the number of injected particles (Table 34.2) appears similarly advisable, at least when significant right-to-left shunting is present and dissemination in the systemic circulation should be avoided or limited to a minimum. Moreover, it prevents a significant increase in pulmonary vascular resistance, even in infants with severe pulmonary hypertension. The total amount of injected particles should not be less than 10,000–20,000, to avoid a significant deterioration of image quality [41].

Lung perfusion scintigraphy does not require specific patient preparation and sedation is not routinely indicated, at least for standard acquisition. Right-to-left shunting, even complete mixing in a univentricular heart, is not a contraindication per se to the perfusion scanning, particularly if particle number reduction is adopted, as previously described. The examination should be postponed when a concomitant disease can interfere with tracer distribution, as in the case of bronco-pulmonary infections. Even low-grade bronco-constriction can produce significant redistribution of pulmonary blood flow [42], which can be related mistakenly to cardiac malformation, therefore it is advisable to wait for the resolution of respiratory symptoms before performing a lung perfusion scan.

The tracer is administered via a peripheral vein, using standard venepuncture technique, avoiding whenever possible injection in a venous line, which can lead to "hot spot" artifacts. The site of administration is not relevant when normal atrial mixing is present and both lungs are perfused through a common blood supply. These conditions are not met in some complex malformations or, more frequently, after some types of surgical repair, as in the staged Fontan procedure, which represents probably the most common of such situations. After bidirectional superior vena cava-to-pulmonary artery anastomosis (hemi-Fontan procedure), lung perfusion can be assessed only by tracer injection in a peripheral vein draining in SVC (arm injection); a foot or leg injection would display only the systemic distribution of the radio-pharmaceutical, due to the persistent right-to-left shunt. After complete correction the dose must be split between arm and leg injection, on two separate days, to evaluate the contribution of SVC and IVC to pulmonary blood flow. A single injection in this situation would give a falsely asymmetric distribution, with a preferential flow to the right lung from the SVC and a prevalent flow to the left lung after leg injection [43, 44]. Therefore MRI imaging can give more reliable results when a complete Fontan circulation is present [45].

Static images are acquired shortly after injection, in posterior and anterior view, on a 256 × 256 matrix, using a standard parallel hole high-resolution collimator. Acquisition zoom varies with patient size. A total of 200,000–500,000 counts are collected for each projection and oblique views are obtained when necessary, to clarify dubious findings.

Relative lung perfusion is usually computed drawing left and right region of interest (ROI), using geometric mean counts from anterior and posterior images. Calculations based on the single posterior projection have been shown to differ only slightly from values based on geometric mean [46]. Therefore it is possible to acquire only the posterior view, without losing significant clinical data, with evident simplification of the acquisition in infants and uncooperative children. Moreover, data obtained from the anterior projection can be misleading, since it is significantly influenced by the heart location [47]. Background ROIs are not required routinely, because extra-pulmonary tracer is usually negligible. Background subtraction can be carefully applied in a few selected patients presenting significant right-to-left shunting and extremely hypoperfused lung. In this case, the contribution to lung ROI counts from extra-pul-

Table 34.2 Suggested numbers of injected particles for lung perfusion scintigraphy in children. (Further reduction is needed when right-to-left shunting is present)

< 5 kg	6–15 kg	16–20 kg	21–35 kg	> 35 kg
10,000–50,000	50,000–100,000	100,000–200,000	200,000–300,000	300,000

monary tissue should be accounted for by background subtraction, and care must be taken to adopt the same approach in the follow-up studies.

Normal pulmonary blood flow distribution is usually defined in the 45–55% range for the single lung (right + left = 100%) and the ROI-based calculation is highly reproducible.

Diffuse unilateral reduction of relative blood flow is the most frequent abnormality observed in congenital heart disease, sustained in most cases by a stenosis of the left or (less frequently) right pulmonary artery. However, the same pattern can be determined by multiple peripheral stenoses of the main arterial branches or by diffuse vascular involvement affecting the whole lung, therefore scintigraphic imaging represents only a step toward a definite diagnosis.

Focal hypoperfusion is a less frequent finding, usually related to a single peripheral stenosis. Of particular interest is the apical hypoperfusion, which can be observed in some cases on the same side of a Blalock–Taussig shunt, probably due to vascular distortion as a consequence of the surgical procedure [48, 49]. This kind of abnormality is usually definitive and will persist even after removing the shunt, but has a small impact on the global distribution of the blood flow to the affected lung. A functioning Blalock–Taussig shunt can lead to underestimation of the blood flow to the ipsilateral lung through a dilution effect of the systemic blood on the radiolabelled particles arriving via the pulmonary artery. The same dilution mechanism underlies the focal hypoactivity of lung segments perfused by persistent aortopulmonary connections, often observed in pulmonary atresia [50].

The initial work-up of congenital heart disease relies on echocardiography and cardiac catheterization. Lung perfusion scintigraphy plays a role in selected cases, in this early phase of clinical management, to confirm a dubious finding in a complex malformation or to obtain information on pulmonary blood flow when angiography is felt unnecessary.

The need for a non-invasive evaluation of lung perfusion distribution is typical of the follow-up after surgical palliation or correction. An imbalance in lung perfusion may arise, without any clinical sign, even after successful uncomplicated one-stage correction of mild anomalies [43]. Ultrasound can evaluate only the most proximal tract of pulmonary arteries and repeated angiographic studies are too invasive for simple follow-up purposes, but lung perfusion scintigraphy is the ideal counterpart for the echography. A similar combined approach allows a prolonged follow-up with little biological cost.

Even more relevant is the role of perfusion scanning in the follow-up of complex malformations, which often require staged surgical repair. In this case, lung perfusion scintigraphy documents the effect of each surgical procedure on pulmonary blood flow distribution.

Residual stenosis of the pulmonary arteries is frequently observed in many malformations, for instance in tetralogy of Fallot. This condition can be effectively studied by a combination of serial echographic and scintigraphic studies. Limiting the use of cardiac catheterization, which can be employed only when angioplasty is required, allows a significant reduction of radiation exposure and invasivity.

In conclusion, lung perfusion scintigraphy can play a critical role in the management of congenital heart disease as a safe and reproducible technique, and the increasing success of early surgical correction will expand its role in the prolonged follow-up of this group of patients.

References

1. Ljung B (1998) The child in diagnostic nuclear medicine. Eur J Nucl Med 24:683–690.
2. Piepsz A, Gordon I, Hahn K (1991) Paediatric nuclear medicine. Eur J Nucl Med 1:41–66.
3. Smith T, Gordon I (1998) An update of radiopharmaceutical schedules in children. Nucl Med Commun 11:1023–1036.
4. Okada R, Glover D (1988) Myocardial kinetics of Technetium 99mhexakis-2-methoxy-isobutyl-isonitrile. Circulation 77:491–498.
5. Piepsz A, Hahn K, Roca I et al. (1990) A radiopharmaceutical schedule for imaging in paediatrics. Eur J Nucl Med 17:127–129.
6. Gould KL (1978) Noninvasive assessment of coronary stenoses by myocardial perfusion imaging during pharmacologic coronary vasodilatation, I: physiologic basis and experimental validation. Am J Cardiol 41:267–278.
7. Gould KL, Westcott RJ, Albro PC et al. (1978) Noninvasive assessment of coronary stenoses by myocardial imaging during pharmacologic coronary vasodilatation, II: clinical methodology and feasibility. Am J Cardiol 41:279–287.
8. Albro PC, Gould KL, Westcott RJ et al. (1978) Noninvasive assessment of coronary stenoses by myocardial imaging during pharmacologic coronary vasodilatation, III: clinical trial. Am J Cardiol 42:751–760.
9. Nguyen T, Heo J, Ogilby JD et al. (1990) Single photon emission computed tomography with thallium-201 during adenosine-inducedcoronary hyperemia: correlation with coronary arteriography, exercise thallium imaging and two-dimensional echocardiography. J Am Coll Cardiol 16:1375–1383.
10. Verani MS, Mahmarian JJ, Hixson JB et al. (1990) Diagnosis of coronary artery disease by controlled coronary

vasodilation with adenosine and thallium-201 scintigraphy in patients unable to exercise. Circulation 82:80–87.
11. Parodi O, Marcassa C, Casucci R et al. (1991) Accuracy and safety of technetium-99m hexakis 2-methoxy-2-isobutyl isonitrile (Sestamibi) myocardial scintigraphy with high dose dipyridamole test in patients with effort angina pectoris: a multicenter study. Italian Group of Nuclear Cardiology. J Am Coll Cardiol 18:1439–1444.
12. Klocke FJ, Baird MG, Lorell BH et al. (2003) ACC/AHA/ASNC guidelines for the clinical use of cardiac radionuclide imaging – executive summary: a report of the American College of Cardiology/American Heart Association Task Force on Practice Guidelines (ACC/AHA/ASNC Committee to Revise the 1995 Guidelines for the Clinical Use of Cardiac Radionuclide Imaging). Circulation 108:1404–1418.
13. Lapeyre AC III, Goraya TY, Johnston DL, Gibbons RJ (2004) The impact of caffeine on vasodilator stress perfusion studies. J Nucl Cardiol 11:506–511.
14. Ford PV, Chatziioannou SN, Moore WH, Dhekne RD (2001) Overestimation of the LVEF by quantitative gated SPECT in simulated left ventricles. J Nucl Med 42:454–459.
15. Hurwitz RA, Randall LC, Girod DA, Brown J, King H (1989) Clinical and hemodynamic course of infants and children with anomalous left coronary artery. Am Heart J 118:1176–1181.
16. Finley JP, Howman-Giles R, Gilday DL, Olley PM, Rowe RD (1978) Thallium-201 myocardial imaging in anomalous left coronary artery arising from the pulmonary artery. Applications before and after medical and surgical treatment. Am J Cardiol 42:675–680.
17. Vogel M, Smallhorn JF, Gilday D, Benson LN, Ash J, Williams WG, Freedom RM (1991) Assessment of myocardial perfusion in patients after the arterial switch operation. J Nucl Med 32:237–241.
18. Hayes AM, Baker EJ, Kakadeker A et al. (1994) Influence of anatomic correction for transposition of the great arteries on myocardial perfusion: radionuclide imaging with technetium-99m 2-methoxy isobutyl isonitrile. J Am Coll Cardiol 24:769–777.
19. Lubiszewska B, Gosiewska E, Hoffman P et al. (2000) Myocardial perfusion and function of the systemic right ventricle in patients after atrial switch procedure for complete transposition: long-term follow-up. J Am Coll Cardiol 36:1365–1370.
20. Weindling SN, Wernovsky G, Colan SD et al. (1994) Myocardial perfusion, function and exercise tolerance after the arterial switch operation. J Am Coll Cardiol 23:424–433.
21. Rabinovitch M, Fischer KC, Treves S (1981) Quantitative thallium-201 myocardial imaging in assessing right ventricular pressure in patients with congenital heart defects. Br Heart J 45:198–205.
22. Bjorkhem G, Evander E, White T, Lundstrom NR (1990) Myocardial scintigraphy with 201thallium in pediatric cardiology: a review of 52 cases. Pediatr Cardiol 11:1–7.
23. Miyagawa M, Mochizuki T, Murase K, Tanada S, Ikezoe J, Sekiya M, Hamamoto K, Matsumoto S, Niino M (1998) Prognostic value of dipyridamole-thallium myocardial scintigraphy in patients with Kawasaki disease. Circulation 10:990–996.
24. Jan SL, Hwang B; Fu YC; Lee PC; Kao CH; Liu RS; Chi CS (2000) Comparison of 201Tl SPET and treadmill exercise testing in patients with Kawasaki disease. Nucl Med Commun 21:431–445.
25. Fu YC, Kao CH, Hwang B, Jan SL, Chi CS (2002) Discordance between dipyridamole stress Tc-99m sestamibi SPECT and coronary angiography in patients with Kawasaki disease. J Nucl Cardiol 9:41–46.
26. [26] Fukuda T, Ishibashi M, Yokoyama T, Otaki M; Shinohara T, Nakamura Y, Miyake T, Kudoh T, Oku H (2002) Myocardial ischemia in Kawasaki disease: evaluation with dipyridamole stress technetium 99m tetrofosmin scintigraphy. J Nucl Cardiol 9:632–667.
27. Ogawa S, Ohkubo T, Fukazawa R, Kamisago M, Kuramochi Y, Uchikoba Y, Ikegami E, Watanabe M, Katsube Y (2004) Estimation of myocardial hemodynamics before and after intervention in children with Kawasaki disease. J Am Coll Cardiol 43:653–661.
28. Newburger JW, Takahashi M, Gerber MA et al. (2004) Diagnosis, treatment, and long-term management of Kawasaki disease: a statement for health professionals from the Committee on Rheumatic Fever, Endocarditis, and Kawasaki Disease, Council on Cardiovascular Disease in the Young, American Heart Association. Pediatrics 114:1708–1733.
29. Bengel FM, Hauser M, Duvernoy et al. (1998) Myocardial blood flow and coronary flow reserve late after anatomical correction of transposition of the great arteries. J Am Coll Cardiol 32(7):1955–1961.
30. Yates RW, Marsden PK, Badawi RD et al. (2000) Evaluation of myocardial perfusion using positron emission tomography in infants following a neonatal arterial switch operation. Pediatr Cardiol 21(2): 111–118.
31. Rickers C, Sasse K, Buchert R, Stern H, van den Hoff J, Lubeck M, Weil J (2000) Myocardial viability assessed by positron emission tomography in infants and children after the arterial switch operation and suspected infarction. J Am Coll Cardiol 36(5):1676–1683.
32. Singh TP, Humes RA, Muzik O, Kottamasu S, Karpawich PP, Di Carli MF (2001) Myocardial flow reserve in patients with a systemic right ventricle after atrial switch repair. J Am Coll Cardiol 37(8):2120–2125.
33. Oskarsson G, Pesonen E, Munkhammar P, Sandstrom S, Jogi P (2002) Normal coronary flow reserve after arterial switch operation for transposition of the great arteries: an intracoronary Doppler guidewire study. Circulation 106(13):1696–1702.

34. Hauser M, Bengel FM, Hager A, Kuehn A, Nekolla SG, Kaemmerer H, Schwaiger M, Hess J (2003) Impaired myocardial blood flow and coronary flow reserve of the anatomical right systemic ventricle in patients with congenitally corrected transposition of the great arteries. Heart 89(10):1231–1235.
35. Hernandez-Pampaloni M, Allada V, Fishbein MC, Schelbert HR (2003) Myocardial perfusion and viability by positron emission tomography in infants and children with coronary abnormalities: correlation with echocardiography, coronary angiography, and histopathology. J Am Coll Cardiol 41(4):618–626.
36. Hwang B, Liu RS, Chu LS, Lee PC, Lu JH, Meng LC (2000) Positron emission tomography for the assessment of myocardial viability in Kawasaki disease using different therapies. Nucl Med Commun 21(7):631–636.
37. Oskarsson G (2004) Coronary. Acta Paediatr Suppl 93(Suppl 446):20–25.
38. Yamakawa Y, Takahashi N, Ishikawa T (2004) Clinical usefulness of ECG-gated 18F-FDG PET combined with ^{99m}Tc-Mibi gated spect for evaluating myocardial viability and function. Ann Nucl Med 18(5):375–383.
39. Friedman WF, Braunwald E, Morrow AG (1968) Alterations in regional pulmonary blood flow in patients with congenital heart disease studied by radioisotope scanning. Circulation 37:747–758.
40. Tong EC, Liu L, Potter RT, Sackler JP, Rabinowitz JG (1973) Macroaggregated Risa lung scan in congenital heart disease. Radiology 106(3):585–592.
41. Gainey MA (1994) Ventilation and perfusion studies of the lung. In: Miller JA, Gelfand M (eds) Pediatric Nuclear Imaging. Philadelphia, PA: W.B. Saunders Company, pp. 65–82.
42. Potchen EJ, Evens RG (1971) The physiologic factors affecting regional ventilation and perfusion. Semin Nucl Med 1(2):153–160.
43. Boothroyd AE, McDonald EA, Carty H (1996) Lung perfusion scintigraphy in patients with congenital heart disease: sensitivity and important pitfalls. Nucl Med Commun 1(17):33–39.
44. Pruckmayer M, Zacherl S, Salzer-Muhar U, Schlemmer M, Leitha T (1999) Scintigraphic assessment of pulmonary and whole-body blood flow patterns after surgical intervention in congenital heart disease. J Nucl Med 40:1477–1483.
45. Fratz S, Hess J, Schwaiger M, Martinoff S, Stern HC (2002) More accurate quantification of pulmonary blood flow by magnetic resonance imaging than by lung perfusion scintigraphy in patients with Fontan circulation. Circulation 106(12):1510–1513.
46. Fleming JS, Whalley DR, Skrypniuk et al. (2004) UK audit of relative lung function measurement from planar radionuclide imaging. Nucl Med Commun 25(9):923–934.
47. Hashimoto K, Nakamura Y, Matsui M, Kurosawa H, Arai T (1992) Alteration of pulmonary blood flow in tetralogy of Fallot: pre- and postoperative study with macroaggregates of 99mtc-labeled human serum albumin. Jpn Circulation J 56(10):992–997.
48. Alderson PO, Boonvisut S, McKnight RC, Hartman AFJ (1976) Pulmonary perfusion abnormalities and ventilation-perfusion imbalance in children after total repair of Tetralogy of Fallot. Circulation 53(2):332–337.
49. Del Torso S, Milanesi O, Bui F (1988) Radionuclide evaluation of lung perfusion after the Fontan procedure. Int J Cardiol 20(1):107–116.
50. Neches WH, Weiss FH, Park SC, Lenox CC, Zuberbuhler JR, Carroll RG (1977) Pulmonary perfusion defect and bronchial artery collateral blood flow. J Am Med Assoc 238(17):1842–1844.

Cardiac Adrenergic Imaging

Chapter 35

Shinichiro Fujimoto, Shohei Yamashina and Junichi Yamazaki

Contents

35.1	Introduction and History	409
35.2	Principle	410
35.3	Technique	411
35.3.1	MIBG Imaging Method	411
35.3.2	MIBG Analysis and Evaluation Methods	411
35.3.3	Factors that Influence the MIBG Test Method	412
35.4	Clinical Application	413
35.4.1	Ischemic Heart Disease	413
35.4.2	Heart Failure	413
35.5	Discussion	415
35.6	Future Trends	416

35.1 Introduction and History

The sympathetic nervous system, which complements the parasympathetic nervous system, plays an important role in the physiological adjustment of circulation kinetics. The control center for the sympathetic nervous system is located in the medulla oblongata, but its activity can also be adjusted by input from the upper centers and the periphery, such as baroreceptors. Norepinephrine (NE) is secreted from sympathetic nerve endings with stimulation of the sympathetic nervous system, and this neurotransmitter acts on α and β receptors to initiate physiological activity specific to each organ. However, results are not always as intended. On the negative side, the sympathetic nerve can also play a role in pathological generation and modification as well as function as a sort of prognosis-limiting factor in circulatory disease. Various types of heart disease are associated with abnormal function of the sympathetic nerve. Sympathicotonia is seen in ischemic heart disease and heart failure [1, 2] and is associated with hypertension and cardiac hypertrophy [3]. Abnormal or lack of sympathetic nerve distribution has been suggested to be a potential cause of arrhythmia and sudden death. The measurement of plasma NE concentration and a record of the sympathetic nerve activity in muscle are used to evaluate sympathetic nerve activity. However, since these do not directly reflect the NE kinetics at work in cardiac sympathetic nerve distribution and in sympathetic nerve endings, development of an imaging method that can record sympathetic nerve activity in the heart was required.

Research on this imaging method was conducted initially for experimentation purposes only, using H-labeled NE, and was not developed to the extent that it could be used in pathological analysis. The complexity of the technique made it impossible to use clinically. However, a metaiodobenzylguanidine method was developed by Wieland et al. of Michigan University that enabled one to describe and evaluate the aortic sympathetic nerve activity [4, 5]. Although C-11 meta-hydroxyephedrine and F-18 6-fluorodopamine with PET are currently used for clinical application [6], I-MIBG myocardial scintigraphy (hereafter referred to as MIBG) is the most popular. With MIBG, the clinical pathology of numerous diseases and the participation of the sympathetic nervous system have been gradually clarified. MIBG, which is currently the most widely used technique for sympathetic nerve imaging, is described below.

35.2 Principle

At the cardiac sympathetic nerve ends, NE is synthesized from tyrosine, an amino acid, through dopamine, and is stored in the synaptic vesicle (NE storage granules). Exocytosis of NE from the nerve ending occurs with stimulation of the sympathetic nerve, however, the majority (approximately 80%) of NE is taken into the nerve ending again through an active re-absorption mechanism, called uptake-1, so NE can be recycled. A part of the NE combines with the receptor of the cardiomyocyte membrane (chiefly the β-receptor), and the other part of the remaining NE enters the blood (spillover) where it is promptly decomposed by monoamine oxidase (MAO) and catechol-O-methyltransferase (COMT) [7] (Fig. 35.1) In animal experiments, it was found that MIBG was taken into non-neural tissue (this uptake process is referred to as uptake-2), however, this is not the case in humans since MIBG does not accumulate in the heart after transplant [8, 9]. MIBG is an analogue of NE that is stored in the nerve ending follicle through uptake-1, as is the case with NE, and secreted according to nerve stimulation. In contrast to NE, MIBG does not combine with the heart muscle receptor, and it is not inactivated by MAO and COMT. Therefore, as the majority (80–90%)

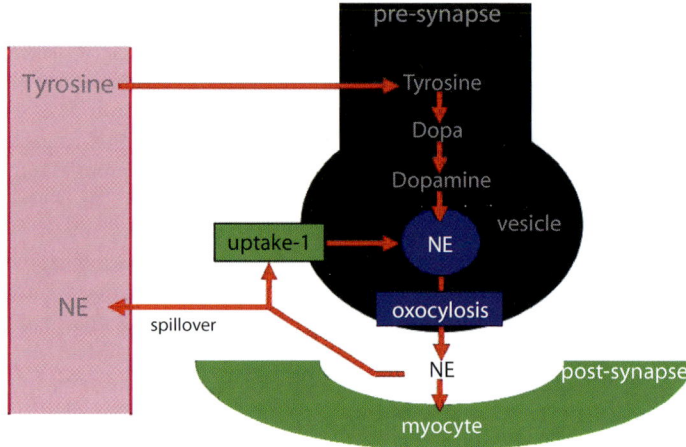

Fig. 35.1 Pharmacodynamics of norepinephrine (NE) at the cardiac sympathetic nerve ending

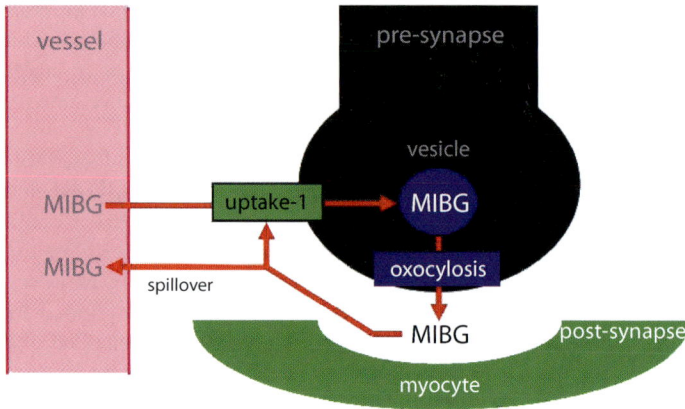

Fig. 35.2 Pharmacodynamics of MIBG at the cardiac sympathetic nerve ending

of MIBG released into the synaptic cleft is reabsorbed through the uptake-1 process, accumulation in the nerve ending can be maintained for a long time, making it an ideal labeled tracer of NE metabolism (Fig. 35.2). MIBG accumulation in the heart muscle has been confirmed in many animal experiments. In normal heart muscle, MIBG uptake occurs in a very short time, with an accumulation rate during its initial circulation of approximately 80%, and 1–2% of the entire dosage accumulates in heart muscle. In the normal heart muscle, MIBG stays for several hours. Washout from the heart muscle quickens as sympathetic nerve activity rises and spillover of NE increases due to heart failure, etc. Therefore, an early image taken right after MIBG administration shows the situation of sympathetic nerve end distribution, while a delayed image taken after several hours reflects the increase of nerve activity in addition to sympathetic nerve distribution. It is also reported that MIBG washout from the heart muscle positively correlates with NE concentration in the blood [10].

35.3 Technique

35.3.1 MIBG Imaging Method

In the resting state, 111–148 MBq of MIBG is intravenously injected. An early image is taken after 15–20 minutes, and a delayed image is taken 3–4 hours after administration. Drugs that influence MIBG accumulation, such as tricyclic antidepressants, labetalol, reserpine, and guanethidine, should be discontinued before the examination. Evaluation by a Planar image only is general, so when SPECT imaging is also required, it is preferable to use a SPECT camera with more than two heads and a visual field that at least covers most of the heart and chest. The energy window should be set at 159 keV ± 10% using the collimator for low energy or exclusively for I. Generally, to take the planar image, three directions (front image, left anterior oblique (LAO) 35–45°, and LAO 70° – left side) have to be imaged for about 3–5 minutes. Each direction has a matrix size of 128 × 128 or 256 × 256. The standard SPECT image is a collection of 360° × 60 directions taken in 6° increments with the matrix size set at 64 × 64, and taken for 30–60 seconds in each direction.

35.3.2 MIBG Analysis and Evaluation Methods

The region of interest (ROI) in the heart and superior mediastinum is established based on the planar image. The index of heart muscle accumulation and the index of washout from the heart are calculated as the H/M ratio = H/M (H: average count value in the heart, M: that in the superior mediastinum) and washout rate (%) = [(H in early image − M in early image) − (H in delayed image − M in delayed image)]/(H in early image − M in early image) × 100, respectively (Fig. 35.3).

The SPECT image is also useful to evaluate local sympathetic nerve distribution. Even in a normal MIBG image, accumulation in the posterior inferior wall is low, that is, 70% of the front wall, and this becomes more pronounced in the elderly and in cases where there is a lot of accumulation in the liver. Therefore, interpretation should be conducted carefully. Using the polar map, which is displayed as one circular map, the SPECT short axis view being imaged as a concentric circle, the extent score, which shows the extent of the decrease of

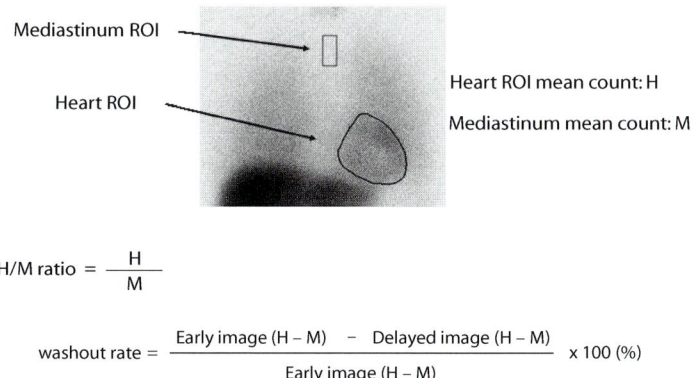

Fig. 35.3 Calculation of H/M (heart to mediastinum ratio) and WR (washout rate) using MIBG planar images (ROI, region of interest)

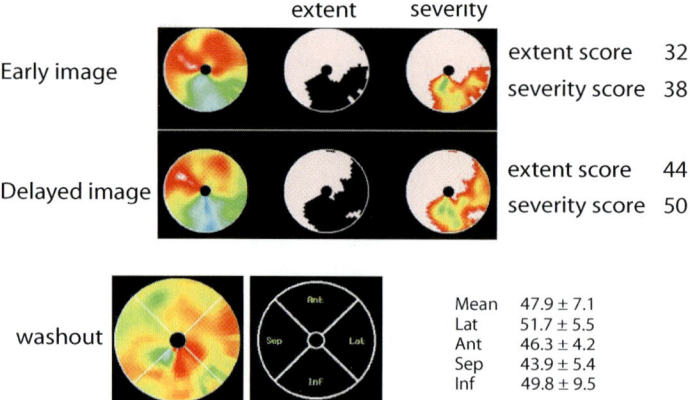

Fig. 35.4 Calculation of extent score, severity score and washout rate using SPECT polar maps. Polar maps are constructed by deploying concentrically the marginal count profile curves compiled using images in short axis tomography of myocardial SPECT obtained from slices from the apex to the base of the heart. Extent maps display blackout of pixel count smaller than −2SD when compared with normal files, and extent score represents the percentage of blackout in the whole. Severity maps display in color the severity of decreased accumulation in the area of blackout, and the severity score is the value of the total of the difference in pixel count between blackouts and the normal area divided by the total pixel count. Washout rate (WR) can be obtained both for the mean washout rate of the total circumference of the left ventricle and by each region. In the present study, tetrameric WR is expressed with mean ±SD

accumulation, and the severity score, which shows the severity of symptoms, can be calculated through comparison with a normal file taken from a healthy person. This type of imaging also has the advantage that there are no effects of background on washout rate (WR) (Fig. 35.4).

35.3.3
Factors that Influence the MIBG Test Method

In imaging and radiographic interpretations of MIBG, it is necessary to consider the following factors. In terms of basic problems, there are differences between the planar image and the SPECT image (washout rate for SPECT is lower than that for the planar image) and in the effects of the ROI settings as well as the presence/absence of background corrections. Moreover, depending on the time at which the delayed image is taken in patients, a correction for time decay may also be necessary. Also, careful attention to H/M change caused by differences between various kinds of collimators is required. Accumulation in the heart increases by increasing the specific activity of I and reducing the amount of MIBG, which then causes H/M to rise. Accumulation in the lung field and the liver is also an influential factor that must be taken into consideration, especially, in the case of SPECT imaging, the influence of artifacts associated with liver accumulation is great. Although it is said that MIBG accumulation tends to decrease in the elderly and in women, significant differences were not found during examinations conducted at the authors' facilities. Drugs that can influence the accumulation of MIBG are: (1) drugs that inhibit sodium-dependent uptake (uptake-1), such as labetarol and tricyclic antidepressants including imipramine and desipramine; (2) drugs that inhibit transportation to storage granules, such as reserpine; (3) drugs that compete with the transportation to storage granules, such as guanethidine; (4) drugs that dry out the content of storage granules, such as reserpine, phenylpropanolamine, amphetamine, etc.; and (5) calcium channel blockers such as verapamil etc. [11]. Factors affecting the images and the parameters of MIBG are summarized in Table 35.1.

Table 35.1 Factors affecting MIBG images and parameters

H/M	1. Types of imaging instrument employed (especially that of collimator)
	2. Methods of setting up ROI (location, form and size)
	3. High accumulation in the liver and lungs
WR	1. Presence or absence of background correction
	2. Time to start photographing delayed images
	3. Presence or absence of decrement correction of ^{123}I due to physical half-life
Images in general	1. Age and sex
	2. Effects of drugs

H/M, heart to mediastinum ratio; WR, washout rate

35.4 Clinical Application

35.4.1 Ischemic Heart Disease

Sympathetic nerve activity in the heart muscle can easily be damaged by ischemia, and even after the remission of ischemia, several weeks to several months are required to resume normal function. It is said that the recovery process in general begins with the improvement of accumulation in early images, but an abnormal increase of washout continues and the improvement of accumulation in the delayed image is delayed This method can be useful for ischemia detection and the identification of responsible blood vessels in cases of unstable angina and coronary vasospastic angina [12, 13]. However, with reperfusion after acute myocardial infarction, the decrease of MIBG accumulation becomes more wide-ranging than blood flow agents, and mismatched findings are often seen; such findings are expressed as "denervated but viable" and are considered to correspond to the risk area [14–16]. Also, because the image quality of MIBG is inferior to that of blood flow agents and BMIPP, and the diagnosis accuracy in the inferior wall area is poor, application to ischemic heart disease is on the decrease.

35.4.2 Heart Failure

After Merlet et al. found in 1992 that delayed H/M was more useful to evaluate the prognosis of chronic heart failure than left ventricular ejection fraction (LVEF) [17], there were some reports of MIBG's usefulness in predicting prognosis of heart failure. While one report indicated that delayed H/M was the most useful factor [18], another stated that WR was the most useful indicator [19]. Thus, a consistent opinion of which factor is actually the most useful as a prognostic prediction tool has not been reached. In truth, both delayed H/M and WR can reflect the severity of symptoms related to heart failure [20], and it is currently considered that both LVEF and BNP are useful prognostic prediction factors of heart failure if imaging is conducted once the symptoms of heart failure have settled down.

35.4.2.1 Hypertrophic Cardiomyopathy (HCM)

In MIBG, decreased accumulation in the apex, posterior inferior wall, and septal inferior area, and increased WR are often found. Abnormalities are observed, especially in the enlarged area of the apical hypertrophic cardiomyopathy, and the range of loss is greater than that of blood flow scintigraphy. MIBG is thought to reflect heart muscle damage due to HCM, and it has been reported that delayed H/M is the most useful parameter for forecasting heart failure [21]. However, the usefulness of MIBG in cases of HCM has not been established, differing from that in cases of DCM.

35.4.2.2 Dilated Cardiomyopathy (DCM)

With respect to DCM, MIBG findings tend to show a decrease in the accumulation in entire areas, especially the inferior wall area, and an increase of WR. As these indices often correlate with heart function, MIBG is useful in evaluating the severity of DCM symptoms [22]. Moreover, it is reported that delayed H/M and WR are helpful for predicting the prognosis of DCM [23, 24]. MIBG seems to be most clinically useful at forecasting and evaluating the effect of β-blocker therapy in cases of

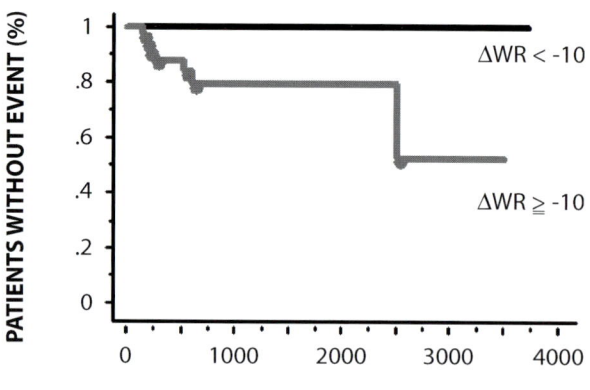

35.5 Kaplan–Meier analysis for the occurrence of cardiac events (quoting from Reference [28]). When the optimal threshold of ΔWR (WR, washout rate) was set at −10 in the calculation of mean −0.25 SD, no cardiac event was recognized in the group of ΔWR<−10

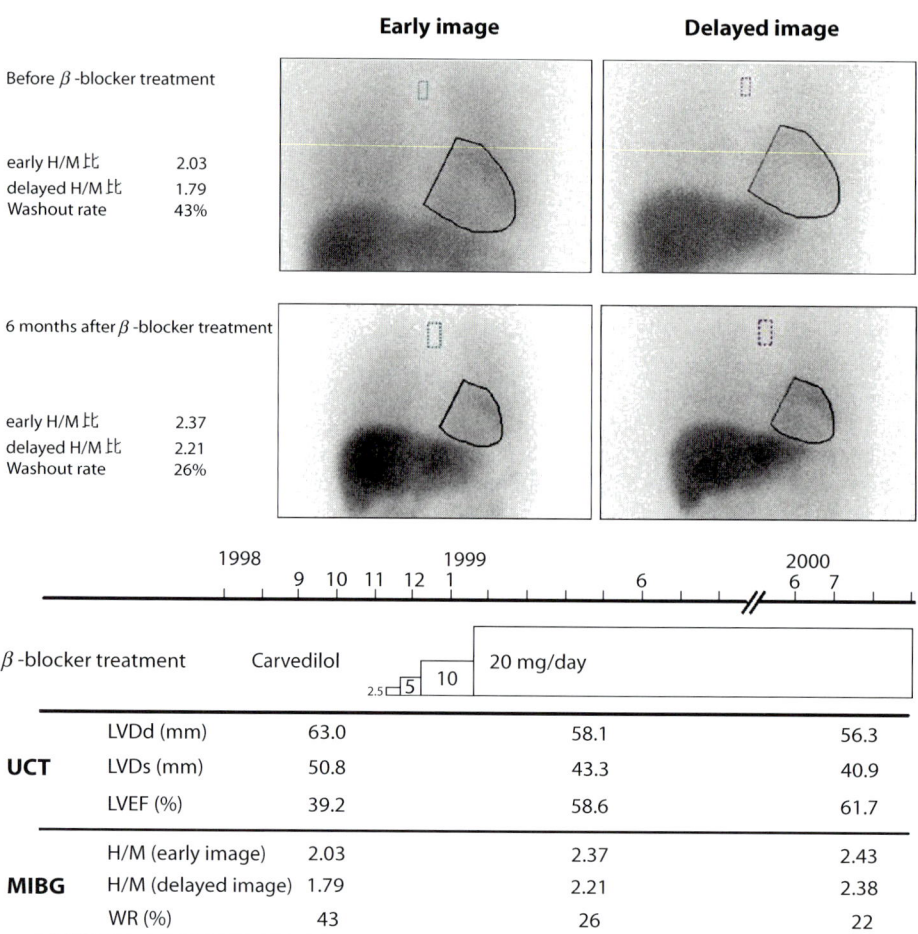

Fig. 35.6 and 35.7 62-year-old male with heart failure was diagnosed with dilated cardiomyopathy. The images show successive changes before and after treatment with beta-blockers. MIBG scan was performed pre and 6 months post therapy with beta-blockers. The LVEF was 39% pre treatment with beta-blockers and the H/M (heart to mediastinum ratio) in early images was maintained relatively well, while WR (washout rate) was elevated. The H/M in delayed images was lower. Six months on beta-blockers, the LVEF improved markedly from 39% to 58% and WR in MIBG improved to 26%

DCM. The usefulness of β-blocker therapy in the event of DCM has been proven by a large-scale clinical trial in recent years [25–27]. The principal underlying mechanism works to normalize the excessive sympathetic nerve activity associated with DCM. It is reasonable that MIBG, which can reflect the state of cardiac sympathetic nerve activity, can provide a forecast and evaluation of the effect of β-blocker therapy. MIBG was executed before and after the introduction of β-blocker therapy in DCM patients who responded successfully to the introduction of β-blocker therapy. Reportedly, the improvement rate of WR with MIBG is a stronger prediction factor of cardiac events than the improvement rate of LVEF, and WR is remarkably improved by the introduction of β-blocker therapy when an early image from MIBG prior to β-blocker therapy is kept for comparison [28] (Fig. 35.5) Moreover, no parameter that can predict prognosis prior to therapy for the time period after the successful introduction of β-blocker therapy has been established. To date, the strongest prediction factor is the continued decrease of MIBG accumulation in the delayed image [29]. Thus, it is clinically very useful to take an MIBG image before and after the introduction of β-blocker therapy in cases of DCM. (Figs. 35.6 and 35.7).

There are some reports that MIBG improves with the administration of other drugs such as angiotensin-converting enzyme inhibitor, angiotensin receptor blocker, and spironolactone; however, more in-depth examination is required [30–32].

35.4.2.3 Arrhythmia

If the sympathetic nerve of the heart muscle is denervated, the effective refractory period shortens to cause a lack of uniformity of the refractory period of the surrounding area, and ventricle tachycardia becomes a concern. Abnormal MIBG findings are reported in cases of arrhythmia with myocardial infarction and cardiomyopathy, idiopatic ventricle tachycardia, arrhythmogenic right ventricular cardiomyopathy [33], Brugada syndrome, and congenital prolonged QT; however, the usefulness has not been properly established. It was previously reported that WR of the MIBG was the most useful prediction factor of cardiac death, including sudden death, by cardiomyopathy [34]. MIBG may, therefore, also be capable of forecasting fetal arrhythmia.

35.4.2.4 Other Diseases

Sympathetic nerve disorder is often present in patients with diabetes mellitus, however, the clinical usefulness of MIBG has yet to be established. Previous reports have

Table 35.2 Indications of MIBG

Ischemic heart disease
Heart failure
Hypertrophic cardiomyopathy (HCM)
Dilated cardiomyopathy (DCM)
Cardiac transplantation
Diabetes mellitus
*Arrhythmia [with myocardial infarction, cardiomyopathy, idiopatic ventricle tachycardia, arrhythmogenic right ventricular cardiomyopathy, Brugada syndrome, and congenital prolonged QT]
*Sick Sinus Syndrome

* Less established

suggested an improvement in MIBG findings when Epalrestat and Mecobalamin were administered to patients with diabetes mellitus [35, 36]. Therefore, we expect further examination will be conducted in the future.

In recent years, in cases of Parkinson's disease, the accumulation of MIBG decreased from the early image, and the extent of the decrease was thought to reflect the symptom severity [37]. We expect to see future research in this area as well.

Indications of MIBG are summarized in Table 35.2.

35.5
Discussion

In recent years, the clinical application of MIBG has become widespread. It appears to be most useful in cases of heart failure and cardiomyopathy. The norepinephrine kinetics have been fully studied in patients with heart failure by Eisenhofer et al. [7]. As for the state of cardiac sympathetic nerve activity in cases of heart failure and cardiomyopathy, there are two states of progress in general. One is the state in which the sympathetic nerve is overstrained and spillover is increased, even though degeneration of the heart muscle is mild. In terms of MIBG parameters, although the accumulation in the early image is comparatively maintained, increased WR and decreased accumulation in the delayed image are seen in many cases. If a β-blocker is introduced in these cases, prognosis improvement can be expected. In the second state, degeneration of the heart muscle has progressed, and the storage granules in the sympathetic nerve end are highly disordered. This second state represents an organic and advanced abnormality in the non-compensatory stage in which degeneration, such as necrosis, dropouts and interstitial fiberization of heart muscle, is usually far advanced. In many instances, in terms of MIBG parameters, accumulation in both the early and delayed image is decreased. During the second state, improvement by β-blocker administration cannot be expected and the prognosis is bad.

Overall, evaluation of both the early image and delayed image of MIBG can provide useful information for the prognosis of heart failure and cardiomyopathy, and a prediction and evaluation of the effect of β-blocker therapy.

35.6
Future Trends

To date, MIBG is being applied clinically to various diseases. While MIBG seems to be most useful at evaluating heart failure and cardiomyopathy, most reports have investigated only a small number of cases/subjects within a single facility. Therefore, there is not sufficient evidence. Different facilities also tended to produce different quantity values for MIBG. H/M and WR obtained from the planar image are generally used as the indices of MIBG, however, the value of H/M fluctuates greatly according to the imaging equipment, especially if a collimator is used. It is believed that the main reason for H/M fluctuation is that the amount of scattered elements with 529 keV gamma rays that mix with data from 159 keV in I-123 differs according to the collimator. Because the permeation rate of 529 keV gamma rays is high, the influence of deteriorating image quality due to scattered radiation increases with use of the collimator at low energy, which is the equipment and setting widely used in examining the heart. The use of a collimator that is especially improved for I-123 and a collimator for use at mid-energy is advocated to avoid the deterioration of image quality; however, only limited facilities carry this type of equipment. The I-123 dual window (IDW) method, which does not require special hardware, has been developed to remove the scattered radiation that originates in 529 keV gamma rays [38, 39]. The authors believe that it is important to execute a large-scale clinical trial in the future to establish more conclusive evidence [40].

Part IV Management of Coronary Artery Disease and Ischaemic Heart Disease

Prevention of Coronary Heart Disease

Firas A Ghanem and Assad Movahed

Contents

36.1	Introduction	419
36.2	Smoking	419
36.3	Dyslipidemia	420
36.4	Hypertension	420
36.5	Diabetes	420
36.6	Obesity and the Metabolic Syndrome	421
36.7	Diet and Nutrition	421
36.8	Exercise	421
36.9	Pharmacological Prevention	421
36.10	Conclusion	422
	References	422

36.1 Introduction

Coronary heart disease (CHD) is a leading cause of death in the USA, and a burden that is estimated to overtake all other causes of mortality worldwide by the year 2020 [1]. Marked advances have been made in recent years to better understand the pathophysiology of CHD and to develop scoring systems that can integrate risk factors to estimate an individual's risk of future cardiovascular (CV) events. Risk factors for CHD are divided into modifiable (smoking, hypertension, lipid abnormalities, diabetes, sedentary lifestyle) and non-modifiable (age, male gender, genetic factors, ethnicity). Interventions aimed at prevention can be divided into primary (disease prevention in patients without overt cardiovascular disease) as opposed to secondary, when dealing with those with known cardiovascular disease (CVD). The following is an overview of interventions aimed at prevention of CHD.

36.2 Smoking

Cigarette smoking is the leading modifiable risk factor for CHD. Smoking accelerates the progression of atherosclerosis, an association that was found stronger for pack-years of smoking than current versus past smoking [2]. A cohort study in 21 countries showed a five-fold increase in the risk of non-fatal myocardial infarction among smokers aged 35–39 years compared with non-smokers [3]. Light smokers, especially women, remain at high risk for CHD even when smoking as little as 3–5 cigarettes a day [4]. Among nonsmokers, exposure to smoke from spouses can cause a 30% excess risk of ischemic heart disease compared with those whose spouses do not smoke [5]. The single most important intervention in preventive cardiology remains the termination of tobacco consumption. Cessation, rather than reduction should be the aim of the counselling physician as the latter has showed no reduction in mortality [6]. Data from the Nurses' Health Study established a progressive reduction in the risk of CHD following smoking cessation.

The excess risk returned to the level of those who never smoked in 10 to 14 years [7]. In patients with established CHD, smoking cessation is associated with a substantial reduction in risk of all-cause mortality regardless of age, sex or the type of cardiac event [8]. Physicians should discuss smoking cessation with their patients at every visit and offer nicotine replacement therapy as well as pharmacological therapy, such as sustained-release bupropion hydrochloride [9].

36.3
Dyslipidemia

Serum total cholesterol is predictive of CHD morbidity and mortality, with clear benefits demonstrated in primary and secondary prevention by dietary and pharmacological therapy [10]. Adult treatment panel III (ATP III) recommends screening fasting lipid profile in all adults > 20 years old and the use of LDL cholesterol as the primary aim of therapy. Using risk factors from the Framingham Heart Study (Table 36.1), projections of a 10-year absolute CHD risk score can be obtained (available online at www.nhlbi.nih.gov/guidelines/cholesterol) [11]. The number of risk factors, together with the risk scores can be further used to shape lipid-lowering intensity. Patients with existing CHD or a CHD risk equivalent (diabetes, peripheral arterial disease or 10-year CHD risk > 20%) should have the most aggressive LDL reduction (< 100 mg/dL). In patients without CHD and two or more risk factors (or a 10-year CHD risk < 20%), the LDL target is < 130 mg/dL. Patients with lower risk should be treated assuming a target LDL < 160 mg/dL.

Table 36.1 Major risk factors (exclusive of LDL cholesterol) that modify LDL goals [11]

Cigarette smoking
Hypertension (BP ≥ 140/90 mmHg or on antihypertensive medication)
Low HDL cholesterol (< 40 mg/dL)†
Family history of premature CHD (CHD in male first degree relative < 55 years; CHD in female first degree relative < 65 years)
Age (men ≥ 45 years; women ≥ 55 years)

Diabetes is regarded as a CHD risk equivalent. LDL indicates low-density lipoprotein; HDL, high-density lipoprotein.

† HDL cholesterol ≥ 60 mg/dL counts as a "negative" risk factor; its presence removes one risk factor from the total count.

Low HDL cholesterol is a strong independent predictor of CHD although ATP III does not specify a goal for raising HDL. For triglycerides > 200 mg/dL, non-HDL cholesterol (total cholesterol minus HDL cholesterol) becomes a secondary target. In the latter two cases, consideration should be given to raising HDL using drugs like fibrates or nicotinic acid [11].

36.4
Hypertension

Hypertension is the most common risk factor for CVD, accounting for 65 million individuals in the USA [12]. For individuals 40–70 years of age, each increment of 20 mmHg in systolic blood pressure BP (BP) or 10 mmHg in diastolic BP doubles the risk of cardiovascular disease across the entire BP range from 115/75 to 185/115 mmHg [13]. A recent meta-analysis of 27 trials, showed the efficacy of systolic blood pressure reduction on lowering cardiovascular events across different classes of antihypertensive drugs [14]. The Seventh Joint National Committee (JNC 7) recognizes that most patients with hypertension will require two or more antihypertensive medications to achieve goal blood pressure (< 140/90 mmHg, or < 130/80 mmHg for patients with diabetes or chronic kidney disease). It also recommends initiating therapy with two agents (one of which a thiazide-type diuretic) if blood pressure is > 20/10 mmHg above goal blood pressure [13].

36.5
Diabetes

Diabetes is a major risk factor for CVD, with both men and women dying from CVD related events [15]. The UK Prospective Diabetes Study revealed that improvement in A1c was associated with decreased incidence of both microvascular and macrovascular complications [16]. ATP III recommends aggressive lipid management in diabetics (LDL < 100 mg/dL) as diabetes confers a high risk of new CHD within 10 years [11]. The American Diabetes Association (ADA) recommends a rigid blood pressure-lowering target of < 130/80 mmHg using angiotensin-converting enzyme (ACE) inhibitors, angiotensin receptor blockers (ARBs), beta blockers and diuretics, as they show efficacy in decreasing coronary events and heart failure and in reducing the progression of renal disease [17]. The ADA also recommends aspirin (75–162 mg/day) as a primary and secondary strategy to prevent CV events [18]. Multifactorial risk management is often needed in patients with diabetes. Intensified intervention with behavior modification and pharmacologic therapy that targets hyperglycemia, hypertension, dyslipidemia, and microalbuminuria, along with aspirin, greatly reduces the risk of cardiovascular and microvascular events [19].

36.6
Obesity and the Metabolic Syndrome

Obesity has reached epidemic proportions in the western world. According to the National Health and Nutrition Examination Survey (2001–2002), the prevalence of overweight and obesity in the USA was 65.7% and 30.6%, respectively [20]. Obesity is an independent risk factor for CVD and may affect the heart through its influence on known risk factors such as dyslipidemia, hypertension, glucose intolerance, inflammatory markers, obstructive sleep apnea/hypoventilation, and the prothrombotic state [21]. Intentional weight loss can improve or prevent many of the obesity-related risk factors for CHD although no data on mortality or CVD events is available from randomized controlled clinical trials [21]. The metabolic syndrome is a common metabolic disorder that results from the increasing prevalence of obesity and insulin resistance [22]. It is defined as the presence of three or more of the following: abdominal obesity (waist size > 40 inches for men or > 35 inches women); blood pressure > 130/85 mm Hg; HDL < 40 mg/dL for men or < 50 mg/dL for women; triglycerides > 150 mg/dL; and fasting blood sugar > 110 mg/dL [11]. The metabolic syndrome identifies subjects at increasing risk of developing both CHD and type 2 diabetes mellitus. With insufficient evidence for use of drugs that target the underlying causes, treatment is directed towards life style interventions followed by drug therapies for of individual risk factors [22].

36.7
Diet and Nutrition

There is a wealth of information from observational prospective cohort studies that support a diet high in fruits, vegetables, fiber, mono and polyunsaturated fats and low in saturated fats and trans-fatty acids in order to decrease CHD risk [22]. Similar observational data showed that diets rich in antioxidants (vitamins C, E and beta-carotene) decrease CVD risk, although this could merely reflect a healthy life style. In fact, in a meta-analysis of the available data from randomized trials of vitamin E and beta-carotene, no benefit was found in total mortality, CVD death or stroke [23]. With regard to alcohol, moderate drinking has been linked to a decreased risk of myocardial infarction [24]. In the absence of randomized trials and the linkage of alcohol to the development of hypertension, drinking should be limited, to no more than two drinks per day in most men and to no more than one drink per day in women and lighter weight persons [13, 25]. Finally, fish consumption (possibly through long-chain omega-3 polyunsaturated fatty acids) was inversely associated with fatal CHD in observational studies supporting fish consumption once per week or more [25].

36.8
Exercise

Epidemiological data support physical inactivity as an independent risk factor for the development of CHD [25]. Starting and maintenance of an exercise program is associated with decreased all cause as well as CVD mortality [26]. Recommendations from the Centers for Disease Control and Prevention/American College of Sports Medicine require adults to engage in 30 minutes or more of moderate-intensity physical activity on most (preferably all) days of the week [27]. The American Heart Association (AHA) stresses the importance of exercise training in managing selected CAD risk factors and the need for exercise testing before vigorous exercise in selected patients with cardiovascular disease and other patients with symptoms or those at high risk [28]. A meta-analysis of 48 randomized trials of ≤6 months' duration compared the effectiveness of exercise-based cardiac rehabilitation in CHD patients with usual medical care. Cardiac rehabilitation was associated with reduced all-cause mortality and cardiac mortality; greater improvement in lipid profile and systolic blood pressure; and lower rates of self-reported smoking [29].

36.9
Pharmacological Prevention

Several highly effective pharmacological interventions are considered appropriate for the prevention of cardiovascular disease. Evidence mainly supports aspirin, beta-blockers, ACE inhibitors and HMG-CoA reductase inhibitors (statins). In a meta-analysis of 5580 randomized participants, aspirin was associated with a statistically significant 32% reduction in the risk of a first MI and a significant 15% reduction in the risk of all important vascular events [30]. The AHA recommends aspirin in persons with CHD risk ≥10% per 10 years [31]. In patients with prior CVD, a significant 25% reduction ($P < 0.00001$) in vascular events (nonfatal MI, stroke, vascular death) was seen with ASA (mostly 75–325 mg/day) independently of age or gender [32].

Despite the lack of a clear indication for beta-blockers in patients with uncomplicated hypertension, beta blockade plays a key role in reduction of mortality and morbidity in patients after myocardial infarction [33]. ACE inhibitors exert favorable effects on patients with coronary artery disease, left ventricular dysfunction, or post-MI, irrespective of concomitant use of aspirin [34]. ARBs are thought, in general, to have a similar effect to ACE inhibitors [35]. Multiple statin trials have confirmed the benefit of cholesterol-lowering therapy for secondary as well as primary prevention in patients with multiple CVD risk factors [11]. In primary prevention, the addition of a statin to aspirin therapy becomes more cost-effective when the patient's 10-year CHD risk before treatment is higher than 10% [36]. The recent modification of the ATP III guidelines recommended an optional goal LDL below 70 mg/dL for very high risk patients defined by the presence of CVD plus (1) multiple major risk factors (especially diabetes), (2) severe and poorly controlled risk factors (especially continued cigarette smoking), (3) multiple risk factors of the metabolic syndrome (especially high triglycerides ≥ 200 mg/dL plus non-HDL-C ≥ 130 mg/dL with low HDL-C [< 40 mg/dL]), and (4) patients with acute coronary syndromes [37]. More recently, in a case-control study, statin and beta-blocker use was associated with lower odds of presenting with an acute myocardial infarction than with stable angina [38].

36.10
Conclusion

Both primary and secondary prevention of CHD have contributed tremendously to the reduction in CHD mortality rates. Identification of risk factors can help to identify subjects at higher risk for cardiovascular disease for more aggressive therapy. A multidisciplinary approach is often needed with therapeutic lifestyle changes and, if not adequate, the addition of pharmacological interventions. Judicious implementation of evidence-based medicine through careful blending of science and art should have overwhelming benefit in preventing heart disease in both women and men.

References

1. Murray CJ, Lopez AD (1997) Alternative projections of mortality and disability by cause 1990-2020: Global Burden of Disease Study. Lancet 349:1498–1504.
2. Howard G, Wagenknecht LE, Burke GL et al. (1998) Cigarette smoking and progression of atherosclerosis: The Atherosclerosis Risk in Communities (ARIC) Study. J Am Med Assoc 279(2):119–124.
3. Mahonen MS, McElduff P, Dobson AJ et al. (2004) Current smoking and the risk of non-fatal myocardial infarction in the WHO MONICA Project populations. Tob Control 3(3):244–250.
4. Prescott E, Scharling H, Osler M, Schnohr P (2002) Importance of light smoking and inhalation habits on risk of myocardial infarction and all cause mortality. A 22 year follow up of 12 149 men and women in The Copenhagen City Heart Study. J Epidemiol Community Health 56(9):702–706.
5. Law MR, Wald NJ (2003) Environmental tobacco smoke and ischemic heart disease. Prog Cardiovasc Dis 46(1):31–38.
6. Godtfredsen NS, Holst C, Prescott E et al. (2002) Smoking reduction, smoking cessation, and mortality: A 16-year follow-up of 19,732 men and women from The Copenhagen Centre for Prospective Population Studies. Am J Epidemiol 156:994.
7. Kawachi I, Colditz GA, Stampfer MJ et al. (1994) Smoking cessation and time course of decreased risks of coronary heart disease in middle-aged women. Arch Intern Med 154(2):169–175.
8. Critchley JA, Capewell S (2003) Mortality risk reduction associated with smoking cessation in patients with coronary heart disease: a systematic review. J Am Med Assoc 290(1):86–97.
9. A clinical practice guideline for treating tobacco use and dependence: A US Public Health Service report (2000) The Tobacco Use and Dependence Clinical Practice Guideline Panel, Staff, and Consortium Representatives. J Am Med Assoc 283(24):3244–54.
10. Kuller LH (2006) Prevention of coronary heart disease and the National Cholesterol Education Program. Circulation 113(5):598–600.
11. Expert Panel on Detection, Evaluation, and Treatment of High Blood Cholesterol in Adults (2001) Executive Summary of The Third Report of The National Cholesterol Education Program (NCEP) Expert Panel on Detection, Evaluation, And Treatment of High Blood Cholesterol In Adults (Adult Treatment Panel III). J Am Med Assoc 285(19):2486–2497.
12. American Heart Association (2005) Heart and Stroke Statistics – 2005 Update. Dallas, Texax, American Heart Association.
13. Chobanian AV, Bakris GL, Black HR et al. (2003) The seventh report of the Joint National Committee on Prevention, Detection, Evaluation and Treatment of High Blood Pressure: the JNC 7 report. J Am Med Assoc 289(19):2560–2572.
14. Staessen JA, Wang JG, Thijs L (2001) Cardiovascular protection and blood pressure reduction: a meta-analysis. Lancet 358(9290):1305–1315.
15. Geiss LS, Herman WH, Smith PJ (1995) National Diabetes Data Group. Diabetes in America. Bethesda, Md: National Institutes of Health, National Institute of Diabetes and Digestive and Kidney Diseases, pp. 233–257.

16. Stratton IM, Adler AI, Neil HA, Matthews DR, Manley SE, Cull CA et al. (2000) Association of glycaemia with macrovascular and microvascular complications of type 2 diabetes (UKPDS 35): prospective observational study. Br Med J 321:405–412.
17. Arauz-Pacheco C, Parrott MA, Raskin P (2002) (American Diabetes Association). Hypertension management in adults with diabetes. Diabetes Care 25(1):134–147.
18. Colwell JA (2004) American Diabetes Association. Aspirin therapy in diabetes. Diabetes Care 27 Suppl 1:S72–S73.
19. Gaede P, Vedel P, Larsen N, Jensen GV, Parving HH, Pedersen O (2003) Multifactorial intervention and cardiovascular disease in patients with type 2 diabetes. N Engl J Med 348(5):383–93.
20. Hedley AA, Ogden CL, Johnson CL, Carroll MD, Curtin LR, Flegal KM (2004) Overweight and obesity among US children, adolescents, and adults, 1999-2002. J Am Med Assoc 291:2847–2850.
21. Poirier P, Giles TD, Bray GA et al. (2006) American Heart Association; Obesity Committee of the Council on Nutrition, Physical Activity, and Metabolism. Obesity and cardiovascular disease: pathophysiology, evaluation, and effect of weight loss: an update of the 1997 American Heart Association Scientific Statement on Obesity and Heart Disease from the Obesity Committee of the Council on Nutrition, Physical Activity, and Metabolism. Circulation 113(6):898–918.
22. Yancy WS Jr, Westman EC, French PA, Califf RM (2003) Diets and clinical coronary events: the truth is out there. Circulation 107(1):10–6.
23. Vivekananthan DP, Penn MS, Sapp SK, Hsu A, Topol EJ (2003) Use of antioxidant vitamins for the prevention of cardiovascular disease: meta-analysis of randomised trials. Lancet 361(9374):2017–23.
24. Mukamal KJ, Conigrave KM, Mittleman MA et al. (2003) Roles of drinking pattern and type of alcohol consumed in coronary heart disease in men. N Engl J Med 348:109–118.
25. Berlin JA, Colditz GA (1990) A meta-analysis of physical activity in the prevention of coronary heart disease. Am J Epidemiol 132:612–628.
26. Blair SN, Kohl HW 3d, Barlow CE, Paffenberger RS Jr, Gibbons LW, Macera CA (1995) Changes in physical fitness and all-cause mortality. A prospective study of healthy and unhealthy men. J Am Med Assoc 273:1093–1098.
27. Pate RR, Pratt M, Blair SN et al. (1995) Physical activity and public health: a recommendation from the Centers for Disease Control and Prevention and the American College of Sports Medicine. J Am Med Assoc 273:402–407.
28. Thompson PD, Buchner D, Pina I et al. (2003) Exercise and physical activity in the prevention and treatment of atherosclerotic cardiovascular disease: a statement from the Council on Clinical Cardiology (Subcommittee on Exercise, Rehabilitation, and Prevention) and the Council on Nutrition, Physical Activity, and Metabolism (Subcommittee on Physical Activity). Circulation 107:3109–3116.
29. Taylor RS, Brown A, Ebrahim S et al. (2004) Exercise-based rehabilitation for patients with coronary heart disease: systematic review and meta-analysis of randomized controlled trials. Am J Med 116:682–692.
30. Eidelman RS, Hebert PR, Weisman SM, Hennekens CH (2003) An update on aspirin in the primary prevention of cardiovascular disease. Arch Internal Med 163(17):2006–2010.
31. Pearson TA, Blair SN, Daniels SR et al. (2002) AHA guidelines for primary prevention of cardiovascular disease and stroke: 2002 update: consensus panel guide to comprehensive risk reduction for adult patients without coronary or other atherosclerotic vascular diseases. American Heart Association Science Advisory and Coordinating Committee. Circulation 106:388–391.
32. Antiplatelet Trialists' Collaboration (1994) Collaborative overview of randomised trials of anti platelet therapy – I: Prevention of death, myocardial infarction, and stroke by prolonged antiplatelet therapy in various categories of patients. Br Med J 308:81–106.
33. Freemantle N, Cleland J, Young P, Mason J, Harrison J (1999) β Blockade after myocardial infarction: systematic review and meta regression analysis. Br Med J 318:1730–1737.
34. Teo KK, Yusuf S, Pfeffer M et al. (2002) Effects of long-term treatment with angiotensin-converting-enzyme inhibitors in the presence or absence of aspirin: a systematic review. Lancet 360:1037–1043.
35. Pfeffer MA, Swedberg K, Granger CB et al. (2003) Effects of candesartan on mortality and morbidity in patients with chronic heart failure: The CHARM-Overall programme. Lancet 362:759–766.
36. Pignone M, Earnshaw S, Tice JA, Pletcher MJ (2006) Aspirin, statins, or both drugs for the primary prevention of coronary heart disease events in men: a cost-utility analysis. Ann Internal Med 144(5):326–336.
37. Grundy SM, Cleeman JI, Bairey Merz CN et al. (2004) For the Coordinating Committee of the National Cholesterol Education Program. Implications of recent clinical trials for the National Cholesterol Education Program Adult Treatment Panel III guidelines. Circulation 110:227–239.
38. Go AS, Iribarren C, Chandra M et al. (2006) Statin and beta-blocker therapy and the initial presentation of coronary heart disease. Ann Internal Med 144(4):229–238.

Cardiovascular Medications: Pharmacokinetics and Pharmacodynamics

Jaffar Ali Raza, Wayne Kreeger and Assad Movahed

Contents

37.1	Introduction	425
37.2	Hypertension	425
37.2.1	Angiotensin-Converting Enzyme Inhibitors	426
37.2.2	Angiotensin II Receptor Antagonists	427
37.2.3	Beta-Blockers	428
37.2.4	Calcium-Antagonist Drugs	429
37.2.5	Diuretics	430
37.3	Heart Failure	431
37.3.1	Digoxin	432
37.3.2	Nitrates	432
37.3.3	Nesiritide	433
37.4	Dyslipidemia	434
37.4.1	Bile Acid Sequestrants	434
37.4.2	Ezetimibe	435
37.4.3	Fibric Acid	435
37.4.4	Niacin	436
37.4.5	Statins	437
37.5	Anti-thrombotic Agents	438
37.5.1	Direct Thrombin Inhibitors	438
37.5.2	Fibrinolytic Agents	439
37.5.3	Glycoprotein IIb-IIIa Inhibitors	440
37.5.4	Heparin	441
37.5.5	Low-Molecular-Weight Heparins	442
37.5.6	Thienopyridines	443
37.5.7	Warfarin	444
37.5.8	Ximelagatran	445
37.6	Conclusion	445
	References	445

37.1 Introduction

Cardiovascular diseases (CVD) have reached epidemic proportions in developed countries, and are the leading cause of morbidity and mortality. An estimated 16.7 million – or 29.2% of total global deaths – result from the various forms of CVD, many of which are preventable by healthy diet, regular physical activity, and smoking cessation [1]. CVD is no longer the disease of the developed world: some 80% of all CVD deaths worldwide took place in developing, low and middle-income countries and these countries also account for 86% of the global CVD disease burden. By 2010, CVD will be the leading cause of death in developing countries. The rise in CVD reflects a significant change in diet habits, physical activity levels, and tobacco consumption worldwide as a result of industrialization, urbanization, economic development and food market globalization. To deal with this changing situation, an extraordinary array of new cardiovascular therapies continues to become available. These drugs and therapies are efficacious and are better tolerated than their predecessors, not only in the management but also in prevention of CVD. This results in ever more difficulty for the practitioners of medicine in understanding the mechanism of action of these medications and also in deciding the proper medication for their patients. This chapter is a concise presentation of the pharmacology of cardiovascular medications.

37.2 Hypertension

Worldwide prevalence estimates for hypertension (HTN) may be as much as 1 billion individuals, and approximately 7.1 million deaths per year may be attributable to hypertension [1]. The World Health Organization reports that suboptimal BP (>115 mmHg systolic blood pressure (SBP) is responsible for 62% of cerebrovascular disease and 49% of ischemic heart disease. Suboptimal blood pressure is the number one attributable risk for death throughout the world. The relationship between HTN and risk of CVD events is consistent, and independent of other risk factors. The higher the HTN, the greater is the chance of heart attack, HF, stroke, and kidney diseases. Hence adequate treatment of HTN is essential.

37.2.1
Angiotensin-Converting Enzyme Inhibitors

Renin Angiotensin Aldosterone System (RAAS) activated in response to myocardial injury plays a critical role in blood pressure regulation and in the process of cardiac remodeling. The diminished left ventricular ejection fraction seen in congestive heart failure (CHF) leads to the production and release of renin from the kidneys. In turn, renin converts angiotensinogen to angiotensin I (AI), which is subsequently converted to angiotensin II (AII), through the actions of angiotensin-converting enzyme (ACE). AII is a potent vasoconstrictor that also promotes the reabsorption of sodium and the release of the antidiuretic hormone aldosterone. AII has been shown to directly promote left-ventricular hypertrophy and remodeling in cardiac tissue [2]. Angiotensin-converting enzyme inhibitors (ACEI) competitively inhibit the enzyme responsible for the conversion of AI to angiotensin II and have become a mainstay in the treatment of heart failure. In a review of three large published trials in patients with CHF, the use of an ACEI alone resulted in an approximately 20% reduction in 1-year mortality, while adding a beta-blocker to ongoing ACEI therapy produced a striking 35% reduction in mortality [3].

37.2.1.1 Pharmacokinetics

There are currently more than 15 ACEI in clinical use. Each drug has a unique structure that determines its potency, tissue receptor binding affinity, metabolism, and prodrug compound, but they have remarkably similar clinical effects [4]. They are classified into sulfhydryl (captopril), carboxyl (Benazepril), or phosphinyl (Fosinopril) categories based on the ligand that binds to the ACE-zinc moiety. The absorption is highly variable among ACEI (25–75%) and food either has no effect or reduces the rate, but not the extent of absorption. Captopril has about 75% bioavailability after oral administration with a half-life of 2 hours. Food may decrease captopril absorption and 30% of captopril is protein bound. Captopril is partially metabolized in the liver into an inactive captopril-cysteine disulfide compound; 95% of the parent compound and metabolites are eliminated in the urine within 24 hours [5]. Most of the carboxyl ACEI except Benazepril and lisinopril are given as prodrugs that undergo biotransformation in the liver into the active compounds. The peak plasma drug concentrations are reached 1–4 h after ingestion. They have an elimination half life that varies from 3 hours to 24 hours. These agents are excreted primarily in the urine by the kidneys. Hence the dosage should be reduced by 25% to 50% in patients with renal failure [6]. Fosinopril sodium is the only available phosphinyl agent in market. It has a bioavailability of approximately 36% : 85% of fosinopril is hydrolyzed in the liver and intestines into the active compound, fosinoprilat, the remainder into inactive metabolites. The elimination half-life of fosinoprilat is 11.5 to 12 hours. All metabolites are excreted in both the urine and feces thus necessitating dose reduction in patients with renal failure [7].

37.2.1.2 Pharmacodynamics

ACEI lower blood pressure mainly by reducing peripheral resistance with little effect on heart rate, cardiac output, or body fluid volumes [8]. Captopril was the first synthesized inhibitor of the angiotensin converting enzyme that breaks the peptidyldipeptide bond in AI, thus preventing the enzyme from attaching to and splitting the AI structure. Since then various agents have been available in the market. As AI is inactive, the renin-angiotensin system is paralyzed, thereby removing the effects of AII as both a vasoconstrictor and a stimulant to aldosterone synthesis [9]. Because the same enzyme that converts AI to AII is also responsible for inactivation of the vasodilating hormone bradykinin, by inhibiting the breakdown of bradykinin, ACEI also causes vasodilation and improvement in insulin sensitivity. ACE inhibitors may also vasodilate by increasing levels of vasodilatory prostaglandins and decreasing levels of vasoconstricting endothelins [10] (Table 37.1). Additional mechanisms include improvement of nitric oxide-mediated endothelial function, reversal of vascular hypertrophy, decrease in aldosterone secretion that causes natriuresis, augmentation of renal blood flow to induce natriuresis, blunting of sympathetic nervous system activity, inhibition of central AII-mediated sympathoexcitation, norepinephrine synthesis, and arginine vasopressin release, inhibition of centrally controlled baroreceptor reflexes, which results in increased baroreceptor sensitivity, and decrease in vasoconstrictor endothelin-1 levels [11].

Table 37.1 Effects of ACE-inhibitors (derived from Expert consensus document on angiotensin converting enzyme inhibitors in cardiovascular disease: The Task Force on ACE-inhibitors of the European Society of Cardiology. *Eur Heart Journal* 2004; 25: 1454–1470 [15])

1) Haemodynamic effects

- Lower peripheral vascular resistances
- Promote natriuresis
- Increase venous capacitance and arterial vasodilatation
- Increase renal blood flow
- Decrease sympathetic tone
- Improve cardiac relaxation and distensibility
- Increase bradykinin level that causes an increased NO level resulting in vasodilation.
- Neurohormonal effects
- Decrease in angiotensin-II and aldosterone levels
- Reduce the plasma levels of epinephrine, norepinephrine and vasopressin
- Increase production of bradykinin, which exhibits vasodilator properties

2) Antiproliferative effects

- Reducing ventricular preload/afterload
- Prevent the proliferative effects of AII and sympathetic nervous system
- Inhibit the aldosterone-induced cardiac hypertrophy
- Reduce formation of superoxide anions and pro-oxidants
- Reduce the oxidation of lipids
- Reduce markers of inflammation like IL-6, chemotactic proteins and adhesion molecules

3) Reverse cardiac hypertrophy in hypertensive patients

4) Reduce endothelial dysfunction

5) Reduce platelet aggregation and adhesion

6) Anti-atherogenic effect by causing the inhibition of angiotensin-II formation, bradykinin potentiation and increased NO release

37.2.1.3 Adverse Effects

ACEI may cause rash, loss of taste, and leukopenia. They may also cause a hypersensitivity reaction with angioneurotic edema or a cough [12]. The increased plasma kinin levels are also responsible for this most common and bothersome side effect of their use, the dry, hacking cough. The removal of the high levels of AII that the kidneys produce may deprive the stenotic kidney of the hormonal drive to its blood flow, thereby causing a marked decline in renal perfusion. Thus, patients with solitary kidneys or bilateral renal artery stenosis may develop acute renal failure [13]. They can also cause fetal or neonatal injury or death when used during the second and third trimesters of pregnancy [14].

37.2.2 Angiotensin II Receptor Antagonists

Angiotensin II receptor antagonists (ARBs) represent a new class of drugs that provide a site-specific blockade of the effects of AII. ACEI are well tolerated, and are used in the treatment of hypertension and heart failure. However, they have two important adverse effects as a class, cough (common) and angioedema (rare) [16]. Search for other approaches to pharmacologically interrupt the renin-angiotensin-aldosterone cascade without these adverse effects has led to the development of the A-II type 1 (AT$_1$) receptor antagonists [17]. Losartan potassium, the first compound of this new drug class, and since then several others have been released for clinical use (candesartan, eprosartan, irbesartan, olmesartan, telmisartan, valsartan) [18]. ARBs are currently used in the treatment of both hypertension and CHF.

37.2.2.1 Pharmacokinetics

AT$_1$ receptor antagonists are chemically classified into biphenyl or nonbiphenyl tetrazoles and non-heterocyclic compounds [19]. These drugs are given in the oral form and have varying degrees of absorption. The bioavailability of the individual ARBs are quite variable. Losartan, candesartan and olmesartan are given as prodrugs that are converted into active metabolites in the body [20]. The ARBs are highly protein bound, in the excess of 90%. All these drugs undergo significant hepatic metabolism, and eliminated in the urine. Losartan, olmesartan and candesartan undergo less hepatic metabolism and are predominantly excreted by the kidneys [20].

37.2.2.2 Pharmacodynamics

AII exerts its effects by stimulating the specific receptors on the membrane of various target organ cells (blood vessel, heart, adrenal cortex) [21]. At least two principal receptor types have been identified by using radioligand binding studies and have been labeled AT_1 and AT_2 receptors. Although both receptor types are seen in various organs, the cardiovascular effects of A-II are mediated by the AT_1 receptor [22]. ARBs block the actions of AII and causes reversal of vasoconstriction, myocardial and vascular hypertrophy, and inhibition of aldosterone secretion. Since the ARBs displace AII from its receptor sites competitively, the circulating levels of angiotensin may actually rise in response to ARBs [17].

37.2.2.3 Adverse Effects

ARBs have an excellent side effect profile with various studies having demonstrated that side effects with ARBs are no greater than with a placebo. Unlike ACEI, ARBs do not cause a cough, although some cases of angioneurotic edema have been reported. As with ACEI, ARBs should be avoided in pregnancy. ARBs therapy should be introduced cautiously in volume depleted or high renin patients and should be avoided in patients with bilateral renal artery stenosis or stenosis of a solitary kidney.

37.2.3
Beta-Blockers

Beta blockers are competitive antagonists of endogenous or exogenous beta agonists. They are widely used in the treatment of hypertension, angina pectoris, supraventricular arrhythmias, acute phase of myocardial infarction, postmyocardial infarction, and heart failure. They show beneficial effects on clinical end points in the management of stroke, coronary heart disease prevention and mortality, and are well established in improving exercise tolerance and diminish the number and duration of anginal attacks in patients with angina pectoris. Based on clinical trials showing reduced morbidity and mortality, beta-blockers are the cornerstone of therapy in CHF and myocardial infarction. Several multicenter double-blind randomized controlled trials have demonstrated that therapy with certain beta-blockers can provide additional survival benefit in systolic heart failure patients who are already receiving ACE inhibitors [23, 24].

Beta-blockers are classified into three classes based on the specific interaction with the ß-1, ß-2, and α-adrenoreceptors (ARs). Drugs that antagonize both ß-1ARs and ß-2ARs are considered *nonselective* antagonists (propranalol, timolol, sotalol, nadolol); while those that inhibit ß-1-ARs predominantly are considered ß-*1-selective* or cardioselective (e.g., atenolol, metoprolol) [25]. The third group of ß-adrenoceptor antagonists are those that block both ß-ARs and α-ARs. This group includes labetalol and carvedilol. Some of the drugs (pindolol, acebutalol) also possess partial agonist properties (intrinsic sympathomimetic activity (ISA). At high concentration, ß-AR antagonists demonstrate a membrane stabilizing property that is separate from their ß-adrenergic blocking property.

37.2.3.1 Pharmacokinetics

The pharmacokinetic profile of a drug is largely based on its lipid solubility, and ß-blockers are no exception. More lipid-soluble drugs (e.g., propranolol, metoprolol, timolol) are readily absorbed, heavily metabolized by the liver, widely distributed to more tissue, readily cross the blood–brain barrier, and have shorter half-lives [26]. The water-soluble drugs (e.g., atenolol, esmolol) are less readily absorbed, less metabolized by the liver, and/or excreted virtually unchanged by the kidney. They have longer half-lives, with decreased ability to cross the blood–brain barrier. Atenolol, nadolol, and sotalol undergo renal clearance; hence their dosage should be decreased in patients with renal insufficiency and in the elderly [27]. Metoprolol, pindolol and propranolol are cleared by the liver and hence their dosage should be decreased in significant liver dysfunction or portacaval shunts.

37.2.3.2 Pharmacodynamics

When selecting a ß-blocker for a specific patient, efficacy, tolerability, product formulation and duration of action, and the presence or absence of specific properties such as ß₁-selectivity or ISA must be considered. ß-adrenergic antagonists have a significant physiological impact on the cardiovascular system. They cause a 10% to 35% reduction in heart rate. The decrease in cardiac output seen with ß blockers is thought to be predominantly due to the decrease in heart rate. Both classes of ß-AR antagonists decrease coronary blood flow (CBF) by 10% to 20% due to the unopposed action of alpha-AR. However, this decrease in CBF is thought to be due to decreased myocardial oxygen demand [28]. ß blockers slow the sinus rate, prolong the sinoatrial and AV nodal conduction time, and prolong the effective refractory period of the AV node and can worsen heart block [29] (Table 37.2).

Table 37.2 Mechanisms of action of beta-blockers* [34]

1) Prevention of the cardiotoxic effects of catecholamines.

2) Antihypertensive action
- Decreases in cardiac output
- Inhibition of the release of renin and production of angiotensin II
- Blockade of presynaptic beta-adrenoceptors that increase the release of norepinephrine.
- Decreases of central vasomotor activity

3) Anti-ischemic action
- Decreases myocardial oxygen demand
- Reduces heart rate
- Decreases cardiac contractility
- Decreases systolic blood pressure

4) Cardioprotective effect
- Improves left ventricular structure and function
- Reduces heart rate and hence prolonging diastolic filling
- Prolongs coronary diastolic perfusion time
- Reduces myocardial oxidative stress
- Improves myocardial energetics by inhibiting catecholamine-induced release of free fatty acids
- Upregulates beta-adrenergic receptors

5) Antiarrhythmic effect
- Reduced heart rate
- Decreased spontaneous firing of ectopic pacemakers
- Slowed conduction and increased refractory period of AV node
- Reduces the sympathetic drive and myocardial ischaemia
- Improves baroreflex function
- Prevents catecholamine-induced hypokalemia

6) Antioxidant properties (Carvedilol)

7) Inhibition of cardiac apoptosis

37.2.3.3 Adverse Effects

In the ß-Blocker Heart Attack Trial Research Group (BHAT), the most common complaints in patient's taking propranolol were tiredness, bronchospasm, diarrhea, and cold extremities [30]. The CVD side effects include worsening heart failure, hypotension, dizziness, or bradycardia. Nonselective ß-blockers such as propranolol could cause a modest increase in triglyceride levels and, in some patients, decreases in high-density lipoprotein (HDL) cholesterol levels [31]. Non-selective ß-blockers may inhibit catecholamine-induced glycogenolysis and glucose mobilization, and these effects may prolong an episode of hypoglycemia in patients with diabetes and mask the symptoms of hypoglycemia [32]. Both non-selective and cardioselective ß-blockers can precipitate bronchoconstriction in patients with obstructive airways disease, so ß-blockers should be avoided in these patients. The effects on pulmonary function generally are not as pronounced with beta$_1$-selective agents as with nonselective agents, especially when administered in low doses [33].

37.2.4 Calcium-Antagonist Drugs

Calcium antagonists or calcium-channel blockers (CCBs) introduced into clinical medicine in the 1960s are now among the most frequently prescribed drugs for the treatment of hypertension [35]. These drugs have also proved to be effective in patients with angina pectoris, supraventricular arrhythmias, and left ventricular diastolic dysfunction. They act by blocking the transmembrane flow of calcium ions through voltage-gated L-type (slowly inactivating) channels [36]. The CCBs are classified into phenylalkylamines (verapamil), benzothiazepines (diltiazem), and the dihydropyridines (nifedipine) based on the three separate receptor sites they bind to on the L-type Ca^{2+} channels [37].

37.2.4.1 Pharmacokinetics

CCBs are nearly completely absorbed with oral administration. However, their bioavailability varies depending on first-pass metabolism in the intestinal wall and liver [38]. They are oxidized to less active metabolites in the liver by predominantly the cytochrome P-450 CYP3A subgroup of the cytochrome P-450 family, and to a lesser extent by other members of this enzyme family [39]. With the exception of diltiazem and nifedipine, CCBs are administered as racemic mixtures, with one active and one inactive stereoisomer with respect to blockade of L-type calcium channels. The cytochrome P-450 metabolizes each isomer at different rates, resulting in stereoselective drug clearance [40]. The half-life of these agents varies from 1.3 hours to 64 hours [41]. CCBs demonstrate age-dependent pharmacokinetic changes in association with age-related reductions in hepatic blood flow, leading to increases in C_{max}, AUC and bioavailability and decreases in systemic clearance [42].

37.2.4.2 Pharmacodynamics

CCBs inhibit the voltage dependant Ca^{2+} channels resulting in vasodilation and lowering of blood pressure [43]. The relative potency of CCBs as vasodilators varies with nifedipine being more potent as compared to verapamil or diltiazem. In vitro, several CCBs bind with some selectivity to the L-type calcium channel in blood vessels as opposed to verapamil which binds equally well to both cardiac and vascular L-type calcium channels [44]. All classes of CCBs depress sinus-node activity, slow atrioventricular (AV) conduction and decreases in myocardial contractility in vitro [45]. However, only verapamil and diltiazem have these effects in vivo.

37.2.4.3 Adverse Effects

Adverse effects of all CCBs include hypotension, peripheral edema, depression of cardiac function, and constipation. Headache, flushing, and dizziness can also occur. Verapamil and diltiazem should not be used in patients with bradycardia, atrioventricular dissociation, atrioventricular block, and sinus node dysfunction [46]. Bepridil can increase QT interval resulting in polymorphous ventricular tachycardia [47].

37.2.5
Diuretics

Diuretics are widely used for the treatment of patients with heart failure and hypertension. Among these drugs, loop diuretics such as furosemide are perhaps the most frequently prescribed in patients with CHF and thiazides in the treatment of hypertension. Other diuretics available are the carbonic anhydrase inhibitors (actazolamide), osmotic diuretics (mannitol), and potassium sparing diuretics (spironolactone).

37.2.5.1 Pharmacokinetics

A high degree of protein binding (>95%) limits glomerular filtration, of furosemide, even in patients with hypoalbuminemia [48]. About 50% of a dose of furosemide is excreted in unchanged form into the urine; the other 50% is conjugated to glucuronic acid in the kidneys thus the half life is prolonged in patients with renal insufficiency [49]. Bumetanide and torsemide are largely metabolized by the liver and therefore, their half-lives are not prolonged in patients with renal insufficiency [50]. Some thiazide diuretics are metabolized primarily by the liver (indapamide) and others are primarily excreted in unchanged form in the urine (chlorthalidone, hydrochlorothiazide). Amiloride is excreted by the kidneys and hence renal disease prolongs its plasma half-life [51]. Triamterene is converted to an active metabolite by the liver, and the metabolite is then secreted into the tubules. Hence the amount of metabolite that reaches the tubular fluid is also reduced in patients with liver and kidney disease [52]. Spironolactone is converted to numerous active metabolites that are active [53]. The plasma half-life of a diuretic determines the frequency of administration. Thiazide and distal diuretics have sufficiently long half-lives that they can be administered once or twice a day. The plasma half-lives of loop diuretics range from about one hour for bumetanide, three to four hours for torsemide and one and a half to two hours for furosemide [54].

37.2.5.2 Pharmacodynamics

Loop diuretics block the sodium–potassium–chloride transporter. Thiazide diuretics block the electroneutral sodium–chloride transporter. Spironolactone is an aldosterone antagonist, while amiloride and triamterene block sodium-proton exchanger in the distal and collecting tubules [55]. The relation between the arrival of a diuretic at its site of action (determined on the basis of the rate of urinary excretion) and the natriuretic response determines the pharmacodynamics of the drug [56]. There is a threshold quantity of loop diuretic that must be achieved at the site of action in order to elicit a response. The diuretic must therefore be titrated in each patient in order to determine the dose that will deliver enough drugs to the site of action in order to achieve maximum response. Mannitol exerts a diuretic effect at the proximal tubules and loop of Henle. Acetazolamide prevents the carbonic anhydrase that is present in the proximal tubules to reabsorb the sodium bicarbonate, and the thiazides inhibit the sodium chloride transportation in the distal convoluted tubules, and triamterene inhibits the transportation of the sodium in the renal

Table 37.3 Site and mechanism of action of diuretics* [63]

Class	Examples	Site of action	Mechanism of action
Carbonic Anhydrase Inhibitors	Acetazolamide	Proximal convoluted tubule	Inhibits the enzyme carbonic anhydrase. Decreases the ability to exchange Na^+ for H^+ resulting in mild diuresis. Weak diuretic.
Loop or High Ceiling Diuretics	Bumetanide Furosemide Ethacrynic Acid	Ascending limb of the loop of Henle	Inhibit the $Na^+/K^+/2Cl^-$ co-transport system, decreasing their reabsorption. Abolishes hyper tonicity of the medulla, preventing concentration of urine. Highest efficacy. Bumetanide is more potent. Ethacrynic acid has a steeper dose response curve.
Thiazides	Chlorthiazide, Hydrochlorthiazide Chlorthalidone	Distal convoluted tubule	Inhibit Na^+/Cl^- co transporter, decreasing their reabsorption. Most widely used agents. Must be excreted into the tubular lumen to be effective, thus less effective in decreased renal function. Newer Thiazide analogs can be used even in advanced renal failure.
Thiazide Analogs	Indapamide, Metolazone		
Potassium sparing diuretics	Spironolactone	Collecting duct	Synthetic aldosterone antagonist prevents Na^+ reabsorption and therefore K^+ and H^+ secretion. Particularly effective in hyper-aldosteronism.
	Triamterene Amiloride	Collecting duct	Block Na^+ transport channels independent of aldosterone.
Osmotic Diuretics	Mannitol, Urea	Throughout the tubule	Filtered through glomerulus but not reabsorbed resulting in water diuresis. Not useful in conditions with Na^+ retention.

epithelial cells in the distal tubules and the collecting ducts [57, 58]. Spironolactone is an aldosterone antagonist competitively inhibits the binding of aldosterone to the mineralocorticoid receptor that is present in the epithelial cells of the distal tubules and the collecting ducts and in turn increases the resorption of sodium and the excretion of potassium [59, 60] (Table 37.3).

37.2.5.3 Adverse Effects

The most important adverse effects of diuretics are abnormalities in fluid and electrolyte homeostasis. Both loop and thiazide diuretics cause loss of potassium and magnesium in the urine, and when administered in combination, they may result in substantial depletion of these cations. However, while the loop diuretics increase urinary calcium excretion; thiazide diuretics cause urinary calcium retention [61]. Other adverse effects are skin reactions and interstitial nephritis with the use of thiazides and loop diuretics; and ototoxicity with loop diuretics. Spironolactone can also cause gynecomastia, impotence, decreased libido, hirsutism and menstrual irregularities due to its steroid structure [62]. Potassium sparing diuretics can result in life threatening hyperkalemia; therefore patients who are on concomitant ACEI therapy should be closely watched.

37.3 Heart Failure

Congestive heart failure (CHF) is a common condition associated with significant morbidity and mortality, and its incidence and prevalence are increasing [64]. Approximately 5 million individuals in the US have CHF, and furthermore, it is estimated that 0.4–2% of the general European population have symptomatic heart failure [65]. Globally, atherosclerosis and coronary artery disease are expected to increase across the world in the next two decades as the levels of obesity, diabetes, and hypertension increase. In addition, more patients are surviving acute myocardial infarction but with damaged hearts, and life expectancy is predicted to increase [66]. Hence, the number of individuals, community, health care, and economic burden of heart failure will continue to rise. Beta-blockers, ACEI, ARBs, diuretics, aldosterone blockers (aldosterone, eplerenone), digoxin, and nitrates are all used in the treatment of heart failure.

37.3.1
Digoxin

Withering, in 1785 published an account of digitalis (dried leaves of the purple foxglove) and some of its medical uses [67]. Since then it has been one of the commonly used drug in the treatment of cardiovascular diseases. Digoxin is a cardiac glycoside containing asteroid nucleus with an unsaturated lactone that is present on the C-17 position. All cardiac glycoside have a particular effect on the myocardium, by their potent and highly selective inhibition of the active transport of Na and K across the cell membrane. They achieve this inhibition by binding to a specific site on the extracytoplasmic face of the alpha sub-unit of Na, K ATPase [68].

37.3.1.1 Pharmacokinetics

The times to onset of pharmacologic effect and to peak effect of preparations of Lanoxin, range from 5–30 minutes for IV to 0.5 to 2 hours for oral preparation. It is concentrated in skeletal muscle and adipose tissues and therefore has a large apparent volume of distribution. Digoxin crosses both the blood-brain barrier and the placenta. Only a small percentage (16%) of a dose of digoxin is metabolized and the rest (50–70%) is excreted unchanged by the kidneys [84]. The clearance rate is proportional to the GFR. In healthy people with normal renal function, digoxin has a half-life of 1.5–2.0 days. The half-life in anuric patients could be prolonged to 3.5–5 days. Digoxin is not effectively removed from the body by dialysis, exchange transfusion, or during cardiopulmonary bypass because most of the drug is concentrated in the tissues.

37.3.1.2 Pharmacodynamics

Digoxin inhibits sodium-potassium ATPase that leads to an increase in the intracellular concentration of sodium [69]. This in turn increases the intracellular calcium content by affecting sodium–calcium exchange across the sarcolemmal membrane through the sodium–calcium exchange channel, producing an enhancement of cardiac contractility [70]. In addition to the direct actions on cardiac muscle, digoxin exerts indirect actions on the cardiovascular system by its effects on the autonomic nervous system [71]. The autonomic effects include: (1) a vagomimetic action, responsible for the effects of digoxin on the sinoatrial and atrioventricular (AV) nodes; and (2) baroreceptor sensitization, which results in increased afferent inhibitory activity and reduced activity of the sympathetic nervous system and renin-angiotensin system for any given increment in mean arterial pressure [72]. These effects are seen clinically as (a) an increase in the force and velocity of myocardial systolic contraction (positive inotropic action); (b) a decrease in the degree of activation of the sympathetic nervous system and renin-angiotensin system (neurohormonal deactivating effect); and (c) slowing of the heart rate and decreased conduction velocity through the AV node (vagomimetic effect). The effects of digoxin in heart failure are mediated by its positive inotropic and neurohormonal deactivating effects, whereas the effects of the drug in atrial arrhythmias are related to its vagomimetic actions.

37.3.1.3 Adverse Effects

In the 1970s digitalis intoxication was reported to be around 23% in patients admitted to the hospital [73] but has now diminished to less than 6% [74]. Digoxin has a narrow therapeutic window. Worsening renal function and increasing age are independent predictors of digoxin toxicity [75]. The main manifestations of digoxin toxicity include cardiac arrhythmias (ectopic and reentrant cardiac rhythms and heart block), gastrointestinal tract symptoms (anorexia, nausea, vomiting and diarrhea) and neurologic symptoms (visual disturbances, headache, weakness, dizziness and confusion). Conditions such as hypokalemia, hypomagnesemia or hypothyroidism may predispose patients to have adverse reactions even at lower serum digoxin concentrations [76].

37.3.2
Nitrates

In 1879 Murrell reported that a 1% solution of nitroglycerin administered orally relieved angina and prevented subsequent attacks [77]. Further basic investigations showed the role of nitrous oxide in the vasodilation produced by the nitrates. The nitrates are prodrugs and are biodegraded to have therapeutic effects. This biotransformation involves denitration of the nitrate, with the subsequent liberation of nitric oxide. Nitric oxide stimulates guanylyl cyclase, which leads to the conversion of guanosine triphosphate to cyclic guanosine monophosphate, which in turn causes vasodilation [78]. The administration of nitrates can result in reduced platelet adhesion and aggregation [79], improved endothelial function and vascular growth through nitrous oxide [80]. Nitrates are widely used in the management of patients with coronary artery disease including unstable angina, printzmetal angina, acute myocardial infarction, and heart failure. The commonly used organic nitrates are nitroglycerin (glyceryl trinitrate), isosorbide dinitrate, and isosorbide mononitrate.

37.3.2.1 Pharmacokinetics

Nitrates are rapidly absorbed from the intravenous, gastrointestinal tract, skin, and mucous membranes [81]. Isosorbide dinitrate and nitroglycerin undergo extensive first-pass hepatic metabolism when given orally. The biotransformation of the nitrates takes place in the liver by the enzymes glutathione organic nitrate reductase that causes reductive hydrolysis [82]. The resulting denitrated metabolites, though metabolically active are less potent than the parent nitrates. The half-life of the nitrates varies depending on the preparation, with the nitroglycerin being the shortest and mononitrates having the longest and dinitrates in between.

37.3.2.2 Pharmacodynamics

The hemodynamic and antianginal actions of the organic nitrates are mediated through vasodilatation of capacitance veins and conductive arteries, reducing ventricular volume, preload and after load [83]. Nitrates also dilate the epicardial coronary arteries, including stenotic segments, which could relive angina. By their actions on the systemic circulation, nitrates reduce the myocardial oxygen demand. A major limitation of the use of nitrates is the development of tolerance, defined as the loss of hemodynamic and antianginal effects during sustained therapy. The mechanism of nitrate tolerance has been the subject of intense debate but remains poorly understood. Co-administration of nitrates and sildenafil can cause life-threatening hypotension [84]. The common adverse effect with the use of nitrates is headache. Other adverse effects include hypotension, presyncope, syncope, and rarely, bradycardia.

37.3.3
Nesiritide

Nesiritide (Natrecor) is a recombinant form of human B-type (brain) natriuretic peptide that has beneficial vasodilatory, natriuretic, diuretic and neurohormonal effects [85]. The drug is administered intravenously for the management of patients with decompensated congestive heart failure (CHF).

37.3.3.1 Pharmacokinetics

Nesiritide has a distribution half-life of about 2 minutes [86]. The recommended dosage is an intravenous bolus of 2 μg/kg followed by a continuous infusion of 0.01 μg/kg/min. Nesiritide has various routes of elimination [87]. Mechanisms contributing to the clearance of BNP include: binding to the cell surface receptor (natriuretic peptide receptor C) where it is internalized and enzymatically degraded; hydrolysis by neutral endopeptidase 24.11; and renal filtration. Nesiritide has a mean terminal elimination half-life of approximately 18 minutes. Clearance of the drug is proportional to bodyweight.

37.3.3.2 Pharmacodynamics

Nesiritide is structurally and pharmacologically indistinguishable from human B-type (brain) natriuretic peptide (BNP) [88]. The vasodilatory, natriuretic and diuretic effects of nesiritide appear to be primarily mediated by its interaction with natriuretic peptide receptor A on target cells and organs (vascular smooth muscle cells, endothelial cells, kidney and adrenal gland) [89]. It exerts its physiologic actions by binding to receptors coupled to guanylate cyclase, which leads to increase in cyclic GMP in the target cells [90]. The drug reduces pulmonary capillary wedge pressure (PCWP) and right atrial pressure (RAP) thus decreases preload [91]. It also reduces the systemic vascular resistance (SVR) thus causing a reduction in afterload and increases cardiac index (CI) [92]. Nesiritide also reduces systemic arterial pressure without causing reflex tachycardia.

37.3.3.3 Adverse Effects

The most common adverse events reported include general pain, abdominal pain, catheter-related pain, headache, nausea, asymptomatic and symptomatic hypotension, nonsustained ventricular tachycardia and angina pectoris [93]. Most episodes of symptomatic hypotension resolved spontaneously or after an intravenous volume challenge.

37.4
Dyslipidemia

Obesity is the most common and costly nutritional problem in the developed countries. In the USA alone, it affects approximately 33% of adults with health care costs directly attributable to obesity amount to approximately $68 billion per year [94]. This has led to a marked increase in the metabolic syndrome, a clustering of atherosclerotic cardiovascular disease risk factors characterized by visceral adiposity, insulin resistance, low HDL cholesterol (HDL-C), and a systemic proinflammatory state [95]. Age-adjusted overall prevalence of metabolic syndrome by the Third National Health and Nutrition Examination Survey (NHANES) ranges from 23.9 to 25.1% [96]. Dyslipidemia is a hallmark of the metabolic syndrome and is characterized by increased triglyceride-rich lipoproteins; low high-density lipoprotein cholesterol; small, dense low-density lipoprotein particles; increased postprandial lipemia; and abnormal apolipoprotein A1 and B metabolism [97]. All these lipoprotein disturbances accelerate atherosclerosis in these patients. Epidemiologic, angiographic and postmortem studies have documented a causal relationship between elevated serum cholesterol levels and the genesis of coronary heart disease [98]. Various randomized controlled trials have demonstrated the efficacy of antilipidemic drugs particularly statins for reducing low-density lipoprotein cholesterol (LDL-C) levels and thus the risk of coronary heart disease (CHD) [99]. The primary target of pharmacologic treatment is to lower LDL and VLDL and increase HDL, with the major objective being prevention of atherosclerotic plaques that lead to myocardial infarction, stroke, and peripheral vascular disease.

37.4.1
Bile Acid Sequestrants

These agents also called resins include cholestyramine, colesevelam and colestipol. They decrease the serum cholesterol level by disrupting the enterohepatic circulation of the bile acids [100]. The binding of these agents to the bile acids leads to the increased secretion of hepatic cholesterol leading to depletion of the cellular hepatic cholesterol, leading to increased hepatic LDL-receptor population. Thus, there is a reduction in the blood LDL and eventually the total cholesterol levels [101]. Currently resins are mostly used as an adjunctive to statins in the treatment of hyperlipidemia. While doubling the dose of statins result only in about 6% further reduction in LDL-C, adding a small dose of resins can lower LDL-C levels by about 12–16% [102].

37.4.1.1 Pharmacokinetics

The resins are a hydrophilic, water-insoluble polymer that is not hydrolyzed by digestive enzymes and is not absorbed. The systemic absorption after oral doses is negligible and hence therapeutic concentrations (peak blood concentrations, tissue concentrations, etc.) are expected to be irrelevant. They are excreted in the stool bound to bile acids [103].

37.4.1.2 Pharmacodynamics

During normal digestion, the major portion of bile acids that are secreted in the intestines are reabsorbed from and returned to the liver via enterohepatic circulation. Bile acid sequestrants, being highly positively charged bind to the negatively charged bile acids in the intestinal lumen [103]. This interrupts the enterohepatic circulation, and increase the excretion of bile acids from the body. This decreases the bile acid pool and stimulates hepatic synthesis of bile acids from cholesterol. Cholesterol is drawn from the bloodstream, resulting in a reduction of blood cholesterol concentration. Depletion of the hepatic pool of cholesterol results in increased cholesterol biosynthesis and an increase in the number of LDL receptors on the hepatocyte membrane. These compensatory effects result in increased clearance of LDL-C from the blood, resulting in decreased serum LDL-C levels.

37.4.1.3 Adverse Effects

The major adverse effect of the resins is gastrointestinal upset. In the Lipid Research Clinics–Coronary Primary Prevention Trial (LRC-CPPT) 68% of these patients reported at least one gastrointestinal side effect, 39% had constipation, 32% had abdominal gas, and 27% had heartburn [104]. The TGL levels may be raised with bile acid sequestrant therapy by about 5% to 20% which tend to be transient and are related to high baseline TG levels or dysbetalipoproteinemia.

37.4.2
Ezetimibe

The level of plasma cholesterol is influenced not only by de novo biosynthesis but also by the absorption of dietary cholesterol and the removal of cholesterol from the blood. Recent evidence supports the presence of a specific transporter that facilitates the movement of cholesterol from bile acid micelles into the brush border membrane of enterocytes, which has been exploited as a therapeutic target in the development of new drugs such as ezetimibe [105]. Ezetimibe belongs to the new class of 2-azetidinones which were initially designed as Acyl-coenzyme A:cholesterol O-acyl transferase (ACAT) inhibitors. Ezetimibe is a potent and selective inhibitor of cholesterol absorption in the intestines thus reducing the overall delivery of cholesterol to the liver, thereby promoting the synthesis of LDL receptors, with a subsequent reduction of serum LDL-C [106]. Interrupting the absorption of cholesterol is an important target for lowering serum cholesterol levels.

37.4.2.1 Pharmacokinetics

Ezetimibe has rapid absorption and undergoes rapid and extensive glucuronidation in the intestinal wall and the liver [107]. The elimination half-life for ezetimibe and ezetimibe-glucuronide is approximately 22 hours, which allows for once-daily dosing. Ezetimibe has no effect on the activity of drug metabolism enzymes, such as cytochrome P450 or N-acetyltransferase in the liver. The pharmacokinetics of ezetimibe does not depend on sex, age, and renal or hepatic function. However ezetimibe is not recommended in patients with moderate or severe liver dysfunction. It is predominantly excreted in the feces (78%) and the rest in the urine (12%) as glucuronide conjugate [105].

37.4.2.2 Pharmacodynamics

Ezetimibe localizes at the brush border of small intestinal enterocytes and inhibits the dietary and biliary cholesterol absorption at the brush border of the intestine without affecting vitamin or triglyceride absorption, thus reducing the decreases LDL levels. Clinical studies have shown that ezetimibe inhibited cholesterol absorption by 54% relative to placebo [108]. Its mechanism of action is different from that of other intestinal-acting lipid-altering agents such as phytosterols/phytostanols, resins, and polymers [109]. Ezetimibe can cause an increase in hepatic cholesterol synthesis [110]. However, statins can reduce the compensatory increase in the hepatic cholesterol synthesis induced by ezetimibe, thus the combination of ezetimibe and statins results in an incremental lowering of LDL cholesterol concentrations. Several recent trials have shown that the combination of ezetimibe with statins produces an incremental reduction of LDL cholesterol in the range of 12% to 15% [111, 112].

37.4.2.3 Adverse Effects

The tolerability of ezetimibe is excellent and there were no serious clinical adverse events or critical laboratory elevations of liver enzymes are seen during ezetimibe treatment [108]. Fatigue, diarrhea, and abdominal pain were the most frequently reported side effects, but they occurred in less than 5% of patients.

37.4.3
Fibric Acid

Beginning with the description of clofibrate in 1962, derivatives of fibric acid (fibrates) have been used clinically to treat dyslipidemias. Subsequently, gemfibrozil, fenofibrate, benzafibrate, ciprofibrate and long-acting forms of gemfibrozil, fenofibrate and benzafibrate have been developed. Although it is not a fibric acid derivative, gemfibrozil shares many of the properties of this class of drugs and has the same clinical indications; it is also being discussed here. These agents are lipid regulating agents that decrease serum triglycerides and very low density lipoprotein (VLDL) cholesterol, and increases high density lipoprotein (HDL) cholesterol.

37.4.3.1 Pharmacokinetics

Fibrates are completely absorbed after oral administration, reaching peak plasma concentrations 1–2 hours after dosing. The pharmacokinetics is affected by the timing of meals relative to time of dosing with both the rate and extent of absorption being significantly increased when administered half hour before meals. The plasma half-life of the parent compound ranges from around 1.5 hours for bezafibrate and gemfibrozil and 81 hours for ciprofibrate. Fibrates are metabolized by the hepatic cytochrome P450 (CYP) 3A4. Gemfibrozil mainly undergoes oxidation of its methyl ring to become hydroxymethyl and a carboxyl metabolite. About 70% of the administered dose is excreted in the urine, as the glucuronide conjugate and less than 2% is excreted unchanged [113].

37.4.3.2 Pharmacodynamics

The mechanisms of action of fibrates are not well established. They have been shown to inhibit peripheral lipolysis and to decrease the hepatic extraction of free fatty acids, thus reducing hepatic triglyceride production. They also inhibit the synthesis and increase clearance of VLDL carrier apolipoprotein B, leading to a decrease in VLDL production [114]. They enhance lipoprotein lipase (LPL) enhanced catabolism of VLDL. The major role of fibrates in atherogenic dyslipidemia is its ability to decrease the TGL levels. Recent research has shown the fibrates to be agonist for the nuclear transcription factor, peroxisome proliferator-activated receptor (PPAR)-alpha. The hypotriglyceridemic actions of fibrates seem to involve PPAR mechanism with increased hydrolysis of plasma triglycerides due to induction of LPL and reduction of apoC-III expression [115]. They also stimulate cellular fatty acid uptake and conversion to acetyl-CoA derivatives. They also increase the PPAR mediated activation of apolipoprotein AI gene and downregulate the apolipoprotein CIII gene [116]. Fibrates exert their hypolipidemic effect by enhancing the catabolism of triglyceride-rich particles and reducing secretion of VLDL particles. Increased risk of CVD seen with elevated fibrinogen level is reduced by fibrates like benzafibrate and fenofibrate by decreasing the fibrinogen levels.

37.4.3.3 Adverse Effects

Fibrates are generally well tolerated by patients. The common side effects are usually gastrointestinal symptoms like diarrhea, abdominal pain, constipation, and dyspepsia. These drugs also increase the lithogenecity of the bile and may result in the formation of gall stones [117]. Fibrates should be cautiously used in combination with statins, due to increased risk of myopathy and rhabdomyolysis [118].

37.4.4
Niacin

Niacin or nicotinic acid, a 3-pyridinecarboxylic acid is a water-soluble B complex vitamin and antihyperlipidemic agent. Nicotinic acid is most effective in preventing CVD by decreasing the hyperlipidemia when give in combination with resins, fibrates or statins. Niacin favorably modifies all aspects of the lipoprotein profile; it raises high-density lipoprotein cholesterol (HDL-C) levels, lowers triglyceride, low-density lipoprotein cholesterol (LDL-C) and lipoprotein (a) levels and reduces atherogenic small dense LDL particles [119].

37.4.4.1 Pharmacokinetics

Niacin is rapidly absorbed from the gastrointestinal tract. It reaches peak level in thirty to sixty minutes with a short plasma elimination half-life [120]. At a 1 g dose, peak plasma concentrations of 15–30 µg/mL are reached within 30–60 minutes. The plasma elimination half-life of nicotinic acid ranges from 20–45 minutes. The primary route of metabolism is via methylation to N-methy nicotinamide which is further oxidized to N-methyl-2- and 4-pyridone carbozyamides. Approximately 88% of an oral pharmacologic dose is eliminated by the kidneys as unchanged drug or as nicotinuric acid (conjugation of nicotinic acid and glycine), its primary metabolite.

37.4.4.2 Pharmacodynamics

Niacin inhibits the mobilization of free fatty acids from the peripheral tissues and hence reduces the synthesis of TGL [121]. It also inhibits the secretion of VLDL and the conversion of VLDL to LDL. One of the important effects of niacin in the treatment of lipid disorders is its ability to increase the HDL-C. Niacin is the also the only anti-hyperlipidemic drug that has been shown to lower elevated levels of lipoprotein (a) [Lp(a)], which has been shown to increase risk for CVD [122]. Niacin blocks free fatty acid from adipose tissue and suppresses hepatic assembly and release of VLDL, which in turn reduces triglyceride levels and the number of small, dense LDL particles. Niacin may block a catabolic receptor for intrahepatic degradation of HDL, increasing the effective HDL half-life and HDL concentration [123]. The mechanism by which nicotinic acid decrease TGL may be also due to decreasing the esterification of hepatic triglycerides. Recent studies done with the Coronary Drug Project have shown that niacin can reduce total mortality and myocardial infarction significantly in patients with metabolic syndrome [124].

37.4 4.3 Adverse Effects

The major disadvantage in the use of niacin is its adverse effects [125]. Niacin causes significant flushing and pruritis that leads to discontinuation of niacin. Other adverse effects include gastrointestinal complaints like nausea, dyspepsia, flatulence, vomiting, diarrhea, and activation of peptic ulcer disease. Hyperuricemia and gout can occur and hyperglycemia may worsen in patients with diabetes [126]. Hepatotoxicity has been reported. Liver enzymes need to be monitored periodically in patients who take nicotinic acid compounds.

37.4.5
Statins

The 3-hydroxy-3-methylglutaryl (HMG) coenzyme A reductase inhibitors commonly known as statins are the most often prescribed agents for the treatment of hyperlipidemia in the developed countries. Recent clinical trials using statins to treat low density lipoprotein (LDL-C) have demonstrated beyond reasonable doubt that coronary events can be prevented by decreasing LDL-C levels [127]. One of the most significant advances in the field of cardiovascular disease prevention has been the introduction of statins. Given alone for primary or secondary prevention of heart disease, these drugs can reduce the incidence of coronary artery disease by 25 to 60% and reduce the risk of death from any cardiovascular disease by about 30% [128].

Table 37.4 Beneficial effects of statins in preventing CVD* [136]

Lipid effects
• Decreases LDL-C level.
• Lowers TGL levels.
• Increases HDL-C and apolipoprotein A-I (apoA-I).
• Decreases oxidation of LDL-C.
Vascular effects
• Increases endothelium-dependent vasodilator response.
• Activates endothelial NO synthesis.
• Promotes plaque stabilization.
• Blocks the accumulation of cholesterol in macrophages.
• Reduces monocyte adhesion to endothelial cells.
• Antiproliferative effects on smooth-muscle cells.
• Suppresses neointimal thickening.
Antithrombotic effects
• Reduces thromboxane synthesis.
• Reduces platelet aggregation.
• Reduces Tissue factor/extrinsic pathway inhibitor (EPI) production.
• Decreases plasma fibrinogen concentrations.
• Improves whole blood and plasma viscosity.
• Reduces plasminogen activator inhibitor-1 (PAI-1) activity.
Other effects
• Reduces C-reactive protein levels.
• Greater reduction in mean blood pressure when used with ACEI.
• Decreases Proteniuria.
• Anti-oxidant effect.

CVD: cardiovascular disease; LDL-C: low density lipoprotein cholesterol; HDL-C: high density lipoprotein cholesterol; TGL: triglycerides; NO: nitric oxide; ACEI: angiotensin converting enzyme inhibitor.

37.4.5.1 Pharmacokinetics

Statins are well tolerated by oral intake. They undergo extensive first pass metabolism by the liver and less than 20% of the administered drug reaches the general circulations [129]. Some of the statins are administered as prodrugs (lovastatin and simvasatin) and are converted to their active metabolite in the liver. However, because the rate of endogenous cholesterol synthesis is higher at night, statins are best when given in the evening. The predominant route of excretion of all the statins is through the bile, after hepatic transformation. Hence, patients with liver disease should be given lower doses.

37.4.5.2 Pharmacodynamics

Statins are structurally similar to HMG-coenzyme A, which is a precursor to cholesterol and competitively inhibit the HMG-coA reductase that is the last step in the synthesis of cholesterol [130]. Statins also up regulate the LDL-C receptor activity and decrease the entry of LDL-C into the circulation resulting in low serum LDL-C concentration [131]. Pleiotropic effects of statins include improvement of endothelial dysfunction, increased nitric oxide bioavailability, antioxidant properties, inhibition of inflammatory responses, and stabilization of atherosclerotic plaques [132]. The mechanism of the non-lipid-lowering actions of HMG-CoA reductase inhibitors may also be due to reduced formation or availability of mevalonic acid within endothelial cells [133] (Table 37.4).

37.4.5.3 Adverse Effects

Statins are well tolerated with no known differences in safety among the various statins. The most important adverse effects are liver and muscle toxicity. The incidence of transaminase increases greater than three-fold is about 1% for all statins and is usually dose related [134]. If this occurs, the drug should be stopped and the transaminase levels usually return to baseline within 2 to 3 months. Myopathy, defined as muscle pain or weakness associated with creatine kinase (CK) levels higher than 10 times the upper limit of normal occurs with statin monotherapy in about 1 in 1000 patients and is dose related. Symptoms may include fever and malaise, and cases have been associated with elevated serum statin drug levels. Rhabdomyolysis and acute renal failure may result if myopathy is not recognized and the drug is continued. If recognized promptly and the drug is stopped, the myopathy is reversible, and acute renal failure could be prevented [135]. Other reported side effects of the statins are gastrointestinal upset, loss of concentration, sleep disturbance and peripheral neuropathy.

37.5 Anti-thrombotic Agents

Thrombosis is an important complication of atherosclerosis. Recent years have seen the introduction of a number of new antithrombotic agents, each offering a unique profile of benefits and potential drawbacks. These agents are used in the treatment and management of acute coronary syndromes, venous thrombosis, acute ischemic strokes, patients undergoing percutaneous coronary interventions, and to prevent the development of thrombus in patients with atrial fibrillation and prosthetic heart valves [137, 138]. There are three classes of agents used in the treatment of thrombotic disorders. They are classified as: anticoagulant agents, antiplatelet agents and thrombolytic agents. The first two prevents the development of thrombus and the third lyses existing thrombus. Bleeding is the major complication of anticoagulant therapy [139].

37.5.1 Direct Thrombin Inhibitors

Direct thrombin inhibitors include hirudin, bivalirudin, and argatroban. Bivalirudin is the most widely used of these agents and is a semisynthetic, 20-amino acid derivative of hirudin formed from residues 53 to 64 of the hirudin molecule, with the addition of a sulfated tyrosine at position 63 [140]. Bivalirudin has been studied in the setting of coronary angioplasty, unstable angina, and acute myocardial infarction and has shown some promise in many of these settings, particularly in preventing complications of percutaneous coronary interventions. The limitations of heparin treatment, such as unpredictable anticoagulant response, frequent laboratory monitoring, and a relatively short half-life, the risk of heparin-induced thrombocytopenia and the inability of the drug to bind to fibrin-bound thrombin; are best minimized or eliminated by these newer anticoagulants, i.e., direct thrombin inhibitors [141].

37.5.1.1 Pharmacokinetics

Bivalirudin is given IV with peak concentrations are seen 15 to 19 minutes after infusion. Bivalirudin has a short half-life about 30 minutes as a result of slow cleavage of the Arg-Pro bond on the amino terminal of bivalirudin after binding with thrombin [142]. The binding of bivalirudin to thrombin is reversible resulting in recovery of thrombin active site functions after cleavage of the Arg-Pro bond. Approximately 20% of bivalirudin is renally excreted. The clearance of bivalirudin decreases with renal impairment and dosage adjustment is necessary [143].

37.5.1.2 Pharmacodynamics

Thrombin (coagulation factor IIa) is a vital component of intravascular clot formation and is produced in response to vascular injury. Thrombin is also the most potent known platelet activator. It binds to receptors on the surface of platelets, ultimately contributing to platelet activation and aggregation [144]. Direct thrombin inhibitors have the ability to inhibit both free and clot-bound thrombin that result in an effective anticoagulation. Substrate binding to thrombin occurs on two different sites: an active site, which cleaves susceptible chemical bonds (e.g., those in fibrinogen); and a site termed exosite 1, which configures substrates in an appropriate orientation [145]. Since the fibrin binds to thrombin via exosite 1, bivalirudin, which also bind to exosite 1, competitively inhibit the ability of fibrin to bind to thrombin. The structure of bivalirudin increases its affinity for thrombin, with the addition of a D-Phe-Pro-Arg-Pro-(Gly)$_4$ sequence to its amino terminal to impart the ability to bind to the active site of thrombin while maintaining the ability to bind to exosite 1 [146]. Bivalirudin directly inhibits thrombin by specifically binding both to the catalytic site and to the anion-binding exosite of circulating and clot-bound thrombin, hence the name bivalirudin. The binding of bivalirudin to the active site of thrombin is only transient and hence needs to be given by continuous intravenous (IV) infusion.

37.5.1.3 Adverse Effects

The major adverse effect is bleeding complications. Bivalirudin is contraindicated in patients with active major bleeding and hypersensitivity to bivalirudin or its components.

37.5.2
Fibrinolytic Agents

Atherosclerotic coronary artery disease is the major cause of death, in men and women, in the USA and in much of the Western world. MIs result from the superimposition of a thrombus over an underlying ruptured or eroded plaque [147]. During the natural evolution of atherosclerotic plaques, especially those that are lipid laden, an abrupt and catastrophic transition may occur, characterized by plaque rupture. After plaque ruptures, there is exposure of substances that promote platelet activation and aggregation, thrombin generation, and, ultimately, thrombus formation [148]. These agents like plasminogen-activator inhibitor type 1 (PAI-1) and increased plasma concentrations of factor VII, fibrinogen, and von Willebrand factor suppresses fibrinolysis and are associated with the development of myocardial infarction [149]. Timely fibrinolytic therapy can re-establish coronary flow in this setting and salvage jeopardized myocardium [150]. Large randomized clinical trials (RCTs) have clearly demonstrated a statistically significant mortality benefit with thrombolytic therapy over placebo in the setting of acute MI [151]. Streptokinase was used for treatment of patients with acute MI appeared in 1958 [152] and since then newer agents have been introduced that binds to fibrin with a greater affinity than streptokinase.

37.5.2.1 Pharmacokinetics

The fibrinolytics are given in the intravenous form, and their half-life varies anywhere from 3–8 minutes for t-PA to 70–120 minutes for Anistreplase. The derivatives of tPA (rPA, nPA, TNK-tPA) have a reduced plasma clearance and a prolonged half-life compared with tPA. Lanoteplase and TNK-tPA are administered as a single bolus and have hepatic excretion, whereas rPA is administered as a double bolus (30 minutes apart) and is excreted by both renal and hepatic routes. Tenecteplase is the most fibrin-specific, reducing systemic fibrinogen and plasminogen levels by only 3% and 13% respectively, at 1 hour after administration [153].

37.5.2.2 Pharmacodynamics

All these agents function by their ability to convert plasminogen to plasmin which then degrades fibrin, the major structure in the thrombus formation. The agents can be grouped into direct and indirect plasminogen activators [154]. The relatively nonspecific agents include streptokinase, anistreplase, and urokinase. The newer plasminogen activators include recombinant tissue-type plasminogen activator (rt-PA) (alteplase) and several variants of tissue-type plasminogen activator: reteplase (r-PA), tenecteplase (TNK-tPA), and lanoteplase (n-PA). The nonspecific agents like streptokinase activates both circulating and fibrin-bound plasminogen to plasmin producing systemic plasminemia with resultant depletion of fibrinogen, plasminogen, and factors V and VIII

Table 37.5 Characteristics of fibrinolytic agents

Agents	Source	Fibrin selective	Metabolism	Half-life, min	Plasminogen binding	Antigenic	Dosing	Other properties
Streptokinase	Group A streptococci	–	Hepatic	18–23	Activator complex	Yes	1-h infusion	NA
Urokinase	Recombinant, human fetal, kidney	–	Hepatic	14–20	Direct	No	1-h infusion	NA
Anistreplase	Group A streptococci plasminogen, anisoylated	–	Hepatic	70–120	Direct	Yes	10-min single bolus	NA
t-PA (alteplase)	Recombinant, human	++	Hepatic	3–8	Direct	No	Bolus, 90-min infusion	↑ fibrin binding
r-PA (reteplase)	Recombinant, human mutant t-PA	+	Renal/Hepatic	15–18	Direct	No	Double bolus	↓ fibrin binding
TNK-tPA (tenecteplase)	Recombinant plus mutation	+++	Hepatic	18–20	Direct	No	Single bolus	Resistance to PAI-1
n-PA (lanoteplase)	Recombinant plus mutation	+	Hepatic	30–45	Direct	No	Single bolus	↓ fibrin binding

[155]. Tissue-type plasminogen activators are naturally occurring, serine proteases that are physiologically identical to the endogenous plasminogen activator in humans and are produced by recombinant DNA technology [156]. They are highly fibrin specific and have the ability to lyse more highly cross-linked fibrin (Table 37.5).

37.5.2.3 Adverse Effects

The main complication of fibrinolytic therapy is bleeding, with the most dreaded complication being intracranial hemorrhage. In their overview of nine trials that randomized 58,600 patients the Fibrinolytic Therapy Trialists' Collaborative Group reported an excess of 3.9 strokes per 1000 patients treated with fibrinolysis versus placebo [151]. The fibrin specific agents have less bleeding events compared to the non-fibrin specific agents [151]. Patients who receive streptokinase can develop antistreptococcal antibodies and may have allergic reactions. Hence, it has been suggested that patients should not receive a second dose of streptokinase within 1 year of initial therapy [154].

37.5.3
Glycoprotein IIb-IIIa Inhibitors

Platelet-mediated coronary thrombosis is an important pathophysiologic mechanism of acute coronary syndromes and acute complications of percutaneous coronary intervention (PCI). Standard antithrombotic therapy for these disorders includes aspirin and heparin. Antagonists of the platelet receptor glycoprotein (GP) IIb-IIIa are a novel class of antithrombotic agents that provide a more comprehensive platelet blockade than the combination of aspirin and heparin. In addition to the chimeric antibody (abciximab), GP IIb/IIIa antagonists currently available for intravenous use include small organic molecules (tirofiban), and a cyclic oligopeptide (eptifibatide). These agents are widely used in the treatment of acute coronary syndromes and in patients undergoing PCIs [158].

37.5.3.1 Pharmacokinetics

Plasma concentration of these drugs is proportional to the administered dose of both bolus and infusion doses. Peak plasma levels are established shortly after the bolus dose, and slightly lower concentrations are subsequently maintained throughout the infusion period; plasma concentrations decrease rapidly after the infusion is discontinued. Approximately 25% of eptifibatide and 65% of tirofiban are bound to plasma proteins [159]. The plasma half-life of tirofiban and eptifibatide are approximately 2 hours and 2.5 hours, respectively. The primary route of clearance of these agents is renal. After the intravenous administration of the bolus dose, the majority of abciximab molecules are bound to GP IIb-IIIa within minutes, and free drug is rapidly eliminated from plasma. Abciximab with high affinity and a slow dissociation rate from the GP IIb/IIIa platelet receptor has a short plasma half-life of 10 to 30 minutes, but a long biologic half-life due to its strong affinity to the GP IIb/IIIa receptor. It is also cleared by the kidneys [160]. The return to normal values for both receptor occupancy and turbidimetric platelet aggregation after discontinuation of therapy is slow [161]. Platelet-associated abciximab can be detected in circulation for more than 14 days after the infusion is stopped [162].

37.5.3.2 Pharmacodynamics

GP IIb-IIIa agents inhibit the platelet receptor glycoprotein (GP) IIb-IIIa mediated final common pathway of platelet aggregation. The cyclic heptapeptide eptifibatide and tyrosine derivative tirofiban are specific for the platelet receptor GP IIb-IIIa integrin. The GP IIb-IIIa integrin specificity of eptifibatide is conferred by the Lys-Gly-Asp (KGD) sequence, a variation on the more common Arg-Gly-Asp (RGD) sequence [163]. The nonpeptide GP IIb-IIIa inhibitor tirofiban affinity is based on the RGD integrin recognition domain found in the GP IIb-IIIa ligands [164]. Their affinity for GP IIb-IIIa is lower than that of abciximab, and their dissociation from the receptor (off-rate) occurs more rapidly [165]. These "small-molecule" GP IIb-IIIa inhibitors binding on GP IIb-IIIa involves the receptor pocket that also mediates the interaction of GP IIb-IIIa with fibrinogen and von Willebrand factor [166]. Because of their small size, the potential of these agents to induce an antibody response is significantly lower than that of abciximab. The mechanism of the GP IIb-IIIa binding of abciximab is qualitatively different from the other two agents. The interaction between GP IIb-IIIa and abciximab can occur even if the binding pocket is occupied by Arg-Gly-Asp (RGD) peptides [167]. It has been proposed that the inhibitory effect of abciximab may be due to steric hindrance of ligand access [167]. The affinity of abciximab for GP IIb-IIIa is very high.

37.5.3.3 Adverse Effects

Since pathologic thrombosis and physiologic hemostasis share common mechanisms, the separation of beneficial (antithrombotic) from detrimental (antihemostatic) effects of these agents is difficult to achieve. Treatment with these agents is accompanied by a substantial increase in bleeding complications and thrombocytopenia [168]. Risk of bleeding can be reduced by the use of low-dose adjunctive heparin, early sheath removal, and meticulous post-procedure care of the vascular access site [169]. The treatment of thrombocytopenia associated with administration of GP IIb/IIIa antagonists requires stopping the drug. Severe thrombocytopenia (platelet count $< 20,000/\mu L$) occurs in 0.1 to 0.5% of patients treated with these agents necessitating platelet transfusion [170]. Abciximab has also been shown to elicit an antibody response, particularly after readministration, most likely due to its large size and murine origin. On subsequent administration, this antigenicity of abciximab may increase the risk of severe thrombocytopenia [171].

37.5.4
Heparin

Heparin was discovered by McLean in 1916. More than 20 years later, it was found that heparin requires a plasma cofactor for its anticoagulant activity which was named antithrombin III, now referred to simply as antithrombin (AT) (172). Heparin is heterogeneous with respect to molecular size, anticoagulant activity, and pharmacokinetic properties. Its molecular weight ranges from 3000 to 30,000 Da, with a mean molecular weight of 15,000 Da [173]. The major effect of heparin is on the interaction of AT and thrombin, to inhibit the thrombin-induced platelet aggregation.

37.5.4.1 Pharmacokinetics

The anticoagulant effect of SC heparin is delayed for 1 to 2 hours. After administration, unfractionated heparin (UFH) binds to endogenous plasma proteins, endothelial cells, platelet factor 4, and high-molecular-weight multimers of von Willebrand factor [174]. Binding to plasma proteins reduces its anticoagulant activity, due to less availability of free drug to interact with antithrombin. This causes an unpredictable anticoagulant response of heparin. Some of these heparin-binding proteins are acute-phase reactants, the concentrations of which increases in sick patients, and factors like platelet factor 4 and von Willebrand factor are released during the clotting process. Because of the unpredictable anticoagulant response, careful laboratory monitoring is essential when UFH is given to patients. UFH is eliminated in two phases in a dose-dependent fashion: a rapid, saturable phase reflecting binding to endothelial cell receptors and macrophages that undergoes hepatic uptake, and a slower phase corresponding to renal clearance [175]. Clearance of heparin is also influenced by the chain length, with the higher-molecular-weight species cleared from the circulation much more rapidly than the lower-molecular-weight species.

37.5.4.2 Pharmacodynamics

Only about one-third of the administered dose of heparin binds to AT, and is responsible for its anticoagulant effect [176]. Heparins exert their anticoagulant activity by activating AT. Their interaction with AT is mediated by a unique pentasaccharide sequence that is randomly distributed along the heparin chains. Binding of the pentasaccharide to AT causes a conformational change in AT that accelerates its interaction with thrombin and activated factor X (factor Xa) by about 1000 times [177]. The heparin-AT complex inactivates a number of coagulation enzymes, including thrombin factor (IIa) and factors Xa, IXa, XIa, and XIIa [177]. For inhibition of thrombin, heparin must bind to both the coagulation enzyme and AT. Molecules of heparin with fewer than 18 saccharides do not bind simultaneously to thrombin and AT and therefore are unable to catalyze thrombin inhibition. By inactivating thrombin, heparin not only prevents fibrin formation but also inhibits thrombin-induced activation of factor V and factor VIII [178]. Heparin also binds to platelets can either induce or inhibit platelet aggregation [179]. In addition to anticoagulant effects, heparin increases vessel wall permeability, suppresses the proliferation of vascular smooth muscle cells, and suppresses osteoblast formation and activates osteoclasts, effects that promote bone loss.

37.5.4.3 Adverse Effects

The main adverse effect on the use of heparin is bleeding. There is an increased risk of heparin-induced hemorrhage in patients with subacute bacterial endocarditis or hematological disorders such as hemophilia, hepatic disease, or gastrointestinal or genitourinary ulcerative lesions. Platelet abnormalities may paradoxically predispose towards heparin thrombosis, characterized by a "white clot" [180]. Some patients may be resistant to heparin, and in such patients administration of high-dose heparin with aPTT monitoring every 4 hours is advised. Heparin can occasionally cause allergy. Heparin can also cause osteopenia with prolonged use as a result of binding of heparin to osteoblasts [181].

37.5.5
Low-Molecular-Weight Heparins

A major advance in the use of heparin has been in the development of low-molecular-weight heparins (LMWH), which combine factor IIa and factor Xa inhibition, thus inhibiting both the action (anti-IIa action) and generation (anti-Xa action) of thrombin. As compared with UFH that has nearly equal anti-IIa (thrombin) and anti-Xa activity, LMWH have increased ratios of anti-Xa to anti-IIa activity. LMWH are glycosaminoglycans consisting of chains of alternating residues of d-glucosamine and uronic acid, either glucuronic acid or iduronic acid [177]. These agents are about one-third of the molecular weight of heparin. They are a heterogeneous mixture of polysaccharide chains ranging in molecular weight from about 3000 to 30,000 produced by enzymatic or chemical depolymerization of the unfractionated heparin [182]. Both unfractionated heparin and low-molecular-weight heparins exert their anticoagulant activity by activating antithrombin (previously known as antithrombin III). However, the ability of LMWH to inhibit and neutralize factor Xa relatively selectively provides them with therapeutic and safety advantages over unfractionated heparin [183]. LMWH has various other benefits as compared to standard heparin [184]: (1) they can inhibit platelet-bound factor Xa and therefore are more effective anticoagulant; (2) LMWH binds less readily to plasma proteins and vascular and blood cells; (3) LMWH are more resistant to neutralization by platelet factor 4, thus have a longer plasma half-life and more predictable bioavailability; and (4) LMWH has less pronounced effects on platelet function and vascular integrity. LMWH is generally preferred to UFH because of its convenience to use, eliminates the need for aPPT monitoring, and avoids the problem of intravenous site infections.

37.5.5.1 Pharmacokinetics

When LMWH are given subcutaneously, the recovery of anti-factor Xa activity approaches 100% [185]. LMWH has less affinity for plasma proteins and endothelium, thus have better bioavailability. They have less hepatic and renal clearance due to its reduced binding to macrophages, thereby accounting for the longer plasma half-life of LMWH. The better bioavailability, dose-independent clearance, and decreased affinity for heparin-binding proteins make the anticoagulant response to LMWH more predictable than UFH [138].

37.5.5.2 Pharmacodynamics

Like UFH and LMWH exert their anticoagulant activity by activating antithrombin. The chief difference between UFH and LMWH is in their relative inhibitory activity against factor Xa and thrombin [186]. Unlike UFH, which has equivalent activity against factor Xa and thrombin, LMWH have greater activity against factor Xa. The ratio of LMWH binding to antithrombin III and inhibition of factor Xa:IIa (where IIa is activated prothrombin) varies with each agent (2:1 with dalteparin and 3:1 with enoxaparin) [187].

37.5.5.3 Adverse Effects

Adverse effects of LMWH are similar to UFH. However, LMWH are associated with a lower incidence of major bleeding complications, immune-mediated heparin induced thrombocytopenia (HIT) and osteoporosis as compared to UFH [138].

37.5.6
Thienopyridines

The thienopyridines ticlopidine and clopidogrel are inhibitors of platelet function. Ticlopidine was the first agent developed in this class. However, the use of ticlopidine has rapidly fallen out of favor because of the high incidence of adverse side effects including severe and sometimes fatal blood dyscrasias. Clopidogrel has similar pharmacological activity but produces fewer side effects. They are effective antiplatelet agents and are useful in the prevention of stroke, myocardial infarction, vascular death in patients with vascular disease; and are used to prevent the thrombotic complications after coronary stent placement [188, 189].

37.5.6.1 Pharmacokinetics

Clopidogrel bioavailability is not affected by food while ticlopidine bioavailability is increased by food and decreased by antacids [190]. Clopidogrel is 98% protein bound and has an elimination half-life of approximately 8 hours. Both these agents are inactive prodrugs that require in vivo oxidation by the hepatic and/or intestinal cytochrome CYP3A4 isoenzyme to active metabolite [191, 192]. The active metabolite is highly reactive and binds rapidly and irreversibly to platelets. The onset of action on platelets occurs within hours after a single oral dose, but steady-state inhibition is only found between 3 and 7 days. Giving loading dosage will help attain early platelet inhibition. A 600 mg loading dose of clopidogrel achieves maximal inhibition of platelets approximately in 2 hours while a 300 mg loading dose does not achieve maximal platelet inhibition until after 24 to 48 hours [193]. The kinetics of these agents is nonlinear, with a markedly decreased clearance on repeated dosing. After being largely metabolized by the liver, they undergo renal excretion.

37.5.6.2 Pharmacodynamics

The thienopyridines inhibit ADP-induced inhibition of adenylate cyclase, prevent the ADP-induced inhibition of the cytoskeletal associated protein VASP (vasodilator-stimulated phosphoprotein) phosphorylation, and prevent the association of labeled G proteins with the platelet membrane [194]. Thus they selectively inhibit ADP-induced platelet aggregation by directly inhibiting the binding of ADP to its receptor on the platelet, thereby affecting ADP-dependent activation of the glycoprotein IIb/IIIa complex. However, inhibition of adenylate cyclase does not alter their platelet inhibitory effect of these agents, which implicates other mechanisms of action. Thus even though thienopyridines appear to act through the ADP receptor, the precise mechanism for their platelet inhibitory effects has not yet been clearly identified [195]. By inhibiting the effects of ADP released from platelet, they also inhibit platelet aggregation induced by other agonists, including thromboxane analogues, platelet activating factor, collagen, and thrombin [196]. Because of these actions, they prolong bleeding time, inhibit platelet aggregation, and delay clot retraction. They produce dose- and time-dependent inhibition of platelet aggregation, reaching a maximum of 40% to 60% inhibition of ADP-induced aggregation after 3 to 5 days. The recovery of platelet function is delayed after discontinuation of these agents, occurring slowly over 3 to 5 days [197].

37.5.6.3 Adverse Effects

Ticlopidine has high incidence of adverse side effects as compared to clopidogrel [194]. Gastrointestinal problems like diarrhea, nausea, and vomiting are common.

Skin rash, cholestatic jaundice, elevated levels of liver enzymes has been reported. The most serious side effect reported with ticlopidine is hematological. Neutropenia, bone marrow aplasia and thrombotic thrombocytopenic purpura can occur with the use of ticlopidine. Thus full blood counts should be performed every 2 weeks during the first 3 months and periodically afterwards during therapy to identify these potential complications. Clopidogrel has a more favorable side-effect profile and fatal complications have not been reported. Gastrointestinal problems are the commonest side effect and skin rash has also been reported.

37.5.7
Warfarin

Coumarins are vitamin K antagonists with anticoagulant property that interferes with the cyclic interconversion of vitamin K to its 2, 3 vitamin K epoxide. Coagulation factors (factors II, VII, IX, and X) require γ-carboxylation for their biological activity [198]. Vitamin K is a cofactor for the posttranslational carboxylation of glutamate residues to γ-carboxyglutamates on the N-terminal regions of these vitamin K-dependent proteins [199]. Warfarin also exerts its anticoagulant effect by inhibiting the vitamin K conversion cycle, thereby causing hepatic production of partially carboxylated and decarboxylated proteins with reduced procoagulant activity [200]. Oral anticoagulants are effective for primary and secondary prevention of venous thromboembolism, for prevention of systemic embolism in patients with tissue or mechanical prosthetic heart valves or AF, for prevention of AMI in patients with peripheral arterial disease, for prevention of stroke, recurrent infarction, or death in patients with AMI, and for prevention of myocardial infarction (MI) in men at high risk [201].

37.5.7 1 Pharmacokinetics

After oral administration warfarin is rapidly absorbed from the GI tract, and reaches maximal blood concentrations in 90 min (200). It has high bioavailability and circulates bound to the plasma proteins (mainly albumin). It accumulates in the liver where the two isomers are metabolically transformed by different pathways [202]. Warfarin undergoes metabolism by oxidation by the cytochrome P450 enzymes [203]. The inactive form of warfarin is excreted in the urine and feces [204]. The medications that affect CYP-450 system significantly affect warfarin metabolism resulting in increase or decrease in its therapeutic effect. Some of the commonly used drugs that increase the international normalized ratio (INR) are alcohol, amiodarone, aspirin, propafenone, propranolol, cephalosporins, tetracycline, trimethoprim-sulfamethoxazole, statins, omeprazole, cimetidine, metronidazole, macrolides, NSAIDs, and azole anti-fungals. Nafcillin, rifampin, griseofulvin, cholestyramine, barbiturates, carbamazepine, chlordiazepoxide, sucralfate, and high vitamin K content food decrease the effect of warfarin. Phenytoin raises the INR initially but lowers it later [205].

37.5.7.2 Pharmacodynamics

As mentioned above, warfarin exerts its anticoagulant effect by inhibiting the coagulant proteins that are dependant on vitamin K. Therapeutic doses of warfarin can decrease the total amount of each vitamin K dependant coagulant factors made by the liver by 30–50% [204]. Coumarins produce their anticoagulant effect by inhibiting the vitamin K conversion cycle, thereby causing hepatic production of partially carboxylated and decarboxylated proteins with reduced procoagulant activity. In addition to their anticoagulant effect, warafin also inhibits carboxylation of the regulatory anticoagulant proteins C and S and therefore have the potential to exert a procoagulant effect. The anticoagulant effect and the antithrombotic effects of warfarin are dissociated during the induction phase of treatment. The antithrombotic effect of warfarin requires 6 days of treatment, whereas an anticoagulant effect was observed after 2 days [206]. The reduction of prothrombin, with a relatively long half-life of about 96 h is more important for the antithrombotic effect of warfarin than reduction of factors VII and IX with half-lives of 6 and 24 h, respectively [207]. Since the antithrombotic effect of warfarin reflects its ability to lower prothrombin levels, overlapping heparin with warfarin during treatment of patients with thrombosis, until the PT/INR has been prolonged into the therapeutic range is essential [208].

37.5.7.3 Adverse Effects

Bleeding complications are the most frequent adverse effects of warfarin [209]. When the INR exceeds the therapeutic range, discontinuing or reducing the dose of warfarin is usually sufficient. If more rapid reversal of warfarin effect is required because of bleeding, vitamin K can be administered orally or parenterally. Major life-threatening bleeding may require immediate treatment with cryoprecipitate or fresh frozen plasma (FFP) to normalize the INR and achieve immediate hemostasis. Skin necrosis is a very rare complication that occurs in patients with underlying protein C or protein S deficiency started on warfarin [210]. Warfarin is teratogenic and should not be used in pregnancy [211].

37.5.8
Ximelagatran

Vitamin K antagonists are effective oral anticoagulants, but they have limitations related to a narrow therapeutic range, food and drug interactions, slow onset of action and the need for routine coagulation monitoring. Ximelagatran is a novel, oral direct thrombin inhibitor (oral DTI) that is rapidly converted to melagatran, its active form, following absorption. Melagatran has been shown to be a potent, rapidly binding, competitive inhibitor of human thrombin [212]. In experimental animals, Ximelagatran and melagatran have been shown to be effective in the prevention and treatment of venous thromboembolism (VTE), in preventing carotid artery thrombosis, cerebral artery thrombosis, coronary artery thrombosis, and as an adjuvant in coronary artery thrombolysis.

37.5.8.1 Pharmacokinetics

Ximelagatran was derived from melagatran by ethylation of the carboxylic acid group and hydroxylation of the amidine group. It is given orally and is converted to the metabolically active melagatran. These groups act as a protecting agent and converts the highly hydrophilic and charged melagatran molecule into ximelagatran, which is more lipophilic than melagatran and uncharged at intestinal pH [212]. After oral administration of ximelagatran, the volume of distribution of melagatran is larger and its plasma half-life increased to approximately 2.5–3.5 h [213]. Melagatran is not metabolized and is mainly (approximately 80%) eliminated by renal excretion. In various clinical trials, patients treated long term with ximelagatran had an elevated serum transaminase levels. Serum alanine aminotransferase levels peaked after 60–120 days and returned to normal within 60–90 days whether treatment was continued or stopped [214].

37.5.8.2 Pharmacodynamics

Melagatran produces similar inhibition of fluid-phase thrombin and of thrombin bound to either fibrin clots or fibrin monomers, and it is significantly more active against clot-bound thrombin than the larger direct thrombin inhibitor, hirudin [215]. It also inhibits thrombin complexed with thrombomodulin and activation of Protein C effectively [216]. In vitro studies have shown that melagatran effectively inhibits both thrombin generation and thrombin activity [217]. Melagatran also inhibits thrombin's ability to activate protease-activated receptors on platelets [214]. Melgatran does not effect the inhibition of t-PA-induced fibrinolysis within its estimated therapeutic plasma concentration range [219].

37.6
Conclusion

The future value of cardiovascular drugs in clinical medicine with prospective drugs in development is highly promising. Some of the new agents that are in the development stage are: cholesteryl ester transfer protein (CETP) and acyl-coenzyme A transferase (ACAT) inhibitors in the treatment of hyperlipedemia; vasopeptidase inhibitors, vasopressin antagonists, and matrix metalloproteinase (MMP) inhibitors in the treatment of hypertension and heart failure; potassium channel openers, partial fatty acid oxidation (pFOX) inhibitors in the treatment of myocardial ischemia [220]. As our armamentarium of cardiovascular agents grows, the process of choosing the most appropriate regimen becomes increasingly complex. Cost, convenience, safety, and efficacy all need to be taken into account by the physician in the myriad situations requiring these agents.

Acknowledgement

The authors thank Ms Malak Atut for her help with manuscript preparation.

References

1. http://www.who.int/dietphysicalactivity/publications/facts/cvd/en. Accessed January 2004.
2. Paradis P, Dali-Youcef N, Paradis FW, Thibault G, Nemer M (2000). Overexpression of angiotensin II type I receptor in cardiomyocytes induces cardiac hypertrophy and remodeling. Proc Natl Acad Sci 972: 931–936.
3. McMurray JJ (1999) Major beta blocker mortality trials in chronic heart failure: A critical review. Heart 82:14–22.
4. Salvetti A (1990) Newer ACE inhibitors. A look at the future. Drugs 40:800–828.
5. Heel RC, Brogden RN, Speight TM, Avery GS (1980) Captopril: A preliminary review of its pharmacological properties and therapeutic efficacy. Drugs 20:409–452.
6. Aronoff GR, Bernes JS, Brier ME (1999) Drug Prescribing in Renal Failure: Dosing Guidelines for Adults. American College of Physicians, Philadelphia, pp. 1–176.
7. Duchin KL, Waclawski AP, Tu JI et al. (1991) Pharmacokinetics, safety, and pharmacologic effects of fosinopril sodium, an angiotensin-converting enzyme inhibitor in healthy subjects. J Clin Pharmacol 31:58–64.
8. Grassi G, Turri C, Dell'Oro R et al. (1998) Effect of chronic angiotensin converting enzyme inhibition on sympathetic

nerve traffic and baroreflex control of the circulation in essential hypertension. J Hypertens 16:1789.
9. Lin C, Frishman WH (1996) Renin inhibition: A novel therapy for cardiovascular disease. Am Heart J 131:1024–1034.
10. Ferri C, Laurenti O, Bellini C, Faldetta MR, Properzi G, Santucci A, De Mattia G (1995) Circulating endothelin-1 levels in lean noninsulin-dependent diabetic patients. Influence of ACE-inhibition. Am J Hypertens 8:40–47.
11. Weir RM, Hanes DS, Klassen DK (2004) Antihypertensive drugs, in Brenner & Rector's The Kidney, 7th edn. Elsevier, pp. 2387–2452.
12. Wood R (1995) Bronchospasm and cough as adverse reactions to the ACE inhibitors captopril, enalapril, lisinopril. Br J Clin Pharmacol 39:265–270.
13. van de Ven PJ, Beutler JJ, Kaatee R, Beek FJ, Mali WP, Koomans HA (1998) Angiotensin converting enzyme inhibitor–induced renal dysfunction in atherosclerotic renovascular disease. Kidney Int 53:986–993.
14. Cunniff C, Jones KL, Phillipson J, Benirschke K, Short S, Wujek J (1990) Oligohydramnios sequence and renal tubular malformation associated with maternal enalapril use. Am J Obstet Gynecol 162:187–189.
15. The Task Force on ACE-inhibitors of the European Society of Cardiology (2004) Expert consensus document on angiotensin converting enzyme inhibitors in cardiovascular disease. Eur Heart J 25:1454–1470.
16. Chu TJ, Chow N (1993) Adverse effects of ACE inhibitors. Ann Internal Med 118:314.
17. Timmermans PBMWM, Wong PC, Chiu AT et al. (1993) Angiotensin II receptors and angiotensin II receptor antagonists. Pharmacol Rev 45:205–251.
18. Conlin PR, Spence JD, Williams B et al. (2000) Angiotensin II antagonists for hypertension: Are there differences in efficacy? Am J Hypertens 13:418–426.
19. Wexler RR, Greenlee WJ, Irvin JD et al. (1996) Nonpeptide angiotensin II receptor antagonists: the next generation in antihypertensive therapy. J Med Chem 39:625–656.
20. Sica DA, Gehr TWB, Frishman WH (2003) The renin-angiotensin axis: Angiotensin converting enzyme inhibitors and Angiotensin receptor blockers. In Frishman WH, Sonnenblick EH, Sica DA (eds). Cardiovascular Pharmacotherapeutics, 2nd edn. McGraw-Hill, pp. 131–156.
21. Timmermans PBMWM, Chiu AT, Herblin WF, Wong PC, Smith RD (1992) Angiotensin II receptor subtypes. Am J Hypertens 5:406–410.
22. Griendling KK, Alexander RW (1993) The angiotensin (AT sub 1) receptor. Semin Nephrol 13:558–566
23. Packer M, Bristow MR, Cohn JN et al. (1996)The effect of carvedilol on morbidity and mortality in patients with chronic heart failure. U.S. Carvedilol Heart Failure Study Group. N Engl J Med 334:1349–1355
24. MERIT-HF (1999) Effect of metoprolol CR/XL in chronic heart failure: Metoprolol CR/XL Randomized Intervention Trial in Congestive Heart Failure (MERIT-HF). Lancet 353:2001–2007.
25. Meyer J, Lawson N (1999) Adrenergic inhibitors. In: Cardiovascular Drugs in Perioperative Period. Philadelphia, Lippincott-Raven, pp. 84–109.
26. Hoffman BB (2001) Catecholamines, sympathomimetic drugs, and adrenergic receptor antagonists. In Hardman JG, Limbird LE (eds) Goodman and Gillman's the Pharmacological Basis of Therapeutics, 10th edn. McGraw Hill Publishers, pp. 215–268.
27. Arthur MJ, Tanner AR, Patel C et al. (1985) Pharmacology of propranolol in patients with cirrhosis and portal hypertension. Gut 26:14–19.
28. Vanhees L, Aubert A, Fagard R et al. (1986) Influence of beta 1-versus beta 2-adrenoceptor blockade on left ventricular function in humans. J Cardiovasc Pharmacol 8:1086–1091.
29. Frischman WH (2003) Alpha and beta adrenergic blocking drugs. In: Frischman WH, Sonnenblick EH, Sica DA (eds) Cardiovascular Pharmacotherapeutics, 2nd edn. McGraw Hill Publishers, pp. 67–98.
30. Beta-Blocker Heart Attack Trial Research Group (1982) A randomized trial of propranolol in patients with acute myocardial infarction, I: mortality results. J Am Med Assoc 247:1707–1714.
31. Ames RP (1986) The effects of antihypertensive drugs on serum lipids and lipoproteins. II. Non-diuretic drugs. Drugs 32:335–357.
32. Lager I, Blohme G, Smith U (1979) Effect of cardioselective and non-selective beta-blockade on the hypoglycemic response in insulin-dependent diabetics. Lancet 1:458–462.
33. Yedinak KC (1993) Formulary considerations in selection of beta-blockers. Pharmacoeconomics 4:104–121
34. Lopez-Sendon J, Swedberg K, McMurray J, Tamargo J, Maggioni AP, Dargie H, Tendera M, Waagstein F, Kjekshus J, Lechat P, Torp-Pedersen C (2004) Task Force On Beta-Blockers of the European Society of Cardiology. Expert consensus document on beta-adrenergic receptor blockers. Euro Heart J 25:1341–1362.
35. Freher M, Challapalli S, Pinto JV, Schwartz J, Bonow RO, Gheorgiade M (1999) Current status of calcium channel blockers in patients with cardiovascular disease. Curr Probl Cardiol 24:236–240.
36. McDonald TF, Pelzer S, Trautwein W, Pelzer DJ (1994) Regulation and modulation of calcium channels in cardiac, skeletal, and smooth muscle cells. Physiol Rev 74:365–507.
37. Hockermon GH, Peterson BZ, Johnson BD, Catterall WA (1997) Molecular determinants of drug binding and action on L-type calcium channels. Annu Rev Pharmacol Toxicol 37:361–396.

38. Zhang Y, Benet LZ (2001) The gut as a barrier to drug absorption: Combined role of cytochrome P450 3A and P-glycoprotein. Clin Pharmacokinet 40:159–168.
39. Kroemer HK, Gautier J-C, Beaune P, Henderson C, Wolf CR, Eichelbaum M (1993) Identification of P450 enzymes involved in metabolism of verapamil in humans. Naunyn Schmiedebergs Arch Pharmacol 348:332–337.
40. Kroemer HR, Echizen H, Heidemann H, Eichelbaum M (1992) Predictability of the in vivo metabolism of verapamil from in vitro data: contribution of individual metabolic pathways and stereoselective aspects. J Pharmacol Exp Ther 260:1052–1057.
41. Kerins DM, Robertson, RM, Robertson, D (2001) Drugs used for the treatment of myocardial ischemia. In Hardman JG, Limbird LE (eds). Goodman and Gillman's the Pharmacological Basis of Therapeutics, 10th edn. McGraw Hill Publishers, pp. 843–870.
42. Kelly JG, O'Malley K (1992) Clinical pharmacokinetics of calcium antagonists. Clin Pharmacokinet 22:416–433.
43. Schwartz A (1992) Molecular and cellular aspects of calcium channel antagonism. Am J Cardiol 70:6F–8F.
44. Morel N, Buryi V, Feron O, Gomez J-P, Christen M-O, Godfraind T (1998) The action of calcium channel blockers on recombinant L-type calcium channel alpha1-subunits. Br J Pharmacol 125:1005–1012.
45. Henry PD, Perez JE (1984) Clinical pharmacology of calcium antagonists. Cardiovasc Clin 14:93–109.
46. Bremner AD, Fell PJ, Hosie J, James IG, Saul PA, Taylor SH (1993) Early side-effects of antihypertensive therapy: comparison of amlodipine and nifedipine retard. J Hum Hypertens 7:79–81.
47. Singh BN (1992) Safety profile of bepridil determined from clinical trials in chronic stable angina in the United States. Am J Cardiol 69:68–74.
48. Odlind B, Beermann B (1980) Renal tubular secretion and effects of furosemide. Clin Pharmacol Ther 27:784–790.
49. Pichette V, du Souich P (1996) Role of the kidneys in the metabolism of furosemide: its inhibition by probenecid. J Am Soc Nephrol 7:345–349.
50. Schwartz S, Brater DC, Pound D, Greene PK, Kramer WG, Rudy D (1993) Bioavailability, pharmacokinetics, and pharmacodynamics of torsemide in patients with cirrhosis. Clin Pharmacol Ther 54:90–97.
51. Sahn H, Reuter K, Mutschler E, Gerok W, Knauf H (1987) Pharmacokinetics of amiloride in renal and hepatic disease. Eur J Clin Pharmacol 33:493–498.
52. Knauf H, Möhrke W, Mutschler E (1983) Delayed elimination of triamterene and its active metabolite in chronic renal failure. Eur J Clin Pharmacol 24:453–456.
53. Overdiek HWPM, Hermens WAJJ, Merkus FWHM (1985) New insights into the pharmacokinetics of spironolactone. Clin Pharmacol Ther 38:469–474.
54. Jackson EK (2001) Diuretics. In: Hardman JG, Limbird LE (eds) Goodman and Gillman's the Pharmacological Basis of Therapeutics, 10th edn. McGraw Hill Publishers, pp. 757–788.
55. Brater DC (1998) Drug therapy: diuretic therapy N Engl J Med 339:387–395.
56. Brater DC, Chennavasin P, Day B, Burdette A, Anderson S (1983) Bumetanide and furosemide. Clin Pharmacol Ther 34:207–213.
57. Cogan MG, Maddox DA, Warnock DG, Lin ET, Rector FC (1979) Effect of acetazolamide on bicarbonate reabsorption in the proximal tubule of the rat. Am J Physiol 237:447–454.
58. Costanzo LS, Windhager EE (1978) Calcium and sodium transport by the distal convoluted tubule of the rat. Am J Physiol 235:492–506.
59. Marver D, Stewart J, Funder JW, Feldman D, Edelman IS (1974) Renal aldosterone receptors: studies with (3H)aldosterone and the anti-mineralocorticoid (3H)spirolactone (SC-26304). Proc Natl Acad Sci USA 71:1431–1435.
60. Weber KT (2001) Aldosterone in congestive heart failure. N Engl J Med 345:1689–1697.
61. Cooperman LB, Rubin IL (1973) Toxicity of ethacrynic acid and furosemide. Am Heart J 85:831–834.
62. Rose LI, Underwood RH, Newmark SR, Kisch ES, Williams GH (1977) Pathophysiology of spironolactone-induced gynecomastia. Ann Intern Med 87:398–403.
63. Raza JA. Movahed A (2002) Use of cardiovascular medications in the elderly. Int J Cardiol 85:203–215.
64. Massie BM, Shah NB (1997) Evolving trends in the epidemiologic factors of heart failure: rationale for preventive strategies and comprehensive disease management. Am Heart J 133:703–712.
65. Remme WJ, Swedberg K (2001) Guidelines for the diagnosis and treatment of chronic heart failure. Eur Heart J 22:1527–1560.
66. Murray CJL, Lopez AD (1997) Alternative projections of mortality and disability by cause 1990–2020: global burden of disease study. Lancet 349:1498–1504.
67. Withering W (1983) An account of the foxglove and some of its medical uses, with practical remarks on dropsy and other diseases. In: Willius FA, Keys TE (eds). Classics of Cardiology: a Collection of Classic Works on the Heart and Circulation with Comprehensive Biographic Accounts of the Authors. Malabar, FL, Krieger.
68. Ooi H, Colucci W (2001) Pharmacological treatment of heart failure. In: Hardman JG, Limbird LE (eds). Goodman and Gillman's the Pharmacological Basis of Therapeutics, 10th edn. McGraw Hill Publishers.
69. Smith TW (1988) Digitalis: mechanisms of action and clinical use. N Engl J Med 318:358–365.
70. Eisner DA, Smith TW (1991) The Na-K pump and its effectors in cardiac muscle. In Fozzard HA, Haber E, Jennings RB, Katz AM, Morgan HE (eds). The Heart and Cardiovascular System, 2nd edn. New York, Raven Press, pp. 863–902.

71. Gheorghiade M (1996) Neurohumoral effects of digoxin: a target for further investigation. Cardiologia 41:967–972.
72. Newton GE, Tong JH, Schofield AM, Baines AD, Floras JS, Parker JD (1996) Digoxin reduces cardiac sympathetic activity in severe congestive heart failure. J Am Coll Cardiol 28:155–161.
73. Howard D, Smith CI, Stewart G (1973) A prospective survey of the incidence of cardiac intoxication with digitalis in patients being admitted to hospital and correlation with serum digoxin levels. Aust NZ J Med. 3:279–284.
74. Howanitz PJ, Steindel SJ (1993) Digoxin therapeutic drug monitoring practices. A College of American Pathologists Q-probes study of 666 institutions and 18,679 toxic levels. Arch Pathol Lab Med 117:684–690.
75. Martin-Suarez A, Lanao JM, Calvo MV et al. (1993) Digoxin pharmacokinetics in patients with high serum digoxin concentrations. J Clin Pharm Ther 18:63–68.
76. Steiner JF, Robbins LJ, Hammermeister KE, Roth SC, Hammond WS (1994) Incidence of digoxin toxicity in outpatients. West J Med 161:474–8.
77. Murrell W (1879) Nitroglycerine as a remedy for angina pectoris. Lancet 1:80–81, 113
78. Fung HL, Chung SJ, Bauer JA, Chong S, Kowaluk EA (1992) Biochemical mechanism of organic nitrate action. Am J Cardiol 70:4–10.
79. Loscalzo J (1985) N-acetylcysteine potentiates inhibition of platelet aggregation by nitroglycerin. J Clin Invest 76:703–708.
80. Kelly RA, Balligand JL, Smith TW (1996) Nitric oxide and cardiac function. Circ Res 79:363–380
81. Bogaert MG (1988) Pharmacokinetics of organic nitrates in man: an overview. Eur Heart J 9:Suppl A:33–37.
82. Grobecker H (1990) Pharmacology and clinical pharmacology of organic nitrates. Euro J Clin Pharmacol 38:1:S3–S7.
83. Abrams J, Frischman WH (2003) The organic nitrates and nitroprusside. In Frischman WH, Sonnenblick EH, Sica DA (eds). Cardiovascular Pharmacotherapeutics, 2nd edn. McGraw Hill Publishers, pp. 203–214.
84. Cheitlin MD, Hutter AM Jr, Brindis RG et al. (1999) ACC/AHA expert consensus document. Use of sildenafil (Viagra) in patients with cardiovascular disease. American College of Cardiology/American Heart Association. J Am Coll Cardiol 33:273–82.
85. Colucci WS. Elkayam U. Horton DP et al. (2000) Intravenous nesiritide, a natriuretic peptide, in the treatment of decompensated congestive heart failure. Nesiritide Study Group. New Engl J Med 343:246–253.
86. Scios Inc. Data on file (accessed December 2004)
87. Mills RM, Hobbs RE (2003) Nesiritide in perspective: evolving approaches to the management of acute decompensated heart failure. Drugs of Today 39:767–774.
88. Levin ER, Gardner DG, Samson WK (1998) Natriuretic peptides. New Eng J Med 339:321–328.
89. Koller KJ, Goeddel DV (1992) Molecular biology of the natriuretic peptides and their receptors. Circulation 86:1081–1088.
90. Kambayashi Y, Nakao K, Kimura H et al. (1990) Biological characterization of human brain natriuretic peptide (BNP) and rat BNP: species-specific actions of BNP. Biochem Biophys Res Commun 173:599–605.
91. Hobbs RE, Miller LW, Bott-Silverman C et al. (1996) Hemodynamic effects of a single intravenous injection of synthetic human brain natriuretic peptide in patients with heart failure secondary to ischemic or idiopathic dilated cardiomyopathy. Am J Cardiol 78:896–901
92. Mills RM, LeJemtel TH, Horton DP et al. (1999) Sustained hemodynamic effects of an infusion of nesiritide (Human b-type natriuretic peptide) in heart failure. J Am Coll Cardiol 34:155–162.
93. Young JB, Abraham WT, Stevenson LW et al. (2002) Intravenous nesiritide vs nitroglycerin for treatment of decompensated congestive heart failure: a randomized controlled trial. J Am Med Assoc 287: 1531–1540.
94. Long-term pharmacotherapy in the management of obesity: National Task Force on the Prevention and Treatment of Obesity (1996). J Am Med Assoc 276:1907–1915.
95. Ford ES, Giles WH, Dietz WH (2002) Prevalence of the metabolic syndrome among US adults: findings from the third National Health and Nutrition Examination Survey. J Am Med Assoc 287:356–359.
96. Grundy SM, Howard B, Smith S et al. (2002) AHA conference proceedings prevention conference VI: diabetes and cardiovascular disease executive summary. Circulation 105:2231–2239.
97. Ginsberg HN, Huang LS (2000) The insulin resistance syndrome: impact on lipoprotein metabolism and atherothrombosis. J Cardiovasc Risk 7:325–331.
98. Superko HR, Krauss RM (1994) Coronary artery disease regression. Convincing evidence for the benefit of aggressive lipoprotein management. Circulation 90:1056–1069.
99. McKenney JM (2004) Optimizing LDL-C lowering with statins. Am J Therap 11:54–59.
100. Shepherd J, Packard CJ, Bicker S, Lawrie TDV, Morgan HG (1980) Cholestyramine promotes receptor-mediated low-density-lipoprotein catabolism. N Engl J Med 302:1219–1222.
101. Schectman G, Hiatt J (1993) Evaluation of the effectiveness of lipid-lowering therapy (bile acid sequestrants, niacin, psyllium, and lovastatin) for treating hypercholesterolemia in veterans. Am J Cardiol 71:759–765.
102. Knapp HH, Schrott H, Ma P, Knopp R, Chin B, Gaziano JM, Donovan JM, Burke SK, Davidson MH (2001) Efficacy and safety of combination simvastatin and colesevelam in patients with primary hypercholesterolemia. Am J Med 110:352–360.
103. Talbert RL (1999) Hyperlipidemia. In: DiPiro JT, Talbert RL, Yee GC et al. (eds) Pharmacotherapy: A Pathophysi-

ologic Approach, 4th edn. Stamford, CT, Appleton and Lange, pp. 350–361.
104. Lipid Research Clinics Program (1984) The Lipid Research Clinics Coronary Primary Prevention Trial results. I. Reduction in incidence of coronary heart disease. J Am Med Assoc 251:351–364.
105. Detmers PA, Patel S, Hernandez M et al. (2000) A target for cholesterol absorption inhibitors in the enterocyte brush border membrane. Biochim Biophys Acta 20: 243–252.
106. Knopp RH, Gitter H, Truitt T et al. (2001) Ezetimibe reduces low-density lipoprotein cholesterol: results of a phase III, randomised, double blind, placebo-controlled trial. Atherosclerosis 2: 38. Abstract.
107. Sudhop T, Von Bergmann K (2002) Cholesterol absorption inhibitors for the treatment of hypercholesterolemia. Drugs 62:2333–2347.
108. Sudhop T, Lutjohann D, Kodal A et al. (2002) Inhibition of intestinal cholesterol absorption by ezetimibe in humans. Circulation 106:1943–1948.
109. Law M (2001) Plant sterol and stanol margarines and health. Br Med J 320: 861–864
110. Davis HR, Pula KK, Alton KB et al. (2001) The synergistic hypocholesterolemic activity of the potent cholesterol absorption inhibitor, ezetimibe, in combination with 3-hydroxy-3-methylglutaryl coenzyme a reductase inhibitors in dogs. Metabolism 50:1234–1241.
111. Kosoglou T, Seiberling M, Statkevich P et al. (2001) Pharmacodynamic interaction between the new selective cholesterol absorption inhibitor ezetimibe and atorvastatin. J Am Coll Cardiol 37(suppl): 229A.
112. Kosoglou T, Meyer I, Cutler DL et al. (2000) Pharmacodynamic interaction between the selective cholesterol absorption inhibitor ezetimibe and lovastatin. In Program and Abstracts of the Third International Congress on Coronary Artery Disease: From Prevention to Intervention. Lyon, France, p. 101.
113. Miller DB, Spence JD (1998) Clinical pharmacokinetics of fibric acid derivatives (fibrates). Clin Pharmacokinet 34:155–162.
114. Ide T, Oku H, Sugano M (1982) Reciprocal responses to clofibrate in ketogenesis and triglyceride and cholesterol secretion in isolated rat liver. Metabolism 31:1065–1072.
115. Auwerx J, Schoonjans K, Fruchart JC, Staels B (1996) Regulation of triglyceride metabolism by PPARs: fibrates and thiazolidinediones have distinct effects. J Atheroscler Thromb 3:81–89.
116. Fruchart JC, Brewer HB, Leitersdorf E (1998) Consensus for the use of fibrates in the treatment of dyslipoproteinemia and coronary heart disease. Fibrate Consensus Group. Am J Cardiol 81:912–927.
117. Palmer RH (1987) Effects of fibric acid derivatives on biliary lipid composition. Am J Med 83: 37–43.
118. Hunston PD, Horn JR (1998) Drug interactions with HMG Co A reductase inhibitors. Drug Interact Newsl 1998:103–106.
119. Guyton JR (2004) Extended-release niacin for modifying the lipoprotein profile. Expert Opin Pharmacotherapy 5:1385–1398.
120. Sirtori CR, Torreggiani D, Fumagalli R (1975) Mechanism of action of hypolipidemic drugs. Adv Exper Med Biol 63:123–133.
121. Knopp RH, Ginsberg J, Albers JJ et al. (1985) Contrasting effects of unmodified and time-release forms of niacin on lipoproteins in hyperlipidemic subjects: clues to mechanism of action of niacin. Metab Clin Exper 34:642–650.
122. Illingworth DR, Stein EA, Mitchel YB et al. (1994) Comparative effects of lovastatin and niacin in primary hypercholesterolemia. A prospective trial. Arch Internal Med 154:1586–1595.
123. Grundy SM, Vega L, McGovern ME et al. (2002) Efficacy, safety, and tolerability of once-daily niacin for the treatment of dyslipidemia associated with type 2 diabetes. Arch Intern Med 162:1568–1576.
124. Canner PL, Furberg C, Terrum ML et al. (2003) Niacin decreases MI and total mortality in patients with metabolic syndrome: results from the coronary drug project. J Am Coll Cardiol 41:291A.
125. Gibbons LW, Gonzalez V, Gordon N, Grundy S (1995) The prevalence of side effects with regular and sustained-release nicotinic acid. Am J Med 99: 378–385.
126. Elam MB, Hunninghake DB, Davis KB et al. (2000) Effect of niacin on lipid and lipoprotein levels and glycemic control in patients with diabetes and peripheral arterial disease: the ADMIT study: a randomized trial. Arterial Disease Multiple Intervention Trial. J Am Med Assoc 284:1263–1270.
127. Scandinavian Simvastatin Survival Study Group (1994) Randomized trial of cholesterol lowering in 4444 patients with coronary heart disease. Lancet 344:1383–1389.
128. Knopp RH (1999) drug therapy: drug treatment of lipid disorders. N Engl J Med 341:498–511.
129. Mahley RW, Bersot TP (2001) Drug therapy for hypercholesterolemia and dyslipidemia. In Hardman JG, Limbird LE (eds). Goodman and Gillman's the Pharmacological Basis of Therapeutics, 10th edn. McGraw Hill Publishers, pp. 971–1002.
130. Davignon J, Montigny M, Dufour R (1992) HMG-CoA reductase inhibitors: a look back and a look ahead. Can J Cardiol 8:843–864.
131. Reihner E, Rudling M, Stahlberg D et al. (1990) Influence of pravastatin, a specific inhibitor of HMG-CoA reductase, on hepatic metabolism of cholesterol. N Engl J Med 323:224–228.
132. Davignon J (2004) Beneficial cardiovascular pleiotropic effects of statins. Circulation 109:39–43.

133. Stalker TJ, Lefer AM, Scalia R (2001) A new HMG-CoA reductase inhibitor, rosuvastatin, exerts anti-inflammatory effects on the microvascular endothelium: the role of mevalonic acid. Br J Pharmacol 133: 406–412.
134. Bradford RH, Shear CL, Chremos AN et al. (1991) Expanded clinical evaluation of lovastatin (EXCEL) study results, I: efficacy in modifying plasma lipoproteins and adverse event profile in 8245 patients with moderate hypercholesterolemia. Arch Internal Med 151:43–49.
135. Pierce LR, Wysowski DK, Gross TP (1990) Myopathy and rhabdomyolysis associated with lovastatin-gemfibrozil combination therapy. J Am Med Assoc 264:71–75.
136. Raza JA, Babb JD, Movahed A (2004) Optimal management of hyperlipidemia in primary prevention of cardiovascular disease. Int J Cardiol 97:355–366.
137. Levine GN, Ali MN, Schafer AI (2001) Antithrombotic therapy in patients with acute coronary syndromes. Arch Int Med 161:937–948.
138. Brogan GX (2003) Update on acute coronary syndromes and implications for therapy. Exp Opin Invest Drugs 12:1971–1983.
139. Levine MN, Raskob G, Beyth RJ, Kearon C, Schulman S (2004) Hemorrhagic complications of anticoagulant treatment: the Seventh ACCP Conference on Antithrombotic and Thrombolytic Therapy. Chest 2126:287S–310S.
140. Nawarskas JJ. Anderson JR (2001) Bivalirudin: a new approach to anticoagulation. Heart Disease 3:131–137.
141. Hirsh J, Warkentin TE, Raschke R et al. (1998) Heparin and low-molecular-weight heparin. Mechanisms of action, pharmacokinetics, dosing considerations, monitoring, and safety. Chest 114:489S–510S.
142. Witting JI, Bourdon P, Brezniak DV et al. (1992) Thrombin-specific inhibition by and slow cleavage of hirulog-1. Biochem J 283:737–743.
143. Fox I, Dawson A, Loynds P et al. (1993) Anticoagulant activity of Hirulog, a direct thrombin inhibitor, in humans. Thromb Haemost 69:157–163.
144. Tideman PA (1999) Antithrombins and the importance of good control. Aust NZ J Med 29:444–451.
145. Bates SM, Weitz JI (1998) Direct thrombin inhibitors for treatment of arterial thrombosis: potential differences between bivalirudin and hirudin. Am J Cardiol 82:12P–18P
146. Maraganore JM, Bourdon P, Jablonski J et al. (1990) Design and characterization of hirulogs: a novel class of bivalent peptide inhibitors of thrombin. Biochemistry 29:7095–7101.
147. Shah PK (2002) Pathophysiology of coronary thrombosis: role of plaque rupture and erosion. Prog Cardiovasc Dis 44:357–368.
148. Davies MJ (2000) The pathophysiology of acute coronary syndromes. Heart 83:361–366.
149. Thompson SG, Kienast J, Pyke SDM, Haverkate F, van de Loo JCW (1995) Hemostatic factors and the risk of myocardial infarction or sudden death in patients with angina pectoris. N Engl J Med 332:635–641.
150. Reimer KA, Lowe JE, Rasmussen MM et al. (1977) The wavefront phenomenon of ischemic cell death:Myocardial infarct size vs duration of coronary occlusion in dogs. Circulation 56:786–794.
151. Fibrinolytic Therapy Trialists' (FTT) Collaborative Group (1994) Indications for fibrinolytic therapy in suspected acute myocardial infarction: collaborative overview of early mortality and major morbidity results from all randomised trials of more than 1000 patients. Lancet 343:311–322.
152. Fletcher AP, Alkjaersig N, Smyrinotis FE (1958) Treatment of patients suffering from early, myocardial infarction with massive and prolonged streptokinase therapy. Trans Assoc Am Physicians 71:287–296.
153. Cannon CP, McCabe CH, Gibson CM et al. (1997) TNK-tissue plasminogen activator in acute myocardial infarction. Circulation 95:351–356.
154. Ohman EM, Harrington RA, Cannon CP et al. (2001) Intravenous thrombolysis in acute myocardial infarction. Chest 119:253S–277S.
155. Yusuf S, Collins R, Peto R et al. (1985) Intravenous and intracoronary fibrinolytic therapy in acute myocardial infarction: overview of results on mortality, reinfarction and side-effects from 33 randomized controlled trials. Eur Heart J 6:556–585.
156. Pennica D, Holmes WE, Kohr WJ et al. (1983) Cloning and expression of human tissue-type plasminogen activator cDNA in E coli. Nature 301:214–221.
157. Berkowitz SD, Granger CB, Pieper KS et al. (1997) Incidence and predictors of bleeding after contemporary thrombolytic therapy for myocardial infarction. Circulation 95:2508–2516.
158. EPIC Investigators (1994) Use of a monoclonal antibody directed against the platelet glycoprotein IIb/IIIa receptor in high-risk coronary angioplasty. N Engl J Med 330:956–961.
159. Barrett JS, Murphy G, Peerlinck K et al. (1994) Pharmacokinetics and pharmacodynamics of MK-383, a selective non-peptide platelet glycoprotein-IIb/IIIa receptor antagonist, in healthy men. Clin Pharmacol Ther 56:377–388.
160. Kleiman NS, Raizner AE, Jordan R et al. (1995) Differential inhibition of platelet aggregation induced by adenosine diphosphate or a thrombin receptor-activating peptide in patients treated with bolus chimeric 7E3 Fab: implications for inhibition of the internal pool of GP IIb/IIIa receptors. J Am Coll Cardiol 26:1665–1671.
161. Tcheng JE, Ellis SG, George BS et al. (1994) Pharmacodynamics of chimeric glycoprotein IIb/IIIa integrin antiplatelet antibody Fab 7E3 in high-risk coronary angioplasty. Circulation 90:1757–1764.
162. Mascelli MA, Lance ET, Damaraju L et al. (1998) Pharmacodynamic profile of short-term abciximab treatment

demonstrates prolonged platelet inhibition with gradual recovery from GP IIb/IIIa receptor blockade. Circulation 97:1680–1688.
163. Phillips DR, Scarborough RM (1997) Clinical pharmacology of eptifibatide. Am J Cardiol 80:11–20.
164. Deckelbaum LI, Sax FL, Grossman W (1997) Tirofiban, a nonpeptide inhibitor of the platelet glycoprotein IIb/IIIA receptor. In Sasahara AA, Loscalzo J (eds) New Therapeutic Agents in Thrombosis and Thrombolysis. Marcel Dekker, New York, pp. 355–365.
165. Bachelot C, Rendu F, Gulino D (1995) Anti-GP IIb/IIIa antibodies: powerful tools to investigate function and regulation of an integrin. Semin Thromb Hemost 21:23–36.
166. Scarborough RM, Rose JW, Naughton MA et al. (1993) Characterization of the integrin specificities of disintegrins isolated from American pit viper venoms. J Biol Chem 268:1058–1065.
167. Jordan RE, Wagner CL, Mascelli MA et al. (1996) Preclinical development of c7E3 Fab: a mouse/human chimeric monoclonal antibody fragment that inhibits platelet function by blockade of GP IIb/IIIa receptors with observations on the immunogenicity of c7E3 Fab in humans. In Horton MA (ed.) Adhesion Receptors as Therapeutic Targets. CRC Press, Boca Raton, FL, pp. 281–305 .
168. Llevadot J, Coulter SA, Giugliano RP (2000) A practical approach to the diagnosis and management of thrombocytopenia associated with glycoprotein IIb/IIIa receptor inhibitors. J Thromb Thrombolysis 9:175–180.
169. Ferguson JJ, Kereiakes DJ, Adgey AA et al. (1998) Safe use of platelet GP IIb/IIIa inhibitors. Am Heart J 135:S77–S89.
170. Coller BS: Blockade of platelet GpIIb/IIIa receptors as an antithrombotic strategy. Circulation 92:2373–2380.
171. Tcheng JE, Kereiakes DJ, Lincoff AM et al. (2001) Abciximab readministration: results of the ReoPro Readministration Registry. Circulation 104:870–875.
172. Hirsh J, Anand SS, Halperin JL, Fuster V (2001) American Heart Association. Guide to anticoagulant therapy: Heparin: a statement for healthcare professionals from the American Heart Association. Circulation 103:2994–3018.
173. Andersson LO, Barrowcliffe TW, Holmer E et al. (1979) Molecular weight dependency of the heparin potentiated inhibition of thrombin and activated factor X: effect of heparin neutralization in plasma. Thromb Res 5:531–541.
174. Weitz JI (1997) drug therapy: low-molecular-weight heparins. N Engl J Med 337:688–699.
175. Bjornsson TO, Wolfram KM, Kitchell BB (1982) Heparin kinetics determined by three assay methods. Clin Pharmacol Ther 31:104–113.
176. Lam LH, Silbert JE, Rosenberg RD (1976) The separation of active and inactive forms of heparin. Biochem Biophys Res Commun 69:570–577.
177. Rosenberg RD, Bauer KA (1994) The heparin–antithrombin system: a natural anticoagulant mechanism. In: Colman RW, Hirsch J, Marder VJ, Salzman EW (eds). Hemostasis and Thrombosis: Basic Principles and Clinical Practice, 3rd edn. Philadelphia, JB Lippincott, pp. 837–860.
178. Beguin S, Lindhout T, Hemker HC (1988) The mode of action of heparin in plasma. Thromb Haemost 60:457–462.
179. Kelton JG, Hirsh J (1980) Bleeding associated with antithrombotic therapy. Semin Hematol 17:259–291.
180. Hunter J, Lonsdale RJ, Wenham PW, Frostick SP (1993) Heparin induced thrombosis: an important complication of heparin prophylaxis for thromboembolic disease in surgery. Br Med J 307:53–55.
181. Bhandari M, Hirsh J, Weitz JI et al. (1998) The effects of standard and low molecular weight heparin on bone nodule formation in vitro. Thromb Haemost 80:413–417.
182. Schafer AI (1996) Low-molecular-weight heparin—an opportunity for home treatment of venous thrombosis. N Engl J Med 334:724–725.
183. Kearon C, Hirsh J (1996) Anticoagulation in venous thromboembolism. In Smith TW (ed.) Cardiovascular Therapeutics. Philadelphia, WB Saunders, pp. 442–455.
184. Kaul S, Shah PK (2000) Low molecular weight heparin in acute coronary syndrome: Evidence for superior or equivalent efficacy compared with unfractionated heparin? J Am Coll Cardiol 35:1699–1712.
185. Antman EM. Cohen M. Radley D et al. (1999) Assessment of the treatment effect of enoxaparin for unstable angina/non-Q-wave myocardial infarction. TIMI 11B-ESSENCE meta-analysis. Circulation 100:1602–1608.
186. Harenberg J (1990) Pharmacology of low molecular weight heparins. Semin Thromb Hemost 16:12–18.
187. Armstrong P (1997) Heparin in acute coronary disease: requiem for a heavyweight? N Engl J Med 337:492–494.
188. CAPRIE Steering Committee (1996) A randomized, blinded trial of clopidogrel versus aspirin in patients at risk of ischemic events (CAPRIE). Lancet 348:1329–1339.
189. The Clopidogrel in Unstable Angina to Prevent Recurrent Events Trial Investigators (2001) Effects of clopidogrel in addition to aspirin in patients with acute coronary syndromes without ST-segment elevation. N Engl J Med 345:494–502.
190. Desager JP (1994) Clinical pharmacokinetics of ticlopidine. Clin Pharmacokinet 26:347–355.
191. Lau WC, Gurbel PA, Watkins PB et al. (2004) Contribution of hepatic cytochrome P450 3A4 metabolic activity to the phenomenon of clopidogrel resistance. Circulation 109:166–171.
192. Savi P, Combalbert J, Gaich C et al. (1994) The antiaggregating activity of clopidogrel is due to a metabolic activation by the hepatic cytochrome P450-1A. Thromb Haemost 72:313–317.

193. Müller I, Seyfarth M, Rudiger S, Wolf B, Pogatsa-Murray G, Schomig A, Gawaz M (2001) Effect of a high loading dose of clopidogrel on platelet function in patients undergoing coronary stent placement. Heart 85:92–93.
194. Quinn MJ, FitzGerald DJ (1999) Ticlopidine and clopidogrel. Circulation. 100:1667–72.
195. Savi P, Pflieger AM, Herbert JM (1996) cAMP is not an important messenger for ADP-induced platelet aggregation. Blood Coagul Fibrinolysis 7:249–252.
196. Heptinstall S, May JA, Glenn JR, Sanderson HM, Dickinson JP, Wilcox RG (1995) Effects of ticlopidine administered to healthy volunteers on platelet function in whole blood. Thromb Haemost 74:1310–1315.
197. Boneu B, Destelle G (1996) Platelet anti-aggregating activity and tolerance of clopidogrel in atherosclerotic patients. Thromb Haemost 76:939–943.
198. Whitlon DS, Sadowski JA, Suttie JW (1978) Mechanisms of coumarin action: significance of vitamin K epoxide reductase inhibition. Biochemistry 17:1371–1377.
199. Choonara IA, Malia RG, Haynes BP et al. (1988) The relationship between inhibition of vitamin K 1,2,3-epoxide reductase and reduction of clotting factor activity with warfarin. Br J Clin Pharmacol 25:1–7.
200. Malhotra OP, Nesheim ME, Mann KG (1985) The kinetics of activation of normal and gamma carboxy glutamic acid deficient prothrombins. J Biol Chem 260:279–287.
201. The Medical Research Council's General Practice Research Framework (1998) Thrombosis prevention trial: randomised trial of low-intensity oral anticoagulation with warfarin and low-dose aspirin in the primary prevention in ischemic heart disease in men at increased risk. Lancet 351:233–241.
202. O'Reilly RA (1986) Warfarin metabolism and drug-drug interactions. In Wessler S, Becker CG, Nemerson Y (eds) The New Dimensions of Warfarin Prophylaxis (vol. 214): Advances in Experimental Medicine and Biology. New York, Plenum, pp. 205–212.
203. Aithal GP, Day CP, Kesteven, PJ et al. (1999) Association of polymorphisms in the cytochrome P450 CYP2C9 with warfarin dose requirement and risk of bleeding complications. Lancet 353:717–719.
204. Majerus PW, Tollefsen DM (2001) Anticoagulant, thrombolytic, and antiplatelet drugs. In Hardman JG, Limbird LE (eds). Goodman and Gillman's the Pharmacological Basis of Therapeutics, 10thy edn. McGraw Hill Publishers, pp. 1519–1538.
205. Gage BF, Fihn SD, White RH (2000) Management and dosing of warfarin therapy. Am J Med 109:481–488.
206. Wessler S, Gitel SN (1984) Warfarin: from bedside to bench. N Engl J Med 311:645–652.
207. Zivelin A, Rao VM, Rapaport SI (1993) Mechanism of the anticoagulant effect of warfarin as evaluated in rabbits by selective depression of individual procoagulant vitamin-K dependent clotting factors. J Clin Invest 92:2131–2140.
208. Furie B, Diuguid CF, Jacobs M et al. (1990) Randomized prospective trial comparing the native prothrombin antigen with the prothrombin time for monitoring anticoagulant therapy. Blood 75:344–349.
209. Levine MN, Raskob G, Landefeld S et al. (1995) Hemorrhagic complications of anticoagulant treatment. Chest 108:276–290.
210. Sallah S, Thomas DP, Roberts HR (1997) Warfarin and heparin-induced skin necrosis and purple toe syndrome: Infrequent complications of anticoagulant treatment. Thromb Haemost 78:785–790.
211. Hall JG, Pauli RM, Wilson KM (1980) Maternal and fetal sequelae of anticoagulation during pregnancy. Am J Med 68:122–140.
212. Gustafsson D, Nyström J, Carlsson S et al. (2001) The direct thrombin inhibitor melagatran and its oral prodrug H 376/95: intestinal absorption properties, biochemical and pharmacodynamic effects. Thromb Res 101:171–181.
213. Johansson LC, Frison L, Logren U, Fager G, Gustafsson D, Eriksson UG (2003) Influence of age on the pharmacokinetics and pharmacodynamics of ximelagatran, an oral direct thrombin inhibitor. Clin Pharmacokinet 42:381–392.
214. Francis CW (2004) Ximelagatran: a new oral anticoagulant. Best Practice Res Clin Haematol 17:139–152.
215. Klement P, Carlsson S, Rak J et al. (2003) The benefit-to-risk profile of melagatran is superior to that of hirudin in a rabbit arterial thrombosis prevention and bleeding model. J Thromb Haemostasis 1:587–594.
216. Mattsson C, Menschik-Lundin A, Nylander S et al. (2001) Effect of different types of thrombin inhibitors on thrombin/thrombomodulin modulated activation of protein C in vitro. Thrombosis Res 104:475–486.
217. Boström SL, Hansson GFH, Kjaer M, Sarich TC (2003) Effects of melagatran, the active form of the oral direct thrombin inhibitor ximelagatran, and dalteparin, on the endogenous thrombin potential in venous blood from healthy male subjects. Blood Coagul Fibrinolysis 14:457–462.
218. Nylander S, Mattsson C (2003) Thrombin-induced platelet activation and its inhibition by anticoagulants with different modes of action. Blood Coagul Fibrinolysis 14:159–167.
219. Gustafsson D, Antonsson T, Bylund R et al. (1998) Effects of melagatran, a new low-molecular-weight thrombin inhibitor, on thrombin and fibrinolytic enzymes. Thromb Haemost 79:110–118.
220. Pimanda JE, Lowe HC, Hogg PJ, Chesterman CN, Khachigian LM (2003) Novel and emerging therapies in cardiology and haematology. Current Drug Targets - Cardiovasc Haematol Disorders 3:101–123.

Anti-Arrhythmic Drugs: Pharmacokinetics and Pharmacodynamics

R. Wayne Kreeger, Jaffar Ali Raza and Assad Movahed

Contents

38.1	Introduction	453
38.2	Class I Agents	454
38.2.1	Quinidine	454
38.2.2	Procainamide	454
38.2.3	Disopyramide	455
38.2.4	Lidocaine	455
38.2.5	Mexiletine	455
38.2.6	Tocainide	455
38.2.7	Phenytoin	455
38.2.8	Flecainide, Propafenone, and Encainide	455
38.3	Class II Agents	456
38.4	Class III Agents	456
38.4.1	Amiodarone	456
38.4.2	Sotalol	456
38.4.3	Dofetilide	457
38.4.4	Ibutilide	457
38.4.5	Bretylium	457
38.5	Class IV – Calcium Channel Blockers	457
38.6	Cardiac Glycosides (Digoxin)	458
38.7	Adenosine	458
38.8	Magnesium	458
38.9	Atropine	458
38.10	Isoproterenol	459
	References	459

38.1 Introduction

The goals of antiarrhythmic drug therapy are to control heart rate, abolish tachyarrhythmias, suppress ectopic beats, and to restore and maintain normal sinus rhythm. The selection of appropriate agents is a match between the common antiarrhythmic drugs, the condition and age of the patient, the urgency of treatment, the potential long-term side effects, and especially the drug's proven efficacy on the arrhythmia in question [1]. This chapter will discuss the pharmacokinetics and pharmacodynamics of the commonly utilized and marketed antiarrhythmic drugs.

Pharmacokinetics is the study of the metabolism and action of drugs, especially on the time for absorption, mode of administration, distribution in the body, duration of action based upon steady state and half-life, their metabolites, and the mechanisms of elimination or metabolism and clearance from the body [2, 3]. Pharmacodynamics refers to the study of the mechanisms of actions of drugs. In the case of antiarrhythmic agents, it is their interaction with ion channels that determine their biochemical and electrophysiological therapeutic effects on the cardiovascular system and the entire body.

Antiarrhythmic drugs are commonly classified into four main classes plus a separate unclassified category. Based upon a drug's electrophysiologic effects, the Vaughn Williams classification scheme provides groupings of drugs with similar effects on ion channels or receptors blocked. The Vaughan Williams classification of antiarrhythmic drugs was developed based upon their variability of electrophysiologic actions [4, 5]. Depolarization is affected by block of sodium channels whereas repolarization is affected by block of the potassium channels [6–8]. The Class I drugs are divided into three subgroups, IA, IB, and IC. They act by blocking the fast sodium channel responsible for the rapid upstroke of the action potential [9]. The subgroups are based on their kinetics and effects on depolarization and repolarization [10]. They exhibit use-dependent blockade of the sodium channel meaning their potency is enhanced at faster rates in contrast to reverse use-dependence (more potency at slower rates) of Class III agents. Drugs may have overlap within subgroups as well as manifest electrophysiologic actions of more than one class [11, 12].

Class IA drugs moderately slow conduction, and prolong the action potential duration and repolarization, lengthening the QRS complex and the QT interval. This category includes quinidine, procainamide, and disopyramide [13]. The Class IB drugs have the lowest sodium channel blocking effects, minimally slow conduction, shorten repolarization and exert little if any effect on action potential duration. Class IB drugs include lidocaine, mexiletine, tocainide, and phenytoin [14]. Class IC drugs, flecainide, encainide (not currently marketed), and propafenone are, however, the most potent sodium channel blockers but have little effect on repolarization, although they may prolong the PR interval and QRS duration. Class IC drugs markedly slow conduction and only minimally prolong the action potential duration [15, 16]. Moricizine remains an undefined Class I drug having characteristics of Class IA and IB but since the CAST study is not utilized. The Class II drugs are the anti-sympathetic or beta-adrenergic receptor blockers, with non-selective and cardioselective varieties. Class III drugs such as amiodarone, bretylium, sotalol, dofetilide, and ibutilide have a complicated mechanism of action in blocking potassium ion channels responsible for Phase 2 and 3 of the action potential [17]. They prolong action potential duration and repolarization, but have little effect on rate of depolarization. They also exert a characteristic of "reverse use-dependence" meaning more potent activity at slower not faster rates, the opposite you would favor for treatment of tachycardias. Use-dependence is that drugs bind more avidly to the more active the channels are, i.e. at faster rates ideal for treatment of tachyarrhythmias. Reverse use-dependence in contrast is when drugs bind more avidly to resting channels such that the effect is more prominent during slower rates. These drugs have a higher propensity to torsades de pointes, the least potential being amiodarone.

Class IV agents are the calcium channel antagonists, blocking primarily the L-type calcium channels particularly involved in AV nodal conduction [18]. They are useful in reentrant arrhythmias within the AV node and rare forms of ventricular tachycardias. The miscellaneous group includes drugs such as digoxin (cardiac glycoside), adenosine, magnesium, and not to forget the parasympatholytic agent atropine and the sympathomimetic beta-agonist, isoproterenol.

The drawbacks to the Vaughan Williams classification scheme of antiarrhythmic drugs include the facts that most of the currently available antiarrhythmic agents have multiple class actions, and their metabolites may augment antiarrhythmic actions or even produce opposite actions or delayed clearance side effects.

38.2
Class I Agents

Class I agents are the sodium channel blockers and include IA drugs (quinidine, procainamide, disopyramide), IB drugs (lidocaine, mexiletine, tocainide, phenytoin), and IC drugs (flecainide, propafenone) and moricizine [19]. Class I agents are effective in suppressing impulse generation and are useful in reentrant arrhythmias both supraventricular and ventricular. Whereas Class IA agents prolong the action potential duration wherein lies the QT prolongation and torsade de pointes risk, Class IB agents shorten the action potential duration and Class IC agents have little to no effect on action potential duration. Class IB agents shorten refractoriness, and decrease automaticity but have little effect on conduction velocity, being most effective on ventricular arrhythmias. The Class IC drugs have intermediate effects between Class IA and IB drugs.

38.2.1
Quinidine

Quinidine is the oldest antiarrhythmic agent extracted and used as the quinine in 1848 from cinchona tree bark [20]. Quinidine and procainamide are used in the cardioversion of atrial fibrillation/flutter, to maintain sinus rhythm and to prevent recurrences of supraventricular and ventricular tachycardias. It has vagolytic effects thus enhancing AV node conduction so that the ventricular response of atrial fibrillation may paradoxically accelerate if not given concomitantly with an AV node blocker such as digoxin or a beta-blocker. Quinidine is metabolized in the liver with a half life of 4–17 hours. The main side effects are diarrhea, cramping, headache, and cinchonism symptoms with decreased hearing, tinnitus, and blurred vision. Proarrhythmic effects such as heart block and torsades also occur with a three-fold increase in mortality compared with placebo. Quinidine may increase digoxin levels by competing for protein binding sites so dosage adjustments are necessary when they are concomitantly used.

38.2.2
Procainamide

Procainamide usage began around 1951. It has similar effects to quinidine, but no parasympatholytic effects [21]. It decreases conduction velocity in atrial, His-Purkinje, and ventricular tissue. It is available for oral and IV use but IV usage is limited by hypotension and negative ionotropic effects. It undergoes hepatic metabolism to an acetylated metabolite, NAPA, which also has antiarrhythmic properties and undergoes renal elimination. N-acetylprocainamide has Class III antiarrhythmic activity [22]. The half-life of procainamide is 3–5 hours. Procainamide's main side effects are GI, torsades, development of a lupus-like syndrome with antinuclear antibodies, rash, fever, agranulocytosis, myalgias, pleuritis, and even pericarditis.

38.2.3
Disopyramide

Disopyramide was approved for use in 1977 and has similar vagolytic effects to quinidine [23]. It is a potent negative inotrope to be avoided in patients with LV dysfunction. It prolongs repolarization. Its elimination half-life is 6–9 hours. The prominent anticholinergic side effects dry eyes, dry mouth, constipation and urinary retention especially in the presence of prostatism limit its usefulness.

38.2.4
Lidocaine

Lidocaine, a Class IB drug, is probably the most widely used [24]. It has little effect on conduction velocity in normal tissue but slows conduction in ischemic tissue. It has no significant effect on atrial tissue and is primarily indicated for ventricular arrhythmias. Elimination is via hepatic metabolism to active metabolites that are renally cleared with the elimination half-life being 1.5–2 hours. Dose adjustments need to be made in the setting of congestive heart failure, hepatic or renal disease. The primary side effects are CNS with drowsiness, altered sensorium, and even seizures at high doses.

38.2.5
Mexiletine

Mexiletine is a lidocaine congener available only orally [25]. It can be used alone or in combination with a Class IA or III drug for ventricular tachyarrhythmias [26]. It is metabolized in the life with an elimination half-life of 8–17 hours. Main side effects include lightheadedness, dizzy sensations, GI distress, tremor, unsteady gait, and even ataxia [27].

38.2.6
Tocainide

Tocainide, also a Class IB drug, has had limited usefulness, having been removed from the market in Europe due to blood dyscrasias [28]. It is metabolized both in the liver and kidneys with half-life 8–20 hours. Ethmozine or Moricizine is an ill-defined Class I antiarrhythmic, which reduces fast inward sodium current, shortens repolarization and decreases action potential duration. It has been shown to increase mortality in the post-infarct patient treated for ventricular arrhythmias with limited usefulness [29, 30].

38.2.7
Phenytoin

Phenytoin is a Class IA and IB drug with anticonvulsant activity but has been used in the past for arrhythmias associated with digitalis toxicity and in the pediatric population. Its half-life is 16–24 hours with primarily hepatic metabolism.[31]

38.2.8
Flecainide, Propafenone, and Encainide

Flecainide, propafenone, and encainide are Class IC drugs [27, 32. Encainide was removed from the market due to enhanced mortality risk in the coronary patient post-infarct. Flecainide was approved by the FDA in 1985 and gained approval for supraventricular tachycardia treatment in 1991. It prolongs atrial refractoriness and terminates atrial fibrillation. It may have a slowing effect on atrial flutter and allow 1:1 AV conduction thereby needing to administer it concomitantly with an AV node blocking medication. Flecainide markedly decreases conduction velocity is utilized primarily for atrial and ventricular arrhythmias though in the setting of normal or preserved left ventricular function due to its profound negative inotropic effects. It should be avoided in severe LV dysfunction, prior infarct, or history of CHF. It is renally excreted with a half-life of 20 hours. CNS effects include blurred vision, headache, and ataxia. In the Cardiac Arrhythmia Suppression Trial (CAST), flecainide and encainide increased mortality compared to placebo in a randomized trial of ventricular arrhythmia suppression after myocardial infarction [30].

Propafenone is similar to flecainide and was approved in 1989 [33, 34]. It has nonselective beta-adrenergic blocking effects as well as mild calcium channel blocking effects. It is useful in the treatment of atrial fibrillation with less negative inotropic effects than flecainide or disopyramide and also can be utilized in treating ventricular arrhythmias, less so in the presence of left ventricular dysfunction. It is hepatic metabolized with an elimination half-life of 3–8 hours. Its main side effects are CHF exacerbation, GI, metallic taste, bronchospasm, and dizziness.

38.3
Class II Agents

The beta-adrenergic receptor blocking agents block catecholaminergic or sympathetic effects, slow the heart rate, decrease myocardial contractility and blood pressure, increase the refractory periods in tissues, and reduce excitability of myocardial cells via membrane stabilizing (anti-fibrillatory) effects [35–37]. There are a myriad of different beta-blockers falling into three categories, nonselective beta1 + beta2 antagonists (nadolol, pindolol, propranolol, sotalol, timolol), cardioselective beta1 antagonists (acebutolol, atenolol, esmolol, metoprolol) and the combined alpha1 and beta-adrenergic antagonists (carvedilol, labetalol) [38, 39] (Table 38.1).

38.4
Class III Agents

The Class III drugs, amiodarone, sotalol, bretylium, dofetilide, and ibutilide are unique in that they block the outflow of potassium ions, which are operative during Phase 2 and 3 of the action potential, thereby prolonging the action potential duration and increasing the repolarization time (increased QT interval) [40, 41]. They suppress ventricular ectopic activity and except for bretylium are also useful in atrial arrhythmias. Amiodarone also has beta-adrenergic and calcium channel blocking activity and sotalol has beta-blocking activity [42].

38.4.1
Amiodarone

Amiodarone was developed as an antianginal coronary vasodilator over 30 years ago, and approved for use in 1986 [43–47]. It has crossover properties of all four antiarrhythmic classes. It has been described as the most effective but most toxic, having an array of dangerous side effects. It is utilized in life threatening arrhythmias intravenously but is also available for oral use. It is useful for treatment of ventricular arrhythmias, ventricular tachycardia and fibrillation refractory to other therapies, and also atrial dysrhythmias in small doses

Table 38.1 Hemodynamic effects of beta-adrenergic blocking drugs

1. Heart rate reduction by sinus node suppression
2. Decreased systolic blood pressure
3. Decreased cardiac output
4. Renin release blocked with decreased angiotensin II production
5. Reduced myocardial oxygen consumption
6. Prolonged diastolic filling by bradycardia
7. Increased calcium loading into sarcoplasmic reticulum, augmenting contractility
8. Beta-2 blockade produces vasodilation and bronchodilation
9. Up-regulation of cardiac Beta-1 receptors in CHF, increasing catecholamine responsiveness

when they are refractory to lesser therapies. It has a large volume of distribution with a very long duration of action and an active metabolite. It has unique pharmacokinetics with a long half-life of 50–110 days [48]. It is highly lipid soluble, requires a long loading period and undergoes hepatic metabolism. Hypotension may occur with intravenous therapy [49]. Once loaded there is a substantial drug reservoir since it is fat soluble. It is 37% iodine being chemically similar to thyroxine and triodothyronine. It suppresses conversion of T4 to T3 and so it can trigger either hypothyroidism or hyperthyroidism. Regular surveillance labs for liver function tests and thyroid studies are recommended. A major benefit is it is safe in moderate and even severe LV dysfunction. However, it has a lengthy side effect profile including pulmonary toxicity progressing to fibrosing alveolitis and fibrosis, corneal microdeposits, slate-gray-blue skin discoloration, photosensitivity, reversible liver function test abnormalities, peripheral neuropathy, tremor, and QT prolongation though its action potential prolongation effects minimize the risk of torsades.

38.4.2
Sotalol

Sotalol was approved for ventricular arrhythmias in 1992 and atrial arrhythmias in 2000 [50–52]. Sotalol in addition to increasing the APD by blocking potassium channels, also is a non-selective beta-adrenergic receptor antagonist. In the ESVEM trial, sotalol when compared to Class I agents was shown to decrease the recurrence of arrhythmias and sudden death and total cardiovascular mortality in VT/VF patients [53]. It is a racemic mixture of d- and l-isomers. The Class III and beta-blocking actions are mainly the l-isomer. It exerts reverse-use-dependence of Class III drugs (greater pharmacologic effects at slower heart rates) and is useful in atrial fibrillation and ventricular tachyarrhythmias. A beneficial side effect of sotalol is its capacity to lower defibrillation thresholds of defibrillators in contrast to most other antiarrhythmic drugs raising them. It is excreted unchanged in the urine and dosages have to be adjusted in renal insufficiency. The half-life is 10–20 hours. The main side effects are the beta-blocker effects of bronchospasm, fatigue, and torsades especially in the setting of renal failure and hypokalemia. D,L-sotalol has been shown to be safe in coronary disease patients but d-sotalol enhanced mortality (SWORD trial) [54].

38.4.3
Dofetilide

Dofetilide was approved in 1999 and has been utilized in conversion of atrial fibrillation and sinus rhythm maintenance even in the face of LV dysfunction or cardiomyopathy [55, 56]. It also exhibits reverse-use-dependence. It prolongs the action potential duration in atria and ventricles, mainly atria and blocks the delayed rectifier potassium channel. It is metabolized renally and strict dosage adjustment guidelines based on creatinine clearance and in hospital monitoring are required. It can prolong the QT interval and enhance the risk of torsades and should be avoided in conjunction with other QT-prolonging drugs as well as verapamil and thiazide diuretics. Dofetilide is effective in maintaining sinus rhythm and its long-term use has not been associated with increased mortality in the CHF or previous infarct patient [57, 58]. In-hospital monitoring during initiation or dosage changes is required.

38.4.4
Ibutilide

Ibutilide is the newest injectable agent for termination of atrial flutter and atrial fibrillation [59, 60]. It was introduced as an IV agent for the termination of atrial fibrillation and of reentrant atrial tachyarrhytmias such as atrial flutter. Its most adverse effect is polymorphic VT in association with excess QT prolongation. Unlike other Class III agents, it increases action potential duration, enhances slow inward sodium current rather than blocking outward potassium currents [61]. It is given as a 1 mg infusion over 10 minutes, repeating as needed 0.5–1.0 mg once. It lowers defibrillation threshold for atrial fibrillation and can be used with cardioversion to enhance likelihood of success. Half-life is 6–9 hours and it undergoes hepatic and renal clearance. However, continuous monitoring after administration is required for 4 hours during the window of enhanced torsades risk since torsades has been reported up to 8%.

38.4.5
Bretylium

Bretylium is the longest utilized Class III antiarrhythmic in the USA [62]. Its primary uses were for lidocaine or defibrillation refractory ventricular tachycardia or ventricular fibrillation. It is only available IV. Usage is limited by variable hemodynamic effects including initial increase and subsequent decrease in heart rate and BP related to norepinephrine release and subsequent inhibition with hypotension being prominent. It is renally excreted with a half-life of 4–16 hours.

38.5
Class IV – Calcium Channel Blockers

The calcium channel blockers, mainly verapamil and diltiazem with antiarrhythmic effects, slow the inward calcium current during Phase 2 and 3 of the action potential. Calcium channels however contribute significantly to depolarization in SA nodal and AV nodal tissue. CCB's increase the action potential duration, and have a pronounced effect on AV nodal and less so SA nodal conduction. They are useful in reentrant tachycardias predominantly involving the atria and AV nodal tissue [63–65].

Calcium channel antagonists are now among the most frequently prescribed drugs for the treatment of hypertension. These drugs have also proved to be effective in patients with angina pectoris as coronary vasodilators, and left ventricular diastolic dysfunction. They act by blocking the transmembrane flow of calcium ions through voltage-gated L-type (slowly inactivating) channels [2]. The CCBs are classified into phenylalkylamines (verapamil), benzothiazepines (diltiazem), and the dihydropyridines (nifedipine) based on the three separate receptor sites they bind to on the L-type Ca^{2+} channels [66, 67, 68].

CCBs are nearly completely absorbed with oral administration. However, their bioavailability varies depending on first-pass metabolism in the intestinal wall and liver. They are oxidized to less active metabolites in the liver by predominantly the Cytochrome P-450

CYP3A enzyme subgroup. With the exception of diltiazem and nifedipine, CCBs are administered as racemic mixtures, with one active and one inactive stereoisomer with respect to blockade of L-type calcium channels. The cytochrome P-450 metabolizes each isomer at different rates, resulting in stereoselective drug clearance. The half-life of these agents varies from 1.3 hours to 64 hours [10] with verapamil and diltiazem having a half-life of 3–7 hours. CCBs demonstrate age-dependent pharmacokinetic changes in association with age-related reductions in hepatic blood flow, leading to changes in bioavailability and slowing of systemic clearance.

CCBs cause vasodilation and hence the resulting antihypertensive effects. The relative potency of CCBs as vasodilators varies with nifedipine being more potent as compared to verapamil or diltiazem. In vitro, several CCBs bind with some selectivity to the L-type calcium channel in blood vessels as opposed to verapamil which binds equally well to both cardiac and vascular L-type calcium channels [69]. All classes of CCBs depress sinus node activity, slow atrioventricular (AV) conduction and decrease myocardial contractility in vitro [70, 71] (Table 38.2).

Adverse effects of all CCBs include hypotension, peripheral edema, depression of cardiac function, and constipation. Headache, flushing, and dizziness can also occur. Verapamil and diltiazem should not be used in patients with bradycardia, atrioventricular dissociation, atrioventricular block, and sinus node dysfunction unless pacing back-up is readily available.

38.6
Cardiac Glycosides (Digoxin)

Digoxin inhibits the sodium/potassium ATPase [72–74]. This leads to decreased intracellular potassium, increased phase 4 slope of spontaneous depolarization and decreased conduction velocity [75]. The effects are also vagotonic with slowing AV node conduction and increasing the AV nodal refractory period [76]. Its main side effects are GI and CNS but more prominent concerns are the capability of triggering arrhythmias such as ventricular ectopy, junctional tachycardia, and heart block [77]. Digoxin is renally cleared with a half-life of 36–48 hours.

38.7
Adenosine

Adenosine is an endogenous nucleoside. Its effects are similar to acetylcholine [78, 79]. It decreases AV node conductivity. It is primarily used to break AV nodal re-

Table 38.2 Hemodynamic effects of calcium channel blockers

Vasodilatation of coronary and peripheral arteries and negative inotropic effects:
1. Decreased vascular resistance
2. Blood flow improvement
3. Peripheral: Nifedipine > Verapamil > Diltiazem
4. Coronary: Nifedipine = Diltiazem > Verapamil
5. Negative inotropic effects: Verapamil > Nifedipine > Diltiazem
6. AV nodal conduction slowing: Verapamil > Diltiazem >>> negligible Nifedipine contribution

entrant tachycardia although it can be diagnostic and therapeutic in clarifying any AV node-dependent arrhythmia by creating transient heart block by its rapid bolus administration. Its half-life is so short (10–30 seconds) that it can clarify atrial tachycardia, atrial flutter or terminate arrhythmias where the AV node is an obligatory part of the perpetuated circuit [80, 81]. Its main side effect is transient chest discomfort and bronchospasm. Its short half-life is ideal for treating AV node reentrant tachycardias since they can be quickly terminated without prolonged residual drug effect. It is also used as an infusion for pharmacologic stress nuclear studies since it is a strong coronary vasodilator.

38.8
Magnesium

Magnesium slows the rate of SA nodal impulse and prolongs conduction time. It is also used in treatment of torsades as well as prophylaxis for ectopic beats [82]. Deficiency of magnesium may cause a variety of arrhythmias including VT/VF, long QT with torsades de pointes, and atrial and ventricular ectopy [83]. Oral magnesium and potassium supplementation may suppress ventricular ectopy as in the study by Zehender [84]. Its mechanism of action is related to maintaining intracellular potassium as well as being linked with calcium metabolism.

38.9
Atropine

Atropine works as an anticholinergic/parasympatholytic agent, blocking the action of acetylcholine in the parasympathetic nervous system [85, 86]. It is useful for symptomatic bradycardias and asystole. It produces an increase in heart rate and inhibition of secretions, pupillary dilatation with blurred vision, and urinary retention and hesitancy. It is given as bolus IV injections and is frequently used for vagal reactions associated with hypotension and bradycardia [1].

38.10
Isoproterenol

Isoproterenol (Isuprel) stimulates beta1 and beta2 receptors and increases heart rate and cardiac contractility. It is a sympathomimetic amine structurally similar to epinephrine. It is used as an intravenous infusion for treatment of torsades and also atropine-resistant bradycardias until temporary pacing support is achieved [87]. It also produces bronchodilation, increased BP, and CNS excitability [88]. It is also used as a vasopressor in profound hypotension and shock.

References

1. Armstrong W, Clapham DE (2005) Pharmacology of cardiac rhythm. In Golan DE, Tashjian AH Jr, Armstrong EJ et al. (eds). Principles of Pharmacology. The Pathophysiologic Basis of Drug Therapy. Baltimore, MD, Lippincott Williams & Wilkins, pp. 267–284.
2. Atkinson AJ Jr, Kushner W (1979) Clinical pharmacokinetics. Annu Rev Pharmacol Toxicol 19:105–127.
3. Shanks RG (1988) How do pharmacokinetics relate to pharmacodynamics of antiarrhythmic drugs? Eur Heart J 9(Suppl B):51–56.
4. Vaughan Williams EM (1970) Classification of antiarrhythmic drugs. In Sandoe E, Flensted-Jensen E, Olsen KH (eds), Symposium of Cardiac Arrhythmias, Sodertalje, AB Astra, p. 449.
5. Vaughan Williams EM (1984) A classification of antiarrhythmic agents reassessed after a decade of new drugs. J. Clin Pharmacol 24:129–147.
6. Roden DM, Balser JR, George AL Jr, Anderson ME (2002) Cardiac ion channels. Annu Rev Physiol 64:431–475.
7. Whalley DW, Wendt DJ, Grant AO (1995) Basic concepts in cellular cardiac electrophysiology: Part I: Ion channels, membrane currents, and the action potential. PACE 18(8):1556–1574.
8. Whalley DW, Wendt DJ, Grant AO (1995) Basic concepts in cellular cardiac electrophysiology: Part II: Block of ion channels by antiarrhythmic drugs. PACE 18(9 Pt 1):1686–1704.
9. Grant AO (1997) Mechanisms of action of antiarrhythmic drugs: from ion channel blockage to arrhythmia termination. PACE 20(2 Pt 2):432–444.
10. Grant AO (2001) Molecular biology of sodium channels and their role in cardiac arrhythmias. Am J Med 110(4):296–305.
11. Kowey PR, Marinchak RA, Rials SJ, Barucha DB (2000) Classification and pharmacology of antiarrhythmic drugs. Am Heart J 140(1): 12–20.
12. Kowey PR (1998) Pharmacological effects of antiarrhythmic drugs. Arch Internal Med 158(2):325–332.
13. Woosley RL (1991) Antiarrhythmic drugs. Annu Rev Pharmacol Toxicol 31:427–455.
14. Nolan PE Jr (1997) Pharmacokinetics and pharmacodynamics of intravenous agents for ventricular arrhythmias. Pharmacotherapy 17(2 Pt 2):65S–75S.
15. Mehvar R, Brocks DR, Vakily M (2002) Impact of stereoselectivity on the pharmacokinetics and pharmacodynamics of antiarrhythmic drugs. Clin Pharmacokinet 41(8):533–558.
16. Sasyniuk BI, Ogilvie RI (1975) Antiarrhythmic drugs: electrophysiological and pharmacokinetic considerations. Annu Rev Pharmacol 15:131–155.
17. Tristani-Firouzi M, Chen J, Mitcheson JS, Sanguinetti MC (2001) Molecular biology of potassium channels and their role in cardiac arrhythmias. Am J Med 110(1):50–59.
18. Shorofsky SR, Balke CW (2001) Calcium currents and arrhythmias: Insights from molecular biology. Am J Med 110(2):127–140.
19. Roden DM, Woosley RL (1984) Class I antiarrhythmic agents: quinidine, procainamide and N-acetylprocainamide, disopyramide. Pharmacol Therapeutics 23(2):179–191.
20. Grace AA, Camm AJ (1998) Drug therapy. Quinidine. N Engl J Med 338(1):35–45.
21. Giardina EG (1984) Procainamide: clinical pharmacology and efficacy against ventricular arrhythmias. Ann NY Acad Sci 432:177–188.
22. Connolly SJ, Kates RE (1982) Clinical pharmacokinetics of N-acetylprocainamide. Clin Pharmacokinet 7(3):206–220.
23. Siddoway LA, Woosley RL (1986) Clinical pharmacokinetics of disopyramide. Clin Pharmacokinet 11(3):214–222.
24. Roden DM, Woosley RL (1986) Drug therapy. Flecainide. N Engl J Med 315(1):37–41.
25. Benowitz NL, Meister W (1978) Clinical pharmacokinetics of lignocaine. Clin Pharmacokinet 3(3):177–201.
26. Labbe L, Turgeon J (1999) Clinical pharmacokinetics of mexiletine. Clin Pharmacokinet 37(5):361–384.
27. Fenster PE, Comess KA (1986) Pharmacology and clinical use of mexiletine. Pharmacotherapy 6(1):1–9.
28. Kreeger, RW, Hammill SC (1987) New antiarrhythmic drugs: tocainide, mexiletine, flecainide, encainide, and amiodarone. Mayo Clin Proc 62:1033–1050.
29. Roden DM, Woosley RL. Drug therapy. Tocainide. N Engl J Med 315(1): 41–45.

30. Clyne CA, Estes NAM, Wang PJ (19992) Drug therapy. Moricizine. N Engl J Med 327(4):255–260.
31. Echt DS, Liebson PR, Mitchell LB et al. (1991) Mortality and morbidity in patients receiving encainide, flecainide, or placebo. The Cardiac Arrhythmia Suppression Trial (CAST). N Engl J Med 324(12):781–788.
32. Browne TR (1998) Pharmacokinetics of antiepileptic drugs. Neurology 51(Suppl 4): S2–S7.
33. Camm AJ (1984) Cardiac electrophsiology of four new antiarrhythmic drugs–encainide, flecainide, lorcainide and tocainide. Eur Heart J 5(Suppl B):75–79.
34. Funck-Brentano C, Kroemer HK, Lee JT, Roden DM (1990) Drug therapy. Propafenone. N Engl J Med 322(8):518–525.
35. Hii JTY, Duff HJ, Burgess ED (1991) Clinical pharmacokinetics of propafenone. Clin Pharmacokinet 21(1):1–10.
36. Upward JW, Waller DG, George CF (1988) Class II antiarrhythmic agents. Pharmacol Therapeutics 37(1):81–109.
37. Seth SD (1980) Antiarrhythmic action of adrenergic beta-receptor blocking agents. Pharmacol Therapeutics 11(1):159–179.
38. Frishman WH (1981) Drug therapy. Beta-adrenoceptor antagonists: new drugs and new indications. N Engl J Med 305(9):500–506.
39. Mehvar R, Brocks DR (2001) Stereospecific pharmacokinetics and pharmacodynamics of beta-adrenergic blockers in humans. J Pharm Pharmaceut Sci 4(2):185–200.
40. Pritchett AM, Redfield MM (2002) Beta-blockers: new standard therapy for heart failure. Mayo Clin Proc 77:839–846.
41. Woosley RL (1987) Pharmacokinetics and pharmacodynamics of antiarrhythmic agents in patients with congestive heart failure. Am Heart J 114(5):1280–1291.
42. Bauman JL (1997) Class III antiarrhythmic agents: The next wave. Pharmacotherapy 17(2Pt2):76S–83S.
43. Zipes DP, Prystowsky EN, Heger JJ (1984) Amiodarone: electrophysiologic actions, pharmacokinetics and clinical effects. J Am Coll Cardiol 3(4):1059–1071.
44. Kowey PR, Marinchak RA, Rials SJ, Filart RA (1997) Intravenous amiodarone. J Am Coll Cardiol 29(6):1190–1198.
45. Naccarelli GV, Wolbrette DL, Patel HM, Luck JC (2000) Amiodarone: clinical trials. Current Opin Cardiol 15:64–72.
46. Mason JW (1987) Drug therapy. Amiodarone. N Engl J Med 316(8):455–466.
47. Chow MSS (1996) Intravenous amiodarone: pharmacology, pharmacokinetics, and clinical use. Ann Pharmacotherapy 30:637–643.
48. Podrid PJ (1995) Amiodarone: Reevaluation of an old drug. Ann Internal Med 122(9):689–700.
49. Latini R, Tognoni G, Kates RE (1984) Clinical pharmacokinetics of amiodarone. Clin Pharmacokinet 9:136–156.
50. Desai AD, Chun S, Sung RJ (1997) The role of intravenous amiodarone in the management of cardiac arrhythmias. Ann Internal Med 127(4):294–303.
51. Nappi JM, McCollam PL (1993) Sotalol: a breakthrough antiarrhythmic. Ann Pharmacotherapy 27:1359–1368.
52. Hohnloser SH, Woosley RL (1994) Drug therapy. Sotalol. N Engl J Med 331(1): 31–38.
53. Khan MH (2003) Oral class III antiarrhythmics: what is new? Current Opin Cardiol 19:47–51.
54. Mason JW, Marcus FI, Bigger JT et al. (1996) A summary of the findings and conclusions of the ESVEM trial. Prog Cardiovasc Dis 38(5):347–358.
55. Pratt CM, Camm AJ, Cooper W et al. (1998) Mortality in the survival with oral D-sotalol (SWORD) trial: why did patients die? Am J Cardiol 81(7):869–876.
56. Kalus JS, Mauro VF (2000) Dofetilide: A class III-specific antiarrhythmic agent. Ann Pharmacotherapy 34(1):44–56.
57. Mounsey JP, DiMarco JP (2000) Dofetilide. Circulation 102(21):2665–2670.
58. Tsikouris JP, Cox CD (2001) A review of class III antiarrhythmic agents for atrial fibrillation: maintenance of normal sinus rhythm. Pharmacotherapy 21(12):1514–1529.
59. Kowey PR, Marinchak RA, Rials SJ, Bharucha D (1997) Pharmacologic and pharmacokinetic profile of class III antiarrhythmic drugs. Am J Cardiol 80(8A):16G–23G.
60. Howard PA (1999) Ibutilide: An antiarrhythmic agent for the treatment of atrial fibrillation or flutter. Ann Pharmacotherapy 33:38–47.
61. Murray KT (1998) Ibutilide. Circulation 97(5):493–497.
62. Gupta AK, Maheshwari A, Thakur RK, Lokhandwala YY (2001) Newer antiarrhythmic drugs. Indian Heart J 53(3):354–360.
63. Rapeport WG (1985) Clinical pharmacokinetics of bretylium. Clin Pharmacokinet 10(3):248–256.
64. Burgess CD (1981) Antiarrhythmic agents V–calcium blockers. Pharmacol Therapeutics 15(3):553–565.
65. Akhtar M, Tchou P, Jazayeri M (1989) Use of calcium channel entry blockers in the treatment of cardiac arrhythmias. Circulation 80(Suppl IV):IV31–IV39.
66. Abernethy DR, Schwartz JB (1999) Drug therapy: calcium-antagonist drugs. N Engl J Med 341(19):1447–1457.
67. Freher M, Challapalli S, Pinto JV, Schwartz J, Bonow RO, Gheorgiade M (1999) Current status of calcium channel blockers in patients with cardiovascular disease. Curr Probl Cardiol 24:236–240.
68. McDonald TF, Pelzer S, Trautwein W, Pelzer DJ (1994) Regulation and modulation of calcium channels in cardiac, skeletal, and smooth muscle cells. Physiol Rev 74:365–507.
69. Hockerman GH, Peterson BZ, Johnson BD, Catterall WA (1997) Molecular determinants of drug binding and ac-

tion of L-type calcium channels. Annu Rev Pharmacol Toxicol 37:361–396.
70. Kroemer HR, Echizen H, Heidemann H, Eichelbaum M (1992) Predictability of the in vivo metabolism of verapamil from in vitro data: contribution of individual metabolic pathways and stereoselective aspects. J Pharmacol Exp Ther 260:1052–1057.
71. Kelly, JG, O'Malley K (1992) Clinical pharmacokinetics of calcium antagonists. Clin Pharmacokinet 22:416–433.
72. Henry PD, Perez JE (1984) Clinical pharmacology of calcium antagonists. Cardiovasc Clin 14(3):93–109.
73. Mooradian AD (1988) Digitalis. An update of clinical pharmacokinetics, therapeutic monitoring techniques and treatment recommendations. Clin Pharmacokinet 15(2):165–179.
74. Smith TW (1985) Pharmacokinetics, bioavailability and serum levels of cardiac glycosides. J Am Coll Cardiol 5(5):43A–50A.
75. Rosen MR (1985) Cellular electrophysiology of digitalis toxicity. J Am Coll Cardiol 5(5):22A–34A.
76. Fozzard HA, Sheets MF (1985) Cellular mechanism of action of cardiac glycosides. J Am Coll Cardiol 5(5):10A–15A.
77. Hauptman PJ, Kelly RA (1999) Digitalis. Circulation 99(9):1265–1270.
78. Fisch C, Knoebel SB (1985) Digitalis cardiotoxicity. J Am Coll Cardiol 5(5):91A–98A.
79. Lerman BB, Belardinelli L (1991) Cardiac electrophysiology of adenosine. Basic and clinical concepts. Circulation 83(5):1499–1509.
80. Belhassen B, Pelleg A (1984) Electrophysiologic effects of adenosine triphosphate and adenosine on the mammalian heart: clinical and experimental aspects. J Am Coll Cardiol 4(2):414–424.
81. Camm AJ, Garratt CJ (1991) Drug therapy. Adenosine and supraventricular tachycardia. N Engl J Med 325(23):1621–1629.
82. Rankin AC, Brooks R, Ruskin JN, McGovern BA (1992) Adenosine and the treatment of supraventricular tachycardia. Am J Med 92(6):655–664.
83. Piotrowski AA, Kalus JS (20004) Magnesium for the treatment and prevention of atrial tachyarrhythmias. Pharmacotherapy 24(7):879–895.
84. McLean RM (1994) Magnesium and its therapeutic uses: a review. Am J Med 96(1):63–76.
85. Zehender M, Meinertz T, Faber T et al. (1997) Antiarrhythmic effects of increasing the daily intake of magnesium and potassium in patients with frequent ventricular arrhythmias. J Am Coll Cardiol 29:1028–1034.
86. Paraskos JA (1986) Cardiovascular pharmacology. III. Atropine, calcium, calcium blockers, and beta-blockers. Circulation 74(6pt2):IV86–IV89.
87. Gonzalez ER (1993) Pharmacologic controversies in CPR. Ann Emergency Med 22(2Pt2):317–323.
88. Morgan DJ (1990) Clinical pharmacokinetics of beta-agonists. Clin Pharmacokinet 18(4):270–294.
89. Easley RB, Rodbard D (1977) Noninvasive monitoring of beta-adrenergic tone during isoproterenol infusions. Clin Pharmacol Therapeutics 22(6):881–887.

Chapter 39

Coronary Angioplasty and Newer Interventional Strategies

Aravinda Nanjundappa, Pabitra Saha and Assad Movahed

Contents

39.1	History	463
39.2	Principle/Purpose/Technique/Types/ Equipment	464
39.3	The Technique of Angioplasty	464
39.4	Clinical Application/Indications for PTCA/Stent – Patient, Lesion, Device	465
39.5.	PTCA Devices	466
39.5.1	Complications, Follow-Up and Limitations	466
39.6	Newer Devices and Strategies – Atherectomy, Laser, Thrombectomy	469
39.7	Stent Versus Coronary Artery Bypass Graft Surgery	469
39.8	Future Trends	469
	References	469

39.1 History

Cardiac catheterization was initially attempted in cadavers around 400 BC. The first successful cardiac catheterization was carried out by Dr Werner Frossmann on himself in 1929 [1]. A catheter was self-introduced via the left anticubital vein into the right atrium at a small hospital in Eberswald, Germany. Dr Frossmann, an innovator, was clearly ahead of his time. Several decades later in the year 1958, Dr Mason Sones accidentally discovered that coronary arteries could be safely injected with contrast dye and studied [2] the coronary arteries at a Cleveland clinic in Ohio, USA.

Dr Charles T. Dotter, the father of interventional cardiology, pioneered the concept of transluminal angioplasty in 1964 [3]. Dr Dotter, working with Dr Melvin Jedkins at the University of Oregon in Portland, introduced the use of multiple catheters at increasing diameter to improve flow in the peripheral vasculature. This "Dotter technique" paved the way for the future development of coronary artery angioplasty. In 1967, Dr M. Jenkins perfected the transfemoral approach to cardiac catheterization called "Judkins technique" and today this is used worldwide [4]. Dr Andreas Gruntzig performed the first human coronary balloon angioplasty in 1974 [5] and by 1980 over 1000 angioplasties were documented in the registry.

The next decade saw the rapid development of the over-the-wire balloon, brachial guiding catheters, steerable guide wires and coronary atherectomy [6]. In 1986, the first coronary wall stent was implanted in France by Jacques Puel and Ulrich Sigwart [7]. From 1986 to 1993, the cardiology community experienced the invention, trial and perfection of innovative and niche devices in the field of interventional cardiology. Devices were made that attempted to reduce the plaque burden of the atheromatous plaque and improve arterial remodeling. Hot and cool laser ablation of the plaque and instent restenosis were promising technologies, however, they did not fare as well as expected. The rotational atherectomy devices (Rotablator [8]) and intravascular ultrasound [9] (IVUS) found their unique use in calcified arterial vasculature and evaluation of the lumen of the artery, respectively.

The turning point of interventional cardiology was with the introduction of stents and final FDA approval in 1994 [10]. The acute and chronic problems of stenting included subacute thrombosis and in-stent restenosis. Subacute thrombosis carries a high mortality while the in-stent restenosis causes angina, target vessel revascularization (TVR) and repeat procedures [11]. The parallel development of pharmacokinetics saw the rapid change in anti-platelet and anticoagulation therapy. Aspirin and unfractionated heparin has been the mainstay of percutaneous coronary angioplasty and stenting. The roller coaster ride of various combinations of drugs evaluated to deal with stent issues included dipyridamole, cilostazol, warfarin, subcutaneous heparin, ticlopidine and clopidogrel. Clopidogrel proved to be efficacious in reducing subacute thrombosis and in-stent restenosis with fewer side effects. Anticoagulation therapy in the catheterization laboratory also went through different doses of unfractionated heparin, use of low molecular weight heparin, IIb/IIa receptor inhibitors and direct thrombin inhibitors [12].

Despite several advances, the Achilles heel of angioplasty and stenting continued to be in-stent restenosis. Despite the revisit of niche technology like atherectomy, Rotablator, cutting balloon and laser use, restenosis was a nagging issue. Initial trials of brachytherapy showed favorable results, however, it did not turn out to be the mainstay in the treatment of in-stent restenosis.

The paradigm shift in interventional cardiology was the introduction of drug-eluting stents. Dr Eduardo Sousa and colleagues implanted the first human coronary drug-eluting stent in 1999 [13]. Subsequently in 2003 and 2004, FDA approved Sirolimus-eluting stents and tacrolimus-eluting stents. The restenosis rates were in single digits and reduced target vessel revascularization. The future of interventional cardiology involves the use of innovative nanotechnology for drug delivery and the concomitant pharmacology cocktail of antiplatelet and anticoagulants. The use of potent lipid-lowering drugs has shown promising adjunct to angioplasty in reducing the major adverse cardiac events.

39.2
Principle/Purpose/Technique/Types/Equipment

The main principle of angioplasty involves dilatation of the arterial stenosis to provide adequate blood supply in a safe manner to reduce angina and ischemia. The operator should pay very meticulous attention to patient selection, technique, treatment options available, pharmacotherapy and complications.

A thorough history and physical examination of every patient prior to angiogram or angioplasty is quintessential. A thorough history should include risk factors; previous angiogram/angioplasty procedures, list of medications, especially Metformin use, contrast allergy, history of bleed and allergies. The physical examination can help in evaluating fluid status, peripheral vascular disease, baseline neurological status and valvular heart disease. The physician should have access to recent laboratory work especially hematocrit, platelet count, prothrombin time and serum creatinine. A fully informed consent explaining the procedure, risks, benefits and all the possible complications in layman's terms must be explained to the patient and the family.

The pre-catheterization [14] screening should be able to determine the suitability of patients for coronary angiogram. Key issues are aspirin allergy, use of Metformin, and elevated prothrombin time for patients on warfarin, elevated creatinine, and contrast allergy. Aspirin desensitization, premedication for contrast allergy, intravenous fluid therapy with N acetyl cysteine therapy for elevated serum creatinine can help to prepare the patients for coronary angiogram and angioplasty. Diabetic patients who are on Metformin should stop use of Metformin 24 to 48 hours prior to scheduled coronary angiogram. All patients undergoing a diagnostic angiogram should have received aspirin, at least 81 mg.

39.3
The Technique of Angioplasty

Vascular access is best obtained percutaneously from a femoral artery, brachial artery, or radial artery. A modified Seldinger technique is the most commonly used method, and is described elsewhere [15]. The benefits and risks of angioplasty are determined by myocardial ischemic burden, coronary anatomy and patients' condition. An ad-hoc angioplasty or planned angioplasty at a separate time is determined at the end of diagnostic coronary angiogram. All patients scheduled for possible coronary angioplasty will receive a loading dose of 300 mg to 600 mg of clopidogrel [16].

Angioplasty and stenting are performed with six French sheaths in the majority of cases; seven French or eight French sheaths are required for complex cases, such as bifurcation lesions or those with tortuous anatomy. Intravenous heparin [17] is given at a dose of 100 units/kg bolus to achieve an activated clotting time (ACT) of > 300 seconds. An ACT of less than 250 seconds are associated with thrombotic complications while ACT>350 are associated with increased risk of bleeding complications [18].

The guide catheters are selected based on coronary anatomy and are tracked over a 0.035-inch guide wire. The stenoses in the coronary artery are crossed with a 0.014-inch steerable coronary guide wire.

An over-the-wire or rapid exchange balloon catheter is used to cross the lesion with the coronary guide wire positioned firmly in place. The balloon position is confirmed by injecting a small amount of contrast material. The balloon is slowly inflated over the secure guiding wire with a mixture of 50% contrast and 50% saline. The balloon is chosen on an approximation of 1:1 balloon to artery ratio or less [19]. The balloon is deflated and then withdrawn under fluoroscopy into the guiding catheter. A post-balloon angioplasty image will show residual stenosis, dissection, or a flow-limiting lesion. There is a direct correlation between the balloon inflation pressure and the outcomes of angioplasty. A repeat balloon angioplasty can be attempted or the operator may choose stent implantation.

The balloon catheter is withdrawn from the guiding catheter and a stent with 1:1 balloon to stent ratio is inserted over the wire. The length of the stent is determined by the lesion length and type of stent used. A short length bare metal stent is preferable (Fig. 39.1), while a longer length drug-eluting stent (Fig. 39.2) is advantageous to cover the lesion in its entirety. The stent balloon is slowly inflated to the deployment pressure designated by the company stent profile. The post-stent angiogram will show stent to artery ratio residual stenosis, distal flow and any obstruction of side branches by the stent, called "jailing".

Hemodynamic monitoring allows observation of the patient's response to angioplasty, and interrogation of the patient will aid in the demonstration of pain alleviation or worsening of chest pain. The stent, if needed, can be post-dilated to the appropriate size by a non-compliant balloon or a semi-compliant balloon to ensure adequate stent expansion and deployment.

Final angiograms are obtained after withdrawal of the wire, in two orthogonal views. Use of nitroglycerin intra-arterially in doses of 200 mcg is preferable to reduce spasm and improve coronary microcirculation. The angiographer analyzes the final angiograms carefully for edge dissections, loss of side branches, distal vessel perforations and distal flow. Intravascular ultrasound [20] (IVUS) use is optional to interrogate the vessel size, lesion length, severity of lesion, type of lesion, and calcification, and helps in balloon/stent sizing prior to PTCA. IVUS post-angioplasty/stent, can guide adequacy of angioplasty residual stenosis, plaque/atheroma volume, stent apposition and deployment.

The guiding catheters are withdrawn over a 0.035 inch guide wire, and activated clotting time (ACT) is checked. If ACT is <170 seconds the catheters can be safely removed with manual pressure applied to obtain hemostasis. The use of a percutaneous vascular closure device is optional and operator dependent. There is no advantage of a closure device over manual compression in terms of reducing the vascular complications, except for reduced time to mobility [21]. An ACT of >170 seconds requires suturing the sheaths to the skin and removal of sheaths when the ACT is less than 170. Special situations such as groin hematoma, obesity or co-morbid conditions that will prevent the patient being supine will require administration of intravenous Protamine. Protamine will reverse the effects of heparin and allow hemostasis with manual pressure or closure device.

The post-angioplasty orders should clearly indicate at least of 4 to 6 hours of bed rest after sheath removal to ensure hemostasis. Orders must indicate dual antiplatelet therapy with ASA and clopidogrel for all stenting cases, anti hypertensive and lipid lowering therapy. Diabetic patients should not receive Metformin for 48 to 72 hours post-contrast exposure and must have normal or baseline serum creatinine prior to restarting Metformin. Patients with a contrast allergy must continue to receive prednisone and antihistamine for 48 hours. Electrocardiographic changes are evaluated for signs of myocardial ischemia or infarction done post-PCI and at 24 hours. Serial cardiac enzymes at 6 hours and 12 hours post-procedure can identify post-percutaneous myocardial infarction and high-risk patients.

Percutaneous transluminal coronary angioplasty (PTCA) is considered a success [22] based on angiographic, procedural, and clinical criteria. Angiographic criteria mandates a residual of <50% lumen diameter if only balloon angioplasty or atherectomy is used and a <20% if stents are used. The procedural criteria incorporate successful PTCA by angiographic criteria plus no in-hospital major clinical complications (e.g., death, myocardial infarction (MI), emergency coronary artery bypass surgery (CABG)). A post- PTCA or stent patient should have creatinine kinase myocardial sub fraction (CKMB) less than three times the normal limit. Clinical success is based on patients being symptom free.

39.4
Clinical Application/Indications for PTCA/Stent – Patient, Lesion, Device

Coronary lesions have been classified by ACC/AHA [23] as type A, B, and C. The classification helps to determine the patient suitability, outcome and complications of angioplasty. Type A lesions have a high success with PTCA

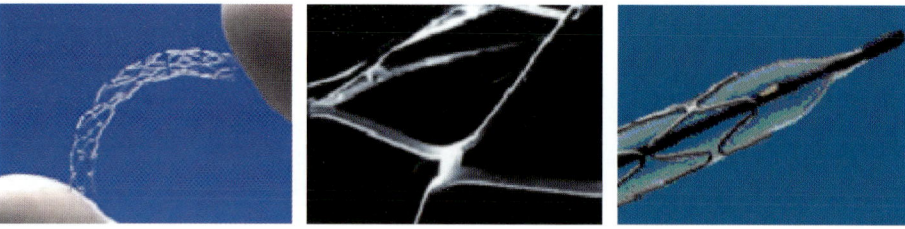

Fig. 39.1 Bare metal stent (Angioplasty.org)

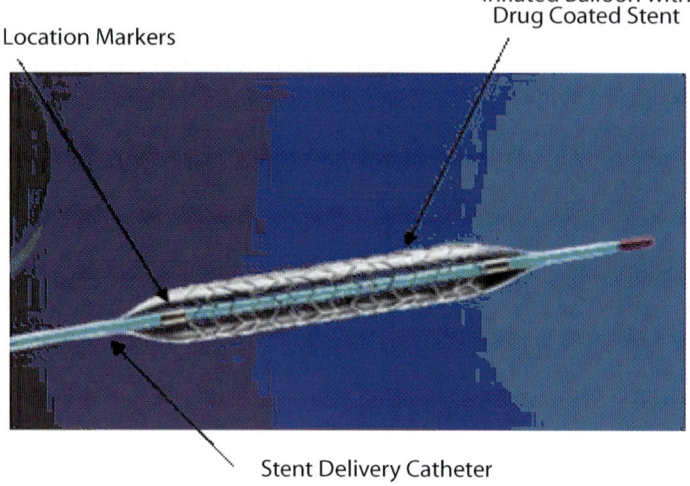

Fig. 39.2 Drug-eluting stent (www.fda.gov/cdrh/MDA/DOCS/p030025.jpg)

and carry low risk. The type B lesions have a moderate success with PTCA and carry moderate risk. The type C lesions have a low success with PTCA and a high risk in terms of complications.

The indications for PTCA [24] are based on several aspects: patient's chief complaint, symptoms, myocardial ischemic burden, severity of coronary lesions and left ventricular function.

1. A large area of viable myocardium involving one or two lesions in one or two coronary arteries and has low risk for PTCA in patients with
   - Asymptomatic ischemia or mild angina
   - Angina Class II to IV or unstable angina.
2. Myocardial infarction: ST segment elevation myocardial infarction (STEMI) presenting < 12 hours after the onset of chest pain:
   a. Primary PTCA has shown reduction in mortality and risk reductions
   b. Patients ineligible for thrombolysis
   c. Rescue PCI for failed thrombolytics
   d. Cardiogenic shock.
3. Non ST segment elevation myocardial infarction (NSTEMI):
   a. Catheterization or PTCA within 24 hours of presentation
   b. Patients who are symptomatic despite medical therapy
   c. Hemodynamically unstable patients.

39.5. PTCA Devices

Currently the management of coronary heart disease has become clearer and the field of modern interventional cardiology really began to take shape with new balloons and stents. Various types of PTCA devices are available (Table 39.1), however, there are advantages and disadvantages to these devices.

39.5.1 Complications, Follow-Up and Limitations

1. Vascular access complications [25, 26]: arterial access complications account for the majority of cardiac catheterization/angioplasty complications (Table 39.2).
   a. Pseudoaneurysm: The vascular puncture site, if accessed below the common femoral artery, po-

Table 39.1 Various PTCA devices

Balloons:
Non-compliant balloon
Semi-compliant balloon
Compliant balloon
Cutting balloon
Over the wire
Rapid exchange
Fixed wire system

Stents
Balloon expandable
Bare metal: open cell and closed cell design
Heparin-coated stents
Drug-eluting stents – sirolimus-eluting and tacrolimus-eluting
Self-expanding: Wall stent
Covered: Jo Med stent
Biodegradable
Atherectomy:
Directional coronary atherectomy (DCA)
Rotational coronary atherectomy (Rotablator)
Transluminal extraction catheter (TEC)
Silver hawk catheter

Laser:
Excimer coronary laser

Thrombectomy devices:
Export catheter
POSIS angiojet
X sizer
PRONTO catheter
Distal protection devices
EZ Filter
Guard wire
Spider Rx

Miscellaneous:
Transit catheter
Vascular coils
Quick cross catheter
Brachytherapy

Types of stents:
1. Balloon expandable
   Bare metal (Fig. 39.1)
   Coated
   Drug eluting – Cypher and Taxus (Fig. 39.2)
2. Self-expanding: Mostly used in peripheral arterial vasculature. Occasional use in saphenous venous grafts. Boston Scientific Magic Wall stent
3. Bioabsorbable stents

The bare metal can further be classified into open cell and closed cell design

---

tentates the occurrence of a pseudo-aneurysm (PSA) that manifests as a hematoma, tenderness and bruit on auscultation. A simple bedside duplex ultrasound will confirm the pseudo-aneurysm. Size of the aneurysm determines the treatment options. PSA smaller than 3 cm can be managed with ultrasound-guided compression. PSA larger than 3 cm warrants percutaneous ultrasound guided injection of thrombin and it can obliterate the PSA. Occasionally very large PSA requires surgical repair.

b. Retroperitoneal hematoma: An arterial puncture above the level of common femoral artery and a puncture that penetrates both the anterior wall and posterior wall of the artery can lead to a retroperitoneal hematoma. Hypotension, back or flank pain and significant decrease in hematocrit are the tell-tale signs of retroperitoneal hematoma. When suspected, aggressive fluid resuscitation, reversal of anticoagulation, type and cross for packed red blood cells and inotropes play a pivotal role

Table 39.2 Complications of PTCA

1. Vascular access complications
   (a) Psuedo-aneurysm
   (b) Vessel rupture
   (c) Groin hematoma
2. Coronary artery dissection
3. Coronary artery spasm
4. Coronary vessel thrombosis
5. Coronary artery occlusion
6. Coronary artery rupture
7. Pericardial effusion/tamponade
8. Myocardial puncture
9. Arrhythmia
10. Cerebrovascular accident and transient ischemic attack
11. Renal failure
12. Hypotension, volume overload and respiratory failure
13. Contrast allergy and anaphylaxis
14. Death
15. Restenosis

in stabilizing patients. Percutaneous evaluation of the arterial puncture site by contra lateral femoral access and balloon tamponade/coil Embolization/ covered stents can be useful in active bleed. If hemodynamically unstable, vascular surgical repair will be mandatory. Computerized tomography scan will demonstrate the presence of hematoma, however imaging should be carried out after the patient is hemodynamically stable.

   c. Vessel rupture: Arterial rupture is rare, however, can be fatal. Ballon tamponade/stent graft placement and surgical repair are life saving.

   d. Groin hematoma: Multiple access attempts, anticoagulation and coagulaopathy predispose occurrence of hematoma. A small size hematoma can be compressed manually and a large size hematoma may require drainage and vascular repair.

   e. Infection: Bacteremia, groin abscess, endocarditis are rare complications. Aggressive antibacterial regimen, endocarditis evaluation, surgical evacuation and repair can be beneficial.

2. Coronary artery dissection: Can result from catheter trauma, coronary guide wire injury, balloon angioplasty, stents and atherectomy devices. Simple dissections without flow limitations can be dealt with by medical management. Complex dissections with limitations of flow can be treated with prolonged balloon inflation, additional stent placement or covered stent use. Surgical bypass is warranted for symptomatic flow limiting dissections that fail percutaneous catheter based options.

3. Coronary artery spasm: The RCA, especially in females, is predisposed to coronary spasm. The consequence of the spasm can be a simple vessel narrowing to symptomatic myocardial ischemia. Various coronary vasodilators such as nitroglycerin, sodium nitroprusside, verapamil and adenosine are used to treat spasm. Rarely, additional stenting or coronary bypass has to be performed.

4. Coronary vessel thrombosis: Acute vessel thrombosis can occur due to vessel trauma, balloon angioplasty, and inadequate anticoagulation and in patients with hypercoagulability. Additional anticoagulation, use of intracoronary thrombolytics, adjunct balloon angioplasty, thrombectomy and aspiration can treat vessel thrombosis.

5. Coronary artery occlusion: Coronary vessel occlusion can occur due to spasm, dissection, vessel thrombosis and emobilization.

6. Coronary artery rupture: Treatment includes placement of covered stent graft with pericardiocentesis, coil, embolization and emergency vessel bypass.

7. Pericardial effusion/tamponade: Pericardiocentesis or surgical window for drainage can be beneficial.

8. Myocardial puncture: The incidence is extremely rare, carries a high mortality, and will need emergency open repair.

9. Arrythmia: Tachycardia, bradycardia, heart blocks, asystole and ventricular tachycardia. Anti arrhythmics, temporary pacemaker, atropine and revascularization can treat arrhythmias.

10. Cerebrovascular accident and transient ischemic attack [27]: Excessive catheter manipulation especially canualting by pass grafts and brachiocephaic vessels predisposes to a stroke. Catheter exchanges over a guide wire and use of five French diagnostic catheters can minimize the risk.

11. Renal failure: Contrast induced and atheroembolism are the leading causes [28]. Minimal use of contrast, adequate pre hydration and use of antioxidants can reduce the occurrence of renal insufficiency

12. Hypotension, volume overload and respiratory failure: Hypotension can result from various conditions, mainly hypovolemia, ischemia, reduced cardiac output, arrhythmias, and medication induced. Care should be taken to keep adequate volume status, evaluate and treat ischemia, manage co-morbid conditions such as aortic stenoses and appropriate treatment of arrhythmias. Volume overload can easily occur in patients with left ventricular dysfunction, ascites and patients with renal failure and those who receive a large quantity of contrast material and intravenous fluids. Judicious use of contrast, saline, inotropes and diuretics can prevent fluid overload. Respiratory failure is seen in patients with heart failure, asthma, allergy to medications, fluid overload and anaphylaxis. A pulse oxygen saturation assessment and close monitoring of respiratory status is mandatory. Use of bronchodilators, diuretics, ventilator support and epinephrine for anaphylaxis are beneficial.

13. Contrast allergy and anaphylaxis [29]: Allergic reactions can present as allergy, itching, rash and wheeze. Serious anaphylaxis manifests as hypotension, laryngeal edema and death can ensue if not promptly recognized and treated. Allergic reaction is treated with steroids, antihistamines and anaphylaxis requires epinephrine, fluids, respiratory support and inotropes.

14. Death: Although the incidence is extremely low, death can occur in elderly patients, those with associated co-morbid conditions especially aortic stenosis, acute myocardial infarction, or mechanical complications such as papillary muscle rupture and ventricular septal defect.

15. Restenosis: Continues to be an important downside of balloon angioplasty and stenting [30]. The rates

of restenosis with plain balloon angioplasty range from 20% to 80%. The rates for bare metal stenting vary from 30% to 50%, while the use of drug-eluting stents has reduced restenosis to <10%.

39.6
Newer Devices and Strategies – Atherectomy, Laser, Thrombectomy

The era of new devices in coronary interventions started in 1990. The following list illustrates a few of the devices available in the market.

Atherectomy: Various atherectomy devices aimed at reducing the plaque burden have been tried as a primary angioplasty tool or adjunct device.

Rotablator (Fig. 39.3): Rotational differential atherectomy

Directional coronary atherectomy

Laser atherectomy

Thrombectomy: Several thrombectomy devices aimed at removal thrombus material are available.

Export catheter: A simple six French compatible catheter, which narrows to a 2.8 mm flexible tip. The proximal tip has a beveled open edge that captures the thrombus, while the distal tip has a 20 cc syringe that is used as suction.

Pronto catheter: Works on the same principle as an export catheter except needs a seven French compatible catheter

Rheolytic thrombectomy: Here a turbulent jet of saline created by a hydraulic pump assists the mechanical thrombus removal and the negative suction vacuum extracts a larger thrombus. Several different sizes are available that can be used in coronaries, saphenous vein bypass grafts, arterial venous fistulas and peripheral arteries.

Rio aspiration catheter: The basic thrombectomy mechanism is similar to export catheter, however the distal tip has a smaller outer diameter and is more flexible.

39.7
Stent Versus Coronary Artery Bypass Graft Surgery

The role of stenting has rapidly expanded since the advent of initial coronary stent use in 1994. The unique role for coronary artery bypass graft surgery (CABG) continues to play a very important role in the care and treatment of patients with coronary artery disease. The most important indications for CABG [31] are:

- Patients with asymptomatic/mild angina/stable angina/unstable angina/ST segment elevation myocardial infarction
- Unprotected left main coronary artery disease
- Two vessel coronary artery disease involving proximal LAD and LCX with LVEF <50%
- Three-vessel coronary artery disease with left ventricular ejection fraction (LVEF) <50% and or large area of ischemia.

For patients with disabling angina despite optimal medical/percutaneous revascularization therapy, CABG can be performed with acceptable risk.

CABG can be used for patients with ST segment elevation myocardial infarctions who have failed angioplasty with persistent pain and hemodynamic instability.

39.8
Future Trends

The future of interventional cardiology is a rapid evolution of several innovative technologies and use of niche devices.

Cell transplantation therapy: Angiogenesis, myogenesis, and cell therapies are being investigated to improve left ventricular function in patients with ischemic cardiomyopathy.

Percutaneous bypass graft surgery: Percutaneous bypass graft surgery has found a place in patients with disabling lower extremity claudication who have failed percutaneous transluminal angioplasty and bypass surgery. A similar methodology for coronary artery disease is being pursued in the research arena.

Use of bioabsorbable stents with or without drug elution promises a novel treatment option without complications of in-stent restenosis and late stent thrombosis. Newer drug-eluting stents to reduce in-stent restenosis and improve long-term potency are being extensively researched. Magnetic resonance guided percutaneous interventions for safe precise angioplasty and stent deployment is underway. This will provide novel drug delivery to the plaque site via nanotechnology, to treat the plaque and reduce future cardiovascular events.

Percutaneous valve repair and valve replacements are being investigated in clinical trials for those patients who are at high risk for traditional open-heart surgery.

References

1. Mueller R, Sanborn T (1995) The history of interventional cardiology. Am Heart J 129:146–172.

2. Myler R, Stertzer S (1993) Coronary and peripheral angioplasty: historic perspective, in Textbook of Interventional Cardiology, Vol. 1, 2nd edn. Topol E (ed). WB Saunders Co., Philadelphia.
3. Dotter CT, Judkins MP (1964) Transluminal treatment of atherosclerotic obstructions: description of a new technique and preliminary report of its applications. Circulation 30:654–670.
4. Judkins MP (1967) Selective coronary angiography: a percutaneous transfemoral technique. Radiology 89:815–824.
5. Gruentzig A (1978) Transluminal dilation of coronary artery stenosis. Lancet 1:263.
6. Bittl JA (1996) Advances in coronary angioplasty. N Eng J Med 93:1621.
7. Sigwart V, Puel J, Mirkovitch V, Joffre F, Kappenberger L (1987) Intravascular stents to prevent occlusions and restenosis after transluminal angioplasty. N Engl J Med 316:701–706.
8. Ellis SG, Popma JJ, Buchbinder M et al. (1994) Relation of clinical presentation, stenosis morphology, and operator technique to the procedural results of rotational atherectomy and rotational atherectomy-facilitated angioplasty. Circulation 89:882–892.
9. Nissen SE, Yock P (2001) Intravascular ultrasound novel pathophysiological insights and current clinical applications Circulation 103:604.
10. Fischman DL, Leon MB, Baim DS et al. (1994) A randomized comparison of coronary-stent placement and balloon angioplasty in the treatment of coronary artery disease. N Engl J Med 331:496–501.
11. Rogers C, Edelman ER (1995) Endovascular stent design dictates experimental restenosis and thrombosis. Circulation 91:2995–3001.
12. Brodison A, Katiraa R, Moreb RS, Chauhana A (2000) Antiplatelet use in interventional cardiology. Postgrad Med J 76:70–79.
13. Sousa JE, Costa MA, Abizaid A et al. (2001) Lack of neointimal proliferation after implantation of sirolimus-coated stents in human coronary arteries: a quantitative coronary angiography and three-dimensional intravascular ultrasound study. Circulation 103:192–195.
14. Nedeljkovic Z, Dhadly M (2004) Introductory guide to cardiac catheterization. Circulation 110: e326.
15. Seldinger SI (1953) Catheter replacement of the needle in percutaneous arteriography, a new technique. Acta Radiol 39:368.
16. Hochholzer W, Trenk D, Frundi D et al. (2005) Time dependence of platelet inhibition after a 600-mg loading dose of clopidogrel in a large, unselected cohort of candidates for percutaneous coronary intervention. Circulation 111:2560–2564.
17. Popma JJ, Weitz J, Bittl JA et al. (1998) Antithrombotic therapy in patients undergoing coronary angioplasty. Chest 114:728S.
18. Wolfe MW, Roubin GS, Schweiger M et al. (1995) Length of hospital stay and complications after percutaneous transluminal coronary angioplasty: clinical and procedural predictors. Circulation 92:311–319.
19. Dirschinger J, Kastrati A, Neumann F-J et al. (1999) Influence of balloon pressure during stent placement in native coronary arteries on early and late angiographic and clinical outcome: a randomized evaluation of high-pressure inflation. Circulation 100:918–923.
20. Nissen SE, Yock P (2001) Intravascular ultrasound: novel pathophysiological insights and current clinical applications Circulation 103:604–616.
21. Applegate RJ, Sacrinty M, Kutcher MA et al. (2006) Vascular complications with newer generations of angioseal vascular closure devices. J Interv Cardiol 19(1):67–74.
22. Detre K, Holubkov R, Kelsey S et al. (1988) Percutaneous transluminal coronary angioplasty in 1985–1986 and 1977–1981: the National Heart, Lung and Blood Institute Registry. N Engl J Med 318:265–270.
23. Ryan TJ, Faxon DP, Gunnar RM et al. (1988) Guidelines for percutaneous transluminal coronary angioplasty. Circulation 78:486–502.
24. Smith SC Jr, Dove JT, Jacobs AK et al. (2001) ACC/AHA Guidelines for Percutaneous Coronary Intervention (Revision of the 1993 PTCA Guidelines). Circulation 103:3019–3041.
25. Popma JJ, Satler LF, Pichard AD et al. (1993) Vascular complications after balloon and new device angioplasty. Circulation 88:1569–1578.
26. Rihal CS, Sutton-Tyrrell K, Guo P et al. (1999) Increased incidence of periprocedural complications among patients with peripheral vascular disease undergoing myocardial revascularization in the bypass angioplasty revascularization investigation. Circulation 100:171–177.
27. Fuchs S, Stabile E, Kinnaird TD et al. (2002) Stroke complicating percutaneous coronary interventions: incidence, predictors, and prognostic implications. Circulation 106:86–91.
28. Rihal CS, Textor SC, Grill DE et al. (2002) Incidence and prognostic importance of acute renal failure after percutaneous coronary intervention. Circulation 105:2259–2264.
29. AHA (2005) AHA guidelines for CPR and emergency cardiovascular care. Part 10.6: Anaphylaxis Circulation, Dec 2005; 112: IV-143 – IV-145.
30. Holmes DR Jr, Vlietstra RE, Smith HC et al. (1984) Restenosis after percutaneous transluminal coronary angioplasty (PTCA): a report from the PTCA Registry of the National Heart, Lung, and Blood Institute. Am J Cardiol 53:77C–81C.
31. Rihal CS, Raco DL, Gersh BJ, Yusuf S (2003) Indications for coronary artery bypass surgery and percutaneous coronary intervention in chronic stable angina: review of the evidence and methodological considerations. Circulation 108:2439–2445.

Coronary Artery Bypass Surgery: Science and Practice

40

Michael W. A. Chu,
W. Randolph Chitwood Jr
and T. Bruce Ferguson

Contents

40.1	Introduction	471
40.2	History	471
40.3	Principles of Surgical Revascularization	472
40.4	Indications and Patient Selection	472
40.5	Preoperative Workup and Management	472
40.6	Surgical Techniques	474
40.6.1	Surgical Approaches	474
40.6.2	Conduit Selection and Preparation	475
40.6.3	"On Pump" Surgery	477
40.6.4	"Off Pump" Surgery	478
40.7	Intraoperative Assessment of Graft Patency	478
40.8	Expected Postoperative Recovery and Follow-Up	480
40.9	Outcomes	480
40.10	CAB vs Other Therapies for Ischemic Heart Disease	480
40.11	Future Trends	481
	References	482

40.1 Introduction

Ischemic heart disease remains the most common cause of death in developed countries. Significant advances have been made in the treatment of coronary artery disease (CAD), resulting in several options for medical, percutaneous and surgical therapies. The goals of treatment must be rigorously upheld when considering the optimal therapy for each patient with CAD, which include anginal relief, improved quality of life, freedom from cardiovascular complications and most importantly, prolonged survival. Despite current trends in percutaneous coronary intervention and the recent popularity of drug-eluting stents, the strongest, most robust evidence with the longest follow-up, still fervently supports coronary artery bypass (CAB) surgery as the gold standard therapy for left main disease, triple vessel disease and two vessel disease with proximal left anterior descending (LAD) artery involvement, especially in patients with diabetes and poor left ventricular (LV) function. Herein, this chapter will review the history of surgical revascularization, along with the clinical indications, preoperative evaluation, surgical techniques, conduit selection, expected postoperative course, complications and future trends in CAB surgery.

40.2 History

Coronary artery surgery is a relatively young field that has been continuously evolving since its inception only 100 years ago. In 1910, future Nobel laureate Alexis Carrel was the first to perform a coronary bypass by creating an anastomosis between the descending aorta and the left coronary artery using a carotid artery in a canine model [1]. Numerous indirect revascularization strategies were described by Claude Beck in the 1930s, which included abrading the epicardial surface of the heart and attaching pericardial, pectoralis or omental flaps to encourage neovascularization, partial ligation of the coronary sinus, and other indirect revascularization methods [2, 3].

In 1946, a Canadian surgeon, Arthur Vineburg, began to implant a pedicled internal thoracic artery (ITA) into tunneled myocardium [4]. This operation gained popularity over the next 20 years because of its success in relieving angina, and angiographic evidence demonstrating communications between the grafted ITA and the coronary vessels [5]. The development of selective coronary angiography by Mason Sones in the early 1960s led to the localization of obstructive atherosclerotic lesions [6] and was an important driving force in the development of direct coronary revascularization.

Over the next decade, a number of individuals, working largely independently from each other, made important contributions to the field of coronary artery surgery. Longmire was the first to report coronary artery endarterectomy without cardiopulmonary bypass (CPB) for ischemic heart disease; however, high mortality rates discouraged its widespread application [7]. The development of the Gibbon cardiopulmonary bypass pump ultimately facilitated the adoption of coronary surgery, which, in conjunction with the development of cardioplegia, created a still bloodless operative field in which fine, delicate anastomoses could be created. Debakey was the first to perform an aorto-coronary bypass with autogenous saphenous vein [8]. Murray and Demikhov did some pioneering work, independently of each other, in constructing ITA bypasses to the LAD artery in animal models. Although many different individuals may have performed the first LITA-LAD anastomosis in humans, most credit Russian surgeon Kolessov with this achievement, which he reported in 1967 [9]. At this point, most coronary surgery was sporadic; however, the pioneering work of Rene Favoloro at the Cleveland Clinic secured its place as 'mainstream' surgery when he began performing routine CAB grafting in 1968 [10–14]. Initially, the reversed saphenous vein graft (SVG) pre-dominated as the bypass conduit of choice because of its easy handling characteristics, availability and ease to harvest. However, important long-term follow-up from Loop, Green and others have consistently demonstrated superior patency rates and improved survival benefits from constructing a direct LITA-LAD anastomosis [15].

40.3
Principles of Surgical Revascularization

The main goal of coronary revascularization is to improve myocardial oxygen supply by increasing coronary blood flow in the setting of obstructive atherosclerotic CAD. Generally, this is accomplished by constructing bypass grafts or conduits that re-route blood from the ascending aorta or its branches, beyond the coronary artery blockages to a distal portion of the coronary vessel. Great care must be taken to perform these operations accurately and expeditiously to achieve the best short and long-term results, with minimal risks of morbidity or mortality. Successful surgical revascularization can result in relief from angina, relief from ischemia, improved quality of life but most importantly, prolonged life expectancy. Ultimately, these expected outcomes should be kept at the forefront when considering modifying current surgical techniques or exploring other methods of coronary revascularization.

40.4
Indications and Patient Selection

There is a wealth of data, including prospective, randomized trials along with observational data over more than 30 years, that support CAB surgery as the principal treatment of choice for extensive CAD [16–21]. In particular, the advantages of CAB surgery have been demonstrated for patients with left main disease, left main equivalent disease, triple vessel disease and two vessel disease with proximal LAD involvement. In addition, the survival benefit is particularly enhanced for patients with diabetes or LVEF < 50%. The most recent American College of Cardiology/American Heart Association (ACC/AHA) guidelines [22] are detailed in Table 40.1. Other contraindications to CAB surgery not listed in the table include ungraftable target vessels (target vessels <1 mm, transplant vasculopathy, etc.), lack of conduit, an actively bleeding diathesis or any other contraindications to systemic heparinization.

40.5
Preoperative Workup and Management

A thorough history and physical examination along with routine blood work, a 12 lead electrocardiogram (ECG), and chest radiography are performed initially to assess the patient's candidacy for CAB surgery. Selective coronary angiography is necessary to define specific lesion patterns and assess distal target adequacy to construct bypass graft anastomoses successfully (minimum target vessel diameter 1–1.25 mm, non-calcified and preferably non-diseased segment; normal or hibernating distal myocardium that would respond to being reperfused). Echocardiography can be substituted for left ventriculography in most cases, which reduces the amount of contrast exposure and decreases the risk of renal insufficiency. Transthoracic echocardiography (TTE) provides superior information regarding global left ventricular (LV) function and segmental wall mo-

Table 40.1 2004 ACC/AHA Guidelines for Coronary Artery Bypass Surgery

Indications	Class
Asymptomatic/mild angina	
Left main disease	I
Left main equivalent disease (proximal LAD, proximal Cx)	I
3VD ± EF < 50% and/or large area of myocardium at risk	I
Proximal LAD disease in 1VD/2VD with EF < 50% ± large area of myocardium at risk	I
Non-proximal LAD 1VD/2VD with large area of myocardium at risk	I
Proximal LAD disease with 1VD/2VD with low risk features	IIa
Non-LAD disease with low risk features	IIb
Stable angina	
Left main disease	I
Left main equivalent disease	I
3VD ± EF < 50% ± large area of myocardium at risk	I
Proximal LAD disease in 2VD with EF < 50% or demonstrable ischemia	I
Non-proximal LAD disease in 1VD/2VD with large area of myocardium at risk	I
Disabling, medically refractory angina	I
Proximal LAD disease in 1VD	IIa
Non-proximal LAD disease in 1VD/2VD with moderate area of myocardium at risk	IIa
Unstable angina	
Proximal LAD disease in 1VD/2VD	I
Non-proximal LAD disease in 1VD/2VD with moderate area of myocardium at risk	I
Persistent ischemia despite maximum medical therapy	I
Previous CAB surgery	
Disabling, medically refractory angina	I
Large area of myocardium at risk	IIa
Ischemic non-LAD territory with patent LITA-LAD graft without aggressive PCI/medical therapy	IIb
Contraindications	
Non-LAD disease in 1VD/2VD without symptoms or demonstrable ischemia	III
Borderline stenosis (50–60%) without demonstrable ischemia	III
Insignificant stenosis < 50%	III

Class I – Conditions for which there is evidence or general agreement that CAB surgery is useful and effective.

Class IIa – Weight of evidence or opinion is in favour of usefulness or efficacy of CAB surgery.

Class IIb – Usefulness and efficacy for CAB surgery is less well established by evidence or opinion.

Class III – Conditions for which there is evidence or general agreement that CAB surgery is not useful and in some cases may be harmful.

tion abnormalities, in addition to ruling out significant valvular or other structural abnormalities. If chest radiography or cardiac catheterization suggest aortic calcification, a non-contrast computed tomographic scan of the thoracic aorta may be helpful in identifying and characterizing the burden of aortic calcification that may complicate aortic cannulation, cross-clamping or other proximal bypass graft anastomoses. This preoperative screening, along with intraoperative epiaortic scanning may help to minimize the risk of perioperative stroke or other atheroembolic events. If a patient has experienced a significant preoperative myocardial infarction, as demonstrated by wall motion abnormalities, viability testing with a thallium scan, FDG-Positron emission tomography, dobutamine stress echocardiography or gadolinium-enhanced magnetic resonance imaging may be helpful to delineate whether revascularization is necessary. This is discussed in detail elsewhere within the textbook. Elective patients with significant pulmonary, gastrointestinal and/or renal disease require preoperative assessment to optimize respective organ function prior to surgery. Typically, all anti-anginal medications are continued to the morning of operation in order to mitigate anesthetic and surgical stresses. Emerging data suggests that statin agents may be protective [23]. Preoperative beta-blockers have been shown to be cardioprotective in CAB patients [24]. Some surgeons discontinue ace inhibitors 2–3 days in advance to minimize problems with vasodilatation when on CPB. Antiplatelet agents other than aspirin are generally held 4 days prior to operation in order to minimize risks of bleeding; aspirin may certainly be continued until the day of operation with little added risk. However, if clopidogrel is administered within 4 days prior to surgery, there is significant increased risk of bleeding, need for blood transfusion and reoperation for bleeding [25–27]. The beneficial effects of prophylactic clopidogrel for urgent patients en route to the cardiac catheterization lab with unknown coronary anatomy in anticipation of percutaneous coronary intervention (PCI) must be weighed against the risks of hemorrhage and its sequelae, if these patients are in fact cardiac surgery candidates.

It is now possible, and indeed highly advisable, to evaluate the perioperative risk of surgical intervention in essentially all potential candidates. The Society of Thoracic Surgeons National Database (http://www.sts.org) has an on-line risk calculator, as does the European Society of Cardiothoracic Surgery (EuroSCORE, http://www.euroscore.org/calc/html).

40.6
Surgical Techniques

Although the goals of CAB surgery are easily stated and clearly understood, the technical details of achieving revascularization can be complex and confusing. There are many different options in performing CAB surgery; however, it is probably best to understand that each patient can have their surgical approach tailored appropriately to their anatomy, left ventricular function, age and co-morbidities, to result in the best possible outcome with the least risk of morbidity and mortality. Modern techniques provide the surgeon with a well equipped arsenal to tackle a wide variety of clinical problems. For example, the best operation for a 45-year-old male with good targets and left main disease may not be the same operation as for an 80-year-old female with diffuse triple-vessel disease, a previous stroke, diabetes and renal failure. This section is subdivided into surgical approaches, conduit selection, 'on pump' and 'off-pump' CAB surgery.

40.6.1
Surgical Approaches

Perioperative anesthetic management has been greatly standardized, and ischemic and/or hemodynamic problems on stable patients are quite uncommon. However, more than 40% of patients in the USA who undergo CAB are classified as unstable based upon preoperative characteristics; thus careful preoperative management of these patients is mandatory to assure an optimal outcome. Standard intraoperative monitoring includes an arterial line, central venous and Swan-Ganz catheters, and often intraoperative TEE.

Standard surgical access to the heart has been through a median sternotomy, as this incision provides safe, simultaneous access to all cardiac chambers, the great vessels, and the epicardial coronary arteries. This approach provides standardized exposure to establish CPB, harvest and prepare the internal thoracic arteries and most importantly, construct the coronary bypasses. The sternotomy approach is by far the most common exposure of the heart performed today; however, modern minimally invasive techniques have been developed utilizing limited incisions that allow for the harvesting and preparation of the internal thoracic artery and exposure of the target vessel of interest through small thoracotomy incisions. A few highly specialized centers have achieved success with totally endoscopic coronary artery bypass (TECAB) techniques, whereby the entire bypass operation is performed with robotic assistance through port-access incisions only.

40.6.2
Conduit Selection and Preparation

There are a number of important considerations when selecting bypass conduits, which can be classified as follows: (1) general patient factors; (2) conduit-specific factors; and (3) coronary target specific factors. Table 40.2 addresses some of these considerations and provides some rationale into graft selection. In general, surgeons select conduits that are available, easy to prepare and use, have superior patency and ideally, improve life expectancy. Bypass conduits are harvested autologously and can be divided into arterial (LITA, RITA, radial arteries and gastroepiploic arteries) and venous (SVG, lesser saphenous vein, brachial or cephalic veins, and cryopreserved allograft veins) grafts. Arterial grafts typically have superior patency rates when compared with venous grafts, which may be attributable to a number of anatomic and physiologic differences between the two conduits.

40.6.2.1 Internal Thoracic Arteries

The internal thoracic artery has little vaso vasorum, but a dense, well defined, non-fenestrated internal elastic lamina and a thin medial layer with few smooth muscle cells. Its endothelium produces much higher concentrations of the vasodilators prostacyclin and nitric oxide than venous grafts. As a result, ITA grafts tend to have high flow reserve with low vasoconstrictor response, and high vasodilator sensitivity in addition to being resistant to oxidative stress and atherosclerosis [28]. Although great care is taken when harvesting the ITA, it is relatively resistant to surgical trauma when compared to venous grafts and is typically a good size match with coronary vessels. Follow-up angiography commonly demonstrates a patent LITA-LAD anastomosis with LITA dilatation to accommodate more flow to the LAD target.

The LITA graft is most commonly harvested in a pedicled manner, where the artery is prepared within a vascular bundle surrounded by endothoracic muscle and fascia. The LITA graft is pedicled on its origin from the inferior aspect of the subclavian artery. After systemic heparinization, it is divided distally beyond its bifurcation into the superior epigastric and musculophrenic arteries and blood flow is assessed. Most surgeons will also administer vasodilators, such as paperverine, to the graft to encourage vasodilatation and protection from spasm. The length of this graft can usually reach the most distal portions of the LAD, any diagonal branches, the ramus intermedius and proximal obtuse marginal artery branches. If the graft is too short to reach the distal target, the ITA can be skeletonized to provide more length, whereby the artery is dissected free of all muscle, fascia and the two associated internal thoracic veins. Some surgeons routinely skeletonize the LITA graft not only for length, but to better preserve chest wall collateral blood flow, which theoretically will encourage better sternal wound healing. If the LITA graft is injured proximally during its preparation, it can be used as a free graft, whereby the proximal end is attached to the aorta or as a side branch off another graft.

The right ITA (RITA) can also be harvested as a pedicled or skeletonized graft in a similar fashion to the LITA graft, and can often reach the proximal right coronary artery (RCA), proximal LAD or proximal circumflex distribution via the transverse sinus. Since the RITA has its best patency as a left sided graft, it is often used as a free graft in order to reach a distal circumflex territory target with the proximal end anastomosed to the LITA, a SVG or the aorta directly.

Evidence regarding the superior patency of ITA grafts over any other conduit or intracoronary revascularization mechanism is clear. Loop and colleagues first demonstrated 10 year patency rates of 90% [15, 29, 30], however, more recent studies suggested higher rates between 95 and 99% patency at 10 years [31–33] and 88% patency at 15 years [31]. The LITA graft is substantially resistant to atherosclerotic disease; thus early failures are usually a result of a technical complication. Late failures ('string signs') are due to poor runoff secondary to native disease, or to competitive flow in the coronary vascular bed. The RITA graft also has excellent patency rates when compared with venous grafts, but this is in part dependent on the territory grafted and the degree of stenosis. At 10 years, the RITA patency rates were 96% to LAD, 90% to circumflex artery territory, and 83% to the RCA territory [31]. In addition, long-term patency was much better when the stenosis was >70% [31,32].

The most persuasive information about the LITA graft is that unlike SVG or coronary stents, the LITA-LAD bypass is the only form of coronary revascularization that has been associated with improved early and late patient survival [15, 34, 35]. More aggressive approaches with bilateral ITA grafting, multi-arterial bypass grafting and total arterial revascularization may further improve the survival benefit of CAB surgery. Bilateral ITA grafting has been performed with excellent perioperative mortality rates [35–41] and retrospective results suggest improved long-term survival with bilateral ITA grafting over single ITA grafting [39, 40]. Controversy exists regarding whether bilateral ITA use is associated with increased sternal wound infections and dehiscence, especially in diabetic, morbidly obese and severe COPD patients. In general, most surgeons reserve bilateral ITA grafting for young, non-diabetic

Table 40.2 Considerations for conduit selection

Factors	Considerations	Ideal Conduit/Scenario
General patient factors		
Age	Young patients with long life expectancy	All arterial grafting – LITA, RITA, radials
Diabetes	May have ↑ risk sternal infections with bilateral ITA	LITA, radials/SVG*
Severe PVD	1) May have used or need SVG for ischemic leg 2) radial arteries may be diseased or inadequate	LITA, RITA, SVG
Previous SVG stripping	No SVG available	LITA, RITA, radials
Cardiogenic shock	Want quickest form of revascularization	SVG**
Aortic atherosclerosis/calcification	1) Risk of embolization with proximal anastamosis 2) calcification may be too dense to construct a proximal anastomosis	Use pedicled arterial grafts (i.e. LITA, RITA, GEA) or Y/T grafts (attach proximal end of free arterial graft to side of pedicled LITA)
Redo CAB	LITA, SVG used previously	RITA, radials/contralateral SVG
Conduit specific factors		
LITA	Best results	Graft to LAD or to largest territory at risk
RITA	May not reach distal Cx/RCA territories	Use as free graft or RITA-LAD, LITA-Cx
Radial artery	Arterial graft, likely requires vasodilators to prevent spasm	Use for Cx or RCA territory lesions with > 90% stenosis
SVG	Easiest for sequential grafting	LITA-LAD, SVG as sequential graft to lateral, posterior or inferior territories
Subclavian stenosis	Inadequate ITA flow & coronary steal	Contralateral ITA, radials/SVG
Size mismatch between conduit and coronary artery	May lead to early graft failure	Use smaller diameter arterial grafts
Coronary target specific factors		
Proximal LAD disease	LITA-LAD graft has best possible outcomes and best life expectancy	LITA
Stenosis > 90%	Can use any graft with good results	LITA, RITA, radials/SVG
Stenosis < 90%	Competitive flow decreases patency rates, especially radial arteries	LITA > RITA > SVG, best to avoid radial artery grafts
Poor targets – diffuse disease, small coronary vessels	Poor graft outflow predisposes to graft failure	ITA grafts most resistant to failure

* There is conflicting evidence on whether bilateral ITA harvesting increases wound infection rates in diabetics.

** This is controversial since there is evidence that supports the use of ITA grafting even in cardiogenic shock because of its life prolonging benefit.

patients with an appropriate body habitus. Total arterial revascularization is gaining popularity and appears to have good early results [41]; however, it is technically more demanding. Because the potential benefits would be derived from both the superior patency rates of ITA grafts and eliminating the poor SVG failure rates, total arterial revascularization patients may experience even better graft patency and further improved long-term survival [31, 33, 41].

40.6.2.2 Radial Arteries

Although early experience with radial artery grafts was unfavorable due to concerns about graft spasm due to the lack of appreciation of the thicker, more vasoactive medial portion within the vessel wall [42, 43], recent experience has been much more positive. Assessment of collateral ulnar flow is mandatory preoperatively to avoid hand ischemia. The radial artery is usually harvested from the non-dominant hand and can be dissected with the adjacent veins as one vascular bundle or can be skeletonized as with the ITA grafts. Modern harvesting techniques exercise great caution to avoid inducing spasm in addition to the routine administration of a vasodilating agent. The radial artery is used as a free arterial graft and is a good choice when considering multi-vessel arterial or total arterial grafting. Retrospective, observational studies have shown mixed mid-term patency results [31, 44, 45]; however, a prospective, randomized trial of 440 patients demonstrated 1 year patency rates of 92% in radial grafts versus 86% in SVG [46]. Further, 7% of the radial grafts did develop angiographic 'string' signs at 1 year. Most importantly, the study identified that radial graft patency was much higher when the bypassed stenosis was ≥ 90%, rather than <90%. Long-term follow-up will be necessary to assess the longevity of the radial graft. In summary, radial artery grafts are generally regarded as a good arterial selection; however, they should be harvested carefully and used to bypass coronary arteries where the native stenosis is ≥ 90%.

40.6.2.3 Saphenous Vein Grafts (SVG)

The reversed SVG was traditionally the graft of choice to perform CAB surgery because of its ubiquitous availability, ease of harvest, and predictability. Laboratory investigations show that SVG have poorly defined internal elastic lamina, a dependence on vaso vasorum, low levels of nitric oxide production and a high sensitivity to oxidative stresses [28]. After arterialization, SVG have poor compliance and are prone to early neo-intimal hyperplasia and the development of late atherosclerosis. In addition, SVG are the most common conduit with size mismatching problems when compared with the coronary target. Modern endoscopic techniques have resulted in the ability to harvest the entire SVG through small, tiny incisions, obviating the long, painful, saphenectomy leg incisions.

PREVENT IV is a recent study of over 3000 patients in the USA undergoing contemporary CAB [47]. This study documented a 26% combined (both arterial and SVG) graft failure rate at 1 year angiographic follow-up in 1800 patients. The adjacated myocardial infarction rate was 9.8%. These two complications were in contrast to the 1- and 2-year survival rates of 1% and 2%, respectively. While it is possible in this study that the graft failure rate was in part due to a Type 1 error in the study design, this 'high' rate may be attributed to technical issues, poor target vessels, poor distal run-off or competitive flow in vessels with <70% stenosis. Overall, historical SVG patency has been reported as approximately 50–60% at 10 years [15, 29–31]. Failure rates appear to be unrelated to the territory grafted, unlike arterial grafts. SVG stenosis or occlusion presents in two phases. The first is a proliferative intimal hyperplasia that tends to present early within the first 2–3 months after surgery. Histologically, it is a concentric, diffuse fibrosis that occurs within the wall of the SVG. The second and later presenting cause for SVG disease is graft atherosclerosis. It begins 3–4 years after surgery, depending on coronary risk factor control. Lipid infiltrates are found in areas of intimal fibroplasia. They are usually very friable and associated with mural thrombi. If these diseased grafts are manipulated with either redo bypass surgery or percutaneous coronary interventions, great caution must be taken to avoid embolization and subsequent myocardial infarction. Aggressive lipid lowering therapy and antiplatelet agents have been demonstrated to help slow the progression of SVG atherosclerosis [48–52], improve overall survival and reduce non-fatal cardiovascular complications following CAB surgery [53–55]. These observations are being tested in the current statin era; with contemporary efforts to use the 'teachable moment' for secondary prevention of CAD [56] these efforts may diminish the effect of vein graft atherosclerosis over time in these patients.

40.6.3 "On Pump" Surgery

In the USA, approximately 80% of CAB surgery is performed with the assistance of the heart lung machine or cardiopulmonary bypass circuit. In brief, cardiopulmonary bypass (CPB) allows the surgeon to operate on a still, non-beating, but metabolically protected heart while keeping the body perfused with oxygenated blood. A right atrial cannula draws blood by gravity into the venous reservoir, which is then pumped through a heater/cooler exchanger, a membrane oxygenator, a series of filters and then returned to the patient via a cannula in the distal ascending aorta. Although the details are outside the scope of this chapter, the conduct of the operation is generally as follows:

1. Establishment of safe general anesthesia and monitoring line placement
2. Conduit harvesting and systemic heparinization
3. Arterial and venous cannulation for CPB
4. Initiation of CPB and mild hypothermia (32–34°C)
5. Visual and manual inspection of the coronary arteries and targets (often the vessels are much more diseased than demonstrated angiographically)
6. Application of the aortic cross-clamp and diastolic cardiac arrest
7. Excellent myocardial protection with ongoing cardioplegia delivery to provide nutrient coronary flow and wash out metabolic waste
8. Construction of the distal coronary anastomosis
9. Construction of proximal anastomosis
10. Weaning from cardiopulmonary bypass when normothermic and recovery of LV function
11. Reversal of systemic heparinization and closure.

40.6.4
"Off Pump" Surgery

Despite continuous improvements in CPB, concerns about the deleterious effects of extracorporeal perfusion on organ function remain. Off pump (OPCAB) surgical techniques were developed to try to mitigate these harmful effects. In particular, major proposed benefits of OPCAB surgery have been decreased risk of neurologic injury including stroke, as a result of less aortic manipulation, and of acute renal failure, as a result of a loss of pulsatile perfusion in patients with hypertensive cardiovascular disease and renal disease [57]. In OPCAB, the heart remains beating and fully supports systemic perfusion; however, the target coronary artery of interest is stabilized and coronary flow is occluded or shunted temporarily at the site of the anastomosis to construct the bypass. In order to reach the posterior or inferior walls, the heart requires displacement out of its anatomic position either by elevating the apex out of the mediastinum or into the right chest. Resulting derangements in venous return, LV filling and subsequent cardiac output require attentive management and coordination with the anesthesia team, but this can usually be routinely accomplished by experienced teams. Contraindications to OPCAB include small diffusely diseased vessels, intramyocardial vessels, significant mitral regurgitation, and inexperienced surgeon and/or anesthesia support. Successful OPCAB surgery requires surgical dexterity, skill, patience, special instruments and successful navigation of a relatively steep learning curve [58].

Critics of OPCAB have argued that less precise anastomoses and incomplete revascularization are significant concerns because of difficulties reaching the posterior wall of the heart. In experienced centers, complete revascularization has not been a problem and early results from prospective, randomized trials have demonstrated similar graft patency and complication rates with OPCAB grafts when compared with conventional techniques [59, 60]. Although many studies have evaluated the beneficial effects of off-pump over on-pump surgery, most were underpowered and had retrospective designs, and when analyzed as a group, produced conflicting results [61]. Early observational studies suggested similar morbidity and mortality rates to conventional techniques [62–65], but more recent studies with results from centers further down the learning curve have suggested lower stroke rates [66,67] and a survival benefit with OPCAB [66–70]. Recently, the AHA suggested that patients can achieve excellent outcomes with either technique. They note that OPCAB is associated with fewer grafts but also with trends towards less blood loss and need for transfusion, less neurocognitive dysfunction and less renal failure [71]. Today, OPCAB is an important technique and may be particularly useful in patients with dense aortic atherosclerosis or pre-existing renal insufficiency.

40.7
Intraoperative Assessment of Graft Patency

Graft patency verification has become increasingly recognized as an important opportunity to improve the short- and long-term outcomes following CAB. Data from PREVENT IV demonstrated an association between perioperative myocardial infarction and less favorable long-term outcomes [72]. Intraoperative technical errors certainly contribute to early graft failures, but until recently use of technologies intraoperatively to evaluate graft patency has been sporadic. The techniques used in contemporary practice have recently been reviewed [73].

Intraoperative angiography in theory would be the 'gold standard' for graft patency, but with the increasing morbidity of patients coming to CAB and for logistic reasons, use of this imaging technology at a point in time where something could technically be done to correct an identified complication is limited. Recently, the use of intraoperative fluorescence imaging has been examined for use in the operating room [74–77]. This technology facilitates imaging of the graft conduit and the anastomosis; early studies have attempted to correlate flow in analogous fashion to TIMI flow in the cath lab. Although this technology cannot yet consistently identify minor, non-occlusive abnormalities, it has been demonstrated to be more sensitive and less susceptible to 'false positive' findings than other techniques. Moreover, excellent correlation of the intraoperative findings with early postoperative angiography has been demonstrated [77]. Finally, and perhaps of greatest interest, is the promise that this intraoperative imaging technology can be used to evaluate coronary perfusion at the regional myocardial level, perhaps quantitatively [78]. This would permit a novel, physiologic assessment of the benefit of surgical revascularization to be performed at the time of the procedure (Fig. 40.1).

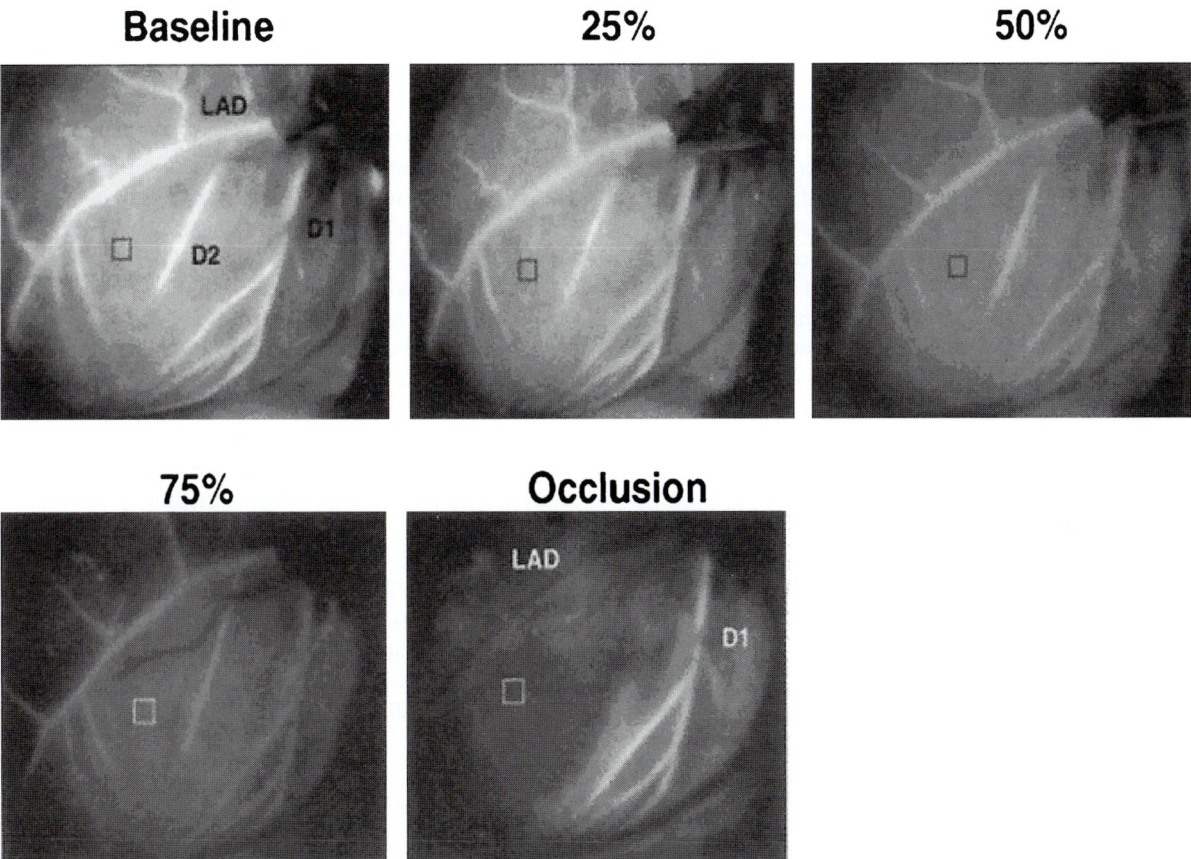

Figure 40.1 Intraoperative fluorescence imaging of the heart. Perfusion of the left ventricular anterior wall by gray scale imaging analyzed with background-subtracted peak fluorescence intensity in a representative animal experiment. The position and size of a typical region of interest used for the analysis are shown. After baseline, the LAD diameter was reduced progressively to produce four graded coronary stenoses (25%, 50%, 75% and 100% flow reduction). Occlusion of the LAD resulted in a total perfusion defect with no fluorescence intensity in the corresponding anterior myocardial wall, whereas the myocardial perfusion of the first diagonal branch D1 was preserved, showing normal perfusion (bottom row, Occlusion). From Detter et al. [78]

40.8
Expected Postoperative Recovery and Follow-Up

As mentioned, attention to postoperative secondary prevention therapy has been recognized as an important quality improvement opportunity in CAB. Antiplatelet therapy is restarted within eight hours of surgery (ASA), and on the first postoperative day for clopidogrel. In addition, B-blocker, Ace-Inhibitor and a statin therapy are indicated in CAB patients without specific contraindications to these agents and are started within 24 hours. Recently, Goyal et al., analyzing data from PREVENT IV, documented that CAB patients who received these four medications, where indicated, had a greater 1-year survival than those patients who did not receive the medication [79]. Strict glycemic control with regular hemoglobin A1c levels is paramount and can affect both early and late mortality.

Most patients can anticipate an overnight convalescence in the cardiac surgery intensive care unit (ICU), where they are recovered from general anesthesia and extubated, usually within 4 hours of surgery. In most patients, all invasive monitoring lines and chest tubes are removed within the first postoperative day. Patients typically experience a 3–4 day stay in a 'step down' unit, where they increase activity and have medications adjusted; however, this is largely dependent on their comorbidities and pre-operative level of physical activity. Most patients are expected to be ambulating well before discharge but are cautioned to observe sternal precautions for a minimum of 1 month to allow for adequate sternal healing.

After discharge, patients are re-evaluated by the cardiac surgery and cardiology teams in 4–6 weeks where a physical examination, chest radiography and 12-lead ECG are performed. Clinical symptoms drive additional investigations, which are typically unusual.

The most important patient-level determinant of long-term outcomes following CAB surgery is coronary risk factor modification. Targeted cholesterol levels and adherence to lipid lowering therapy are important for both graft patency and limiting progression of native coronary atherosclerosis. Blood pressure control is equally important and smoking cessation is imperative. In those patients with poor LV function, B-blocker and Ace-Inhibitor therapy can greatly impact both the symptoms of congestive heart failure and its associated mortality. Indeed, improvement in postop/preop ventricular function has been documented as the mechanism in part for the survival benefit associated with CAB [80]. Cardiac rehabilitation serves as an excellent opportunity to improve physical activity and obtain diet counseling following surgery. In addition, it provides patients with a good support and resource network, and reinforces important coronary risk factor modification as well.

40.9
Outcomes

Despite recent trends that demonstrate the higher risk profiles of patients presenting for CAB surgery, there continues to be a steady decrease in perioperative morbidity and mortality rates [18, 81]. These trends may be directly attributable to improvements in surgical techniques, myocardial preservation, perfusion technology, aortic imaging and perioperative medical care. In hospital mortality rates for isolated CAB surgery are 1–2% in most centers [18, 82], with low risk patients even reaching <1% [33, 57, 83, 84]. Most complications that occur following surgical revascularization tend to be related to advanced age or co-morbid disease, such as COPD, PUD and preoperative renal dysfunction. Other major complications that occur after CAB include perioperative myocardial infarction, stroke and neurocognitive dysfunction, acute renal failure, bleeding requiring re-operation and wound infection. There are risk assessment models for these major complications now available for program quality evaluations in the STS Database, and these complication rates are combined in the National Quality Forum Performance Metric Set for Cardiac Surgery [85]. Minor complications include low cardiac output syndrome and supraventricular arrhythmias. Measures that may help to prevent the devastating complication of stroke include preoperative non-contrast CT scanning, intraoperative TEE and epiaortic scanning, careful selection of arterial cannula, cardioplegia needle and proximal bypass graft locations, soft flow cannulas, non-pulsatile CPB flow and OPCAB techniques. If a stroke develops several days after the operation, it is usually related to uncontrolled paroxysmal atrial fibrillation and embolization of left atrial thrombus.

40.10
CAB vs Other Therapies for Ischemic Heart Disease

There have been a remarkable number of developments in the domain of ischemic heart disease therapy over the past 5 years, virtually all of which impact on CAB. The impact of stenting, and in particular the widespread adoption of drug-eluting stents, has resulted in a decline in the number of CAB cases at most centers between 10 and 20% over the past several years. While a discussion of all aspects of this controversy is beyond the scope of this chapter, several salient points can be made. This can best be discussed in terms of efficacy and effectiveness of alternative therapies. First, the efficacy of PCI vs CAB has been evaluated predominantly by industry-sponsored trials in patients with limited coronary artery disease; these trials assessed endpoints other than patient mortality, and indeed were all underpowered to assess mortality differences [86]. Typically, these trials randomized <10% of eligible patients, and the CAB cohorts from these trials had predicted mortalities of 1% or less (which is what was observed), and for which the benefit of CAB would be difficult to demonstrate (one- or two-vessel disease patients all with normal ventricular function). Second, these trials were unable to account for the rapid adoption of DES into the off-label population of patients with multivessel disease and greater degrees of ventricular dysfunction, which is the patient population in which CAB has been demonstrated to be of greatest benefit. Thus accurate comparisons between these patient cohorts is not supplied by the results of the published RCTs. Third, these trials didn't address the effectiveness of therapy for ischemic heart disease; effectiveness is tested in the real world based on inference from efficacy data; the impact of the COURAGE trial on referral patterns for cardiovascular investigation speaks to this [87]. Finally, data are accumulating from 'real-world' observational studies addressing efficacy that there is a statistically significant survival advantage as early as 1 year post-intervention when multivessel disease patients are compared between PCI and CAB. Data from four highly regarded registries that can statistically compare PCI vs CAB all document an excess of PCI with bare metal stents mortality vs CAB, with an increasing survival benefit out to 7 years [88-91] (Table 40.3). While these PCI cohorts received BMS vs DES, currently no data exist to demonstrate a survival superiority between multivessel disease patients undergoing BMS vs DES. Additional observational studies with DES PCI cohorts are pending.

40.11
Future Trends

These effectiveness comparisons mandate that studies and observational datasets continue to evaluate outcomes from these continually evolving technologies going forward. They also, however, demonstrate that peri-procedural outcomes are insufficient to fully evaluate the impact of these alternative therapies, and that future comparisons cannot forego comparisons across therapeutic domains (including medical therapy alone) in favor of comparisons with an earlier version of the same technology.

In the surgical domain, several important trends are evolving that will shape the future of coronary surgery. Multi-arterial grafting and total arterial revascularization have been performed with excellent in-hospital mortality rates and have demonstrated superior patency rates, which potentially will further improve long-term survival over single ITA grafts, SVG or coronary stents. Better preoperative coronary imaging with multislice computed tomography scans and magnetic resonance imaging may help with preoperative planning and better characterization of coronary disease patterns to plan more expeditious operations and appropriate graft selection. Improvements in perfusion technology, such as heparin-coated circuits, routine use of centrifugal pumps, and elimination of cardiotomy suction, continue to decrease its deleterious effect on organ function. Further work in stem cell therapy and angiogenesis may reveal a therapeutic role for concomitant surgical revascularization and direct interventions that may pro-

Table 40.3 Observational studies comparing long-term mortality in patients with significant coronary artery disease undergoing either PCI or CAB. Excess PCI mortality results from treatment with PCI in the setting where data indicate that CAB therapy would have yielded a better long-term survival. All studies used independent, sophisticated statistical methods to correct for baseline characteristics and propensity (total 32,237 patients).

Study	Excess PCI Mortality	Difference	Patients per 100 treated	Duration of Follow-up
Duke CV Database [88]	Yes	2.3%	2.3 pts / 100 treated	1 year
Cleveland Clinic [89]	Yes	4.3%	4.3 pts / 100 treated	3 years
NY State Registry [90]	Yes	5.1%	5.1 pts / 100 treated	5 years
NNE Consortium [91]	Yes	6.3%	6.3 pts / 100 treated	7 years

mote neovascularization and myocardial repair or regeneration. As the era of the SVG begins to fade, many of these patients will return in the following years with graft atherosclerosis and recurrent ischemia. When considering preoperative CAB surgery, we will have to be ingenious and aggressive about the most appropriate conduits to use in these redo patients to provide them with the best results based on our current knowledge of arterial grafts. As patients continue to seek less invasive alternatives, OPCAB, minimally invasive and totally endoscopic CAB techniques will have increasing roles. Already on the horizon are hybrid operations that take advantage of the superior patency rate and survival benefit of the LITA-LAD anastomosis via limited incisions and combine it with a PCI to a non-LAD lesion [92–94]. It is likely that the ideal therapy for CAD requires a collaborative effort from cardiology and cardiac surgery and must be tailored specifically for each patient, keeping in mind the ultimate goals of relief of symptoms, improved quality of life and prolonged survival.

References

1. Carrel A (1910) On the experimental surgery of the thoracic aorta and the heart. Ann Surg 52:83–95.
2. Beck C (1935) The development of a new blood supply to the heart by operation. Ann Surg 102:801–813.
3. Beck C (1937) Coronary sclerosis and angina pectoris: treatment by grafting a new blood supply upon the myocardium. Surg Gynecol Obstet 64:270–272.
4. Vineberg A (1946) Development of an anastomosis between the coronary vessels and a transplanted internal mammary artery. Can Med Assoc J 55:117–119.
5. Effler DB, Sones FM, Jr., Groves LK, Suarez E (1965) Myocardial revascularization by Vineberg's internal mammary artery implant. Evaluation of postoperative results. J Thorac Cardiovasc Surg 50(4):527–533.
6. Sones FM Jr, Shirey EK (1962) Cine coronary arteriography. Mod Concepts Cardiovasc Dis 31:735–738.
7. Longmire WP Jr, Cannon JA, Kattus AA (1958) Direct-vision coronary endarterectomy for angina pectoris. N Engl J Med 259(21):993–999.
8. Garrett HE, Dennis EW, DeBakey ME (1973) Aortocoronary bypass with saphenous vein graft. Seven-year follow-up. J Am Med Assoc 223(7):792–794.
9. Kolessov VI (1967) Mammary artery-coronary artery anastomosis as method of treatment for angina pectoris. J Thorac Cardiovasc Surg 54(4):535–544.
10. Favaloro RG (1967) Unilateral self-retaining retractor for use in internal mammary artery dissection. J Thorac Cardiovasc Surg 53(6):864–865.
11. Favaloro RG, Effler DB, Groves LK, Sones FM, Jr., Fergusson DJ (1967) Myocardial revascularization by internal mammary artery implant procedures. Clinical experience. J Thorac Cardiovasc Surg 54(3):359–370.
12. Favaloro RG (1968) Double internal mammary artery implants: operative technique. J Thorac Cardiovasc Surg 55(4):457–465.
13. Favaloro RG (1968) Saphenous vein autograft replacement of severe segmental coronary artery occlusion: operative technique. Ann Thorac Surg 5(4):334–339.
14. Favaloro RG, Effler DB, Groves LK, Fergusson DJ, Lozada JS (1968) Double internal mammary artery-myocardial implantation. Clinical evaluation of results in 150 patients. Circulation 37(4):549–555.
15. Loop FD, Lytle BW, Cosgrove DM et al. (1986) Influence of the internal-mammary-artery graft on 10-year survival and other cardiac events. N Engl J Med 314(1):1–6.
16. Hoffman SN, TenBrook JA, Wolf MP, Pauker SG, Salem DN, Wong JB (2003) A meta-analysis of randomized controlled trials comparing coronary artery bypass graft with percutaneous transluminal coronary angioplasty: one- to eight-year outcomes. J Am Coll Cardiol 41(8):1293–1304.
17. Brener SJ, Lytle BW, Casserly IP, Schneider JP, Topol EJ, Lauer MS (2004) Propensity analysis of long-term survival after surgical or percutaneous revascularization in patients with multivessel coronary artery disease and high-risk features. Circulation 109(19):2290–2295.
18. Hannan EL, Racz MJ, Walford G et al. (2005) Long-term outcomes of coronary-artery bypass grafting versus stent implantation. N Engl J Med 352(21):2174–2183.
19. Malenka DJ, Leavitt BJ, Hearne MJ et al. (2005) Comparing long-term survival of patients with multivessel coronary disease after CABG or PCI: analysis of BARI-like patients in northern New England. Circulation 112(9 Suppl):I371–I376.
20. Smith PK, Califf RM, Tuttle RH et al. (2006) Selection of surgical or percutaneous coronary intervention provides differential longevity benefit. Ann Thorac Surg 82(4):1420-1428; discussion 8–9.
21. Taggart DP (2005) Surgery is the best intervention for severe coronary artery disease. Br Med J 330(7494):785–786.
22. Eagle KA, Guyton RA, Davidoff R et al. (2004) ACC/AHA 2004 guideline update for coronary artery bypass graft surgery: a report of the American College of Cardiology/American Heart Association Task Force on Practice Guidelines (Committee to Update the 1999 Guidelines for Coronary Artery Bypass Graft Surgery). Circulation 110(14):e340–e437.
23. Clarke LL, Ikonomidid JS, Crawford FA et al. (2006) Preoperative statin treatment is associated wit reduced postoperative mortality and morbidity in patients undergoing cardiac surgery: an 8-year retrospective cohort study. J Thorac Cardiovasc Surg 131:679–685.
24. Ferguson TB Jr, Coombs LP, Peterson ED (2002) Society of Thoracic Surgeons National Cardiac Database. Preoperative beta-blocker use and mortality and morbicidty following CABG surgery in North America. J Am Med

Assoc 287:2221–2227 (Published correction in J Am Med Assoc 2002, 287:3212).

25. Chu MW, Wilson SR, Novick RJ, Stitt LW, Quantz MA (2004) Does clopidogrel increase blood loss following coronary artery bypass surgery? Ann Thorac Surg 78(5):1536–1541.

26. Yusuf S, Zhao F, Mehta SR, Chrolavicius S, Tognoni G, Fox KK (2001) Effects of clopidogrel in addition to aspirin in patients with acute coronary syndromes without ST-segment elevation. N Engl J Med 345(7):494–502.

27. Mehta RH, Roe MT, Mulgund J et al. (2006) Acute clopidogrel use and outcomes in patients with non-ST-segment elevation acute coronary syndromes undergoing coronary artery bypass surgery. J Am Coll Cardiol 48(2):281–286.

28. Motwani JG, Topol EJ (1998) Aortocoronary saphenous vein graft disease: pathogenesis, predisposition, and prevention. Circulation 97(9):916–931.

29. Fitzgibbon GM, Kafka HP, Leach AJ, Keon WJ, Hooper GD, Burton JR (1996) Coronary bypass graft fate and patient outcome: angiographic follow-up of 5,065 grafts related to survival and reoperation in 1,388 patients during 25 years. J Am Coll Cardiol 28(3):616–626.

30. Goldman S, Zadina K, Moritz T et al. (2004) Long-term patency of saphenous vein and left internal mammary artery grafts after coronary artery bypass surgery: results from a Department of Veterans Affairs Cooperative Study. J Am Coll Cardiol 44(11):2149–2156.

31. Tatoulis J, Buxton BF, Fuller JA (2004) Patencies of 2127 arterial to coronary conduits over 15 years. Ann Thorac Surg 77(1):93–101.

32. Sabik JF, 3rd, Lytle BW, Blackstone EH, Houghtaling PL, Cosgrove DM (2005) Comparison of saphenous vein and internal thoracic artery graft patency by coronary system. Ann Thorac Surg 79(2):544–551; discussion -51.

33. Tatoulis J, Buxton BF, Fuller JA, Royse AG (1999) Total arterial coronary revascularization: techniques and results in 3,220 patients. Ann Thorac Surg 68(6):2093–2099.

34. Dabal RJ, Goss JR, Maynard C, Aldea GS (2003) The effect of left internal mammary artery utilization on short-term outcomes after coronary revascularization. Ann Thorac Surg 76(2):464–470.

35. Cameron A, Davis KB, Green G, Schaff HV (1996) Coronary bypass surgery with internal-thoracic-artery grafts–effects on survival over a 15-year period. N Engl J Med 334(4):216–219.

36. Galbut DL, Traad EA, Dorman MJ et al. (1990) Seventeen-year experience with bilateral internal mammary artery grafts. Ann Thorac Surg 49(2):195–201.

37. Lytle BW, Blackstone EH, Loop FD et al. (1999) Two internal thoracic artery grafts are better than one. J Thorac Cardiovasc Surg 117(5):855–872.

38. Endo M, Nishida H, Tomizawa Y, Kasanuki H (2001) Benefit of bilateral over single internal mammary artery grafts for multiple coronary artery bypass grafting. Circulation 104(18):2164–2170.

39. Stevens LM, Carrier M, Perrault LP et al. (2005) Influence of diabetes and bilateral internal thoracic artery grafts on long-term outcome for multivessel coronary artery bypass grafting. Eur J Cardiothorac Surg 27(2):281–288.

40. Lytle BW, Blackstone EH, Sabik JF, Houghtaling P, Loop FD, Cosgrove DM (2004) The effect of bilateral internal thoracic artery grafting on survival during 20 postoperative years. Ann Thorac Surg 78(6):2005–2012; discussion 12–4.

41. Baskett RJ, Cafferty FH, Powell SJ, Kinsman R, Keogh BE, Nashef SA (2006) Total arterial revascularization is safe: multicenter ten-year analysis of 71,470 coronary procedures. Ann Thorac Surg 81(4):1243–1248.

42. Chardigny C, Jebara VA, Acar C et al. (1993) Vasoreactivity of the radial artery. Comparison with the internal mammary and gastroepiploic arteries with implications for coronary artery surgery. Circulation 88(5 Pt 2):II115–II127.

43. Acar C, Jebara VA, Portoghese M et al. (1991) Comparative anatomy and histology of the radial artery and the internal thoracic artery. Implication for coronary artery bypass. Surg Radiol Anat 13(4):283–288.

44. Acar C, Ramsheyi A, Pagny JY et al. (1998) The radial artery for coronary artery bypass grafting: clinical and angiographic results at five years. J Thorac Cardiovasc Surg 116(6):981–989.

45. Khot UN, Friedman DT, Pettersson G, Smedira NG, Li J, Ellis SG (2004) Radial artery bypass grafts have an increased occurrence of angiographically severe stenosis and occlusion compared with left internal mammary arteries and saphenous vein grafts. Circulation 109(17):2086–2091.

46. Desai ND, Cohen EA, Naylor CD, Fremes SE (2004) A randomized comparison of radial-artery and saphenous-vein coronary bypass grafts. N Engl J Med 351(22):2302–2309.

47. Alexander JA, Hafley G, Harrington RA et al. (2005) Efficacy and safety of edifoligide, an E2F transcription factor decoy, for prevention of vein graft failure following coronary artery bypass graft surgery: PREVENT IV: a randomized control trial. J Am Med Assoc 294:2446–2454.

48. The Post Coronary Artery Bypass Graft Trial Investigators (1997) The effect of aggressive lowering of low-density lipoprotein cholesterol levels and low-dose anticoagulation on obstructive changes in saphenous-vein coronary-artery bypass grafts. N Engl J Med 336(3):153–162.

49. Campeau L, Hunninghake DB, Knatterud GL et al. (1999) Aggressive cholesterol lowering delays saphenous vein graft atherosclerosis in women, the elderly, and patients with associated risk factors. NHLBI post coronary artery bypass graft clinical trial. Post CABG Trial Investigators. Circulation 99(25):3241–3247.

50. Sanz G, Pajaron A, Alegria E et al. (1990) Prevention of early aortocoronary bypass occlusion by low-dose aspirin and dipyridamole. Grupo Espanol para el Seguimiento del Injerto Coronario (GESIC). Circulation 82(3):765–773.

51. Gavaghan TP, Gebski V, Baron DW (1991) Immediate postoperative aspirin improves vein graft patency early and late after coronary artery bypass graft surgery. A placebo-controlled, randomized study. Circulation 83(5):1526–1533.
52. Stein PD, Schunemann HJ, Dalen JE, Gutterman D(2004) Antithrombotic therapy in patients with saphenous vein and internal mammary artery bypass grafts: the Seventh ACCP Conference on Antithrombotic and Thrombolytic Therapy. Chest 126(3 Suppl):600S–8S.
53. Knatterud GL, Rosenberg Y, Campeau L et al. (2000) Long-term effects on clinical outcomes of aggressive lowering of low-density lipoprotein cholesterol levels and low-dose anticoagulation in the post coronary artery bypass graft trial. Post CABG Investigators. Circulation 102(2):157–165.
54. Mangano DT (2002) Aspirin and mortality from coronary bypass surgery. N Engl J Med 347(17):1309–1317.
55. Bhatt DL, Chew DP, Hirsch AT, Ringleb PA, Hacke W, Topol EJ (2001) Superiority of clopidogrel versus aspirin in patients with prior cardiac surgery. Circulation 103(3):363–368.
56. Ferguson TB Jr, DeLong ER, Cowan R et al. (2007) Secondary Prevention Following Coronary Bypass Surgery: A National Randomized Trial. (Abstract). ACC LBCT II, Monday, March 26 2007. New Orleans, LA.
57. Hannan EL, Wu C, Smith CR, Higgins RSD, Carlson RE, Culliford AT, Gold JP, Jones RH (2007) Offpump versus on-pump coronary artery bypass graft surgery. Differences in short-term outcomes and in long-term mortality and need for subsequent revascularization. Circulation 116:1145–1152.
58. Ferguson TB Jr, Shroyer AL, Coombs LP, DeLong ER, Grover FL, Peterson ED (2003) Risk-adjusted mortality, revascularization completeness and the learning curve effect in off-pump CABG. American Heart Association Scientific Sessions 2003; Circulation Supplement 2003.
59. Puskas JD, Williams WH, Mahoney EM et al. (2004) Off-pump vs conventional coronary artery bypass grafting: early and 1-year graft patency, cost, and quality-of-life outcomes: a randomized trial. J Am Med Assoc 291(15):1841–1849.
60. Nathoe HM, van Dijk D, Jansen EW et al. (2003) A comparison of on-pump and off-pump coronary bypass surgery in low-risk patients. N Engl J Med 348(5):394–402.
61. Cheng DC, Bainbridge D, Martin JE, Novick RJ (2005) Does off-pump coronary artery bypass reduce mortality, morbidity, and resource utilization when compared with conventional coronary artery bypass? A meta-analysis of randomized trials. Anesthesiology 102(1):188–203.
62. Cartier R, Brann S, Dagenais F, Martineau R, Couturier A (2000) Systematic off-pump coronary artery revascularization in multivessel disease: experience of three hundred cases. J Thorac Cardiovasc Surg 119(2).221–229.
63. Kshettry VR, Flavin TF, Emery RW, Nicoloff DM, Arom KV, Petersen RJ (2000) Does multivessel, off-pump coronary artery bypass reduce postoperative morbidity? Ann Thorac Surg 69(6):1725–1730; discussion 30-1.
64. Dewey TM, Magee MJ, Edgerton JR, Mathison M, Tennison D, Mack MJ (2001) Off-pump bypass grafting is safe in patients with left main coronary disease. Ann Thorac Surg 72(3):788–791; discussion 92.
65. Aldea GS, Goss JR, Boyle EM, Jr., Quinton RR, Maynard C (2003) Use of off-pump and on-pump CABG strategies in current clinical practice: the Clinical Outcomes Assessment Program of the state of Washington. J Card Surg 18(3):206–215; discussion 16.
66. Racz MJ, Hannan EL, Isom OW et al. (2004) A comparison of short- and long-term outcomes after off-pump and on-pump coronary artery bypass graft surgery with sternotomy. J Am Coll Cardiol 43(4):557–564.
67. Sharony R, Bizekis CS, Kanchuger M et al. (2003) Off-pump coronary artery bypass grafting reduces mortality and stroke in patients with atheromatous aortas: a case control study. Circulation 108 Suppl 1:II15–II20.
68. Magee MJ, Jablonski KA, Stamou SC et al. (2002) Elimination of cardiopulmonary bypass improves early survival for multivessel coronary artery bypass patients. Ann Thorac Surg 73(4):1196-1202; discussion 202–3.
69. Mack MJ, Pfister A, Bachand D et al. (2004) Comparison of coronary bypass surgery with and without cardiopulmonary bypass in patients with multivessel disease. J Thorac Cardiovasc Surg 127(1):167–173.
70. Al-Ruzzeh S, Ambler G, Asimakopoulos G et al. (2003) Off-Pump Coronary Artery Bypass (OPCAB) surgery reduces risk-stratified morbidity and mortality: a United Kingdom Multi-Center Comparative Analysis of Early Clinical Outcome. Circulation 108 Suppl 1:II1–II8.
71. Sellke FW, DiMaio JM, Caplan LR et al. (2005) Comparing on-pump and off-pump coronary artery bypass grafting: numerous studies but few conclusions: a scientific statement from the American Heart Association council on cardiovascular surgery and anesthesia in collaboration with the interdisciplinary working group on quality of care and outcomes research. Circulation 111(21):2858–2864.
72. Magee MJ, Alexander JH, Hafley G et al. (2008) Coronary artery bypass graft failure after on-pump and off-pump coronary artery bypass: findings from PREVENT IV. Ann Thorac Surg 85:494–499.
73. Balacumaraswami L, Taggart DP (2007) Intraoperative imaging techniques to assess coronary artery bypass graft patency. Ann Thorac Surg 83:2251–2257.
74. Taggart DP, Choudhary B, Anastasiadis K et al. (2003) Preliminary technique with a novel intraoperative fluorescence imaging technique to evaluate the patency of bypass grafts in total arterial revascularization. Ann Thorac Surg 75:870–873.

75. Desai ND, Miwa S, Kodama D et al. (2005) Improving the quality of coronary bypass surgery with intraoperative angiography: validation of a new technique. J Am Coll Cardiol 46:1521–1525.
76. Desai ND, Miwa S, Kodama D et al. (2006) A randomized comparison of intraoperative indocyanine green angiography and transit-time flow measurement to detect technical errors in coronary bypass grafts. J Thorac Cardiovasc Surg 132:585–594.
77. Takahashi M, Isikawa T, Higashidani K et al. (2004) SPYTM: an innovative intra-operative imaging system to evaluate graft patency during off-pump coronary artery bypass grafting. Interactive CardioVasc Thorac Surg 3:479–483.
78. Detter C, Wipper S, Russ D et al. (2007) Fluorescent cardiac imaging: a novel itraoperative method for quantitative assessment of myocardial perfusion during graded coronary artery stenosis. Circulation 116:1007–1014.
79. Goyal A, Alexander JH, Jafley GE et al. (2007) Outcomes associated with the use of secondary prevention medications after Coronary Artery Bypass Graft Surgery. Ann Thorac Surg 83:993–1002.
80. Smith PK (2006) Presentation at December 7-8, 2006 FDA Circulatory System Devices Panel of the Medical Devices Advisory Committee (Transcript may be found at http://222.accessdata.fda.gov/scripts/cdrh/efdocs/cfAdvisory/details.cfm?mtg=672,
81. Estafanous FG, Loop FD, Higgins TL et al. (1998) Increased risk and decreased morbidity of coronary artery bypass grafting between 1986 and 1994. Ann Thorac Surg 65(2):383–389.
82. Birkmeyer JD, Siewers AE, Finlayson EV et al. (2002) Hospital volume and surgical mortality in the United States. N Engl J Med 346(15):1128–1137.
83. Taggart DP, Lees B, Gray A, Altman DG, Flather M, Channon K (2006) Protocol for the Arterial Revascularisation Trial (ART). A randomised trial to compare survival following bilateral versus single internal mammary grafting in coronary revascularisation [ISRCTN46552265]. Trials 2006;7:7.
84. Zhang Z, Spertus JA, Mahoney EM et al. (2005) The impact of acute coronary syndrome on clinical, economic, and cardiac-specific health status after coronary artery bypass surgery versus stent-assisted percutaneous coronary intervention: 1-year results from the stent or surgery (SoS) trial. Am Heart J 150(1):175–181.
85. NQF National Voluntary Consensus Standards for Cardiac Surgery (2005) . Washington , DC. NQF.
86. Taggart DP (2006) Coronary artery bypass grafting is still the best treatment for multivessel and left main disease, but patients need to know. Ann Thorac Surg 82:1966–1975.
87. Boden WE, O'Rourke RA, Teo KK et al. (2007) Optimal medical therapy with or without PCI for stable coronary disease. New Eng. J Med 356:1–14.
88. Smith PK, Califf RM ,Tuttle RH, Shaw LK, Lee KL, Delong ER, Lilly RE, Sketch MH, Peterson ED, Jones RH (2006) Selection of surgical or percutaneousl coronary intervention provides differential longevity benefit. Ann Thorac Surg 82:1420–1429.
89. Brener SJ, Lytle BW, Casserly IP, Schneider JP, Topol EJ, Lauer MS (2004) Propensity analysis of long-term survival after surgical or percutaneous revascularization in patients with multivessel coronary artery disease and high-risk features. Circulation 109:2290–2295.
90. Hannan EL, Racz MJ, Walford et al. (2005) Long-term outcomes of coronary artery bypass graft versus stent implantation. N Engl J Med 352:2174–2183.
91. Malenka DJ, Leavitt BJ, Hearne MJ et al. (2005) Comparing long-term survival of patients with multivessel coronary disease after CABG or PCI: analysis of BARI-like patients in Northern New England. Circulation 112: 371–376.
92. Katz MR, Van Praet F, de Canniere D et al. (2006) Integrated coronary revascularization: percutaneous coronary intervention plus robotic totally endoscopic coronary artery bypass. Circulation 114(1 Suppl):I473–I476.
93. Kiaii B, McClure RS, Kostuk WJ et al. (2005) Concurrent robotic hybrid revascularization using an enhanced operative suite. Chest 128(6):4046–4048.
94. Bonatti J, Schachner T, Bonaros N et al. (2005) Treatment of double vessel coronary artery disease by totally endoscopic bypass surgery and drug-eluting stent placement in one simultaneous hybrid session. Heart Surg Forum 8(4):E284–E286.

Minimally Invasive Cardiac Surgery

L. Wiley Nifong and W. Randolph Chitwood Jr

Contents

41.1	Introduction	487
41.2	Evolution of Robotic Cardiac Surgery	488
41.2.1	Level I – Direct Vision and Mini-Incisions	488
41.2.2	Level II – Video-Assisted and Micro-Incisions	489
41.2.3	Level III – Video-Directed and Port Incisions	489
41.2.4	Level IV – Video-Directed and Robotic Instruments	489
41.3	Clinical Applications/Patient Selection	490
41.4	Operative Techniques	491
41.4.1	Mitral Valve Surgery	491
41.4.2	Coronary Artery Bypass Surgery	491
41.5	Clinical Outcomes	493
41.6	Conclusion	493
	References	493

41.1 Introduction

Recently, interest in minimally invasive cardiac surgery has grown exponentially among both cardiac surgeons and their patients. This shift from traditional techniques can be attributed to expanding surgical technical capabilities, excellent clinical results, and expanding communication. Heretofore, traditional cardiac surgery has been performed through a median sternotomy, which provides generous exposure and easy access to all cardiac structures as well as the great vessels. Since the early 1990s, improvements in endoscopic technology and techniques, as well as surgeon education, have resulted in a substantial increase in the number of minimally invasive non-cardiac surgical procedures performed. In many specialties, endoscopic procedures are now standard. Until recently, a median sternotomy and cardiopulmonary bypass were required in most cardiovascular procedures due to the complexity of the operations. However, in the early 1990s, alternative, less traumatic methods for performing cardiothoracic surgery were developed. Initially, the minimally invasive direct coronary artery bypass (MIDCAB) provided a single vessel bypass on the anterior surface of a beating heart through a small anterior thoracotomy. The Port-Access™ (Cardiovations Inc., Somerville, NJ) method involved endoscopic cardiac surgery on an arrested heart using peripheral cardiopulmonary bypass and cardioplegic arrest methods [1, 2] Nevertheless, there were many limitations that precluded the widespread adoption of these methods. For example, standard endoscopic instruments, with only four degrees of freedom, reduced dexterity significantly. Working through fixed entry points (trocars), operators have to reverse hand motions (fulcrum effect) and at the same time, instrument drag induces the need for higher manipulation forces, leading to hand muscle fatigue [3].

Computer-enhanced or robotic systems have been developed to overcome these and other limitations resulting from traditional laparoscopic techniques. Systems can be classified according to the tasks they facilitate. The first group functions as an assisting tool for the surgeon and secures or positions instruments. The Automated Endoscopic System for Optimal Positioning (AESOP™ 3000, Intuitive Surgical, Sunnyvale, CA) is used to guide an endoscope. Using voice-activation, the surgeon can order the robot to hold a specific position within the operative field providing a steady view without tremor. The second group consists of tele-manipulators developed to facilitate fine manipulations by eliminating tremor and providing three-dimensional vision. Currently, there is only one commercially available tele-manipulative system, the da Vinci™ surgical system developed and manufactured by Intuitive Surgical, Inc. (Sunnyvale, CA).

The da Vinci™ surgical system is composed of three components; a surgeon console, a patient-side instrument cart, and a vision tower. The surgeon operates from the console using three-dimensional vision to affect simultaneous, filtered, and scaled movements at the patient side instrument cart that drives the tiny articulated intra-cardiac instruments. The operator becomes immersed in the topography of the heart. Furthermore, the finger and wrist movements of the surgeon are registered digitally, and these actions are transferred to the patient-side instrument cart, which operates the synchronous end-effector instruments. The seven degrees of motion are provided by the combination trocar-positioned "arms" (insertion, pitch yaw) and articulated instrument "wrists" (yaw, pitch, roll, and grip). A clutching mechanism enables re-adjustment of hand-positions to maintain an optimal ergonomic position relative to the visual field. Recently, high definition optics allow for digital zoom and high-power magnification (>15×).

41.2
Evolution of Robotic Cardiac Surgery

To perform minimally invasive cardiac operations, cardiac surgeons need to operate in restricted spaces, requiring assisted vision, and ever more complex instrumentation. Due to concerns over safety and operative quality, most cardiac surgeons have not embraced endoscopic techniques to date. Through our experience we advocate a progression through graded levels of difficulty to a progressive reliance on video assistance (Table 41.1). In this scheme, entry levels of technical complexity are mastered prior to advancing past small incision, direct-vision approaches (Level I), toward more complex video-assisted procedures (Levels II–III), and finally, to robotic cardiac operations (Level IV).

Table 41.1 Minimally invasive cardiac surgery

Level 1
Direct Vision
Mini (10–12 cm) Incisions
Level 2
Video-assisted
Micro (4–6 cm) Incisions
Level 3
Video-directed & Robot-assisted
Micro or Port Incisions (1 cm)
Level 4
Robotic Tele-manipulation
Port Incisions (1 cm)

41.2.1
Level I – Direct Vision and Mini-Incisions

Initially, minimally invasive cardiac valve surgery was based on modifications of previously used incisions and performed under direct vision. Most of these incisions were at least 10 to 12 cm in length. Surgeons found quickly that these incisions provided adequate exposure of the mitral and aortic valve. Using mini-sternal or para-sternal incisions, Cohn, Cosgrove, and Arom independently showed encouraging results with low surgical mortalities (1–3%) and complication rates comparable with conventional mitral valve surgery [4–8]. During the same time period, the first minimally invasive mitral valve replacements were performed by the Stanford group using intra-aortic balloon occlusion, called Port-access™ methods and with cardioplegia (CardioVations, Summerville, NJ). Port-access™ methods were also utilized for coronary artery bypass operations [9, 10]. Both modified sternal and Port-access™ direct vision methods (Level I) have been successful in large numbers of patients. [11–13]. Most Level I operations have been done using modifications of conventional perfusion and instrumentation methods. When intra-aortic balloon occluders are added, significant cost increases have been incurred. Therefore, a transthoracic aortic cross clamp (Scanlan International, Minneapolis, MN) has been the most reasonable solution for economic, safe, limited-access aortic occlusion (Fig. 41.1).

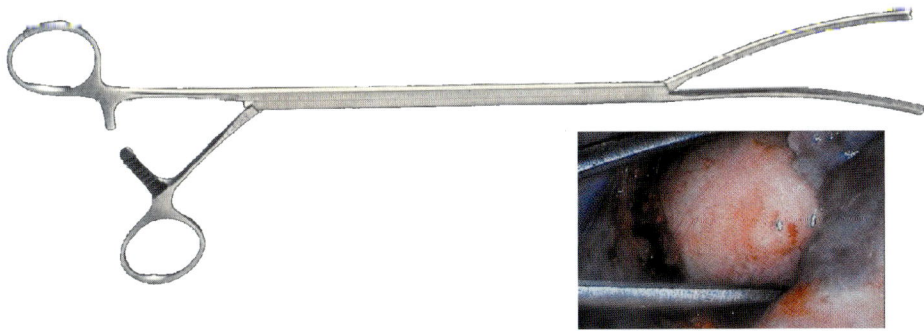

Fig. 41.1 Chitwood transthoracic aortic clamp™ (Scanlan International, Inc. Minneapolis, MN). The instrument is passed through the chest wall in the third intercostal space. Correct orientation is required to avoid injury to vital structures; therefore, the posterior or fixed prong is passed under videoscopic control through the transverse sinus. The anterior prong passes across the anterior aorta

41.2.2
Level II – Video-Assisted and Micro-Incisions

Video assistance implies that 50 to 70% of the operation has been done while viewing a two-dimensional monitor screen, and micro-incisions are considered to be 4 to 6 cm skin incisions. Video assistance was first used for closed chest internal mammary artery harvests and congenital heart operations [14–16]. In February 1996, Carpentier performed the first video-assisted mitral valve repair via a min-thoracotomy using cold ventricular fibrillation [17]. Three months later, the authors' group performed a mitral valve replacement using a micro-incision, videoscopic vision, percutaneous transthoracic aortic clamp, and retrograde cardioplegia. This work demonstrated that mitral valve repairs were possible with no major complications and mortality less than 1% [18–20].

41.2.3
Level III – Video-Directed and Port Incisions

In 1997, with the assistance of AESOP™ 3000 cardiac surgery entered the robotic age and allowed smaller incisions with better mitral valve and subvalvular visualization. In early June of 1998, the authors' group performed the first video-directed mitral operation in the USA using the voice-controlled Aesop 3000™ robot and a Vista™ three-dimensional camera [19]. Visual accuracy was improved by operating surgeon camera voice manipulation. Along with others, we found that camera motion was smoother, more predictable, with no tremor, and that less lens cleaning was required. The addition of voice-activated robotic camera control was responsible for decreased operative, perfusion, and cardiac arrest times [19, 21].

Surgeons began to also use voice-activated robotic camera control to harvest internal mammary arteries with excellent facility and less patient trauma than experienced by conventional means [15]. However, early attempts at coronary revascularization with long instruments through small incisions proved futile. The addition of three-dimensional visualization, robotic camera control, and instrument tip articulation were the next essential steps toward a totally endoscopic procedure where wrist-like instruments and three-dimensional vision could transpose surgical manipulations from outside the chest wall to within the closed mediastinum. With advancing technology toward more computer enhanced tele-manipulative systems, production of voice-activated "holding" devices has now ceased.

41.2.4
Level IV – Video-Directed and Robotic Instruments

In 1998, Carpentier performed the first mitral valve repair using an early prototype of the da Vinci™ surgical system [22]. Two years later [23], the authors' group performed the first complete repair of a mitral valve in North America using the da Vinci™ system. Subsequently, we have performed over 325 mitral valve procedures. Complex mitral repairs can be done with reasonable cross clamp and perfusion times as well as excellent midterm results. Early in our experience simple mitral repairs were done including annuloplasty band insertion and leaflet resections (Fig. 41.2a and 41.2b). After mastering these techniques we progressed to leaflet resections with sliding valvuloplastes and chordal procedures. Further advancement led to the successful repair of both anterior leaflet disease and Barlow's (bileaflet) valves. Most recently, experience has led to development of the "haircut" procedure in which leaflet resections are done at the coapting edge of the posterior mitral leaflet followed by chordal re-attachments. This precludes work at the annular level. Advancements have progressed to a point where totally endoscopic mitral procedures are feasible.

In May of 1998, Mohr and Falk harvested the left internal mammary artery (LIMA) with the da Vinci™ system and performed the first human coronary anastomosis through a small left anterior thoracotomy incision [24, 25]. The first totally endoscopic coronary artery bypass (TECAB) was performed on an arrested heart at the Broussais Hospital in Paris [26] using an early prototype of the da Vinci™ system. The Leipzig group attempted a total closed chest approach for LIMA to left anterior descending coronary artery (LAD) grafting on the arrested heart in 27 patients and were successful in 22 [27]. Furthermore, surgeons in Europe improved the initial da Vinci™ coronary method and eventually were able to complete bilateral internal mammary artery grafts off-pump to the anterior descending and right coronary arteries while working from one side of the chest [28, 29].

41.3
Clinical Applications/Patient Selection

Early in the development of any minimally invasive cardiac surgery program, strict inclusion and exclusion criteria should be followed (Table 41.2). In initial experience with robotic mitral repairs, all patients had isolated mitral insufficiency. Patients with a previous right thoracotomy were excluded from the da Vinci™ procedures; however, we now approach these patients with a video-assisted mitral valve operation. Patients with severely calcified mitral annulus are not candidates. Decalcification requires further instrument development as well as a reliable means to evacuate any calcium that may fall into the left ventricle. Patients with mitral valve stenosis were excluded in the early FDA trials; however, patients treatable by commissurotomy are suitable candidates for robotic repair. The improved visualization of the valve and subvalvular apparatus along with the maneuverability of bladed micro-instruments facilitate performance of a commissurotomy.

As previously discussed, early efforts at totally endoscopic coronary surgery using conventional instruments were discouraging and were hampered with imprecision and two-dimensional visualization. With the development of computer-assisted telemanipulation systems and three-dimensional visualization, TECAB has not only become feasible but has also been demonstrated to be safe as well. Nevertheless, with current technology, these operations are usually performed on single vessel (LAD) disease with either an arrested heart using the Port-Access™ system, or a beating heart using specially designed endoscopic stabilizers. Table 41.3 lists common exclusion criteria for TECAB.

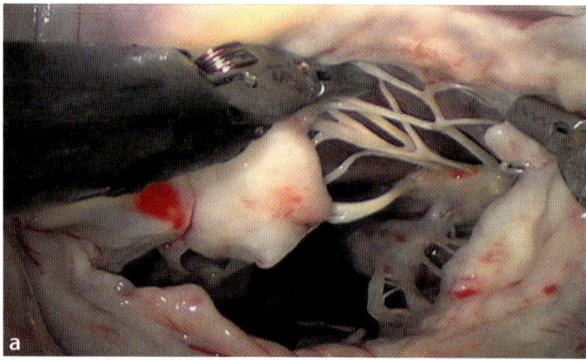
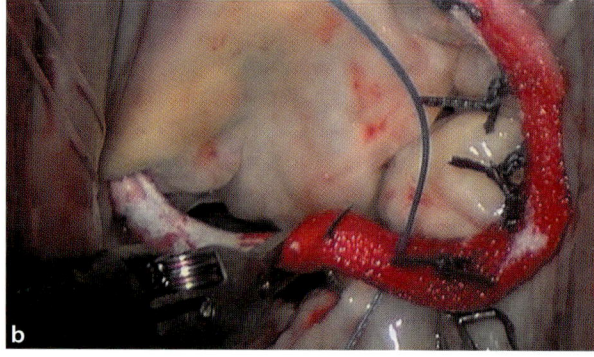

Fig. 41.2 **a** Visualization of chords traversing from papillary muscles within the left ventricular cavity to mitral valve leaflets. **b** Each repair is concluded with an annuloplasty (Cosgrove Annuloplasty™, Edwards LifeSciences, Inc., Irvine, CA). The band is removed from the traditional holder and passed into the left atrium. Furthermore, all knots are tied intracorporeal

Table 41.2 Robotic mitral surgery exclusion criteria

Previous right thoracotomy
- Renal failure
- Liver dysfunction
- Bleeding disorders
- Pulmonary hypertension (PAS > 60 torr)
- Significant aortic or tricuspid valve disease
- Coronary artery disease requiring surgery
- Recent myocardial ischemia (< 30 days)
- Recent stroke (< 30 days)
- Severely calcified mitral valve annulus
- A body mass index (BMI) > 35 kg/m^2

Table 41.3 Robotically assisted coronary artery bypass surgery exclusion criteria

1. Patients older than 80 years.
2. Patients with ejection fraction of 40% or less.
3. Severe noncardiac conditions.
4. Severe peripheral vascular disease.
5. Myocardial infarction within 7 days before procedure.
6. Patients undergoing concomitant surgery, emergency surgery, or who have had previous thoracic surgery.
7. Calcified or diffuse disease in the left anterior descending coronary artery.
8. Patients participating in other investigational device or drug studies.

41.4
Operative Techniques

41.4.1
Mitral Valve Surgery

Pre- and post-operative surface and trans-esophageal echocardiographic (TEE) studies are performed. Cardiopulmonary bypass is established using femoral arterial inflow and venous drainage through the femoral and right internal jugular veins. A 3 cm working incision is made in the 4th intercostal space (ICS) to provide cardiac access and placement of the camera for the robotic system. The pericardium is opened either under direct vision or with the robotic system 2–3 cm anterior to the phrenic nerve. Antegrade cardioplegia is given by an aortic needle/vent placed either under direct vision or videoscopically. To minimize intracardiac air entrainment, the thoracic cavity is flooded continuously with carbon dioxide at 1–2 L/min. A transthoracic aortic cross-clamp (Scanlan International, Inc., Minneapolis, MN) is positioned via a 4 mm incision in the 3rd ICS and intermittent antegrade cold blood cardioplegia maintains cardiac arrest and myocardial protection. Positions for da Vinci™ left and right arm port incisions are determined. The right trocar is placed in the 5th ICS posterior-lateral to the working incision and parallel to the right superior pulmonary vein. The left trocar generally is placed 6 cm cephalad and medial to the right trocar, insuring internal clearance between arms to avoid both external and internal conflicts. Optimal robotic arm convergence avoids left atrial wall tearing during instrument manipulations. The working incision is used as a working port for the assistant. Needles and suture remnants are removed through the working incision.

Operative procedures are performed from the surgeon's console placed approximately ten feet from the operating table but in the same operating room (Fig. 41.3) The patient-side assistant changes instruments as well as supplies and retrieves operative materials. Most often an annuloplasty band (Edwards Lifesciences, LLC, Irvine, CA) has been used to support repairs or provide annular reduction. Each suture is placed and tied intracorporeal. Upon completion of the repair, the left atrium is closed using the robotic system. Standard de-airing and weaning procedures are performed under TEE control. One month after discharge, all patients return for a follow-up visit and a transthoracic echocardiogram.

41.4.2
Coronary Artery Bypass Surgery

Proper port placement is essential for initiating endoscopic mammary artery harvesting. The camera port is placed bluntly in the fifth intercostal space on the anterior axillary line. The chest is insufflated with continuous CO_2 at pressures of 5–10 mm Hg to increase the available space between the heart and sternum. An endoscope is placed into this port and under visual control; two more port sites are placed, usually in the third and seventh intercostal spaces above the anterior axillary line, for both robotic arms. The LIMA is mobilized from the subclavian artery to the distal bifurcation with a 30° endoscope (Fig. 41.4). After LIMA harvesting, the patient is placed on cardiopulmonary bypass through femoral vessel cannulation if the procedure is being performed on an arrested heart. Otherwise, attention is turned to the pericardium, which is opened. (Fig. 41.5). The target vessel (LAD) is identified and sharply dissected free. For beating heart operations, a 1 cm skin incision is created at the subxiphoid area and an endoscopic stabilizer is

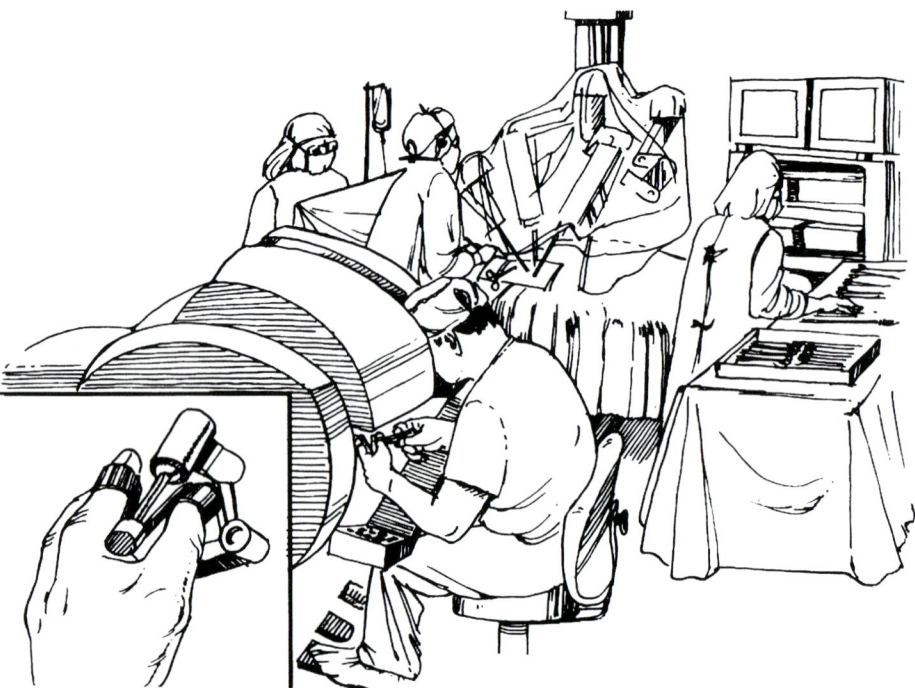

Fig. 41.3 The operating surgeon manipulates the master controls from the surgeon's console. These movements travel via fiber-optics to the patient-side surgical cart emulating precise finger movements deep within the patient's chest. Additional robotic features include tremor filtration, motion scaling and variable needle grip strength

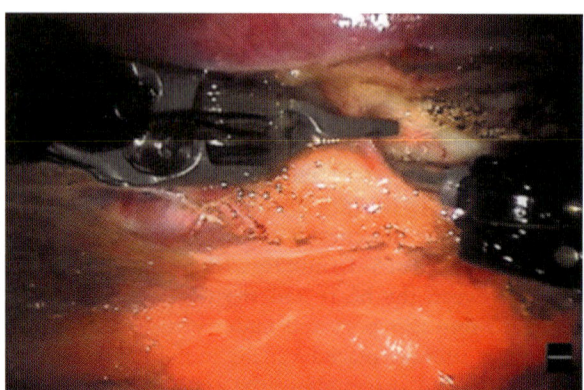

Fig. 41.4 After patient positioning and port placement, the internal mammary artery is harvested using the robotic system. A combination of spatula and bipolar cautery allow safe dissection

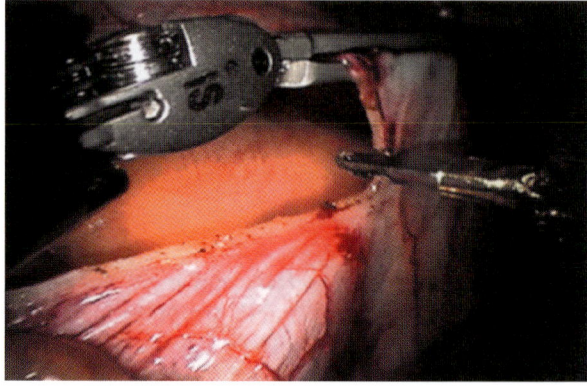

Fig. 41.5 The pericardium must be opened to allow access to the heart. Forceps and cautery are used. Care is taken to avoid injury to the phrenic nerve

introduced. The recent development of an endoscopic stabilizer adapted to the 4th arm of the surgical system will improve both visualization and stabilization. After placing the stabilizer onto the LAD, blood flow through this vessel is temporarily interrupted using silastic loops. After incision of the LAD with the robotic system, the anastomosis is completed on a beating heart using 7-0 polypropylene running suture.

41.5 Clinical Outcomes

A multicenter da Vinci™ trial, enlisting 112 patients for robotic mitral valve repair was completed and demonstrated efficacy and safety in performing these operations by multiple surgeons at various centers, thereby becoming the first robotic tele-manipulation system to become FDA-approved for mitral valve repair surgery [30]. Since FDA approval, others have reported similar good outcomes [31].

To date, we have completed over 325 robotic mitral valve repairs with the da Vinci™ system with good results. Cardiopulmonary bypass and cardiac arrest times have decreased since starting our program, with the average being 2.0 ± 0.6 hours and 2.6 ± 0.7 hours, respectively (mean $\pm$ st. deviation). Intra-operative times vary depending on repair techniques. For example, more complex repairs for Barlow's disease involve leaflet resection, sliding valvuloplasty, chordal transfers and annuloplasty. Therefore, these cases require longer operative times.

Similarly, experience with endoscopic coronary artery bypass surgery has been limited to only a few centers and results are highly controlled. Because the success of coronary surgery depends on multiple, complex steps culminating in the creation of a vascular anastomosis, most clinical series have introduced robotically assisted coronary surgery in a stepwise fashion. Specifically, initial experience is limited to endoscopic LIMA harvesting, followed by a robotically assisted anastomosis through a median sternotomy and finally a total endoscopic procedure performed on an arrested heart followed by a beating heart operation.

Currently, one of the largest published series of TE-CAB is the prospective multicenter trial of robotically assisted TECAB that led to FDA approval of this procedure in the USA [32]. Ninety-eight patients requiring single-vessel LAD revascularization were enrolled at 12 centers. Thirteen patients (13%) were excluded intra-operatively. In the remaining 85 patients who had TE-CAB, cardiopulmonary bypass time was 117 ± 44 minutes, cross-clamp time was 71 ± 26 minutes, and hospital length of stay was 5.1 ± 3.4 days. There were five (6%) conversions to open techniques. Freedom from reintervention or angiographic failure was 91% at 3 months. Kappert [33] described TECAB in 37 patients, of which 29 were performed on a beating heart. Of these 29 patients, three received double vessel bypass using bilateral mammary arteries and the rest were revascularized with a LIMA-LAD. As experience was gained, the duration of surgery decreased noticeably from 280 ± 80.2 to 186 ± 58.6 minutes. An average of 30 ± 6.5 minutes for robotically performed anastomosis versus 12 ± 3 minutes for directly hand-sewn anastomoses was observed. Nevertheless, none of the 37 patients revealed any sign of delayed wound healing but three patients did undergo re-exploration for bleeding.

41.6 Conclusion

Clearly, advances in cardiopulmonary perfusion, intracardiac visualization, instrumentation, and robotic tele-manipulation have hastened a shift toward efficient and safe minimally invasive cardiac surgery. Currently, cardiac surgery, particularly valve surgery done through small incisions, has become standard practice for many surgeons.

With improved optics and instrumentation, incisions are smaller. The placement of wrist-like articulations at the end of the instruments moves the pivoting action to the plane of the operative field. This improves dexterity in tight spaces and allows for ambidextrous movements. Sutures can be placed more accurately because of tremor filtration and high-resolution video magnification. The most recent addition has been high definition vision with digital zoom. Furthermore, robotic systems may serve as educational tools. In the near future, operative simulation systems will be able to model most surgical procedures through immersive technology [34–36]. Thus, a "flight simulator" concept emerges were one may be able to simulate, practice, and perform the operation without a patient. Already, effective curriculums for training teams in robotic surgery exist [37].

Robotic cardiac surgery is an evolutionary process, and even the greatest skeptics must concede that progress has been made. Surgical scientists must continue to evaluate this technology critically. Despite enthusiasm, caution cannot be overemphasized. Surgeons must be careful as indices of operative safety, speed of recovery, level of discomfort, procedural cost, and long-term operative quality have yet to be defined. Traditional cardiac operations still enjoy long-term success with ever-decreasing morbidity and mortality, and remain our measure for comparison.

References

1. Stevens JH, Burdon TA, Peters WS et al. (1996) Port-access coronary artery bypass grafting: a proposed surgical method. J Thorac Cardiovasc Surg 111:567–573.
2. Pompili MF, Stevens JH, Burdon TA et al. (1996) Port-access mitral valve replacement in dogs. J Thorac Cardiovasc Surg 112:1268–1274.
3. Mohr FW, Falk V, Diegeler A et al. (2001) Computer-enhanced "robotic" cardiac surgery: experience in 148 patients. J Thorac Cardiovasc Surg 121:842–853.

4. Cohn LH, Adams DH, Couper GS et al. (1997) Minimally invasive aortic valve replacement. Semin Thorac Cardiovasc Surg 9:331–336.
5. Cosgrove DM, Sabik JF (1996) Minimally invasive approach for aortic valve operations. Ann Thorac Surg 62:596–597.
6. Arom KV, Emery RW (1997) Minimally invasive mitral operations [letter]. Ann Thorac Surg 63:1219–1220.
7. Navia JL, Cosgrove DM (1996) Minimally invasive mitral valve operations. Ann Thorac Surg 62:1542–1544.
8. Cohn LH, Adams DH, Couper GS, Bichell DP, Rosborough DM, Sears SP, Aranki SF (1997) Minimally invasive cardiac valve surgery improves patient satisfaction while reducing costs of cardiac valve replacement and repair. Ann Surg 226:421–426.
9. Ribakove GH, Miller JS, Anderson RV et al. (1998) Minimally invasive port-access coronary artery bypass grafting with early angiographic follow-up: initial clinical experience. J Thorac Cardiovasc Surg 115:1101–1110.
10. Reichenspurner H, Gulielmos V, Wunderlich J et al. (1998) Port-access coronary artery bypass grafting with the use of cardiopulmonary bypass and cardioplegic arrest. Ann Thorac Surg 65:413–419.
11. Cosgrove DM, Sabik JF, Navia J (1998) Minimally invasive valve surgery. Ann Thorac Surg 65:1535–1538.
12. Galloway A C, Shemin RJ, Glower DD, Boyer JH, Groh MA, Kuntz RE, Burdon TA, Ribakove, GH, Reitz BA, Colvin SB (1999) First report of the Port Access Registry. Ann Thorac Surgery 67:51–56.
13. Grossi EA, Galloway AC, Ribakove GH, Zakow PK, Derivaux CC, FG Baumann, Schwesinger S, Colvin SB (2001) Impact of minimally invasive valvular heart surgery: a case-control study. Ann Thorac Surg 71:807–810.
14. Acuff TE, Landrenau RJ, Griffith BP, Mack MJ (1996) Minimally invasive coronary artery bypass grafting. Ann Thorac Surg 61:135–137.
15. Nataf P, Lima L. Regan M, Benarim S, Pavie A, Cabrol C, Gandjbakch I (1996) Minimally invasive coronary surgery with thoracoscopic internal mammary dissection: Surgical technique. J Card Surg 11:228–292.
16. Burke RP, Wernovsky G, van der Velde M et al. (1995) Video-assisted thoracoscopic surgery for congenital heart disease. J Thorac Cardiovasc Surg 109:499–507.
17. Carpentier A, Loulmet D, LeBret E et al. (1996) Chirurgie à coeur ouvert par video-chirurgie et mini-thoracotomie-primer cas (valvuloplastie mitrale) opéré avec succès. Comptes Rendus De L'Academie des Sciences: Sciences de la vie 319:219–223.
18. Chitwood WR, Elbeery JR, Chapman WHH et al. (1997) Video-assisted minimally invasive mitral valve surgery: the "micro-mitral" operation. J Thorac Cardiovasc Surg 113:413–414.
19. Felger JE, Chitwood WR Jr., Nifong LW et al. (2001) Evolution of mitral valve surgery: toward a totally endoscopic approach. Ann Thorac Surg 72:1203–1209.
20. Chitwood WR Jr., Wixon CL, Elbeery JR et al. (1997) Video-assisted minimally invasive mitral valve surgery. J Thorac Cardiovasc Surg 114:773–780.
21. Falk V, Walter T, Autschbach R et al. (1998) Robot-assisted minimally invasive solo mitral valve operation. J Thorac Cardiovasc Surg 115:470–471.
22. Carpentier A, Loulmet D, Aupecle B et al. (1998) Computer assisted open-heart surgery. First case operated on with success. CR Acad Sci II 321:437–442.
23. Chitwood WR Jr., Nifong LW, Elbeery JE et al. (2000) Robotic mitral valve repair: trapezoidal resection and prosthetic annuloplasty with the da Vinci surgical system. J Thorac Cardiovasc Surg 120:1171–1172.
24. Mohr FW, Falk V, Diegeler A et al. (1999) Computer-enhanced coronary artery bypass surgery. J Thorac Cardiovasc Surg 117:1212–1215.
25. Falk V, Fann JI, Grunenfelder J et al. (2000) Endoscopic computer-enhanced beating heart coronary artery bypass grafting. Ann Thorac Surg 70:2029–2033.
26. Loulmet D, Carpentier A, d'Attellis N et al. (1999) Endoscopic coronary artery bypass grafting with the aid of robotic assisted instruments. J Thorac Cardiovasc Surg 118:4–10.
27. Falk V, Diegeler A, Walther T et al. (2000) Total endoscopic coronary artery bypass grafting. Eur J Cardiothorac Surg 17:38–45.
28. Kappert U, Cichon R, Gulielmos V et al. (2000) Robotic-enhanced Dresden technique for minimally invasive bilateral internal mammary artery grafting. Heart Surg Forum 3:319–321.
29. Aybek T, Dogan S, Andressen E et al. (2000) Robotically enhanced totally endoscopic right internal thoracic coronary artery bypass to the right coronary artery. Heart Surg Forum 3:322–324.
30. Nifong LW, Chitwood WR, Pappas PS et al. (2005) Robotic mitral valve surgery: a United States multicenter trial. J Thorac Cardiovasc Surg 129:1395–1404.
31. Murphy DA, Miller JS, Langford DA et al. (2006) Endoscopic robotic mitral valve surgery. J Thorac Cardiovasc Surg 132:776–781.
32. Argenziano M, Katz M, Bonatti J et al. (2006) Results of the prospective multicenter trial of robotically assisted totally endoscopic coronary artery bypass grafting. Ann Thorac Surg 81:1666–1675.
33. Kappert U, Schneider J, Cichon R et al. (2001) Development of robotic enhanced endoscopic surgery for the treatment of coronary artery disease. Circulation 104:I-102–I-107.
34. Meir AH, Rawn CL, Krummel TM (2001) Virtual reality: surgical application- challenge for the new millennium. J Am Coll Surg 192:372–384.

35. Gorman PJ, Meir AH, Krummel TH (1999) Simulation and virtual reality in surgical education: real or unreal. Arch Surg 134:1203–1208.
36. Gorman PJ, Meir AH, Krummel TH (2000) Computer-assisted training and learning in surgery. Comput Aided Surg 5:120–130.
37. Chitwood WR, Nifong LW, Chapman WIIII et al. (2001) Robotic surgical training in an academic institution. Ann Surg 234:475–486.

Transmyocardial Revascularization

Jay Jayakumar, Wai Weng Woon and Peter L. C. Smith

Chapter 42

Contents

42.1	Background	497
42.2	History	497
42.3	Methods of TMR	497
42.4	Hypotheses for TMR Mechanism of Action	498
42.4.1	Patent Channels	498
42.4.2	Angiogenesis	498
42.4.3	Denervation	498
42.4.4	Fibrosis	499
42.5	Pre-Clinical Studies	499
42.5.1	Mechanical vs Laser	499
42.5.2	Comparison Between Lasers	499
42.5.3	TMR Combined with Therapeutic Angiogenesis	499
42.6	Clinical Studies	499
42.6.1	Non-Randomized Studies	499
42.6.2	TMR Alone	500
42.6.3	TMR with CABG	500
42.7	Outcome Analysis	500
42.7.1	Morbidity	500
42.7.1	Mortality	500
42.8	Risk Factors	502
42.9	Surgical Techniques	503
42.10	Peri-Operative Complications	504
42.11	Indications and Contraindications	504
42.12	Clinical Guidelines	505
42.12.1	Recommendations for TMR as Sole Therapy	505
42.12.2	Recommendations for TMR as an Adjunct to CABG	505
42.12.3	Summary of Guidelines	505
42.13	Future Investigations	505
42.14	Summary	506
	References	506

42.1 Background

Treatment of patients with chronic severe angina that is refractory to conventional medical treatment, percutaneous coronary intervention or coronary artery bypass grafting (CABG) can present particular challenges. One possible further treatment option is the use of transmyocardial revascularization (TMR), either alone or combined with CABG, for a certain sub-group of these patients.

42.2 History

Myocardial revascularization by creation of direct channels was initially reported by Sen [1, 2] and Hershey and White [3–6] in the early 1960s, but was overshadowed by the development of CABG. However, interest was revived by Mirhoseini [7, 8] in the early 1980s using a CO_2 laser to create channels in a non-graftable portion of the heart of a patient who was also undergoing salvage CABG to other territories. Interest was dampened until the reports by Frasier and Cooley in the mid 1990s [9]. They showed the beneficial sole use of TMR in 21 patients, leading to alleviation of angina, increased endocardial perfusion (measured by PET), and increased regional contraction. The FDA subsequently approved use of TMR as sole therapy for angina when patients were deemed unsuitable for CABG.

42.3 Methods of TMR

Initially, mechanical punctures using needles was used. Later, lasers were used to create channels spaced 1 cm apart and 1 mm deep [10]. The three main laser types (Table 42.1) are carbon dioxide (CO_2), holmium:yttrium-aluminum garnet (YAG) and xenon-chloride (excimer) [11–14]. The end result is the creation of a channel approximately 1 mm diameter, surrounded by a 1–2 mm

Table 42.1 Main types of lasers used for TMR

	CO$_2$	Holmium:YAG	Xe:CI (Excimer)
Spectrum	Infrared	Infrared	Ultraviolet
Energy level	High	Low	Low
No. pulses/channel	Usually 1	6–8	6–8
Mechanics	Continuous thermal	Pulsed thermal	Continuous cold
Thermal injury	++	+++	+
Fiberoptic	No	Yes	Yes
R-wave sync	Yes	No	No

rim of necrosis and a 1–3 mm zone of myofibril degeneration in the periphery of this rim [15].

CO$_2$ lasers have the advantage of producing high-energy pulses, creating a trans-mural channel with a single pulse, low peak power, and high photonic absorption; compared with other laser types, they minimize structural tissue trauma. Pulses can be synchronized with the R wave of the ECG and delivered during end-diastole, taking 10 to 60 milliseconds to form the channels, minimizing interference with ventricular conduction. The holmium:YAG and excimer lasers are low-energy, require multiple firing for creation of a single channel, but cannot be synchronized with the ECG; however, they have the capacity of being coupled to a fiberoptic catheter for transluminal endocardial delivery [16].

To avoid uncontrolled pericardial hemorrhage, channels created by a percutaneous approach are not transmural; it has been hypothesized that this may lead to less stimulation of subepicardial collateralization and arteriogenesis between normally perfused and collateral-dependent myocardial territories after TMR [16].

42.4
Hypotheses for TMR Mechanism of Action

42.4.1
Patent Channels

TMR does not result in channels of long-term patency. This has been demonstrated by numerous studies and autopsy reports [17, 18]. Channels are now known to be occluded by thrombus within 6–24 hours, followed by organization and neovascularization of the region surrounding the channel, or occluded by scar tissue [19, 20].

42.4.2
Angiogenesis

TMR leads to an increase in density of arterial vessels [21–30]. This may have been stimulated by either a general wound-healing response or by a specific TMR-response. The latter is supported by studies showing a molecular basis for laser-induced TMR angiogenesis, such as an induction of vascular endothelial growth factor (VEGF) gene expression and elevated tissue levels of VEGF mRNA [31]. Both mechanical and laser transmyocardial revascularization can also lead to an increase in the expression of VEGF and fibroblast-growth-factor (FGF-2) [23, 28].

42.4.3
Denervation

Denervation of cardiac sympathetic afferent fibers as a result of TMR may be yet another mechanism that leads to angina relief. Some studies have shown that holmium:YAG TMR leads to visceral afferent signals being interrupted in the subepicardium [32]. However, other studies contradict the role of electrical or chemical activation of sympathetic or parasympathetic efferent neurons in reducing the ventricular contractile response following holmium:YAG TMR [33]. TMR may decrease the chemical response of the intrinsic cardiac nervous pathways, as shown by myocardial PET hydroxyephedrine uptake (a sympathetic innervation marker) in TMR patients [34]. However, as TMR affects less than 1% of total left ventricular mass [35], this mechanism is unlikely to explain all the ischemia-alleviating effects of TMR.

42.4.4
Fibrosis

TMR can lead to fibrosis [22, 36] and the resulting tethering of the left ventricle in diastole may prevent further ischemia and dilation of the ischemic segment, leading to more favorable ventricular remodeling [37].

42.5
Pre-Clinical Studies

42.5.1
Mechanical vs Laser

Investigations have compared various TMR devices (Fig. 42.1) [38] and have shown a statistically significant increase in contractility (from baseline to post-treatment, as measured by echocardiogram) when laser TMR was compared with various needle TMR techniques and control treatment.

42.5.2
Comparison Between Lasers

Investigations have also compared various laser TMR devices (Fig. 42.2) [39]. Significant increase in myocardial blood flow to the lased myocardium following TMR was seen with both holmium:YAG and CO_2 lasers, with no significant change in myocardial blood flow after excimer TMR or sham thoracotomy. There was a significant decrease in peak-stress wall motion score index (WMSI), consistent with a reduction in ischemia following holmium:YAG and CO_2 laser TMR, with no significant change in peak-stress WMSI following excimer TMR or sham thoracotomy.

42.5.3
TMR Combined with Therapeutic Angiogenesis

Some investigations have reported an increased inflammatory response when TMR is combined with VEGF treatment, without the expected increase in angiogenesis [26, 40]. TMR with gene-therapy (e.g., VEGF) has shown mixed results, with some studies showing increased transfection efficiency [41], with others showing decreased transfection together with increased inflammation [42].

42.6
Clinical Studies

42.6.1
Non-Randomized Studies

Many trials have shown that use of holmium:YAG or CO_2 laser leads to increase of Canadian Cardiovascu-

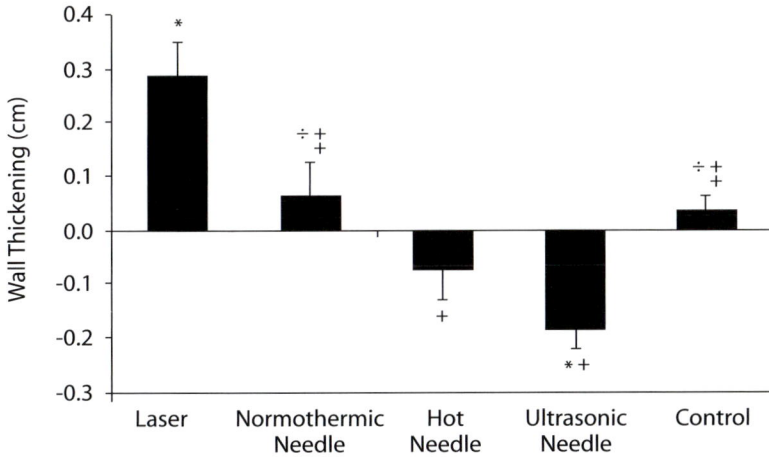

Fig. 42.1 Functional results of treatment of myocardium by various TMR devices or no device (*control*) [change in contractility from baseline to post-treatment]

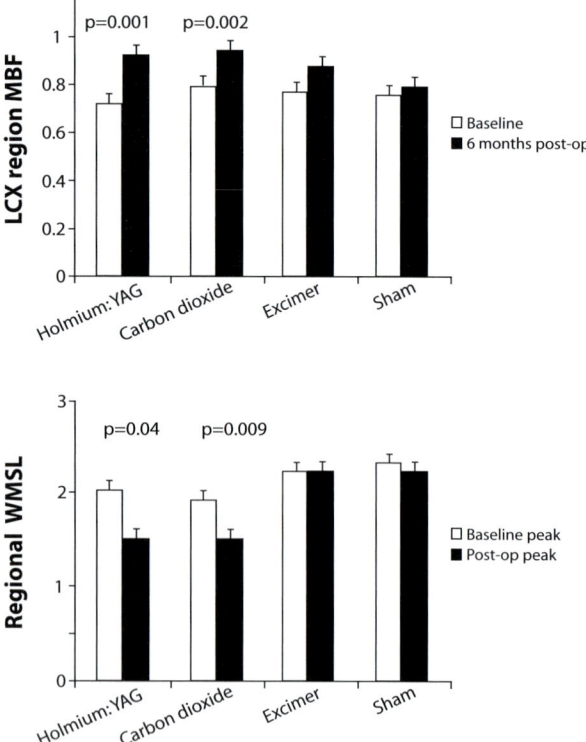

Fig. 42.2 **a** Significant increase in myocardial blood flow to the lased LCX distribution following TMR with both holmium:YAG and CO_2 lasers. **b** Resting regional WMSI by DSE preoperatively and 6 months postoperatively. **c** Peak stress regional WMSI by DSE preoperatively and 6 months postoperatively. **d** Quantitative vascular density analysis. *DSE* = dobutamine stress echocardiography, *LCX* = left circumflex coronary artery, *WMSI* = wall motion score index

lar Society (CCS) scoring of anginal symptoms, including increase in exercise capacity [9, 10, 13, 43–50].

42.6.2
TMR Alone

TMR patients have shown improvement in angina score, compared with medical therapy alone [51], though without a significant survival benefit. A summary of the key results of the most important trials is shown in Table 42.2.

42.6.3
TMR with CABG

Most studies of TMR with CABG do not show a survival benefit when TMR was performed on ungraftable regions of the myocardium [60]. A summary of the key results of the most important trials is shown in Table 42.3.

42.7
Outcome Analysis

42.7.1
Morbidity

Morbidity from TMR may include myocardial infarction, arrhythmias, left ventricular dysfunction, and cerebral micro-embolization [68–71].

42.7.1
Mortality

All the randomized trials excluded patients with ejection fractions less than 0.20 to 0.30 [28, 72–74], possi-

Table 42.2 Summary of best evidence papers for TMR

Author	Key Results
Burns et al. [52]	Mortality/morbidity: 90/932 patients died (9.7%), 29% of patients had a complication, 8% bleeding, 4% MI, 8% LVF. TMR groups improved their exercise test times by mean 1 min 50 s at 12 months (compared to pre-operatively, $P<0.01$). CCS angina score improved by 2 or more classes in 34% of patients at 12 months; NYHA angina score 2 classes in 49 and at 12 months
Burkhoff et al. [70]	Improvement in CCS angina score of 2 or more after 1 year: TMR group 47/77 (61%), Medical management (MM) alone 8/73 (11%) ($P<0.001$). Exercise tolerance: TMR group 65s median increase, MM group 46s drop ($P=0.0001$). Deaths: TMR 5/92 deaths (5%), Medical management 9/90 (10%) ($P<0.001$)
Allen et al. [53]	Improvement in CCS angina score of 2 or more after 5 year: TMR alone 42/48 (88%), MM alone 16/36 (44%) ($P<0.001$). Mean angina class: TMR group at 5 years 1.2 ± 1.1. 5 year survival: TMR alone 33/50 (65%), MM alone 26/49 (52%) ($P=0.03$). Operative mortality 3%
Bridges et al. [54]	Recommendations for TMR as sole therapy. Class I Patients with EF > 30 and CCS III/IV refractory to medical therapy (level A), Class IIB Patients with EF < 30 with or without IABP (level C). Patients with unstable angina requiring intravenous medication (level B). Patients with CCS II angina (level C). Class III Patients with acute MI, cardiogenic shock, VT/SVT, decompensated CHF (level C)
Allen et al [55]	Improvement in CCS angina score of 2 or more after 1 year: TMR 58/76 (76%), MM alone 16/50 (32%) ($P<0.001$). Treatment Failure: TMR 43%, MM 73% ($P<0.001$). Perioperative complications: TMR 7/132 (5%) deaths, 6 non-Q wave MIs, 16 episodes of ventricular arrhythmias
Schofield et al. [56]	Improvement in CCS angina score of 2 or more after 1 year: TMR 18/74 (25%), MM alone 3/78 (4%) ($P<0.001$). 1 year survival: TMR and MM 89%, MM alone 96% ($P=0.14$) Pre-operative mortality 5% (5/94). TMR treadmill exercise time 40 s longer (95% CI –15 to 94 s) ($P=0.152$). TMR 12 min walk distance 33 m further (–7 to 44) ($P=0.108$). 33% of TMR had wound or respiratory infections. 15% LVF
Hattlet et al. [57]	Improvement in CCS angina score of 2 or more after 1 year: Unstable Angina (UA) and TMR 9/37 (24%), Chronic Angina (CA) and TMR 5/15 (33%) ($P=0.001$). Perioperative mortality: UA and TMR 12/76 (16%), CA and TMR 3/91 (5%) ($P=0.005$). Mortality at 1 year: UA and TMR 8/64 (13%), CA and TMR 10/88 (11%) ($P=0.83$)
Aaber et al [58]	Improvement in CCS angina score of 1 or more after 5 years: TMR 23/38 (61%), MM alone 9/37 (24%) ($P=0.01$). Improvement in CCS angina score of 2 or more after 5 years: TMR 24%, MM alone 3% ($P=0.001$). Mortality: TMR 8/38 (22%), MM alone 9/37 (24%) ($P=$ NS). Operative mortality 4%
Frazier et al [59]	Improvement in CCS angina score of 2 or more after 1 year: TMR 72%, MM alone 13%, MM but crossed over to TMR 43% ($P<0.001$). Mortality: TMR 13/91 (12%), MM 22/101 (22%) of which 15 deaths were in the crossover group ($P<0.001$). 3 intraoperative deaths. Complications: TMR patients 7% MI, 11% CCF, 8% VT or VF
Peterson et al. [60]	Mortality for TMR alone: TMR RCT group 25/722 (3.5%), TMR STS group 42/661 (6.4%). Mortality for TMR+CABG: TMR+CABG RCT group 4/263 (1.5%), TMR+CABG STS group 104/2475 (4.2%). CABG alone vs all CABG+TMR: CABG alone 1602/39064 (4.9%), CABG and TMR 19/390 (4.1%) ($P=0.37$)
Hovath [10]	Reduction in angina of 2 classes or more: 117/156 (75%) at 3 months, 70/95 (75%) at 12 months. Morbidity: 2% MI, 1 patient had mitral valve damage requiring repair, 1% bleeding rate, 4% IABP rate. Mortality: 18/200 (9%) died

Table 42.3 Summary of best evidence papers for TMR + CABG

Author	Key Results
Bridges et al. [54]	Class IIA Patients with angina CCS I–IV with CABG as standard of care with area of reversible ischaemia not amenable to revascularization: (level B). Class IIB Patients without angina with CABG as standard of care with diffuse coronary artery disease: (level C)
Peterson et al. [61]	Mortality for TMR alone: TMR RCT group 25/722 (3.5%), TMR STS group 42/661 (6.4%). Mortality for TMR+CABG: TMR+CABG RCT group 4/263 (1.5%), TMR + CABG STS group 104/2475 (4.2%). Mortality for all CABG alone vs all CABG + TMR: CABG alone 1602/39064 (4.9%), CABG and TMR 19/390 (4.1%) ($P=0.37$)
Loubani et al. [62]	CCS angina score at 36 months: TMR+CABG Post-op mean CCS 0.7 ± 0.4, CABG alone Post-op mean CCS 0.8 ± 0.5. Exercise tolerance at 6 months: TMR+CABG Improvement of 199 ± 66 s, CABG alone Improvement of 46.8 ± 20 s ($P<0.0001$). Mortality: No deaths in either group
Stamou [63]	Angina class at 1 year: 7% of patients had CCS grade III or IV angina at 1 year. Complications: 7 patients had re-exploration for bleeding (4%). Mortality: 14 deaths (8%), 85% 1 year survival
Allen [64]	Improvement in CCS angina score of 2 or more after 1 year: CABG+TMR group 5/106 (4.7%), CABG alone 11/98 (11.2%) ($P=0.11$). Survival estimates at 1 year: CABG + TMR 95%, CABG alone 89% ($P=0.05$). Mean angina class at 12 months: CABG + TMR Mean class CCS = 0.5, CABG alone Mean class CCS = 0.6 ($P=0.2$). Operative mortality: CABG TMR 2/132 (1.5%), CABG alone 10/131 (7.6%) ($P=0.02$)
Burns et al. [52]	Mortality/morbidity: 90/932 patients died (9.7%), 29% of patients had a complication, 8% bleeding, 4% MI, 8% LVF. TMR groups improved their exercise test times by mean 1 min 50 s at 12 months compared to pre-operatively ($P<0.01$). CCS angina score improved by 2 or more classes in 34% of patients at 12 months, and NYHA angina score 2 classes in 49 and at 12 months
Trehan et al. [65]	Improvement in CCS angina score after 1 year: CABG+TMR 33/38 (86.8%) were angina free. Mortality: 1/56 (1.78%)
Vincent et al. [66]	CCS grade 0 or 1 at 1 year follow-up: TMR + CABG 85%, TMR alone 42%. Complications: 22 patients returned for bleeding, 34 patients required IABP. Mortality: TMR + CABG 15/127, TMR alone 12/128
Trehan et al. [67]	Improvement in CCS angina score: 22/24 (92%) were angina free at 12 months. Angina score: 50% angina free at 3 months. Mortality: 3/104 (2.88%) 30 d mortality

bly leading to the lower peri-operative mortality rate, when compared with previous retrospective studies [22, 23, 32, 34].

The largest trial was based on The Society of Thoracic Surgeons National Cardiac Database (STS NCD) [60]. A total of 2,475 patients underwent holmium:YAG/CO_2-laser TMR with concomitant CABG, with a peri-operative mortality of 4.2%. In addition, 661 patients underwent holmium:YAG/CO_2-laser TMR alone, with a peri-operative mortality of 6.4%.

42.8
Risk Factors

Patients with unstable angina [57, 70, 75], acute ischemia [76, 77], and low ejection fraction [47] have the highest risk of peri-operative complications from sole-therapy TMR. When TMR is combined with CABG, there is however scarce information on specific benefits or risks.

42.9 Surgical Techniques

TMR can be performed via surgery, when combined with CABG [64, 79–80] or via a separate antero-lateral thoracotomy [78, 81–84], or via a thoracoscopic approach. In essence, a laser-handpiece is used to create one channel per cm² of myocardium (Fig. 42.3 shows LV exposure via thoracotomy for TMR), gated to the ECG R-wave. Hemostasis is achieved as required, and

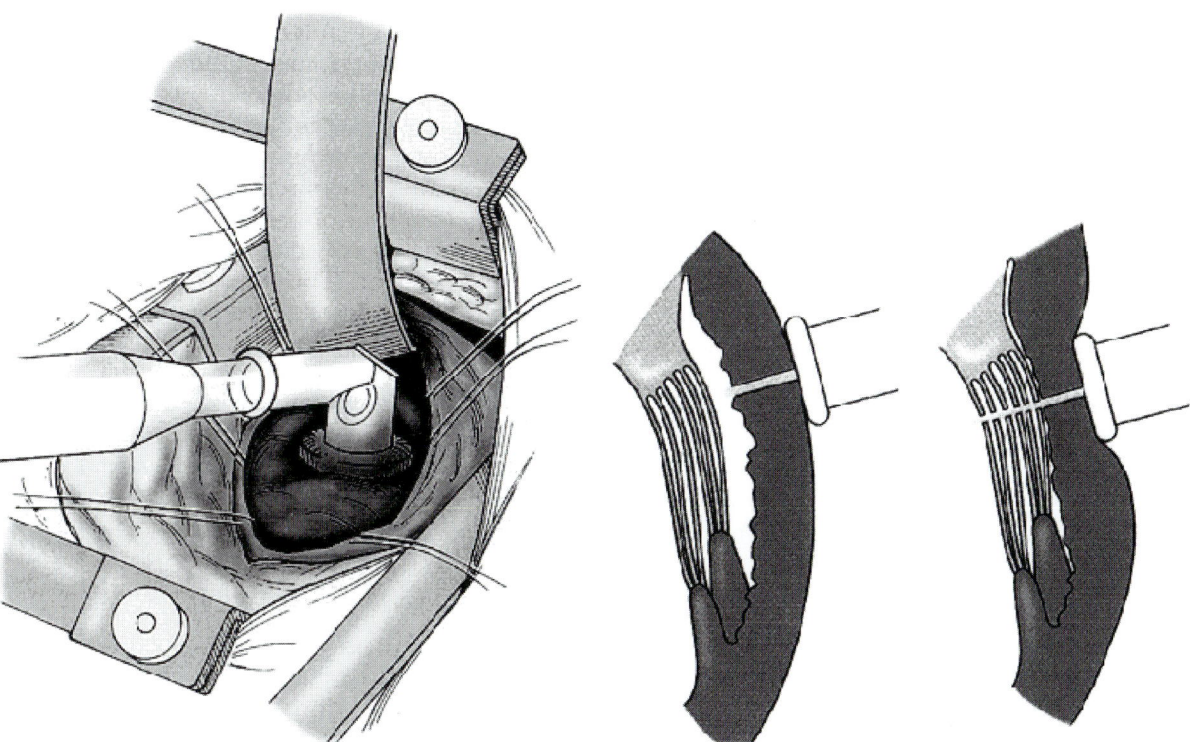

Fig. 42.3 Exposure of the left ventricle for TMR via thoracotomy incision with suspension of pericardium (adapted from [78])

Fig. 42.4 Dissection of epicardial adhesions prevents dimpling of the LV during TMR, reducing potential of damage to the mitral valve chordae lying close to the endocardial surface (adapted from [78])

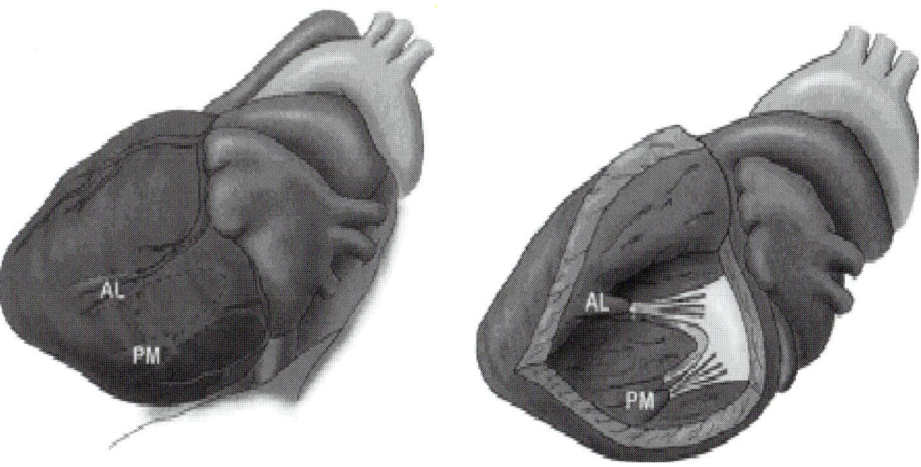

Fig. 42.5 The anterolateral (AL) and posteromedial (PM) papillary muscles should be excluded from the area of myocardium being lased (adapted from [78])

arrhythmias are minimized by minimal tissue handling. Once 30–50 channels are created, careful final hemostasis is followed by approximation of the pericardium. Correct technique will avoid damage to mitral valve chordae (Fig. 42.4) and also reduce papillary muscle damage (Fig. 42.5). TMR can also be performed percutaneously, where a holmium:YAG laser is guided by electro-mechanical mapping to create non-transmural channels in the selected regions [85].

42.10
Peri-Operative Complications

Complications of TMR include myocardial infarction, low cardiac output syndrome, and ventricular arrhythmias (Table 42.4) [66, 86, 87]. Mitral chord rupture and pericardial tamponade require aggressive management in the ICU, possibly with prompt surgical intervention.

Independent risk factors for peri-operative morbidity include poor LVEF (<40%) and unstable angina [70, 86]. However, decreased mortality is associated with prior CABG, good perfusion of remaining myocardium and female patients [75, 76].

Table 42.4 Peri-operative complications of TMR

Myocardial infarction
Low cardiac output syndrome
Pericardial tamponade
Ventricular arrhythmias
Papillary muscle injury
Mitral chordal injury
Cerebrovascular event (micro–air emboli)
Atrial fibrillation

42.11
Indications and Contraindications

Indications and contraindications to TMR are shown in Table 42.5. TMR should be reserved for patients who have severe chronic stable angina but who cannot be treated by conventional revascularization procedures [86]. It should not be used for emergency revascularization or salvage of threatened myocardium, having abysmal results in this sub-group of patients. TMR may be used for relieving unstable angina when weaning IV anti-anginal medications has been unsuccessful, but there is increased peri-operative mortality compared with their use in chronic stable angina [57, 88].

Table 42.5 Potential indications and contra-indications to TMR

Potential indications	Contra-indications
	Malignancy within past 5 years
Chronic stable angina in the presence of ungraftable CAD in a major coronary distribution, with:-	Vascular proliferative lesions:
(a) documentation of ischemia in the ungraftable territory	(a) diabetic retinopathy
(b) evidence of ungraftability (eg previous failed attempts at PTCA or CABG)	(b) arteriovenous malformations
(c) presence of viable myocardium in the ungraftable territory	(c) hemangiomas
	LVEF <30%
	Chronically low BP
	Impaired renal function (FGF-2)

42.12
Clinical Guidelines

Guidelines for diagnostic and therapeutic procedures, based on The Society of Thoracic Surgeons Practice Guidelines Series on TMR [54], are summarized according to (a) Class and (b) Level of evidence:

Class I: evidence that a treatment is useful and effective.
Class II: conflicting evidence on efficacy of a treatment:
　IIA. evidence in favor of efficacy.
　IIB. efficacy is less well established by evidence.
Class III: evidence that the treatment is not useful, or even harmful.

Level of evidence: (A) data derived from multiple randomized clinical trials; (B) data derived from a single randomized trial or several non-randomized studies; (C) consensus expert opinion.

42.12.1
Recommendations for TMR as Sole Therapy

Class I
I. Patients with ejection fraction >0.30 and CCS class III or IV, angina refractory to maximal medical therapy, with reversible ischemia of LV wall and coronary artery disease (CAD) corresponding to regions of myocardial ischemia. The CAD must not be amenable to CABG or percutaneous transluminal angioplasty (PTCA) either as a result of (a) severe diffuse disease, (b) lack of suitable targets for complete revascularization, or (c) lack of suitable conduits for complete revascularization (level of evidence: A).

Class IIB
I. Patients who otherwise have class I indications for TMR but who have either:
　a) Ejection fraction <0.30 with or without insertion of an intraaortic balloon pump (IABP) (level of evidence: C).
　b) Unstable angina or acute ischemia necessitating IV anti-anginal therapy (level of evidence: B).
　c) Patients with class II angina (level of evidence: C).

Class III
I. Patients without angina or with class I angina (level of evidence: C).
II. Acute evolving myocardial infarction or recent transmural or non-transmural myocardial infarction (level of evidence: C).
III. Cardiogenic shock (systolic blood pressure <80 mm Hg or cardiac index <1.8 L min^{-1} m^{-2} (level of evidence: C).
IV. Uncontrolled ventricular or supra-ventricular tachyarrhythmias (level of evidence: C).
V. Decompensated congestive heart failure (level of evidence: C).

42.12.2
Recommendations for TMR as an Adjunct to CABG

Class IIA
I. Patients with angina (class I–IV) in whom CABG is the standard of care who also have at least one accessible and viable ischemic region with demonstrable coronary artery disease that cannot be bypassed either because of (a) severe diffuse disease, (b) lack of suitable targets for complete revascularization, or (c) lack of suitable conduits for complete revascularization (level of evidence: B).

Class IIB
I. Patients without angina in whom CABG is the standard of care, who also have at least one accessible and viable ischemic region with demonstrable CAD that cannot be bypassed either because of (a) severe diffuse disease, (b) lack of suitable targets for complete revascularization, or (c) lack of suitable conduits for complete revascularization (level of evidence: C).

Class III
I. Patients in whom CABG is not the standard of care (level of evidence: C).

42.12.3
Summary of Guidelines

Class I indications exist for TMR as sole therapy, with class IIA indications for TMR as an adjunct to CABG, with levels of evidence A and B, respectively.

42.13
Future Investigations

TMR is being attempted using thoracoscopy [81, 89] and via percutaneous routes (direct myocardial revascularization) [90, 91]. Alternative methods of channel creation include use of ultrasound [47] and radiofrequency ablation [92]. Further studies include investigation of alternative laser wavelengths in order to reduce myocardial damage. Combining these techniques with gene-therapy for administration of various growth factors (VEGF, FGF-2) shows great promise [40, 93].

42.14
Summary

TMR may be used as sole therapy for a subset of patients with refractory angina, and as an adjunct to CABG for a subset of patients with angina who cannot be completely revascularized surgically.

References

1. Sen PK, Udwadia TE, Kinare SG, Parulkar GB (1965) Transmyocardial acupuncture: a new approach to myocardial revascularization. J Thorac Cardiovasc Surg 50:181.
2. Sen PK, Daulatram J, Kinare SG et al. (1968) Further studies in multiple transmyocardial acupuncture as a method of myocardial revascularization. Surgery 64:861.
3. Hershey JE, White M (1969) Transmyocardial puncture revascularization: a possible emergency adjunct to arterial implant surgery. Geriatrics 24:101.
4. Hershey JE (1999) Multiple transmyocardial puncture revascularization. Ann Thorac Surg 68:1890.
5. Hershey JE (2000) Transmyocardial revascularization: could mechanical puncture be more effective than puncture by laser? Tex Heart Inst J 27:80.
6. White M, Hershey JE (1968) Multiple transmyocardial puncture revascularization in refractory ventricular fibrillation due to myocardial ischemia. Ann Thorac Surg 6:557.
7. Mirhoseini M, Cayton MM (1981) Revascularization of the heart by laser. J Microsurg 2:253.
8. Mirhoseini M, Fisher JC, Cayton M (1983) Myocardial revascularization by laser: a clinical report. Lasers Surg Med 3:241.
9. Frazier OH, Cooley DA, Kadipasaoglu KA et al. (1995) Myocardial revascularization with laser. Preliminary findings. Circulation 92: II58.
10. Horvath KA, Cohn LH, Cooley DA et al. (1997) Transmyocardial laser revascularization: results of a multicenter trial with transmyocardial laser revascularization used as sole therapy for end-stage coronary artery disease. J Thorac Cardiovasc Surg 113:645.
11. Yano OJ, Bielefeld MR, Jeevanandam V et al. (1993) Prevention of acute regional ischemia with endocardial laser channels. Ann Thorac Surg 56:46.
12. Whittaker P, Kloner RA, Przyklenk K (1993) Laser-mediated transmural myocardial channels do not salvage acutely ischemic myocardium. J Am Coll Cardiol 22:302.
13. Lee LY, O'Hara MF, Finnin EB et al. (2000) Transmyocardial laser revascularization with excimer laser: clinical results at 1 year. Ann Thorac Surg 70:498.
14. Martin JS, Sayeed-Shah U, Byrne JG et al. (2000) Excimer versus carbon dioxide transmyocardial laser revascularization: effects on regional left ventricular function and perfusion. Ann Thorac Surg 69:1811.
15. Lutter G, Schwarzkopf J, Lutz C et al. (1998) Histologic findings of transmyocardial laser channels after two hours. Ann Thorac Surg 65:1437.
16. Kadipasaoglu KA, Frazier OH (1999) Transmyocardial laser revascularization: effect of laser parameters on tissue ablation and cardiac perfusion. Semin Thorac Cardiovasc Surg 11:4.
17. Fisher PE, Khomoto T, DeRosa CM et al. (1997) Histologic analysis of transmyocardial channels: comparison of CO_2 and holmium:YAG lasers. Ann Thorac Surg 64:466.
18. Kohmoto T, Fisher PE, Gu A et al. (1997) Physiology, histology, and 2-week morphology of acute transmyocardial channels made with a CO_2 laser. Ann Thorac Surg 63:1275.
19. Genyk IA, Frenz M, Ott B et al. (2000) Acute and chronic effects of transmyocardial laser revascularization in the non-ischemic pig myocardium by using three laser systems. Lasers Surg Med 27:438.
20. Gassler N, Wintzer HO, Stubbe HM et al. (1997) Transmyocardial laser revascularization: histological features in human non-responder myocardium. Circulation 95:371.
21. Burkhoff D, Fisher PE, Apfelbaum M, Kohmoto T, DeRosa CM, Smith CR (1996) Histologic appearance of transmyocardial laser channels after 4 1/2 weeks. Ann Thorac Surg 61:1532.
22. Malekan R, Reynolds C, Kelley ST, Suzuki Y, Bridges CR (1998) Angiogenesis in transmyocardial laser revascularization: a non-specific response to injury. Circulation 98(Suppl 2):II62.
23. Chu V, Kuang J, McGinn A, Giaid A, Korkola S, Chiu RC (1999) Angiogenic response induced by mechanical transmyocardial revascularization. J Thorac Cardiovasc Surg 118:849.
24. Kohmoto T, Fisher PE, Gu A et al. (1998) Does blood flow through holmium: YAG transmyocardial channels? Ann Thorac Surg 61:861.
25. Kohmoto T, DeRosa CM, Yamamoto N et al. (1998) Evidence of vascular growth associated with laser treatment of normal canine myocardium. Ann Thorac Surg 65:1360.
26. Fleischer KJ, Goldschmidt-Clermont PJ, Fonger JD, Hutchins GM, Hruban RH, Baumgartner WA (1996) One-month histologic response of transmyocardial laser channels with molecular intervention. Ann Thorac Surg 62:1051.
27. Zlotnick AY, Ahmad RM, Reul RM, Laurence RG, Aretz HT, Cohn LH (1996) Neovascularization occurs at he site

of closed laser channels after transmyocardial laser revascularization. Surg Forum 47:286.
28. Chu VF, Giaid A, Kuang JQ et al. (1999) Thoracic Surgery Directors Association Award. Angiogenesis in transmyocardial revascularization: comparison of laser versus mechanical punctures. Ann Thorac Surg 68:301.
29. Mack CA, Magovern CJ, Hahn RT et al. (1997) Channel patency and neovascularization after transmyocardial revascularization using an excimer laser: results and comparison to non-lased channels. Circulation 96(Suppl 2):II65.
30. Pelletier MP, Giaid A, Sivaraman S et al. (1998) Angiogenesis and growth factor expression in a model of transmyocardial revascularization. Ann Thorac Surg 66:12.
31. Horvath KA, Chiu E, Maun DC et al. (1999) Up-regulation of VEGF mRNA and angiogenesis after transmyocardial laser revascularization. Ann Thorac Surg 68:825.
32. Kwong KF, Kanellopoulos GK, Nickols JC et al. (1997) Transmyocardial laser treatment denervates canine myocardium. J Thorac Cardiovasc Surg 114:883.
33. Hirsch GM, Thompson GW, Arora RC, Hirsch KJ, Sullivan JA, Armour JA (1999) Transmyocardial laser revascularization does not denervate the canine heart. Ann Thorac Surg 68:460.
34. Al-Sheikh T, Allen KB, Straka SP et al. (1999) Cardiac sympathetic denervation after transmyocardial laser revascularization. Circulation 100:135.
35. Massimo C, Boffi L (1857) Myocardial revascularization by a new method of carrying blood directly from the left ventricular cavity into the coronary circulation. J Thorac Surg 34:257.
36. Gassler N, Rastar F, Hentz MW (1999) Angiogenesis and expression of tenascin after transmural laser revascularization. Histol Histopathol 14:81.
37. Laham RJ, Simons M (2000) Laser myocardial revascularization: fact or fiction? Card Vasc Regener 1:70.
38. Horvath KA, Belkind N, Wu J et al. (2001) Functional comparison of transmyocardial revascularization by mechanical and laser means. Ann Thorac Surg 72:1997.
39. Hughes GC, Kypson AP, Annex BH et al. (2000) Induction of angiogenesis after TMR: a comparison of holmium:YAG, CO_2, and excimer lasers. Ann Thorac Surg 70:504.
40. Yamamoto N, Kohmoto T, Roethy W et al. (2000) Histologic evidence that basic fibroblast growth factor enhances the angiogenic effects of transmyocardial laser revascularization. Basic Res Cardiol 95:55.
41. Sayeed-Shah U, Mann MJ, Martin J et al. (1998) Complete reversal of ischemic wall motion abnormalities by combined use of gene therapy with transmyocardial laser revascularization. J Thorac Cardiovasc Surg 116:763.
42. Hughes GC, Annex BH, Yin B et al. (1999) Transmyocardial laser revascularization limits *in vivo* adenoviral-mediated gene transfer in porcine myocardium. Cardiovasc Res 44:81.
43. Cooley DA, Frazier OH, Kadipasaoglu KA et al. (1996) Transmyocardial laser revascularization: clinical experience with twelve-month follow-up. J Thorac Cardiovasc Surg 111:791.
44. Donovan CL, Landolfo KP, Lowe JE, Clements F, Coleman RB, Ryan T (1997) Improvement in inducible ischemia during dobutamine stress echocardiography after transmyocardial laser revascularization patients with refractory angina pectoris. J Am Coll Card 30:607.
45. Horvath KA, Mannting F, Cummings N, Sherman SK, Cohn LH (1996) Transmyocardial laser revascularization: operative techniques and clinical results at two years. J Thorac Cardiovasc Surg 111:1047.
46. Krabatsch T, Tambeur L, Lieback E, Shaper F, Hetzer R (1998) Transmyocardial laser revascularization in the treatment of end-stage coronary artery disease. Ann Thorac Cardiovasc Surg 4:64.
47. Lutter G, Sauerbier B, Nitzsche E (1998) Transmyocardial laser revascularization (TMLR) in patients with unstable angina and low ejection fraction. Eur J Cardiothoracic Surg 13:21.
48. Milano A, Pratali S, Tartarini G et al. (1998) Early results of transmyocardial revascularization with a holmium laser. Ann Thorac Surg 65:700.
49. Horvath KA, Aranki SF, Cohn LH et al. (2001) Sustained angina relief 5 years after transmyocardial laser revascularization with CO_2 laser. Circulation 104(Suppl 1):I81.
50. De Carlo M, Milano AD, Pratali S, Levantino M, Mariotti R, Bortolotti U (2000) Symptomatic improvement after transmyocardial laser revascularization: how long does it last? Ann Thorac Surg 70:1130.
51. Sanni A, Dunning J (2004) Is transmyocardial revascularisation of benefit to people with 'no option' angina? Interact CardioVasc Thorac Surg 3:586.
52. Burns SM, Sharples LD, Tait S, Caine N, Wallwork J, Schofield PM (1999) The transmyocardial laser revascularization international registry report. Eur Heart J 20:31.
53. Allen KB, Dowling RD, Angell WW et al. (2004) Transmyocardial revascularization: 5-year follow-up of a prospective, randomized multicenter trial. Ann Thorac Surg 77:1228.
54. Bridges CR, Horvath KA, Nugent WC et al. (2004) The Society of Thoracic Surgeons Practice Guidelines Series: transmyocardial laser revascularization. Ann Thorac Surg 77:1494.
55. Allen KB, Dowling RD, Fudge TL et al. (1999) Comparison of transmyocardial revascularization with medical therapy in patients with refractory angina. N Engl J Med 341:1029.
56. Schofield PM, Sharples LD, Caine N et al. (1999) Transmyocardial laser revascularisation in patients with refractory angina: a randomised controlled trial [erratum appears in Lancet, 1999 May 15;353(9165):1714]. Lancet 353:519.

57. Hattler BG, Griffith BP, Zenati MA et al. (1999) Transmyocardial laser revascularization in the patient with unmanageable unstable angina. Ann Thorac Surg 68:1203.
58. Aaberge L, Rootwelt K, Blomhoff S, Saatvedt K, Abdelnoor M, Forfang K (2002) Continued symptomatic improvement three to five years after transmyocardial revascularization with CO_2 laser: a late clinical follow-up of the Norwegian randomized trial with transmyocardial revascularization. J Am Coll Cardiol 39:1588.
59. Frazier OH, March RJ, Horvath KA (1999) Transmyocardial revascularization with a carbon dioxide laser in patients with end-stage coronary artery disease. N Engl J Med 341:1021.
60. Sanni A, Dunning J (2004) Is transmyocardial revascularisation of benefit in addition to coronary artery bypass grafting for patients with diffuse coronary disease? Interact CardioVasc Thorac Surg 3:581.
61. Peterson ED, Kaul P, Kaczmarck RG et al. (2003) From controlled trials to clinical practice: monitoring transmyocardial revascularization use and outcomes. J Am Coll Cardiol 42:1611.
62. Loubani M, Chin D, Leverment JN, Galinanes M (2003) Mid-term results of combined transmyocardial laser revascularization and coronary artery bypass. Ann Thorac Surg 76:1166.
63. Stamou SC, Boyce SW, Cooke RH, Carlos BD, Sweet LC, Corso PJ (2002) One-year outcome after combined coronary artery bypass grafting and transmyocardial laser revascularization for refractory angina pectoris. Am J Cardiol 89:1365.
64. Allen KB, Dowling KB, DelRossi AJ, Realyvasques F, Lefrak EA (2000) Transmyocardial laser revascularization combined with coronary artery bypass grafting: a multicentre, blinded, prospective, randomized controlled trial. J Thorac Cardiovasc Surg 119:540.
65. Trehan N, Mishra M, Bapna R, Mishra A, Maheshwari P, Karlekar A (1997) Transmyocardial laser revascularisation combined with coronary artery bypass grafting without cardiopulmonary bypass. Eur J Cardiothorac Surg 12:276.
66. Vincent JG, Bardos P, Kruse J, Maass D (1997) End stage coronary disease treated with transmyocardial CO_2 laser revascularisation: a chance for the inoperable patient. Eur J Cardiothorac Surg 11:888.
67. Trehan N, Mishra M, Kohli A, Bapna R (1996) Transmyocardial laser revascularisation as an adjunct to CABG. Indian Heart J 48:381.
68. Tjomsland O, Aaberge L, Almdahl S et al. (2000) Perioperative cardiac function and predictors for adverse events after transmyocardial laser treatment. Ann Thorac Surg 69:1098.
69. Kadipasaoglu K, Sartori M, Masai T et al. (1999) Intraoperative arrhythmias and tissue damage during transmyocardial laser revascularization. Ann Thorac Surg 67:4230.
70. Hughes GC, Landolfo KP, Lowe JE et al. (1999) Diagnosis, incidence, and clinical significance of early postoperative ischemia after transmyocardial laser revascularization. Am Heart J 137:1163.
71. Hughes GC, Landolfo KP, Lowe JE, Coleman RB, Donovan CL (1999) Perioperative morbidity and mortality after transmyocardial laser revascularization: incidence and risk factors for adverse events. J Am Coll Cardiol 33:1021.
72. Aaberge L, Nordstrand K, Dragsund M et al. (2000) Transmyocardial revascularization with CO_2 laser in patients with refractory angina pectoris. Clinical results from the Norwegian randomized trial. J Am Coll Cardiol 35:1170.
73. Aaberge L, Rootwelt K, Blomhoff S, Saatvedt K, Abdelnoor M, Forfang K (2002) Continued symptomatic improvement three to five years after transmyocardial revascularization with CO_2 laser: a late clinical follow-up of the Norwegian randomized trial with transmyocardial revascularization. J Am Coll Cardiol 39:1588.
74. Burkhoff D, Schmidt S, Schulman SP et al. (1999) Transmyocardial laser revascularization compared with continued medical therapy for treatment of refractory angina pectoris: a prospective randomized trial. Lancet 354:885.
75. Frazier OH, March RJ, Horvath KA (1999) Transmyocardial revascularization with a carbon dioxide laser in patients with end-stage coronary artery disease. N Engl J Med 341:1021.
76. Burkhoff D, Wesley MN, Resar JR, Lansing AM (1999) Factors correlating with risk of mortality after transmyocardial revascularization. J Am Coll Cardiol 34:55.
77. Kraatz EG, Misfeld M, Jungbluth B, Sievers HH (2001) Survival after transmyocardial laser revascularization in relation to non-lasered perfused myocardial zones. Ann Thorac Surg 71:532.
78. March RJ (2000) Laser revascularization of ischemic myocardium. In Naunheim KS (ed). Minimal Access Cardiothoracic Surgery. Philadelphia, WB Saunders, p. 598.
79. Saatvedt K, Dragsund M, Nordstrand K (1996) Transmyocardial laser revascularization and coronary artery bypass grafting without cardiopulmonary bypass. Ann Thorac Surg 62:323.
80. Trehan N, Mishra Y, Mehta Y, Jangid DR (1998) Transmyocardial laser as an adjunct to minimally invasive CABG for complete myocardial revascularization. Ann Thorac Surg 66:1113.
81. Horvath KA (1998) Thoracoscopic transmyocardial laser revascularization. Ann Thorac Surg 65:1439.
82. Milano A, Pietrabissa A, Bortolotti U (1997) Transmyocardial laser revascularization using a thoracoscopic approach. Am J Cardiol 80:538.
83. Milano A, Pietrabissa A, Bortolotti U (1998) Thoracoscopic transmyocardial revascularization. Ann Thorac Surg 65:1510.

84. Milano A, Pratali S, De Carlo M et al. (1998) Transmyocardial holmium laser revascularization: feasibility of a thoracoscopic approach. Eur J Cardiothorac Surg 14(suppl 1): S105.
85. Bortone AS, D'Agostino D, Schena S et al. (2000) Instrumental validation of percutaneous transmyocardial revascularization: follow-up data at one year. Ann Thorac Surg 70:1115.
86. Nagele H, Stubbe HM, Nienaber C, Rodiger W (1998) Results of transmyocardial laser revascularization in non-revascularizable coronary artery disease after 3 years follow-up. Eur Heart J 19:1525.
87. von Knobelsdorff G, Brauer P, Tonner PH et al. (1997) Transmyocardial laser revascularization induces cerebral microembolization. Anesthesiology 87:58.
88. Dowling RD, Petracek MR, Selinger SL, Allen KB (1998) Transmyocardial revascularization in patients with refractory, unstable angina. Circulation 98:II73.
89. Frazier OH, Kadipasaoglu KA, Radovancevic B et al. (1998) Transmyocardial revascularization in allograft coronary artery disease. Ann Thorac Surg 65:1138.
90. Kornowski R, Baim DS, Moses JW et al. (2000) Short- and intermediate-term clinical outcomes from direct myocardial laser revascularization guided by biosense left ventricular electromechanical mapping. Circulation 102:1120.
91. Oesterle SN, Reifart NJ, Meier B, Lauer B, Schuler GC (1998) Initial results of laser-based percutaneous myocardial revascularization for angina pectoris. Am J Cardiol 82:659.
92. Whittaker P, Zheng S, Patterson MJ, Kloner RA, Daly KE, Hartman RA (2000) Histologic signatures of thermal injury: applications in transmyocardial laser revascularization and radiofrequency ablation. Laser Surg Med 27:305.
93. Sayeed-Shah U, Reul RM, Byrne J.G, Aranki SF, Cohn LH (1999) Combination TMR and gene therapy. Semin Thorac Cardiovasc Surg 11:36.

Prevention of Re-Stenosis of Coronary Arteries by Radionuclides

John R. Buscombe

Contents

43.1 Introduction 511
43.2 Edothelial Hypertrophy, Proliferation
and Re-Endothelialisation 512
43.3 Methods of Post-Angioplasty Irradiation 513
43.4 Results of Human Studies 514
43.5 Conclusions 514
References 515

43.1
Introduction

In the developed world heart disease, primarily in the forms of coronary artery disease, vies with all cancers as the biggest cause of premature deaths. Even in the developing world, as many live longer, death rates from heart disease increase and the disease becomes more prominent. The ideal solution would be primary prevention, which would require the control of diet, often from a young age, and the reduction of plasma cholesterol, again from a young age. There is also a need to reduce the rate of diabetes and treat hypertension. Then all one would need to do is stop people from smoking! Indeed, much work has been done in this area and over the past 20 years there has been a fall in the number of deaths from coronary artery disease in both North America and Western Europe.

Once the disease has developed and the vessels are lined with atheroma the next stage is to prevent the disease progressing by introducing the techniques described above and also by timely intervention. Patients presenting with angina or even an MI should now undergo assessment of the coronary arteries and blood flow. This will be done initially by exercise electrocardiography then myocardial perfusion scintigraphy. If evidence for disease is established then an angiogram (direct or indirect) is performed. The identification of significant areas of stenosis will lead to angioplasty or surgery.

In angioplasty a balloon is inflated to a pressure at which the plaque of the atheroma is disrupted and fractured therefore allowing more blood to flow down the artery. Performing a coronary angiogram is a simple procedure for the skilled cardiologist to undertake. Success rates are initially high but re-stenosing can occur within a short period of time, with up to 70% of some arteries subject to re-stenosis within a year [1]. Re-angioplasty is possible but it would be preferable if the re-stenosis could be prevented. One method has been the use of stents, which can be impregnated with chemicals that prevent or reduce re-stenosis [1, 2]. Alternatively it has been found that radiation can reduce re-stenosis rates and good results have been obtained using stents impregnated with a medium energy pure beta emitter such as P-32. This has a long half-life and will provide some irradiation to the wall over time. There are, however, some atheromatous lesions in which stent placement is not possible due to the shape of the artery or the length of the atheroma. Irradiation has been given using iridium wires placed in the artery after angioplasty but these can lead to very irregular radiation fields ([3], Fig. 43.1). There was, therefore, a need for a more versatile method of delivering radiation and this was the genesis of using radionuclides held within an angioplasty balloon immediately after angioplasty.

43.2
Edothelial Hypertrophy, Proliferation and Re-Endothelialisation

If one is treating a clinical problem it is important to know the target: in this case, the cell types that induce re-stenosis. It is important to look at what happens during angioplasty and any subsequent reaction. During angioplasty the vessel is widened by pressure in the balloon. The atheromatous plaque is damaged and crushed. It is a physical insult and results in a damage response. It would be hoped that this is limited to scarring at the site of the damage and re-endothelialisation of the vessel wall to produce a smooth surface to stop more atheroma and thrombus development. In about half of patients this re-endothelialisation tends to occur in a more haphazard way. This can lead to endothelial hypertrophy and proliferation. It would appear that the cells involved in this process are the endothelial progenitor cells (EPCs), which are recruited to the area of damaged blood vessel from the bone marrow. This recruitment appears to be secondary to high levels of granulocyte-macrophage colony stimulating factor (GM-CSF) [4]. The GM-CSF is released as part of the damage signalling that occurs at damage. This is released from inflammatory cells such as granulocytes and granulocytes, which migrate to the cell wall immediately after angioplasty (Fig. 43.2). In many, if not most patients, the re-endothelisation becomes disorganised and results in areas of intimal hyperplasia, which can result in re-stenosis. This could occur within 4–6 weeks of the vascular injury and can result in continued growth for up to 12 months.

The site of this re-endothelialisation is normally at the proximal and distal end of the plaque. The reason for this is unclear but it is proposed that to ensure that the whole plaque is treated, the balloon chosen will be longer than the defect. This will mean that at each end,

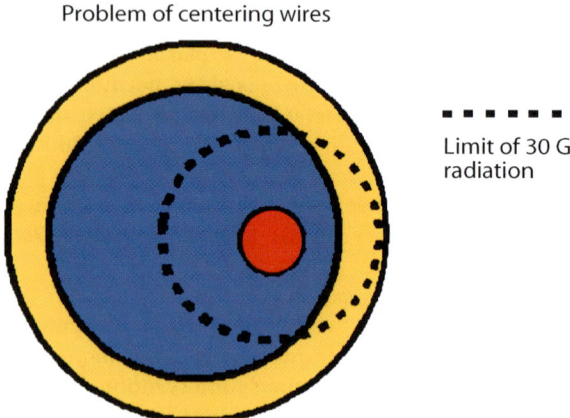

Fig. 43.1 Asymmetric radiation of the vessel wall by a wire placed in the coronary artery

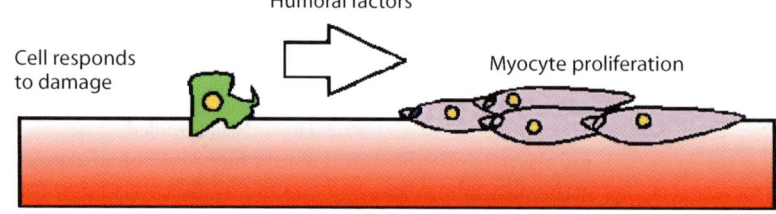

Fig. 43.2 Method of intimal growth after angioplasty showing macrophages would be the ideal target cell

a small amount of normal vessel will be put under pressure and potentially damaged. As this represents normal vessel wall the damage response is greater than that of the abnormal wall and the subsequent release of GM-CSF and migration of inflammatory cells and myoblasts is greater, resulting in a thicker area of intimal hypertrophy. This results in what is called a "candy wrapper" lesion [5]. It is the prevention of this intimal hyperpalsia that irradiation of the vessel wall after angioplasty is addressed. The cells producing this "damage" response will be killed and chemotactic factors such as GM-CSF will not be released. However, sufficient radiation must be delivered to ensure cell death and not just cell damage, which could result in an enhanced damage response.

43.3
Methods of Post-Angioplasty Irradiation

There are three main methods used in post-angioplasty irradiation. The first was the use of iridium wires. These were placed in the vessel for a short period after angioplasty; however, it was very difficult to ensure that the wire was placed centrally, especially in tortuous vessels, resulting in uneven wall irradiation. If an area of wall received less than 11 Gy there was unlikely to be any positive effect of the treatment, while high doses in excess of 60 Gy could lead to damage of the normal vessel wall and subsequent scarring and stenosis.

To ensure more even distribution of the radiation dose two methods have been developed (Fig. 43.3). The first is the use of balloons filled with a radionuclide, which is administered just after angioplasty either to the naked vessel wall or inside a stent. The choice of isotope for this is most important. Ideally it should be a beta emitter; alpha emitters would not pass the balloon substance and gamma emitters would not have a short enough track. The radiation itself must be able to penetrate at least the first 1 mm of the vessel wall. If the radiation is more energetic and able to traverse the whole vessel wall damage to the basement membrane could occur, resulting in vascular failure with resulting occlusion or necrosis. For this reason common beta-emitters such as Y-90 are not appropriate. To date the ideal isotope has been shown to be rhenium-188 (Re-188). This is a generator-produced isotope, the daughter produced from a tungsten-188 generator. It has a 17 hour half-life with a mean energy beta of 2.12 MeV. Within a balloon system this will give a radiation dose primarily to the first 1 mm of the vessel wall.

To determine the dose of radiation to the wall it is necessary to distribute a given activity of Re-188 in a given volume. The radiation dose per unit area is then calculated to deliver 15 Gy at 1 mm. The figure of 15 Gy comes from animal work showing that the maximum protection against re-stenosis was achieved with this dose at 1 mm of vessel wall [6]. Confusingly, some publications refer to 22.5 Gy at 0.5 mm, but this is the dose with 15 Gy at 1 mm. The activity produced is limited by the specific activity of the generator; when fresh it may be possible to obtain 4 GBq per mL but as the parent isotope decays over 6 months this may fall to 1 GBq per mL. Clearly the balloon used has a limited capacity so that it is not possible to just administer more fluid if the specific activity is less. However, radiation dose also depends on time of exposure, therefore radiation dose can be increased by simply increasing the exposure time to the isotope. Clearly there is a physiological limit to the time a balloon can be inflated in a coronary artery before ischaemic damage occurs to the cardiac muscle downstream of the balloon placement. This is normally considered to be 5 minutes. Therefore, if it is necessary to use a longer exposure time the balloon will need to

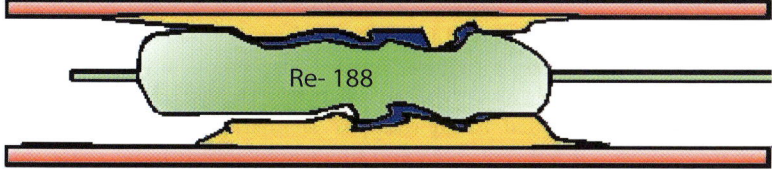

Fig. 43.3 How a balloon filled with RE-188 can "conform" to the vessel shape giving a more equal radiation dose to the cell wall and preventing "candy wrapper" stenosis

be deflated then subsequently re-inflated. This must be done via a leakproof and shielded system to reduce the risk of radiation spillage and exposure to the operator. This means that it is not possible to use this technique without a dose calculation being performed. This can be done if a radiation physicist is present during the procedure but is more commonly done on previously performed angiogram images when the operator has already chosen the volume of balloon to be used, the length and diameter of the stenosis and the specific activity of the Re-188 to be used.

The third method allows radiation of the vessel in a more pre-determined way by the use of radioactive stents. Traditionally these were impregnated with phosphorus-32 (P-32), however, the beta particles from this isotope have a high energy and subsequently caused much intimal damage beyond either end of the stent. This resulted in intimal hyperplasia and the so-called "candy wrapper" effect. There has been recent work by the groups working with Re-188 to produce a Re-188 covered stent. The process is not easy as the stainless steel stent must be heated to 950°C in the presence of Re-188 and hydrogen chloride in a pure vacuum. Results in animals have been encouraging [7], with more even radiation effects and less dependence on plaque length and vessel diameter than with the balloon. In publicised studies vessels treated with Re-188 stents do not appear to suffer from the candy wrapper effect, however, human studies are awaited and there must be doubts about the economics of such a complex preparation method with a short-lived isotope.

43.4
Results of Human Studies

So far the body of evidence for the use of radionuclides in preventing stenosis is limited to the use of Re-188 products administered in a catheter balloon after angioplasty. Phase 1 and 2 studies have shown the most efficacious radiation dose to be 15 Gy at 1 mm and 22.5 Gy at 0.5 mm [8–10]. However, to provide evidence for efficacy it is important to perform a randomised control trial and one such trial has been reported from Dresden [6]. In this study 113/125 patients were assigned to Re-188 therapy after angioplasty. The activity and time of exposure was chosen to provide 22.5 Gy at 0.5 mm. using Re-188 eluted from a generator provided by Oak Ridge in the USA. The specific activity was 3.7 GBq/mL and this was infused into non-compliant balloons used after angioplasty. A single maximum inflation time of 5 minutes was used. If greater times were required, the patient had repeat inflations and deflations until the required inflation time was achieved. The catheter used was 10 mm longer than the catheter used during the angioplasty procedure. The deflation period was normally 2 minutes, and the length of vessel irradiated varied from 20 mm to 90 mm, most being 30–40 mm. The procedure was covered by acetylsalicilate to prevent platelet adhesion and thrombus formation. Re-stenosis was determined angiographically during the follow-up period. There was no angina or ECG changes in the treated group. Most patients were treated using between one and three inflations of 5 minutes but as many as seven were required. The infarct rate over the first year was similar for the two groups; 6.2% in the treated group compared with 4.5% in the control group. The re-stenosis rate in the treated group was 6.3% compared with 27.5% in the non-irradiated group. Only 12.6% needed any further re-vascularisation procedure in the treated group compared with 28.6% in the non-irradiated group. In all those with re-stenosis from the rhenium treated group the re-stenosis was at the edges of the lesion. This was rare in the untreated group (1%), however, the untreated group tended to re-stenose at the site of old atheroma.

In a further German study [11], similar results were obtained in a series of over 200 patients. The re-stenosis rate in the placebo group at 12 months post-angioplasty was 40% compared with 24% in those receiving Re-188 treatment by balloon immediately after angioplasty. It was noted that in diabetics this difference was maintained, with 44% in the control group and 27% in the Re-188 treated group. However, when the patient received both a stent and then Re-188 within a balloon there was very high re-stenosis and thrombotic event and this was found to be due to inadequate re-endothelialisation of the metal stent surface after the procedure, leaving the raw metal exposed and itself becoming thrombogenic. It is not recommended by this group that Re-188 by balloon be combined with placement of stents.

43.5
Conclusions

The use of balloon filled beta-emitting radioisotopes, able to deliver 22.5 Gy to the first 0.5 mm of the endothelial wall provides a relatively inexpensive method of preventing re-stenosis in patients undergoing angioplasty for coronary artery stenosis. It appears the dreaded "candy wrapper" stenosis caused by P-32 stents is not replicated and this would appear to be a safe and efficacious treatment.

References

1. Morice MC, Serruys PW, Sousa JE, Fajadet J, Ban Hayashi E, Perin M, Colombo A, Schuler G, Barragan P, Guagliumi G, Molnar F, Falotico R (2002) RAVEL Study Group. Randomized Study with the Sirolimus-Coated Bx Velocity Balloon-Expandable Stent in the Treatment of Patients with de Novo Native Coronary Artery Lesions. A randomized comparison of a sirolimus-eluting stent with a standard stent for coronary revascularization. N Engl J Med 346:1773–1780.
2. Cutlip DE (2006) Drug-eluting stent era: will we improve 5-year outcomes? Coronary Artery Dis 17:289–292.
3. Marijnissen JP, Coen VL, van der Giessen WJ, de Pan C, Serruys PW, Levendag PC (2004) Optimal source position for irradiation of coronary bifurcations in endovascular brachytherapy with catheter based beta or iridium-192 sources. Radiotherapy Oncol 71:99–108.
4. Cho HJ, Kim HS, Lee MM, Kim DH, Yang HJ, Hur J, Hwang KK, Oh S, Choi YJ, Chae IH, Oh BH, Choi YS, Walsh K, Park YB (2003) Mobilized endothelial progenitor cells by granulocyte-macrophage colony-stimulating factor accelerate reendothelialization and reduce vascular inflammation after intravascular radiation. Circulation 108:2918–2925.
5. Angiolillo DJ, Sabata M, Alfonso F, Macaya C (2004) "Candy wrapper" effect after drug-eluting stent implantation: deja vu or stumbling over the same stone again? Catheter Cardiovasc Interv 61:387–391.
6. Hoher M, Wohrle J, Wohlfrom M, Kamenz J, Nusser T, Grebe OC, Hanke H, Kochs M, Reske SN, Hombach V, Kotzerke J (2003) Intracoronary beta-irradiation with a rhenium-188-filled balloon catheter: a randomized trial in patients with de novo and restenotic lesions. Circulation 107:3022–3027.
7. Tepe G, Dietrich T, Grafen F, Brehme U, Muschick P, Dinkelborg LM, Greschniok A, Claussen CD, Duda SH (2005) Reduction of intimal hyperplasia with Re-188-labeled stents in a rabbit model at 7 and 26 weeks: an experimental study. Cardiovasc Intervent Radiol 28:632–637.
8. Hsieh BT, Hsieh JF, Tsai SC, Lin WY, Huang HT, Ting G, Wang SJ (1999) Rhenium-188-Labeled DTPA: a new radiopharmaceutical for intravascular radiation therapy. Nucl Med Biol 26:967–972.
9. Kim EH, Moon DH, Oh SJ, Choi CW, Lim SM, Hong MK, Park SW (2002) Monte Carlo dose simulation for intracoronary radiation therapy with a rhenium 188 solution-filled balloon with contrast medium. J Nucl Cardiol 9:312–318.
10. Hang CL, Fu M, Hsieh BT, Leung SW, Wu CJ, Ting G (2003) Intracoronary beta-irradiation with liquid rhenium-188 to prevent restenosis following pure balloon angioplasty: results from the TRIPPER-1 study. Chang Gung Med J 26:98–106.
11. Kropp J, Reynen K, Koeckeritz U, Knapp FF (2005) Intracoronary radiation therapy: Placbo controlled study: A report. World J Nucl Med 4:S27–S28.

Cardiac Transplantation: Current Status and Limitations

Sheetal Kaul and Assad Movahed

Contents

44.1	Historical Background	517
44.2	Donor Selection and Management	517
44.3	Recipient Selection	518
44.4	Contraindications	518
44.5	Surgical Technique	518
44.6	Post-Transplant Care	518
44.7	Post-Transplant Complications	519
44.7.1	Rejection	519
44.7.2	Infection	519
44.7.3	Malignancies	521
44.7.4	Transplant Vasculopathy	521
44.8	Future	523
	References	523

44.1 Historical Background

Surgical replacement with an allograft is the definitive therapy for end-stage myocardial disease. Carrel and Guthrie were early pioneers in the field, notably with respect to vascular anastomotic techniques [1]. Further advancements are credited to Mann and his colleagues at Mayo [2] as well as Shumway and Lower at Stanford [3]. Barnard in South Africa (1967) [4] and Shumway at Stanford [1968] were the early successful pioneers in human allograft heart transplantation. The introduction of immunosuppressant therapies in the 1980s was a great boost to this field.

In the years since, improvements in donor and recipient selection, surgical technique, post-surgical care and medical therapy have allowed tremendous improvements in survival and general acceptability of transplantation as the "gold standard" of care for end-stage heart failure refractory to best medical and device-based therapy. Over 300 centers worldwide, half of which are in the USA, transplant over 3000 hearts a year. The perioperative mortality is less than 10%. About 80% of patients survive the first year, after which mortality is about 4% per year. However, the limited availability of donor hearts has led to stagnation in volumes seen in recent years. It is also postulated that with improvements in medical therapy, devices and aggressive revascularization, the pool of "eligible" candidates for transplantation may shrink by 20–50%.

44.2 Donor Selection and Management

The "ideal" donor, who has met criteria for brain death, is preferably under 55 years of age [5]. A history of significant or active cardiac, infectious or malignant disease prior to death is sought and excluded as well as severe chest trauma. Prolonged hemodynamic instability and metabolic derangements such as tissue hypoxia/hypoperfusion are ruled out. Diabetes, dyslipidemia and hypertension are considered relative exclusion criteria. Screening for HIV and hepatitis B and C is carried out.

Frequently, echocardiography and coronary angiography are performed to assess cardiac function and exclude significant coronary artery disease, especially in older donors.

Organ retrieval is usually performed by a team from the nearest transplant center, often as part of a multi-organ harvest. Donor and recipient are matched for ABO compatibility and body size. Meticulous attention to organ preservation and minimization of "cold ischemic time" is critical to maintaining the viability of the donor heart.

44.3 Recipient Selection

The critical shortage of donor hearts compared with the number of terminally ill patients with CHF makes it imperative that patient selection be based on universally accepted criteria. Typically, these patients have an unacceptable prognosis and quality of life despite aggressive medical therapy, appropriate revascularization, removal of reversible causes and treatment of conditions such as giant cell or lymphocytic myocarditis. These candidates are expected to die in a short time despite best therapy unless they receive a transplant but have no other medical condition that would compromise survival or compliance after transplantation [6]. Patients commonly have had prolonged or recurrent admissions for refractory heart failure symptoms and are usually inotrope or device dependant for circulatory support.

44.4 Contraindications

The presence of irreversible pulmonary hypertension (Pulmonary Vascular Resistance PVR > 4 Wood units) is an absolute contraindication to transplantation. This is because the donor heart, being not used to the elevated pressures in the recipient's pulmonary vasulature, often fails in the immediate postoperative period. It is common practice to invasively assess both the PVR and its reversibility with vasodilators such as prostaglandins, nitroprusside, dobutamine, etc. and exclude patients with irreversible pulmonary hypertension.

Patients with malignancies and active serious infections are routinely excluded due to the risk of such conditions worsening with immunosuppressant therapy. Specifically, HIV, disseminated tuberculosis and the B and C subtypes of chronic hepatitis are considered contraindications at many centers.

Severe cerebrovascular disease, compromising functional status post-transplant, is a major contraindication.

Most centers exclude patients with ongoing drug, tobacco and alcohol abuse problems or serious noncompliance with medical care.

Relative contraindications are taken into consideration while assessing the eligibility of candidates for transplantation and include:
- Diabetes mellitus, especially with end-organ damage
- Severe obstructive or restrictive lung disease
- Renal insufficiency
- Cirrhosis with coagulopathy
- Recent pulmonary embolism/infarction
- Extensive peripheral vascular disease
- Poor psychological and social support network

Age has been a moving target in terms of being a contraindication. While most centers historically turned down candidates above 65, there is a trend towards accepting older patients with no other major contraindications or comorbidities who could be expected to have an acceptable improvement in quality or quantity of life with the procedure.

44.5 Surgical Technique

A median sternotomy is used to expose the donor heart, which is then examined for gross evidence of congenital, coronary or myocardial pathology. After systemic heparinization and decompression of the left heart, the aorta is cannulated and cold crystalline cardioplegia instilled. The vena cavae, pulmonary veins, aorta and pulmonary artery are then divided and the heart retrieved. Up to 3 to 4 hours of cold ischemic time often ensue while the organ is transported to a transplant center in an iced preservative solution. The recipient heart is excised after dividing its attachments to the great arteries and inflow veins following the same principles used in the harvesting of the donor organ. The classic "biatrial" technique has given way to the "bicaval" approach, which consists of anastomosing the donor organ to recipient atrial muscle [7]. Advantages of this method include reduced atrioventricular valve regurgitation, reduced sino-atrial node dysfunction and improved atrial mechanical function. The reader is referred to specialized texts for further surgical details.

44.6 Post-Transplant Care

The postoperative care of the transplant patient is similar to that of the usual open-heart patient with two major exceptions. There is a more frequent need for inotropic support and pacing (due to sino-atrial node dysfunction). The second is the institution of immunosuppression. Typically, patients are discharged home in less than 2 weeks unless complications ensue.

Immunosuppressive regimens vary significantly from center to center and are constantly evolving. However, initial therapy almost always includes high-dose steroids in addition to a T-cell inhibitor (such as sirolimus) and a calcineurin inhibitor such as cyclosporine. The intensity of therapy is tapered and customized to individuals based on frequency and severity of rejection episodes, susceptibility to infection and drug side-effects. In addition, some centers use short regimens of induction immunosuppression in the postoperative course when rejection is most common and most serious.

44.7
Post-Transplant Complications

44.7.1
Rejection

Transplant rejection is a common and often recurrent complication of transplantation. Careful surveillance and expeditious treatment with augmented immunosuppressive therapy is paramount. Rejection is the most common cause of death early on but the frequency decreases with time. Most patients have between one and three episodes in the first year alone.

Rejection is suspected on clinical grounds (symptoms or signs of LV dysfunction) or echocardiography but proven by means of a right ventricular biopsy done via the right internal jugular route. The frequency of biopsies is dictated by center preference and the patient's rejection history. A typical schedule includes once-weekly biopsies for 6 weeks, once every 3 months for the rest of the first year and every 6–12 months thereafter.

Noninvasive detection of rejection has not yet matched the test performance of biopsy but many modalities are being studied. Myocardial T2 relaxation time determined by black-blood magnetic resonance imaging sequence has been shown by French investigators to be promising in the detection of acute rejection episodes, with a sensitivity and specificity of about 90% and 70%, respectively [8] (Fig. 44.1). Indium-111 labeled anti-myosin antibody uptake scanning may turn out to be a reliable noninvasive method of detecting rejection in the post-acute phase [9]. Since uptake is abnormal in other conditions such as infarction, contusion, myocarditis, etc., sensitivity is improved by clinical correlation and a high pretest index of suspicion for rejection (Fig. 44.2).

There are multiple classification schemes for the his-

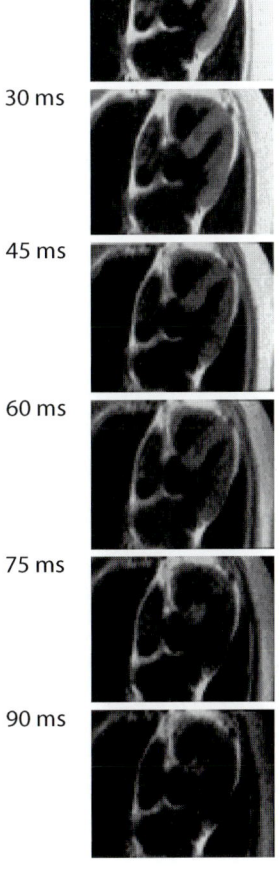

Fig 44.1 Magnetic resonance imaging using black-blood sequence to determine myocardial relaxation time T2 (examples of images obtained using the black blood sequence with echo images 15, 30, 45, 60, 75, 90 ms). The ratios, calculated for each echo image between the myocardial signal from septal wall and the blood signal from the left ventricular cavity, were 9.7 at 15 ms, 5.8 at 30 ms, 3.9 at 45 ms, 3.4 at 60 ms, 2.6 at 75 ms and 2.1 at 90 ms. Reproduced with permission from [8]

tologic grading of rejection. The International Society of Heart and Lung Transplantation nomenclature is reproduced for the reader's reference (Table 44.1). Grades 3 and above warrant augmented therapy, as does grade 2 with symptoms or hemodynamic compromise.

Treatment of early rejection episodes involves high dose steroids or OKT3 and follow-up biopsies to confirm resolution. Rejection episodes more than 3 months out can be treated with oral steroids. Sirolimus, everolimus, anti-thymocyte globulin, total lymphoid irradiation and methotrexate have been used in severe or recurrent cases. As a last resort, retransplanation is the definitive treatment but success rates are not encouraging.

44.7.2
Infection

Increased susceptibility to infections is an unintended but obvious consequence of immunosuppressant ther-

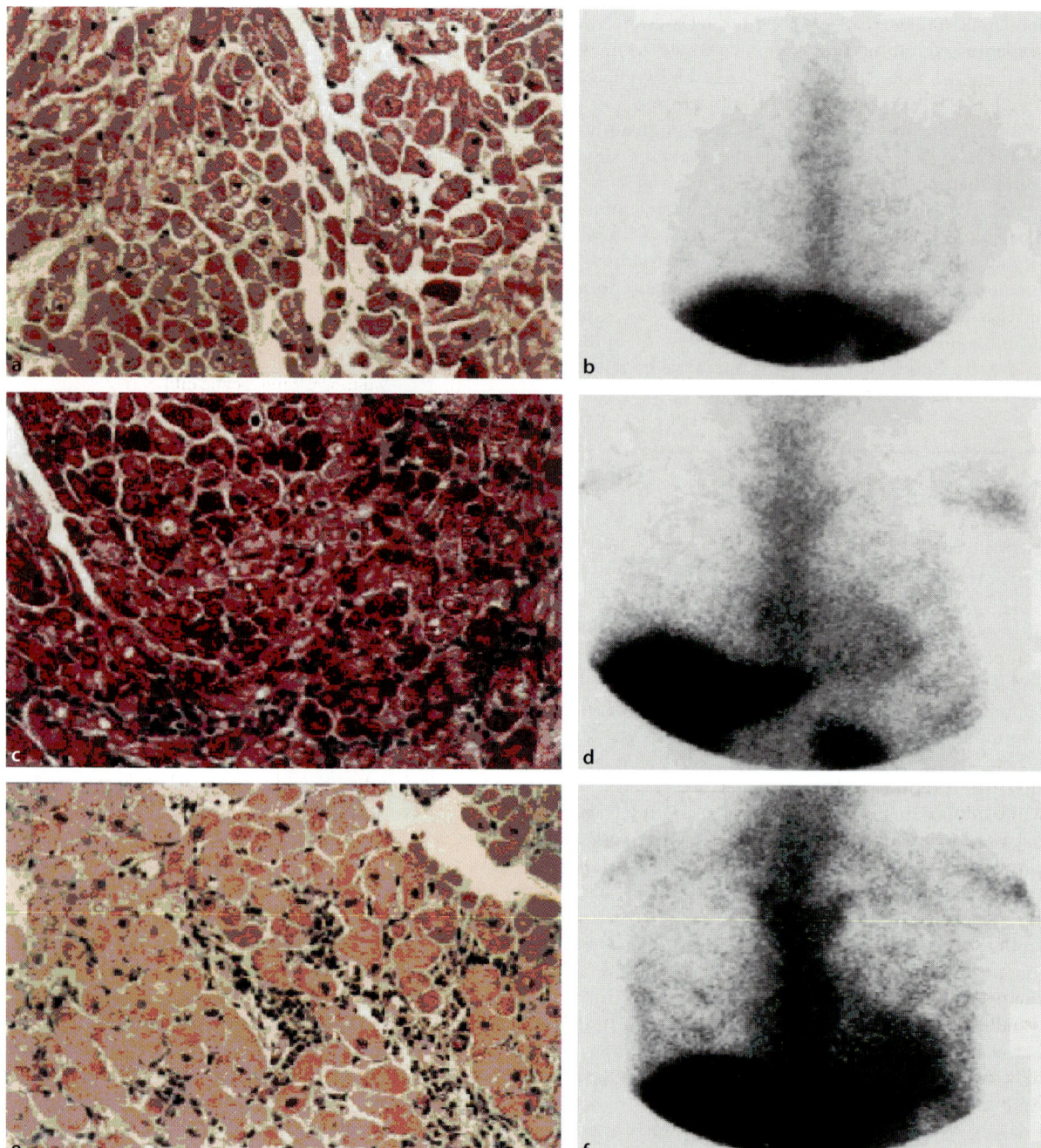

Fig. 44.2a–f Comparison of histologic evidence of rejection with corresponding findings on antimyosin imaging scans. The first pair of images depicts grade 0, the second grade 1B and the third grade 3A. Reproduced with permission from [9]

Table 44.1 The International Society for Heart and Lung Transplantation classification of rejection with histologic correlation, in comparison with an older scheme. Reproduced with permission from [10]

"Old" nomenclature	Grade	"New" nomenclature
No rejection	0	No rejection
Mild rejection	I	A = perivascular or focal interstitial infiltrate without myocyte damage
	I	B = sparse focal interstitial infiltrate without myocyte damage
"Focal" moderate rejection	II	One focus only with activated lymphocytes and myocyte damage
"Low/moderate" rejection	III A	Multifocal lymphocytic infiltrates with myocyte damage
"Borderline/severe" rejection	III B	Diffuse (sometimes polymorphous) inflammatory process
"Severe/acute" rejection	IV	Diffuse polymorphous infiltrate with myocyte necrosis +/- hemorrhage +/- edema +/- vasculitis
"Resolving" rejection	Denoted by a lower grade	Healing tissue with fibroblasts and pigmented macrophages
"Resolved" rejection	0	Mature scar tissue

apy. The titration of drug regimens to avoid rejection while minimizing infectious sequelae is really a balancing act requiring frequent changes in the care plan. Close clinical follow-up and chest radiography are the core elements of surveillance. While the common organisms are Aspergillus, Pneumocystis (PCP), Pneumococcus and Cytomegalovirus (CMV), the list of possible agents is much longer. Antimicrobial prophylaxis directed against candidiasis, Herpes simplex, PCP and CMV are usually implemented. In the case of an actual infection, consultation with infectious disease specialists as well as diligent attempts to reliably identify the agent by culture or immunologic methods is recommended.

44.7.3
Malignancies

An increased incidence of malignancies, particularly lymphoid and dermatologic, is noted after transplantation and is attributed to immunosuppression. In fact, reduction in immunosuppression often leads to regression but is fraught with the consequences of increased rejection. Reactivation of previously treated malignancy in remission is an additional concern. Lesions are usually extra-nodal and respond better to radiotherapy and less to chemotherapy. Surgery is an option when localized. There is increasing interest in the role of the Epstein–Barr virus in the lymphoid malignancies (often termed Post-transplant Lymphoproliferative Disorders) and agents such as acyclovir are sometimes used as part of therapy [11].

44.7.4
Transplant Vasculopathy

While rejection and infection are the common causes of mortality in the early post-transplant period, the main culprit after the first year is transplant vasculopathy, also known as coronary allograft arteriopathy or cardiac allograft vasculopathy (CAV). The pathogenesis is not well understood and is presumed to be related to immunogenic processes, although the use of immunosuppression has not appreciably reduced the incidence or severity of this phenomenon, with the possible exception of everolimus [12].

The features of transplant vasculopathy that differ from classic atherosclerosis are illustrated in Fig. 44.3 and include:

- Uniform, diffuse and predominantly distal nature of disease
- Marked intimal thickening
- Relative lack of thrombosis
- Poor collateralization.

The prevalence of CAV is about 5% in the first year, rising to 40–70% in the fifth year and dipping back down to 20% after the first decade of survival. While most disease is not obstructive, progression is unpredictable. About 20% of those with CAV have angiographically severe disease in one or more epicardial vessels. Survival is inversely proportional to number of vessels affected – only 13% of patients with three vessel disease > 40% severity survive 2 years or more.

Most patients present with arrhythmias, LV dysfunction, silent ischemia or sudden death. On account of denervation, symptoms are rare and atypical. However, some centers have reported correlation between anginal symptoms and demonstration of sympathetic reinnervation by 123 I-metaiodobenzylguanidine (MIBG) imaging [13].

Surveillance for CAV is standard and consists of angiography performed before discharge and annually thereafter. Angiography tends to underestimate the severity of disease due to its uniform nature. It is advisable to visually compare angiographic data from prior studies to reliably assess progression of CAV. The use of intravascular ultrasound (IVUS), coronary flow reserve (CFR) and TIMI frame counts is expanding.

There is currently insufficient evidence to support the replacement of catheterization by noninvasive techniques. Dobutamine stress echocardiography is supported by the largest amount of data with acceptable sensitivity, specificity and prognostic value, especially if serial annual scans depict worsening wall motion abnormalities [14]. Some centers have published data utilizing myocardial perfusion imaging with dobutamine or dipyridamole. Carlsen et al. have demonstrated the excellent negative predictive value of a normal MPI scan in ruling out angiographically treatable lesions [15]. Both thallium-201 and 99m-technetium based myocardial perfusion radiopharmaceuticals have been studied. The Mayo clinic published a series of 13 patients where

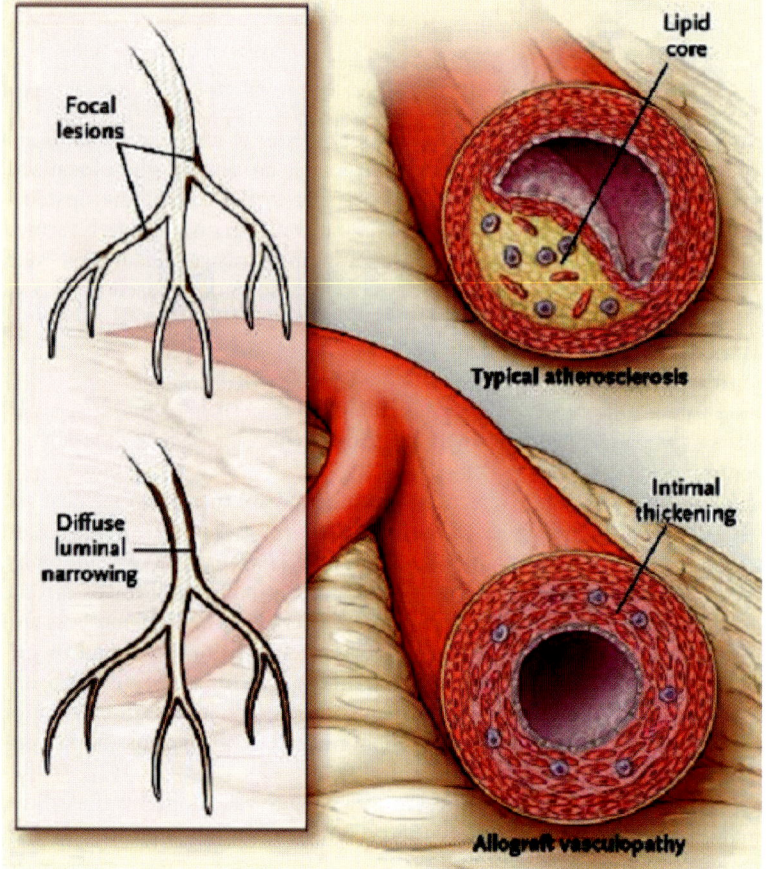

Fig. 44.3 Schematic illustration of the differences between typical coronary atherosclerosis and allograft vasculopathy. Reproduced with permission from Avery RK (2003) Cardiac-allograft vasculopathy. New Eng J Med 9349:829–830. Copyright 2003 Massachusetts Medical Society

201-Tl SPECT imaging had 100% sensitivity in predicting angiographic lesions of at least 70% severity [16]. Wu and his colleagues from Taiwan published a larger series with 89% sensitivity and 96% negative predictive value for the same angiographic endpoints [17]. EBCT and PET are emerging technologies, which hold significant promise.

Treatment of CAV is largely empiric. The use of statins has been shown to reduce frequency and severity of rejection, IVUS indices of atherosclerosis and angiographic disease, and prolong survival. This is in addition to the expected lipid-altering effects. Pravastatin is favored on account of its lack of CYP3A4-based interactions with other therapies such as cyclosporine and tacrolimus [18]. Interestingly, a small series has shown reduction in angiographic progression with the use of diltiazem with some survival benefit [19].

Intensification of immunosuppressant therapy is associated with regression of disease but the risk of infection and lymphoproliferative disease increases significantly. Target Of Rapamycin (TOR) inhibitors such as sirolimus and everolimus are showing promise but are not yet the standard of care in the USA [12] (Everolimus is approved in Europe). PCI is often performed for discrete lesions with noninvasive evidence of ischemia or evidence of LV dysfunction without concomitant evidence of rejection. Retransplantion is the last option and is performed at some centers but reserved for highly selected patients on account of lower survival rates (48–52%).

44.8
Future

There has been a "plateauing" in the volume of transplants performed annually worldwide. This is partially attributed to better medical care of the CHF patient and limited availability of donor hearts. Efforts to make transplantation more feasible and less expensive are required as are improvements in the quality of post-transplant life. Exclusion criteria are being liberalized. The use of novel non-invasive imaging modalities to detect ischemia and rejection may reduce the need for repeated angiography and biopsy and is of particular interest to imaging specialists. Xenotransplantation and mechanical prostheses such as "destination Ventricular Assist Devices" may change the landscape significantly.

References

1. Carrel A, Guthrie CC (1905) The transplantation of veins and organs. Am J Med 10:1101.
2. Mann FC, Priestly JT, Markowitz J, Yater WM (1933) Transplantation of the intact mammalian heart. Arch Surg 26:219–224.
3. Lower RR, Shumway NE (1960) Studies of orthotopic homotransplantation of the canine heart. Surg Forum 11:18–19.
4. Barnard CN (1967) The operation. S African Med J 41:1271–1274.
5. Zaroff JG, Rosengard BR, Armstrong WF et al. (2002) Consensus conference report: Maximizing Use of Organs Recovered from the Cadaveric Donor-Cardiac Recommendations. Circulation 106:836–841.
6. Cimato TR, Jessup M (2002) Recipient selection in cardiac transplantation: contraindications and risk factors for mortality. J Heart Lung Transplant 21:1161–1173.
7. Aziz TM, Burgess M, Khafagy R et al. (1999) Bicaval and standard techniques in orthotopic heart transplantation: Medium-term experience in cardiac performance and survival. J Thorac Cardiovasc Surg 118:115–122.
8. Marie PY, Angioi M, Carteaux JP et al. (2001) Detection and prediction of acute heart transplant rejection with the myocardial T2 determination provided by a black-blood magnetic resonance imaging sequence. J Am Coll Cardiol 37(3):825–831.
9. Ballester M, Bordes R, Tazelaar et al. (1998) Evaluation of biopsy classification for rejection: relation to detection of myocardial damage by monoclonal antimyosin antibody imaging. J Am Coll Cardiol 31:1357–1361.
10. Billingham ME, Carey NRB, Hammond EH et al. (1990) A working formulation for the standardization of nomenclature in the diagnosis of heart and lung rejection: Heart rejection study group. J Heart Transplant 9:587–592.
11. Hanto DW, Frizzera G, Gail-Peczalska KJ et al. (1982) Epstein-Barr virus induced B-cell lymphoma after renal transplantation. N Engl J Med 306:913–918.
12. Eisen HJ, Tuzcu EM, Dorent R et al. (2003) Everolimus for the prevention of allograft rejection and vasculopathy in cardiac-transplant recipients. N Engl J Med 349(9):847–858.
13. Estorch M, Camprecios M, Flotats A et al. (1999) Sympathetic reinnervation of cardiac allograft evaluated by 123I-MIBG imaging. J Nucl Med 40(6):911–916.
14. Spes CH, Klauss V, Mudra H et al. (1999) Diagnostic and prognostic value of serial dobutamine stress echocardiography for noninvasive assessment of cardiac allograft vasculopathy: A comparison with coronary angiography and intravascular ultrasound. Circulation 100:509–515.
15. Carlsen J, Toft JC, Mortensen SA, Arendrup H, Aldershvile J, Hess B (2000) Myocardial perfusion scintigraphy as a screening method for significant coronary artery stenosis in cardiac transplant recipients. J Heart Lung Transplant 19(9):873–878.
16. Howarth DM, Forstrom LA, Samudrala V, Sinak LJ, McGregor CG, Rodeheffer RJ et al. (1996) Evaluation of

201 Tl SPECT myocardial perfusion imaging in the detection of coronary artery disease after orthotopic heart transplantation. Nucl Med Commun 17(2):105–113.

17. Wu YW, Yen RF, Lee CM et al. (2005) Diagnostic and prognostic value of dobutamine thallium-201 single-photon emission computed tomography after heart transplantation. J Heart Lung Transplant 24(5):544–550.

18. Kobashigawa JA, Katznelson S, Laks H et al. (1995) Effects of pravastatin on outcomes after cardiac transplantation. N Engl J Med 333:621–627.

19. Schroeder JS, Gao SZ, Alderman EL et al. (1993) A preliminary study of diltiazem in the prevention of coronary artery disease in heart transplant recipients. N Engl J Med 328:164–170.

Subject Index

A

abciximab 316, 440, 441
accelerated idioventricular rhythm 102
ACD. *see* annihilation coincidence detection
acebutalol 428
ACEI. *see* angiotensin-converting enzyme inhibitor (ACEI)
ACE inhibitor 317, 422, 480
acetate
– carbon-11 (^{11}C) 381
acetylcholine 458
acquisition matrix 327
ACT. *see* activated clotting time
actazolamide 430
actin 13
actin filament 4
actin–myosin cross-bridge 14
actinobacillus 139
action potential (AP) 4, 11
activated clotting time (ACT) 465
acute chest pain 166, 299
acute coronary syndrome (ACS) 26, 31, 35, 77, 232, 299
acute infarction 233
acute ischemia 233, 502
acute phase protein 81
acute rest myocardial perfusion imaging (ARMPI) 300
acyclovir 521
acyl-coenzyme A (CoA) 394
acyl-coenzyme A transferase (ACAT) 445
adaptive array 164
adenosine 25, 26, 182, 192, 232, 238, 245, 247, 253, 292, 313, 328, 402, 458
– infusion 253
adenosine triphosphate (ATP) 253
– hydrolysis 14
adenylate cyclase 10, 16
adrenergic receptor 10
afferent nerve 9
Agaston coronary calcium score 164
AGE. *see* advanced glycation end product
allograft 140, 517
alpha decay 215

alpha emitter 513
ambulatory electrocardiographic (AECG) monitoring 113
amiloride 430
aminophylline 254, 402
amiodarone 454, 456
amphetamine 412
anaerobic glycolysis 381
anaphylaxis 468
angina 131, 312
– cardiac catheterization 156
– pattern 56
– type 56
angina pectoris 24
angioblast 28
angiogenesis 27, 383
angiographic restenosis 277
angioplasty 38, 276, 511, 514
– technique 464
angiotensin converting enzyme (ACE) 316
angiotensin-converting enzyme inhibitor (ACEI) 420, 426
– pharmacodynamic 426
angiotensin II receptor antagonist 427
angiotensin receptor blocker 420
anistreplase 439
annexin-V 209, 383
annihilation coincidence detection (ACD) 365
annular shielding 367
annuloplasty 491, 493
annuloplasty band insertion 490
anomalous pulmonary vein drainage 142
antegrade cardioplegia 491
anti-arrhythmic drug
– pharmacokinetic 453
– Sicilian Gambit classification 149
– Vaughan Williams classification 149
anticoagulant therapy 438
antineutrino 216
antiplatelet therapy 480
antitachycardia pacing 150
antithrombin (AT) 441
anti-thrombotic agent 438
aortic dissection 141

aortic intramural hematoma (AHI)   142
aortic valve replacement (AVR)   142
apex beat   59
apical hypoperfusion   405
apical thinning   339
apoptosis   28, 383
ARB
- adverse effect   428
- pharmacodynamic   428
arbutamine   245, 249
arginine-glycine-aspartate (RGD)   383
ARMPI. *see* acute rest myocardial perfusion imaging
- cost saving   301
- outcome   301
arrhythmia   123, 131, 415, 468, 522
- differential diagnosis   147
- genetic   148
- pharmacological treatment   149
- re-entry   146
- triggered activity   146
arrhythmias   268
arrhythmogenic right ventricular dysplasia (ARVD)   148, 184
arterial baroreceptor   19
arterial graft   475
arterial pressure   18
arterial remodeling   463
arterial switch operation   402
arteriogenesis   27
ASD. *see* atrial septal defect
Aspergillus   521
aspirin   27, 422, 440, 464
asymmetric pulmonary blood flow   404
atenolol   428
atherectomy   464, 469
atherogenesis   25
atheroma   33, 512
atheromatous plaque   463, 512
atherosclerosis   24, 27, 31, 33, 311, 438
- accelerated   46
- pathogenesis   31
atherosclerotic
- AHA classification   32
atherosclerotic cardiovascular disease   18
atherosclerotic coronary artery disease   31
atherosclerotic plaque   171
atherothrombosis   32
- phases   33
athletic amenorrhoea   19
atomic number   214
ATP. *see* adenosine triphosphate
atrial arrhythmia   97, 98, 99
atrial fibrillation   457
atrial fibrillation (AF)   99, 139, 151
atrial flutter   97, 99

atrial hypertrophy   106
atrial septal defect (ASD)   73
atrial systole   17
atrioventricular bundle   146
atrioventricular node (AVN)   6, 146
atropa belladonna   255
atropine   129, 132, 255, 458
attenuation
- correction   335
attenuation artefact   334
attenuation correction   372
- cardiac PET   370
attenuation correction software   294
atypical chest pain   300
Auger electron   215
auscultation   60
automated voxel classification   374
automaticity   146
autonomic neuropathy   311
AV block   100
AV node   11

B

back projection   199
balanced ischaemia   341
balloon angioplasty   277
balloon catheter   465
balloon mitral valvuloplasty (BMV)   141
bare metal stent   466
Barlow's (bileaflet) valve   490
Barlow's disease   493
baroreceptor   16
Bayesian principle   234
Bayes theorem   132
B-blocker   480
Benazepril   426
$beta_2$-receptor stimulation   129, 130
beta blocker   129, 132, 238, 316, 317, 328, 394, 414, 415, 420, 422, 428, 454, 474
- adverse effect   429
- pharmacodynamic   428
- pharmacokinetic   428
beta emission   216
beta emitter   513
beta particle   216
beta receptor agonist   307
Bezold–Jarisch reflex   130
bicycle ergometer   18, 237
bidirectional shunt   358
bile acid   434
bile acid sequestrant
- adverse effect   434
- pharmacodynamic   434
- pharmacokinetic   434
bileaflet tilting disc valve   140

bioabsorbable stent   469
biochemistry   83
bivalirudin   438, 439
biventricular pacing   152
black blood imaging   178, 179
Blalock–Taussig shunt   405
Bland–White–Garland syndrome   341
blood flow   120
– velocity map   180
blood pressure (BP)   129, 288
BMIPP   227, 302
– imaging   392
BMV. *see* balloon mitral valvuloplasty
bradyarrhythmia   147, 151
bradycardia   59, 114
bradykinin   426
breast
– attenuation   332
breast attenuation artefact   269, 292
breast augmentation implant   293
breast cancer   287
breast-feeding   224
bretylium   454, 457
bright blood imaging   179
Bruce protocol   109, 237
Brugada syndrome   147, 148
bumetanide   430
bundle branch block (BBB)   102
bundle of His   4, 146
Butterworth filter   200
bypass conduit   475
bypass-graft patency   180
bypass surgery   128

C

C^{11} palmitate   392
C^{11} sodium acetate   383
CABG. *see* coronary artery bypass graft
CAB surgery
– complications   480
– indication   472
– management   472
– outcome   480
– patient selection   472
– preoperative workup   472
– surgical technique   474
CAD. *see* coronary artery disease
Ca^{++} influx   13
calcified nodule   37
calcineurin inhibitor   519
calcium antagonist   429
calcium-channel blocker (CCB)   238, 429, 457
– adverse effect   430
– pharmacodynamic   430
– pharmacokinetik   429

calcium ion influx   145
calcium scoring   165, 316
camera axis   205
camera–detector configuration   193
cAMP (cyclic adenosine monophosphate)   10, 16
candesartan   427
candy wrapper   513, 514
captopril   426
carbon dioxide   25
carboxyl   426
cardiac
– arrhythmia   146
– automaticity
  –   146
– biomarker   80
– catheterization   463
– cell
  – depolarisation   15
  – repolarisation   15
– chest pain   306
– contractility   432
– contraction   60
– creep   205
– cycle   16, 345
– dysautonomia   291
– magnetic resonance imaging (MRI)   177
– marker   79, 81
– muscle   4, 79
– muscle contraction   13
– neurotransmission imaging   393
– output (CO)   18, 130
– perfusion   180
– plexus   9
– resynchronization   152
– silhouette   68
– skeleton   7
– sudden death   35
– sympathetic nerve   16
– troponin   79
– tumor   122
– valve   7
– vein   6
– viability   180
cardiac allograft vasculopathy (CAV)   521
– treatment   523
cardiac anatomy   155
cardiac beat length acceptance window   262
cardiac beats   263
cardiac catheterization   155
– complications   159
– injection techniques   158
– lesion classification   159
– vascular access   158
– views   158
cardiac death rate   266

cardiac glycoside 458
cardiac hypertrophy 409
cardiac neurotransmission imaging 393
cardiac rehabilitation 480
cardiac surgery
– minimally invasive 488
cardiobacterium hominis 139
cardioembolic disease 123
cardioembolic stroke 140
cardiolite 224
cardiomegaly 73
cardiomyopathy 183, 265, 340, 351
cardioplegia 472, 488, 491
cardiopulmonary bypass (CPB) 472, 477
cardiothoracic ratio 68
cardiotoxic chemotherapy 351
cardiovascular calcification 70
cardiovascular disease (CVD) 234, 306, 419, 425, 478
cardiovascular examination 58
cardiovascular magnetic resonance (CMR) 392
cardiovascular system 11
– aging 19
– circulatory pathway 12
– clinical examination 53
– examination 59
– gender difference 19
– palpation 59
carvedilol 395
catecholamine 24, 247
– radiolabelled 383
catechol-o-methyltransferase (COMT) 248, 410
catheter ablation 151
catheter balloon 514
catheterization 155
CCB. see calcium channel-blocker
cell transplantation therapy 469
centre of rotation (COR) 206, 326
centrifugal pump 481
cerebrovascular accident 468
Chang method 335
characteristic X-ray 215
CHD. see coronary heart disease
CHD risk
– LDL cholesterol 420
chemoreceptor 16, 19
chest pain 77, 122, 173, 300
– cause 55
chest radiography 68, 474
– assessment of adequacy 66
– future trend 74
– normal variant 66
– pitfall 66
– technique 65
chest trauma 517

chlorthalidone 430
cholesterol 288, 434, 435
cholesteryl ester transfer protein (CETP) 445
cholestyramine 434
chronic chest pain syndrome 231
chronic heart failure 413
chronic ischemic heart disease 42
chronic severe angina 497
chronotropy 9, 16
circumflex artery 279
class I agent 454
class II agent 456
class III agent 456
clinical cardiac electrophysiology 145
clinical examination 53
clofibrate 435
clopidogrel 168, 443, 464, 474, 480
CMV. see cytomegalovirus
CNS
– baroreceptor 10
– chemoreceptor 10
CO_2 laser 498
coarse fibrillatory wave 99
coarse ventricular fibrillation 102
coincidence detection 373
cold crystalline cardioplegia 518
cold pressure testing 346
colesevelam 434
colestipol 434
collateral circulation 27
collimator 195, 326, 327
– high resolution 195
color Doppler echocardiography 120
colour-coded image 133
commissurotomy 490
complete heart block 100
Compton scattering 203, 366, 371
computed tomography (CT) 163
– ECG gated 167
computer-assisted telemanipulation system 490
COMT. see catechol-O-methyltransferase
congenital heart disease (CHD) 73, 123, 171
– classification 73
– diffuse unilateral reduction of relative blood flow 405
– radioactive tracer 355
congestive heart failure
– cardiac catheterization 157
congestive heart failure (CGF) 351
congestive heart failure (CHF) 431
constrictive pericarditis 184
continuous mode 198
continuous mode acquisition 199
contraction band necrosis 43

contrast allergy   468
contrast echocardiography   117, 120, 121
contrast nephropathy   157, 158
Copper-62   383
COR. *see* centre of rotation
- image mis-registration   327
coronary
- angiography   309
- angioplasty   128
- anomaly   172
- arteriography   180
- artery   6
  - aneurysm   39
  - bypass graft   181
  - calcification   70
  - congenital abnormality   39
  - spontaneous dissection   39
- artery disease (CAD)   23
- blood supply   8
- calcification   164, 171
- calcium   316
- circulation   6, 17
- collateral   17
- endothelial dysfunction   232
- flow reserve (CFR)   311, 381
- heart disease (CHD)   23, 45
- microcirculation   311
- revascularization   167
- sinus   6
coronary angiogram
- angiography   157
- contraindications   157
coronary angiography. *see also* cadiac catheterization
- indications   156
coronary artery bypass (CAB) surgery   316, 471, 491
coronary artery bypass graft (CABG)   167, 275, 497
- off-pump surgery   171
- stress test   278
coronary artery bypass graft surgery (CABG)   469
coronary artery disease (CAD)   471, 505
- collateral circulation   27
- diabetes   305, 307, 311
- early diagnosis in diabetic women   315
- family history   27
- inflammation   27
- pathology   31
- pathophysiology   24
- pre-test probability   231
- risk factor   55
- risk stratification in diabetic patient   311
- stress MPS   245
- test   307
coronary artery dissection   468
coronary artery occlusion   468

coronary artery rupture   468
coronary artery spasm   468
coronary atherosclerosis   480
coronary heart disease (CHD)
- diet   421
- metabolic syndrome   421
- nutrition   421
- obesity   421
- pharmacological prevention   421
- prevention   419
- risk factor   419
- serum total cholesterol   420
coronary revascularization   472
coronary steal syndrome   381
coronary vasospastic angina   413
coronary vessel thrombosis   468
couer en sabot   68
coumarin   444
count-rate performance   369
COURAGE trial   481
CPB. *see* cardiopulmonary bypass
C-reactive protein (CRP)   27, 47, 81
creatine kinase (CK)   78, 438
creatine kinase (CK)-MB activity   77
creatine kinase–MB   233
CRP. *see* C-reactive protein
CT. *see* computed tomography (CT)
culprit lesion   233
cut-off frequency   200, 201
CVD
- diabetes   420
- diet   421
- hypertension   420
- nutrition   421
- pharmacological prevention   421
cycle   14
cycle ergometer   108, 109
cyclosporine   519, 523
cyclotron   215, 217, 222, 381
cytochrome P-450   429, 457, 458
cytokine   25
Cytomegalovirus (CMV)   27, 521

D

data analysis   346
da Vinci™ system   490, 493
DCM. *see* dilated cardiomyopathy (DCM)
deconvolution technique   358
defibrillation electrode   150
defibrillator   114
delayed after-depolarization (DAD)   146
depolarisation   15
desipramine   412
destination ventricular assist device   523

detection of ischemia in asymptomatic diabetics (DIAD)   313
dextrorotation of the heart   339
d-glucosamine   442
diabetes   290, 305, 420, 511
– abnormal metabolic state   46
– development of CAD   318
– microvessel   48
– noninvasive cardiac imaging modality   317
– screening algorithm   317
– type 1   316
– vascular inflammation   47
diabetes mellitus (DM)   157, 395
– altered cellular function   46
– cardiovascular complication   45
– vascular smooth muscle function   47
diabetic
– nephropathy   48
– retinopathy   48
diacylglycerol   49
diaphragmatic attenuation   334
diastasis   17
digoxin   454, 458
– adverse effect   432
– pharmacodynamic   432
– pharmacokinetic   432
dilatation   68
dilated cardiomyopathy (DCM)   340
– MIBG   413
diltiazem   429, 457, 458
dipyridamole   182, 192, 232, 238, 245, 247, 254, 278, 292, 522
dipyridamole echocardiography   133
dipyridamole MPI   233
dipyridamole stress echocardiography   313
directional coronary atherectomy   469
direct thrombin inhibitor
– adverse effect   439
– pharmacodynamic   439
– pharmacokinetic   438
diseases of the great vessel   123
disopyramide   455, 456
dissecting aneurysm   39
diuretic   420, 430
– adverse effect   431
– pharmacodynamic   430
– pharmacokinetic   430
DM. *see* diabetes mellitus (DM)
dobutamine   192, 238, 245, 255, 292, 328, 346, 351
– low-dose   248
– β2 activity   247
dobutamine–atropine protocol   133
dobutamine echocardiography   124, 391, 392
dobutamine stress   232

dobutamine stress echocardiography (DSE)   127, 182, 248, 255, 522
– analysis   129
– indication   128
– protocol   129
– technique   129
dofetilide   454, 457
donor heart   518
Doppler echocardiography   181
– aliasing   120
– continuous wave (CW)   120
– limitation   120
– pulsed wave (PW)   120
Doppler equation   117
double-vessel disease   132
Down's Syndrome   66
doxorubicin   234, 351
Dressler's syndrome   42
dromotropy   9, 16
drug-eluting stent   464, 465, 466, 480
DSE. *see* dobutamine stress echocardiography (DSE)
dual chamber pacemaker   151
dual-isotope gated SPECT imaging   266
dual isotope protocol   240, 243
Duke treadmill score   291
dysautonomia   393
dysbetalipoproteinemia   434
dysglycemia   318
dyskinesia   129, 185
dyslipidemia   46, 318, 420, 421, 434, 435
dyspnoea   122, 312, 351

E

early after-depolarization (EAD)   146
EBCT. *see* electron-beam CT
Ebsteins anomaly   68, 69
ECG. *see* electrocardiogram
ECG gating   261, 337, 344
ECG stress test   164
echocardiography   163, 472
– clinical application   122
– imaging modality   118
– limitation   121, 124
– M-mode   118
– principles of ultrasound   118
– real-time 3D volume   135
– three-dimensional (3D)   123
– transesophageal. *see there* echocardiography
– two-dimensional   118
echo time   178
ectopic pacemaker   97, 99, 146
edema   122
eicosanoid   25
Eisenmengher's syndrome   73, 74

ejection fraction (EF)   14, 307
- after revascularization   390
electrical cell   13, 14
electrocardiogram (ECG)   17, 77, 191
- abnormality   92, 93
- ambulatory monitoring
  - guideline   115
- analysing   91
- artefact   93
- chest electrode   93
- computerised   107
- gating   164, 180
- interpretation   105
- recording   87
- resting   87
electrocardiography   511
electrode catheter   151
electromagnetic radiation   214
electron   214, 365
- capture   216
electron-beam CT (EBCT)   164
electron donor   48
electronic collimation   365
electrophysiological (EP) study   147
electrophysiologic principle   145
elliptical orbit   198
emory angioplasty versus surgery trial (EAST)   279
Emory Cardiac Toolbox   264
encainide   454, 455
endarterectomy   39
end-diastolic volume   14
endocardium   4
endoscope   488
endothelial dysfunction   46
endothelial progenitor cell (EPC)   512
endothelin-1   383
end-stage heart failure refractory   517
end-stage renal disease (ESRD)   80
energy resolution   369
energy spectrum   364
epicardium   3, 4
Epstein–Barr virus   521
eptifibatide   440, 441
equilibrium radionuclide angiocardiography (ERNA)   343, 346
- CAD   350
- cardiomyopathy   351
- clinical indication   350
- congenital heart disease (CHD)   351
- congestive heart failure   351
- diastolic function   349
- ischemia heart disease   350
- myocardial infarction   350
- myocardial viability   350

- toxicity of doxorubicin (adriamycin)   351
equilibrium radionuclide angiography
- planar gated   346
equilibrium ventriculography   218
ERNA. *see there* equilibrium radionuclide
everolimus   523
excimer laser   498
excitation–contraction coupling   13
exercise ECG   133
exercise echocardiography   133
exercise physiology   18
exercise SPECT thallium imaging   275
exercise stress   237
exercise stress test   105, 107, 108
- interpretation   110
- patient preparation   110
exercise test   127
- equipment   108
- protocol   109
exercise treadmill testing (ETT)   278
export catheter   469
ezetimibe
- adverse effect   435
- pharmacodynamic   435
- pharmacokinetic   435

F
F^{18}-2-fluoro-2-deoxy-D-glucose (FDG)   364, 381, 382, 393
Fallot's tetralogy   68, 69
fan beam collimator   196
fan-beam collimator   403
fast spin echo (FSE)   178
fatty acid
- imaging   391
- metabolism   302
fatty streak   24, 25, 33, 36
FBP. *see* filtered back projection (FBP)
FDG-SPECT   391
fibrate   435
- adverse effect   436
- pharmacodynamic   436
fibric acid
- pharmacokinetic   435
fibrillatory wave (f wave)   99
fibrin deposition   31
fibrinolysis   440
fibrinolytic   439
fibrinolytic agent
- pharmacodynamic   439
- pharmacokinetic   439
fibrinolytic therapy
- adverse effect   440
fibroatheromas   34

fibrocalcific plaque   36
fibrointimal hyperplasia   39
fibrous cap atheromata   36
fibrous cap rupture   37
fibrous plaque   25
fibrous skeleton   4
filling fraction (FR)   349
film-cassette system   65
filtered back projection (FBP)   199, 200, 374
– star artefact   201
first pass angiocardiography study   355
first pass study
– acquisition   356
– left to right shunt   357
– LV function   357
– quality control   357
– radiopharmaceutical   356
FLAP gene   27
flecainide   454, 455, 456
flight simulator concept   493
fluorine-18 labeled deoxyglucose (FDG)   389
fluoro-ammonia   383
flutter wave   99
foam cell   46
focal hypoperfusion   405
Fontan procedure   404
forward projection   202
fosinopril   426
Fourier rebinning   374
Fourier transformation   178, 346
Framingham score   165
Framingham study   24
French sheath   464
FSE. see fast spin echo
fulcrum effect   487
funnel chest   66
furifosmin   225
furosemide   430
F wave   99

G

gag reflex   138
gallium-67   219
Gamma camera   193, 207, 209, 218, 263, 300, 331, 337
– automated count-optimized reconstruction filter   332
– centre of rotation (COR)   326
– collimator   326
– data acquisition   197
– first pass study   356
– image quality   196
– large field-of-view (LFOV)   344
– linearity   326
– non-circular orbit   205
– quality control (QC)   205
– resolution   326
– small field-of-view (SFOV)   344
– spatial resolution   196
– uniformity   326
gamma emitter   513
gamma ray   216, 217
gated blood pool imaging (MUGA)   357
gated equilibrium   344
gated equilibrium angiocardiography   358
gated SPECT
– diagnostic and prognostic value   265
gated-SPECT myocardial perfusion   272
gene therapy   384
giant cell
– lipid-laden   39
Gibbon cardiopulmonary bypass pump   472
glucose   49
glucose intolerance   421
glucose metabolism   395
glucose mobilization   429
glucose transport   381
glucose utilisation   363
glucuronic acid   442
glycogenolysis
– catecholamine-induced   429
glycoprotein IIb/IIIa inhibitor   168, 440
glycopyrrolate   138
glycosaminoglycan   442
GP IIb-IIIa agent
– adverse effect   441
– pharmacodynamic   441
– pharmacokinetic   441
G-protein coupled receptor (GPCR)   253
GRACE study   306
graft failure   477
graft patency verification   478
granulocyte-macrophage colony stimulating factor (GM-CSF)   512
groin hematoma   468
growth factor   25
guanethidine   412
guanylyl cyclase   433
gut uptake   203

H

haemophilus parainfluenza   139
haircut procedure   490
handgrip isometric exercise   346
harmonic imaging   118
HCM. see hypertrophic cardiomyopathy (HCM)
HDL. see high density lipoprotein
heart
– anatomy   3
– autonomic nervous system   16
– block   100

- conduction system 10, 11
- dextrorotation 339
- electrical activity 91
- electrical conduction system 145
- levorotation 339
- murmur 122
- nerve supply 9
- physiological stress 105
- physiology 11
- rate (HR) 18
- standard surgical access 474

Heart disease
- family history 55

heart failure 24, 28, 71, 122, 431
heart rate 90
heart transplantation
- contraindication 518
- donor selection 517
- infection 519
- management 517
- post-transplant care 518
- post-transplant complication 519
- recipient selection 518
- rejection 519
- surgical technique 518

hemidiaphragm 68
hemi-Fontan procedure 404
hemodynamic monitoring 465
hemophilia 442
heparin 440, 464
- adverse effect 442
- pharmacodynamic 442
- pharmacokinetic 441
heparin-coated circuit 481
heparin induced thrombocytopenia (HIT) 443
hepatic cytochrome P450 (CYP) 3A4 435
hepatic triglyceride 436
hepatobiliary clearance 203
heterograft 140
hexokinase 381
hibernating myocardium 43, 122, 182, 350, 364, 383
high density lipoprotein (HDL) 46
high density lipoprotein (HDL) cholesterol 420, 429
high-energy shock 150
hole collimator 239
holmium:YAG laser 498
Holter monitor 113, 114, 115
homograft 140
Hounsfield Units (HU) 163
HTN. see hypertension (HTN)
hybrid imaging 172
hydrochlorothiazide 430
hydrogen ion 25
hydrogen proton 178
hyperaemia 248

hypercholesterolaemia 288
hyperemia 238
hyperglycemia 46, 48, 166, 436
hypertension (HTN) 46, 288, 420, 421, 425
hypertrophic cardiomyopathy (HCM) 135, 148, 183, 184, 340
- MIBG 413
hypertrophic papillary muscle 339
hypertrophy 68, 93
hyperuricemia 436
hypoglycemia 429
hypoinsulinemia 395
hypokalaemia 129
hypokinesia 129
hypotension 468
- dobutamine stress-induced 130
hypovolaemia 142
hypoxia tracer 383

I

I^{123} MIBG imaging 393
ibuprofen 256
ibutilide 454, 457
ICD. see implantable cardiac defibrillator
ICE. see intracardiac echocardiography
ice-pick 118
idiopathic dilated cardiomyopathy 128
idioventricular rhythm (IVR) 100, 102
iduronic acid 442
IHD
- noninvasive stress testing 291
- racial difference 288
- risk factor
  - gender-related difference 288
- women 287
image
- reconstruction 329
image fusion 219
image reconstruction 374
image reorientation 202
image timing 327
- artefact 329
image uniformity 326
imaging protocol
- Tl-201-based 242
imipramine 412
immunosuppressant 517
immunosuppression 519, 521
implantable cardioverter defibrillator (ICD) 71, 149
- contraindication 150
- indication 150
implantable loop recorder 114
indapamide 430
indium-111 219

infarct
- expansion   42
- extension   42
infection   468
infective endocarditis (IE)   122, 139
- prophylaxis   138
inflammation   27, 32
in-stent restenosis   168, 277, 464
insulin resistance   26, 318, 395, 421
insulin resistance syndrome   288
intercalated disc   6
internal mammary artery graft   39
internal thoracic artery (ITA)   472, 475
intimal
- thickening   36
- xanthomata   36
intimal fibroplasia   477
intimal hyperplasia   512
intra-aortic balloon occlusion   488
intra-aortic balloon pump (IABP)   505
intracardiac echocardiography (ICE)   123
intraluminal metallic prosthese   38
intraoperative angiography   478
intraoperative fluorescence   479
intravascular stent   38
intravascular ultrasound (IVUS)   464, 465
iodine-123   219
iodophenylpentadecanoic acid   227
ionisation   214
ion movement   145
ionotropy   9, 16
IPPA. see 123 I-iodophenylpentadecanoic acid
ischaemia
- dipyridamole-induced   254
- exercise-induced   338
ischaemic heart disease (IHD)   18, 107
- pre-test probability   295
- stress MPS   245
ischaemic stroke   139
ischemia   268, 306
- cardiac catheterization   156
ischemic cardiomyopathy   42
- enhanced FDG uptake   390
ischemic cascade   134
ischemic heart disease
- pathology   39
ischemic heart disease (IHD)   299
- life-time risk of IHD   287
ischemic memory   302, 392
ischemic myocardium   309
isoenzyme   78, 79
isomer   215
isomeric transition   216, 218
isoproterenol   459

isotone   215
isotope   215, 240, 363
- positron-emitting   389
isotropic array   164
isovolumetric ventricular contraction   17
isuprel   459
ITA graft   475, 477
iterative reconstruction technique   201
IVR. see idioventricular rhythm (IVR)

J

Jaszczak phantom™   206
Judkins technique   463
jugular venous pressure (JVP)   58, 60
junctional atrioventricular (AV) arrhythmia   99
junctional escape rhythm   100
junctional point   89
junctional rhythm   100

K

Kaplan–Meier analysis   414
Kawasaki disease   39, 181, 402, 403
Kerley B line   69
Kingella   139
Kronos Early Estrogen Prevention Study (KEEPS)   290
k-space   178

L

labetarol   412
lactate dehydrogenase (LDH)   77, 80
lanoxin   432
laser   497
laser ablation   463
laser atherectomy   469
laser-handpiece   503
LDH. see lactate dehydrogenase
LDL. see low density lipoprotein (LDL)
leaflet resection   493
left anterior descending artery (LAD)   6
left atrium (LA)   4
left bundle branch block (LBBB)   104, 128, 337
left circumflex (LCx)   6
left coronary artery (LCA)   6
left internal mammary artery (LIMA)   39
left to right shunt   357
left ventricle (LV)   4
left ventricular ejection fraction (LVEF)   207
- estimation   347
left ventricular hypertrophy (LVH)   17, 128, 394
left ventricular peak filling rate (PFR)   349
lesion
- with thrombi   37
levorotation   339

lidocaine 454, 455
light microscopy 41
LIMA. see left internal mammary artery
linear attenuation coefficient 371
line of response (LOR) 365
lipid core 34
lipid metabolism 32
lisinopril 426
list mode acquisition 345
LITA graft 475
LMWH. see low-molecular-weight heparin
longitudinal magnetization 178
long QT syndrome 71, 148
loop diuretic 430, 431
loop of Henle 430
loop recorder 113, 114
LOR 366, 371. see line of response
losartan 427
lovastatin 438
low cardiac output syndrome 480, 504
low density lipoprotein (LDL) 46, 288
low energy all purpose (LEAP) collimator 239
low energy general-purpose collimator (LEGP) 326
low energy high resolution (LEHR) collimation 326
low energy high resolution (LEHR) collimator 239
low-molecular-weight heparin (LMWH)
– adverse effect 443
– pharmacodynamic 443
– pharmacokinetic 442
lung perfusion scintigraphy (LPS) 405
– infants and children 404
LV dysfunction 390
lymphocytic myocarditis 518

M

macrophage
– foam cell 34
macrovascular disease 314
magnesium 458
magnetic resonance imaging (MRI) 163
– advantage 177
– coronary artery disease 180
– delayed enhancement 182
– disadvantage 177
– myocardial viability 183
– principal concept 178
– technique 178
Maillard reaction 48
Maltz–Treves method 358
mannitol 430
MAO. see monoamine oxidase
Marfan syndrome 66, 123
mastectomy 293
maximum oxygen consumption 19

maximum pulsation 58
MBF. see myocardial blood flow
MDCT 165
– angiography 173
– coronary angiography 168
– enhancement 171
mechanoreceptor 19
median sternotomy 518
mediastinum 3
medulla oblongata 409
melagatran 445
messenger RNA (mRNA) 26
metabolic imaging 394
metabolic syndrome 291, 318, 421, 434
metabolic trapping 392
metformin 160, 464
methylmethacrylate 38
metoprolol 395, 428
mexiletine 454, 455
MFAO. see myocardial fatty acid oxidation
MIBG 227, 409, 410, 522
– accumulation in the heart muscle 411
– analysis 411
– arrhythmia 415
– DCM 413
– evaluation method 411
– HCM 413
– heart failure 413
– imaging method 411
– indication 415
– ischemic heart disease 413
– radiographic interpretation 412
microalbuminuria 312, 316
micro-incision 489
micronized progesterone 290
microvascular disease 311
microvascular ischaemic syndrome 26
MIDCAB. see minimally invasive direct coronary artery bypass
minimally invasive. see there cardiac surgery
minimally invasive cardiac surgery 487
– clinical application 490
– patient selection 490
minimally invasive direct coronary artery bypass (MIDCAB) 487
mini-sternal 488
missense mutation 148
mitochondrial oxidative phosphorylation 40
mitral regurgitation (MR) 134, 141
mitral scoring 141
mitral stenosis 69, 134
mitral valve annulus
– calcification 71
mitral valve prolapse 122

mitral valve prosthese   140
mitral valve stenosis   490
mitral valve surgery   488
molybdenum-99   218
monoamine oxidase (MAO)   410
moricizine   454
MPI. *see* myocardial perfusion imaging
MPI scan
- imaging protocol   192
- resting   192
- stressing   192
MPI SPECT
- acquisition time   199
- gate scan   206
- number of projection   199
- reconstruct scan   203
- wall motion   207
MPS
- SPECT imaging result   243
MRI. *see* magnetic resonance imaging
MUGA. *see there* gated blood pool imaging
MUGA technique
- clinical application   349
multi-arterial grafting   481
multi-detector/multi-slice computed tomography (MDCT/MSCT)   163
multiple coincidence   367
multislice CT   173
multivessel disease   278, 481
murmur   60
muscular contraction   107
myoblast   513
myocardial
- abscess   139
- blood flow   48
- calcification   70
- damage   17
- fatty acid metabolism   209
- functional reserve   133
- glucose utilization (MGU)   394
- hibernation   42
- hypoperfusion   299, 301
- imaging agent   221
- infarction (MI)   24, 80, 300
- injury   78, 79, 276
  - current marker   78
- ischaemia   24, 181
- ischemia   128
- ischemic injury   39
- metabolism   24, 381
- necrosis   77
- oxygen consumption   381
- perfusion   167, 173, 203, 213
  - MRI   181

- SPECT imaging   182
- perfusion imaging (MPI)   231, 299
  - error   325
  - imaging protocol   237
- perfusion scan   28
- perfusion scintigraphy   305
- rupture   42
- stunning   167
- tagging   179
- viability   182, 381, 394
myocardial blood flow (MBF)   363
myocardial cell   13
myocardial contrast echocardiography (MCE)   392
myocardial dysfunction
- cardiac catheterization   156
myocardial fatty acid oxidation (MFAO)   394
myocardial infarction   23, 350, 504
- expansion   41
- extension   41
- location   40
- macroscopic characteristic   40
- microscopic characteristic   41
- pathology   40
myocardial ischemia   129
- diabetes   314
myocardial oxygen   17
myocardial perfusion imaging (MPI)   191, 265, 275, 379
- after coronary artery bypass graft   278
- asymptomatic patient   234
- limitation   234
- paediatric patient   402
- patient movement   331
- SPECT   193
- SPECT image   191
- women   234
myocardial perfusion scintigraphy (MPS)   292, 294, 511
- paediatric patient   403
myocardial PET scanning
- in children   403
myocardial puncture   468
myocardial revascularization   497
myocarditis   70, 185
myocardium   4
- oedema   185
myocyte
- apoptosis   28
myocyte metabolism   389
myocyte necrosis   42
myocytolysis   41
myofibril   4
myoglobin   78, 80, 81
myopathy   436

myosin 13
myosin filament 4

N

N^{13}-ammonia 158, 380, 381, 382
N-acetylprocainamide 455
nadolol 428
nanocolloid
– Tc-99m-labelled 360
narrow-beam geometry 371
natrecor 433
NE. *see* norepinephrine (NE)
– exocytosis 410
– storage granule 410
– uptake-1 410
near-syncope 113
neo-intimal hyperplasia 477
nephropathy 316
nephrotoxity 157
nesiritide
– adverse effect 433
– pharmacodynamic 433
– pharmacokinetic 433
N-ethoxy-N-ethyl-dithiocarbamate nitrido 227
neurological embolic event 123
neutral atom 213
neutrino 216
neutropenia 444
niacin
– adverse effect 436
– pharmacodynamic 436
– pharmacokinetic 436
nicotine replacement therapy 420
nifedipine 429, 457, 458
Nipple shadow 66
nitrate 394, 432
– pharmacodynamic 433
– pharmacokinetic 433
nitric oxide 25, 26, 46, 475
nitroglycerine 256, 351, 394, 465
nitrous oxide 432
noise equivalent counts (NEC) 369
noise-reduction filter 368
non-ischaemic myocardial injury 80
non-occlusive atherosclerosis 295
nonreversible segments (NRS) 280
non-ST-segment elevation myocardial infarction (NSTEMI) 232
non-uniform attenuation correction method 203
non-uniform attenuation correction (NUAC) 208, 209
nonviable myocardium 393
norepinephrine kinetic 415
norepinephrine (NE) 9, 16, 409, 415

NSTEMI 466. *see* non-ST-segment elevation myocardial infarction
nuclear cardiology 213
– development 209
nuclear cardiology software 264
nuclear reactor 215
nuclear transition 216
Nyquist limit 120

O

O^{15}-Water 381, 382
obesity 421, 434
obesity-insulin resistance 395
obstructive sleep apnea 421
obstructive sleep hypoventilation 421
oesophagus 138
oestrogen 288, 289
off pump surgery 478
olmesartan 427
one-day imaging protocol 240
one-day protocol 242, 329
on pump surgery 477
oral direct thrombin inhibitor (oral DTI) 445
orbit
– selection of type 327
osmotic stress
– sorbitol-induced 49
osteopenia 442
oxidative metabolism 363
oxidative stress 48
– hyperglycemia-induced 47
oxygen deficiency 40

P

PAC. *see* premature atrial contraction
pacemaker 71, 72, 114, 332
pacemaker cell 146
paclitaxel 277
PACS. *see* picture archiving and communication system
paediatric imaging
– dual-head system 403
– radiation protection 401
palmitate 364
palpitation 113, 123
pannus 141
paracetamol 256
paradoxical embolism 121
parallel hole collimator 195
para-sternal incision 488
parasympathetic fibre 10, 16
parent nuclide 215
Parkinson's disease 415
paroxysmal atrial tachycardia (PAT) 97
PAT. *see* paroxysmal atrial tachycardia

patent ductus arteriosus (PDA)   73
patent foramen ovale (PFO)   117, 140
P-cell (Pale/Pacemaker-cell)   10
PCI. see percutaneous coronary intervention
PCWP. see pulmonary capillary wedge pressure
PDA. see patent ductus arteriosus
pectus excavatum   66, 67
pencil-beam   163
penetrating aortic ulcer (PAU)   142
pentasaccharide   442
percutaneous bypass graft surgery   469
percutaneous coronary intervention (PCI)   38, 275, 474
percutaneous radio-frequency (RF) catheter ablation   151
percutaneous transluminal coronary angioplasty (PTCA)   38, 43, 276, 465, 505
– complication   467
– device   466
– indication   466
perfusion scintigraphy   128
perfusion SPECT   263
perfusion tracer   191, 383
pericardial calcification   70
pericardial disease
– evaluation   177
pericardial effusion   122, 468
pericardial sac   3
pericardial tamponade   468
pericardiocentesis   468
pericardium   3, 138
peri-infarction ischemia   266
peripheral pruning   73
permanent pacemakers (PPM)   151
peroxisome proliferator-activated receptor (PPAR)-alpha   436
peroxynitrite   48
Perspex cylinder   205
pertechnetate   328
PET. see there positron emission tomography
pharmacological agent
– patient instruction   252
– side effect   252
pharmacological stress   294, 346
pharmacological stress agent   245, 257
pharmacological stress test   238, 263
– adenosine   253
pharmacologic stress echocardiography   128
pharmacologic testing
– in infant and younger children   402
phase contrast angiography   180
phased-array transducer   118
phase image analysis   349
phenylpropanolamine   412
phenytoin   454, 455

phosphinyl   426
photocathode   367
photoelectric absorption   203
photomultiplier tube (PMT)   194, 326, 367
photon attenuation   203, 205, 332
photon beam
– mono-energetic   371
photon flux   221
photopeak   327, 369
photopeak emission energy   337
photostimulable phosphor plate   74
physical exercise   346
physical inactivity   421
physical stress   256
picture archiving and communication system (PACS)   74
piezoelectric crystal   118
pindolol   428
pixel   194
– size   198
planar imaging   193, 239, 278, 332
planar projection   202
planar scintillation camera   380
plaque
– calcification   37
– erosion   35, 37
– fibrocalcific   36
– imaging   171, 181
– localization   32
– prone to thrombose   35
– rupture   35, 37
plasma glucose   46
plasminogen-activator inhibitor type 1 (PAI-1)   439
platelet
– function   47
– microparticle   47
pleural air   72
pleural effusion   69, 70
PMT. see photomultiplier tube
Pneumococcus   521
Pneumocystis (PCP)   521
Pneumothorax   71, 72
Point spread function (PSF)   365
polyol pathway   49
Port-access™ method   488
Port-access™ system   490
port incision   489
positron   365, 388
– annihilation   364
– emission   364
positron emission
– beta decay   216
positron emission tomography (PET)   387
– basic principle   364
– biochemical measurement   388

- clinical application   388
- coincidence event   366
- coronary artery disease   394
- count-rate performance   369
- data acquisition   367
- data processing   370
- detection system   365
- detector scintillator   369
- development   374
- dynamic data acquisition   374
- energy resolution   369
- energy window manipulation   373
- gated acquisition   374
- left ventricular hypertrophy   394
- match   389
- MBF   363
- measurement of myocardial blood flow   317
- metabolism-perfusion mismatch   389
- model-based scatter correction   373
- Monte Carlo calculation   373
- myocardial fatty acid metabolism   394
- myocardial metabolism   363
- myocardial viability   389
- physiological   388
- pre-reconstruction filtering   373
- radiopharmaceutical   379
- ring geometry   367
- scatter fraction   369
- scintillation process   367
- sensitivity   369
- spatial resolution   368
- subtraction operation   373
- tracer   370
- tracer kinetic modelling   374
positronium   365
post-angioplasty irradiation   513
post-balloon angioplasty   465
posterior descending artery (PDA)   6
post-MI syndrome   42
post-symptom recorder   114
post-thrombolysis   233
post-transplant lymphoproliferative disorder   521
potassium   379, 458
potassium ion   14
PPM. *see* permanent pacemaker
pre-excitation syndrome   147
premature atrial contraction (PAC)   97
premature junctional contractions (PJC)   99
premature ventricular contractions (PVCs)   100, 345
pre-symptom recorder   114
presyncope   114
pretest probability   291
procainamide   454
procanamide   89
programmed cell death. *see* apoptosis

prone imaging   205
Pronto catheter   469
propafenone   454, 455
propranalol   428
prostacyclin   475
prostaglandin   25
prosthetic valve endocarditis   124
protein kinase
- activation   49
proteoglycans   34
prothrombin   444
proton   178
P-selectin   47
pseudo-aneurysm (PSA)   42, 466, 467
pseudodefect   340
PSF. *see* point spread function
PTCA. *see* percutaneous transluminal coronary angioplasty
pulmonary arterial hypertension   72
pulmonary blood flow   357
pulmonary capillary wedge pressure (PCWP)   69, 433
pulmonary circulation   11, 121, 355
pulmonary embolism
- in infant and children   404
pulmonary hypertension   105, 518
pulmonary oedema   69, 70
pulmonary plethora   73
pulse repetition frequency (PRF)   120
Purkinje cell   10
Purkinje fibre   11, 145
P-wave   17, 87, 88, 97, 104

Q
QRS complex   87, 88, 89, 90, 100, 102, 454
- axis   93
QT interval   89, 454
quadriceps muscle   108
quantitative gated SPECT; QGS   264
quinidine   89, 454
Q wave   92

R
RAAS. *see* renin angiotensin aldosterone system
radial artery graft   477
radiation
- spillage   514
radiation protection   401
radioactive decay   215, 217
radiofrequency ablation   505
radiofrequency pulse   179
radioisotope   215
radioisotopes   261
radionuclide   213, 513, 514
- angiography (RNA)   343
- first pass study   355

- half-life 217
- ideal property 217
- injection
  - timing 301
- tracer uptake 299
- ventriculography (RVG) 343
radionuclide imaging 134, 163
radionuclide MPI 278
radionuclide myocardial perfusion SPECT imaging 166
radionuclide ventriculography (RVG) 123
radiopharmaceutical 191, 193, 221, 327, 343, 356, 387
- administration 328
- effective half-life 217
- procedure guideline 222
radiotracer 221, 238, 328
ramp filter 199, 200, 201
random coincidence 366
randoms correction 373
Rb^{82}-rubidium chloride 382
rebinning 374
receptor antagonist
- antagonist 427
- pharmacodynamic 428
- pharmacokinetic 427
red blood cell
- TC99m-labelled 379
red blood cell labeling 344
re-endothelialisation 512
re-entrant tachycardia 146, 147
re-entry 146
refractory angina 281
regadenoson 257
regional wall motion abnormality 181
reinjection protocol 242
relative lung perfusion 404
renal disease 478
renal failure 468
renal insufficiency 157
renin angiotensin aldosterone system (RAAS) 426
reperfusion 43
repetition time 178
repolarisation 15
reserpine 412
residual radioactivity 329
resin 434
re-stenosis 281, 468, 511, 512, 514
restrictive cardiomyopathy 184
rest thallium and stress Tc99m dual isotope acquisition protocol 242
retinopathy 316
retransplantion 523
retroperitoneal hematoma 467
re-vascularisation 514

revascularization surgery
- outcomes in woman 291
rhabdomyolysis 436
rheolytic thrombectomy 469
rheumatic fever 70
rheumatic heart disease 71
rib notching 73, 74
right atrium (RA) 4
right bundle branch block (RBBB) 104
right coronary artery (RCA) 6
right to left shunt 360
right-to-left shunting 404
right ventricle (RV) 4
right ventricular ejection fraction (RVEF) 348
Rio aspiration catheter 469
RITA graft 475
robotically assisted anastomosis 493
robotic arm 491
robotic cardiac operation 488
robotic instrument 489
robotic mitral surgery
- exclusion criteria 491
robotic system 487
robotic tele-manipulation 493
ROSETTA Registry 276
rotablator 464, 469
routine stress test
- after revascularization 276
R–R interval 93, 263, 345
ruthenium-99 218
RVG. *see* radionuclide ventriculography
R wave 90, 262

S

S-adenosyl homocysteine 253
saline flushing 329
same day protocol 242
same day rest stress Tc99m- acquisition protocol 242
SA node 12
saphenous vein graft (SVG) 280, 472, 477
- stenosis 477
saphenous venous bypass graft (SVBG) 38
sarcomere 4
scanner sensitivity 369
scar 265
scatter coincidence 366, 370
scatter correction 373
scattered photon 327
scatter fraction 369
scintillation crystal 194, 196, 369
scintillation process in PET 367
scintillator 370
Seldinger technique 156, 464
selective coronary angiography 156

semilunar valve (SL)   17
septa   195
septal hypertrophy   340
septal view   344
sestamibi   203, 219, 220, 223, 231, 239, 242, 262, 329
– salient feature   224
short axis (SA) image   202
short-axis tomogram   340
short septum   338
short-term cardiac monitoring   114
silent CAD
– asymptomatic diabetes   313
silent ischemia   278, 305, 306, 314, 317
silent myocardial infarct   306
silent myocardial infarction   312
silent myocardial ischemia   45
simvasatin   438
single detector camera   197
single isotope protocol   240
single photon emission computed tomography (SPECT)   134, 163, 173, 191, 239
– alignment   332
– attenuation   332
– data   198
– ECG-gated acquisition   307
– ERNA   346
– filtered back projection   199
– gating   337
– image reconstruction   329
– imaging camera   390
– myocardial perfusion imaging   380
– non-Uniform attenuation correction (NUAC)   207
– orbit   327
– patient-related artefact   332
– short axis view   411
single photon imaging technique   363
single-vessel disease   107, 132
sino-atrial node dysfunction   519
sinoatrial node (SA)   94
sinuatrial node (SAN)   145
sinus
– arrest   95
– arrhythmia   95, 96
– bradycardia   94
– rhythm   94, 100
– tachycardia   94, 95
sinus venosus defect   142
sirolimus   277, 519, 523
sirolimus-eluting stent   464
skeletal muscle trauma   81
sliding valvuloplaste   490
sliding valvuloplasty   493
smoking   419
smooth muscle cell   25, 34

sodium iodide scintillation crystal   193
sodium pertechnetate   343
sodium-potassium ATPase   432
soft plaque   171
soft tissue attenuation artefact   265
sorbitol   49
sorbitol dehydrogenase   49
sotalol   428, 454, 456
sound mark   60
spatial distortion   326
spatial linearity   326
spatial resolution   368
SPECT   261. *see* single photon emission computed tomography
– acquisition   262
– "fixed temporal resolution framing" approach   262
– gated   262
– imaging protocols   263
SPECT imaging
– data acquisition   197
– uniformity of response   205
SPECT MPI   232
SPECT stress MPS
– ECG-gated   312
sphingolipid   28
spider view   158
spironolactone   430, 431
splanchnic thoracic nerve   10
SSFP. *see* steady state free precession
stable angina   231, 232, 300
stannous citrate   344
stannous pyrophosphate   344
Staphylococcus aureus   139
statin   421, 422, 437, 480
– adverse effect   438
– pharmacodynamic   438
– pharmacokinetic   438
– pleiotropic effect   438
steady state free precession (SSFP)   179
steal phenomenon   254
STEMI   233, 234, 466. *see* ST-segment elevation myocardial infarction
stenting   464, 469
step and shoot acquisition   199
step and shoot mode   198
sternotomy   487, 493
sternotomy approach   474
strain Doppler echocardiography   124
streptokinase   439
stress ECG testing   291
stress echocardiography   292, 309
stress ERNA   350
stress imaging   232
stress ischemia   307

stress MPS
- optimal frequency   315
stress myocardial perfusion imaging   245
stress myocardial perfusion scintigraphy   307
stress protocol   109, 346
stress radiotracer uptake   317
stress-rest myocardial perfusion assessment   173
stress–rest thallium 201 protocol   242
stress testing   394
string sign   475
stroke volume count   349
stroke volume (SV)   14, 17, 18
strontium-82   379
ST segment   89, 94
- dobutamine stress-induced   131
ST-segment elevation myocardial infarction (STEMI)   232
stunned myocardium   40, 350
subacute thrombosis   464
subendocardial infarct   40
subendocardium   40
subepicardium   40
sulfhydryl   426
summed difference score (SDS)   280
summed rest score (SRS)   280
summed stress score (SSS)   280, 282
supraventricular arrhythmia   480
SVBG. *see* saphenous venous bypass graft
sympathetic nerve   9
- activity   409, 413, 415
- disorder   415
- distribution   409
sympathetic nervous system   409
sympathicotonia   409
syncope   113, 114
syndrome X   26, 166
systemic blood pressure   129
systemic circulation   11
systemic hypertension   123

T

T1 value   178
tachyarrhythmia   147, 454
- differential diagnosis   148
- EAD-induced   148
tachycardia   59, 114, 454
tacrolimus   523
tacrolimus-eluting stent   464
Tangier disease   27
target heart rate (THR)   245, 250
target of rapamycin (TOR) inhibitor   523
target-to-nontarget ratios   263
target vessel revascularization (TVR)   464
Tc99m-diethylenetriamine pentaacetic acid (DTPA)   343

Tc99m-human serum albumin (HSA)   344
Tc99m-labelled
- nanocolloid   360
Tc99m-macroaggregates of albumin (MAA)   360
Tc99m-pertecnetate   343
Tc99m-sestamibi   238, 312
- labelling efficiency   328
Tc99m-tetrofosmin   238
- duodeno-gastric   329
- entero-gastric reflux   329
- labelling efficiency   328
T-cell inhibitor   519
TDE. *see there* tissue Doppler echocardiography
teboroxime   225
TECAB. *see* totally endoscopic coronary artery bypass
tension pneumothorax   72
testosterone   295
tetralogy of Fallot   403, 405
tetrofosmin   203, 219, 220, 223, 224, 231, 239, 242, 329
- biological half-life   225
- salient feature   225
thallium   223, 276
- scintigram   276
- SPECT   277
thallium-201   219, 231, 238
theophylline   254, 402
thiazide   430, 457
thienopyridine
- adverse effect   443
- pharmacodynamic   443
- pharmacokinetic   443
thin cap fibrous atheroma (TCFA)   35, 36
thoracic aorta   141
thoracic splanchnic nerve   9
thoracotomy   503
THR. *see* target heart rate
thrombectomy   469
thrombin   439, 442
thrombocytopenia   441
- heparin-induced   438
thromboembolism   139
thrombosis   26, 32, 34, 39, 438, 441
thrombus   139, 141
ticlopidine   443
time to peak filling rate (tPFR)   349
timolol   428
tirofiban   440, 441
tissue Doppler echocardiography (TDE)   124
tissue Doppler imaging (TDI)   133
TMR. *see* transmyocardial laser revascularization; *see* transmyocardial revascularization
tobacco consumption   419
tocainide   454, 455
TOE. *see* transesophageal echocardiography

tomographic equilibrium blood pool imaging
– gated   346
torsades de pointes   458
Torsedes de pointes   102
torsemide   430
total arterial revascularization   481
totally endoscopic coronary artery bypass (TECAB)   474, 490
total peripheral resistance (TPR)   18
tracer   387
– Tc99m-labelled   220
tracer kinetic   387
tracer kinetic modelling   370, 374
transcatheter closure   142
transesophageal cardioversion   143
trans-esophageal echocardiographic (TEE)   491
transesophageal echocardiography (TOE)   137
– atrial fibrillation   139
– catheter-based procedure   142
– contraindication   138
– endocarditis   139
– indication   138
– intraoperative monitoring   142
– miniaturisation transducer   143
– technological development   137
– thoracic aorta   141
– valvular evaluation   140
transient ischemic attack   468
transient ischemic dilatation (TID)   264
transitional cell   10
transmission measurement   372, 375
transmission scan duration   372
transmission source attenuation correction system   337
transmural infarct   42
transmyocardial revascularization (TMR)   281, 497
– CABG   500
– clinical guideline   505
– combined with VEGF treatment   499
– contraindication   504
– denervation   498
– fibrosis   499
– indication   504
– laser-induced angiogenesis   498
– mechanism of action   498
– method   497
– morbidity   500
– mortality   500
– patent channel   498
– peri-operative complication   504
– risk factor   502
– surgical technique   503
transplant rejection   519
transplant vasculopathy   521
transposition of the great arteries (TGA)   403

transtelephonic monitor   114
transthoracic echocardiography (TTE)   139, 172, 472
treadmill   18, 108, 109, 173, 237
triacylglycerol   395
triamterene   430
tricuspid valve   68
tricuspid valve regurgitation   359
tricyclic antidepressant   411
triglyceride   288
triglyceride-rich lipoprotein   46
triphenytetrazolium chloride (TTC)   40
triple-vessel disease   107
Trisomy 21   66
trocar   487
tropomyosin   4, 13
troponin   4, 79, 80, 301
troponin analysis   233
troponin-C   13
troponin-T   78
TTC. see triphenytetrazolium chloride
T tubules   4
tunneled myocardium   472
T wave   88, 89, 92, 93
two-day imaging protocol   240
two day stress rest Tc99m-protocol   242

U
UA. see unstable angina
ulcerate plaque   142
ultrasound
– transducer   118
– wave   118
unfractionated heparin (UFH)   441
unstable angina
– cardiac catheterization   156
unstable angina (UA)   209, 232, 413, 502
unstable plaque   181
urokinase   439
uronic acid   442
U wave   89
– abnormality   93

V
Valsalva test   314
valvular disease   341
valvular diseases
– cardiac catheterization   157
valvular heart disease   134
vascular endothelial growth factor (VEGF)   27, 383
vascular endothelium   25
vasculogenesis   27
vasoactive autacoid   17
vasodilator   253, 255
vasodilator-stimulated phosphoprotein   443
vectrocardiography   180

VEGF. *see* vascular endothelial growth factor
vein graft atherosclerosis   39
vena cava   6
venous circulation   6
venous pulse
– assessment   58
venous thromboembolism (VTE)   445
ventricle   4
ventricle tachycardia   415
ventricular
– aneurysm   42
– arrhythmia   100
– ectopy   102
– fibrillation   100, 102, 132
– flutter   102
– hypertrophy   105
– infarction   42
– standstill   102
– tachyarrhythmia   151
– tachycardia   100, 102, 131
ventricular aneurysm   347
ventricular arrhythmia   504
ventricular-fibrillation zone   150
ventricular hypertrophy   106
ventricular septal defect (VSD)   42, 73
ventricular tachyarrhythmia   457
ventricular volume   349
verapamil   412, 429, 457
very low density lipoprotein (VLDL)   46
vessel rupture   468
viable myocardium   134, 392
video assistance   489
video-directed mitral operation   489
vitamin K   444
vitamin K antagonist   445
VLDL. *see* very low density lipoprotein
von Willebrand factor   441
VSD. *see* ventricular septal defect (VSD)
vulnerable plaque   181

W

wall motion   347
wall motion abnormality (WMA)   127, 181
wall motion score index (WMSI)   499
wandering at trial pacemaker   99
wandering trail pacemaker   97
warfarin
– adverse effect   444
– pharmacodynamic   444
– pharmacokinetic   444
WMA   129. *see* wall motion abnormality (WMA)
Wolff–Parkinson–White (WPW) syndrome   148, 307
Woman's Ischaemic Syndrome Evaluation (WISE) study   295

X

xenograft   140
xenon detector   163
xenotransplantation   523
ximelagatran
– pharmacodynamic   445
– pharmacokinetic   445
X-ray   65
– angiography   172
– anteroposterior projection   66
– equipment   74
– fan-shaped beam   164
– lateral projection   66
– posteroanterior projection (PA)   65
– transmission data   375
X-ray source   163

Y

Y signal   194

Z

Z line   4, 43
Z resolution   164
Z signal   194